Antimicrobial Therapy in Veterinary Medicine

THIRD EDITION

Antimicrobial Therapy in Veterinary Medicine

THIRD EDITION

Edited by

John F. Prescott
M.A., Vet.M.B., Ph.D.

J. Desmond Baggot
M.V.M., Ph.D., D.Sc., F.R.C.V.S.

Robert D. Walker
M.Sc., Ph.D.

with Thirty Contributors

Iowa State University Press / Ames

John F. Prescott, M.A., Vet.M.B., Ph.D., is Professor in the Department of Pathobiology, University of Guelph, Ontario, Canada.

J. Desmond Baggot, M.V.M., Ph.D., D.Sc., F.R.C.V.S., is formerly Professor of Preclinical Veterinary Studies, Faculty of Veterinary Science, University of Zimbabwe, Harare, Zimbabwe, and currently Visiting Professor of Comparative Pharmacology, Victorian College of Pharmacy, Monash University, Melbourne, Australia.

Robert D. Walker, M.Sc., Ph.D., is formerly Professor in the Animal Health Diagnostic Laboratory, College of Veterinary Medicine, Michigan State University, East Lansing, and currently Director, Division of Animal and Food Microbiology, Center for Veterinary Medicine, U.S. Food and Drug Administration.

Iowa State University Press
2121 South State Avenue, Ames, Iowa 50014
Orders: 1-800-862-6657
Office: 1-515-292-0140
Fax: 1-515-292-3348
Web site: www.isupress.com

∞ Printed on acid-free paper in the United States of America

Authorization to photocopy items for internal or personal use, or the internal or personal use of specific clients, is granted by Iowa State University Press, provided that the base fee of $.10 per copy is paid directly to the Copyright Clearance Center, 222 Rosewood Drive, Danvers, MA 01923. For those organizations that have been granted a photocopy license by CCC, a separate system of payments has been arranged. The fee code for users of the Transactional Reporting Service is 0-8138-0779-4/2000 $.10.

First edition, 1988
Second edition, 1993
Third edition, 2000

Library of Congress Cataloging-in-Publication Data

Antimicrobial therapy in veterinary medicine / edited by John F. Prescott, J. Desmond Baggot, R.D. Walker; with thirty contributors.—3rd ed.
       p. cm
    Includes bibliographical references.
    ISBN 0-8138-0779-4
       1. Anti-infective agents in veterinary medicine. 2. Communicable diseases in animals—Chemotherapy. I. Prescott, John F. (John Francis)   II. Baggot, J. Desmond. III. Walker, R.D. (Robert D.)

SF918.A48 A58 2000   00-036967
636.089'5329—dc21
The last digit is the print number: 9 8 7 6 5 4 3 2

Acknowledgment

Publication of this book was supported by a generous donation from **Pfizer, Inc.,** Animal Health Group, New York, New York.

Further Acknowledgments

Publication of this book was supported in part by a donation from Fort Dodge Animal Health, Overland Park, Kansas.

Dr. John Prescott acknowledges the Ontario Veterinary College for the time to work on this edition and for the monetary support through the Bull Fund to complete this venture.

Contents

Contributors **xi**
Preface **xiv**
Important Notice and Abbreviations **xvi**

1. Antimicrobial Drug Action and Interaction: An Introduction (*Prescott*) **3**

2. Antimicrobial Susceptibility Testing and Interpretation of Results (*Walker*) **12**

3. Antimicrobial Drug Resistance and Its Epidemiology (*Prescott*) **27**

4. Principles of Antimicrobial Drug Bioavailability and Disposition (*Baggot*) **50**

5. Principles of Antimicrobial Drug Selection and Use (*Prescott, Walker*) **88**

6. Beta-lactam Antibiotics: Penam Penicillins (*Prescott*) **105**

7. Beta-lactam Antibiotics: Cephalosporins and Cephamycins (*Prescott*) **134**

8. Other Beta-lactam Antibiotics: Beta-lactamase Inhibitors, Carbapenems, and Monobactams (*Prescott*) **160**

9. Peptide Antibiotics: Polymyxins, Glycopeptides, Streptogramins, and Bacitracin (*Prescott*) **177**

10. Aminoglycosides and Aminocyclitols (*Prescott*) **191**

11. Lincosamides, Macrolides, and Pleuromutilins (*Prescott*) **229**

12. Chloramphenicol, Thiamphenicol, and Florfenicol (*Prescott*) **263**

13. Tetracyclines (*Prescott*) **275**

14. Sulfonamides, Diaminopyrimidines, and Their Combinations
(*Prescott*)   **290**

15. Fluoroquinolones (*Walker*)   **315**

16. Miscellaneous Antibiotics: Ionophores, Nitrofurans,
Nitroimidazoles, Rifamycins, and Others (*Prescott*)   **339**

17. Antifungal Chemotherapy (*Prescott*)   **367**

18. Antiviral Chemotherapy (*Yoo*)   **396**

19. Special Considerations   **416**
    Selected Organ Systems   **416**
        Infections in Bones and Joints (*Prescott*)   **416**
        Infections of the Eyes: Conjunctivitis, Keratitis, and Endophthalmitis
           (*Prescott*)   **418**
        Infections of the Nervous System: Meningitis and Encephalitis (*Prescott*)   **422**
        Urinary Tract Infections (*Rinkardt and Kruth*)   **426**
    Dose Modification   **437**
        Drug Disposition and Dosage in Neonatal Animals (*Baggot*)   **437**
        Antimicrobials and Anthelmintics in Pregnancy (*Baggot*)   **452**
        Renal Impairment (*Riviere*)   **453**
    Selected Bacterial Infections   **458**
        Anaerobes (*Hirsh*)   **458**
        Brucella (*Hirsh*)   **462**
        Atypical Mycobacteria (*Hirsh*)   **463**
        Mycoplasmas (*Hirsh*)   **466**
        Nocardia (*Hirsh*)   **468**
        Leptospira (*Prescott*)   **470**
    Infections Associated with Neutropenia in the Dog and Cat
        (*Abrams-Ogg, Kruth*)   **471**

20. Anthelmintic Chemotherapy (*Rew, McKenzie*)   **490**

21. Antimicrobial Drug Use in Horses (*Giguere, Sweeney*)   **509**

22. Antimicrobial Drug Use in Dogs and Cats (*Watson, Rosin*)   **537**

23. Antimicrobial Drug Use in Cattle (*Bateman*)   **576**

24. Antimicrobial Drug Use in Sheep and Goats (*Menzies*)   **591**

25. Antimicrobial Drug Use in Swine (*Friendship*)   **602**

26. Antimicrobial Drug Use in Companion Birds (*Dorrestein*)   **617**

27. Antimicrobial Drug Use in Poultry (*Tanner*)   **637**

28. Antimicrobial Drug Use in Rodents, Rabbits, and Ferrets
(*Burgmann*)   **656**

29. Antimicrobial Drug Use in Reptiles (*Jacobson*)   **678**

30. Antimicrobial Drug Use in Aquaculture (*Alderman*)   **692**

31. Antimicrobial Drug Use in Bovine Mastitis (*Erskine*)   **712**

32. Growth Promotion and Feed Antibiotics (*Shryock*)   **735**

33. Antimicrobial Drug Residues in Food-producing Animals (*Sundlof, Fernandez, Paige*)   **744**

34. Regulation of Antibiotic Use in Animals (*Miller, Flynn*)   **760**

Index   **773**

Contributors

Chapter numbers are in parentheses.

Dr. A. C. G. Abrams-Ogg (19)
Department of Clinical Studies
Ontario Veterinary College
University of Guelph
Guelph, Ontario N1G 2W1
Canada

Dr. D. J. Alderman (30)
Centre for Environment, Fisheries
    and Aquaculture Science
Weymouth Laboratory
Barrack Road, The Nothe
Weymouth, Dorset DT4 8UB
United Kingdom

Dr. J. D. Baggot (4, 19)
Department of Preclinical
    Veterinary Studies
Faculty of Veterinary Science
University of Zimbabwe
Harare, Zimbabwe

Dr. K. G. Bateman (23)
Department of Population
    Medicine
Ontario Veterinary College
University of Guelph
Guelph, Ontario N1G 2W1
Canada

Dr. P. Burgmann (28)
High Park Animal Clinic
3194 Dundas Street, West
Toronto, Ontario M6P 2A3
Canada

Dr. G. M. Dorrestein (26)
Department of Veterinary
    Pathology
Section of Laboratory and Special
    Animals
Utrecht University
Yalelaan 1, 3584 CL Utrecht
The Netherlands

Dr. R. J. Erskine (31)
Michigan State University
College of Veterinary Medicine
Department of Large Animal
    Clinical Sciences
D-201 Veterinary Medical Center
East Lansing, MI 48824-1314
U.S.A.

Dr. A. H. Fernandez (33)
Center for Veterinary Medicine
U.S. Food and Drug
    Administration
7500 Standish Place
Rockville, MD 20855
U.S.A.

Dr. W. T. Flynn (34)
Office of Surveillance and
    Compliance
Center for Veterinary Medicine
U.S. Food and Drug
    Administration
7500 Standish Place, HFV-100
Rockville, MD 20855
U.S.A.

Dr. R. M. Friendship (25)
Department of Population
    Medicine
Ontario Veterinary College
University of Guelph
Guelph, Ontario N1G 2W1
Canada

Dr. S. Giguere (21)
Department of Large Animal
    Clinical Sciences
College of Veterinary Medicine
University of Florida
P.O. Box 100136
Gainesville, FL 32610-0136
U.S.A.

Dr. D. C. Hirsh (19)
Department of Veterinary
    Microbiology, Pathology,
    Immunology
School of Veterinary Medicine
University of California
Davis, CA 95616
U.S.A.

Dr. E. R. Jacobson (29)
Department of Small Animal
    Clinical Sciences
College of Veterinary Medicine
Box J-126, Health Science Center
Gainesville, FL 32610-0126
U.S.A.

Dr. S. A. Kruth (19)
Department of Clinical Studies
Ontario Veterinary College
University of Guelph
Guelph, Ontario N1G 2W1
Canada

Dr. E. McKenzie (20)
Pfizer, Inc.
Animal Health Group
812 Springdale Drive
Exton, PA 19341-2803
U.S.A.

Dr. P. I. Menzies (24)
Department of Population
    Medicine
Ontario Veterinary College
University of Guelph
Guelph, Ontario N1G 2W1
Canada

Dr. M. A. Miller (34)
Office of Surveillance and
    Compliance
Center for Veterinary Medicine
U.S. Food and Drug
    Administration
7500 Standish Place, HFV-100
Rockville, MD 20855
U.S.A.

Dr. J. C. Paige (33)
Center for Veterinary Medicine
U.S. Food and Drug
    Administration
7500 Standish Place
Rockville, MD 20855
U.S.A.

Dr. J. F. Prescott (1, 3, 5–14, 16, 17, 19)
Department of Pathobiology
University of Guelph
Guelph, Ontario N1G 2W1
Canada

Dr. R. S. Rew (20)
Pfizer, Inc.
Animal Health Group
812 Springdale Drive
Exton, PA 19341-2803
U.S.A.

Dr. N. Rinkardt (19)
Department of Clinical Studies
Ontario Veterinary College
University of Guelph
Guelph, Ontario N1G 2W1
Canada

Dr. J. E. Riviere (19)
College of Veterinary Medicine
North Carolina State University
Box 8401
Raleigh, NC 27606
U.S.A.

Dr. E. Rosin (22) (deceased)

Dr. T. J. Shryock (32)
Elanco Animal Health
2001 West Main Street
P.O. Box 708
Greenfield, IN 46140
U.S.A.

Dr. S. F. Sundlof (33)
Director, Center for Veterinary
    Medicine
U.S. Food and Drug
    Administration
7500 Standish Place
Rockville, MD 20855
U.S.A.

Dr. C. R. Sweeney (21)
Department of Clinical Studies
Section of Medicine
University of Pennsylvania
New Bolton Center
382 West Street Road
Kennett Square, PA 19348
U.S.A.

Dr. A. C. Tanner (27)
Pfizer, Inc.
Animal Health Group
235 E. 42nd Street
New York, NY 10017-5755
U.S.A.

Dr. R. D. Walker (2,5,15)
Center for Veterinary Medicine,
    HFV-530
U.S. Food and Drug
    Adminstration
8401 Muirkirk Road
Laurel, MD 20708
U.S.A.

Dr. A. D. J. Watson (22)
Department of Veterinary
    Clinical Sciences
University of Sydney
New South Wales 2006
Australia

Dr. D. Yoo (18)
Department of Pathobiology
Ontario Veterinary College
University of Guelph
Guelph, Ontario N1G 2W1
Canada

Preface

This third edition of *Antimicrobial Therapy in Veterinary Medicine* is an updated and slightly expanded version of the second edition. We welcome the editorial reinforcement and expertise of Bob Walker for this edition. Besides revising the antimicrobial and species chapters, we have added chapters on the use of antimicrobial drugs in aquaculture (by David Alderman) and regulation of antibiotic use in animals (by Peggy Miller and William Flynn), as well as recruiting Tom Shryock to revise the chapter on growth promotion and feed antibiotics, Ron Erskine on bovine mastitis, and Dongwan Yoo on antiviral therapy. We are grateful to all the contributors for the care and effort they have put into their chapters. More generally, veterinary medicine owes a debt of gratitude to the many scientists who have contributed to the large volume of literature on antimicrobial drug use in animals. Although we do not have space to name these scientists here, some of their work is cited in the bibliography associated with each chapter or section.

We have revised this book against the background of extensive reexamination of the use of feed antibiotics as growth promoters and disease prophylactics in animals, because of the crisis of antibiotic resistance in human medicine. The crisis of resistance reminds all who use antibiotics of the relative fragility of what remain to us "miracle drugs," a source of constant wonder. We hope the message of prudence in their use comes across to each new generation of veterinarians and others entrusted with using antimicrobial drugs in animals.

We thank the Animal Health Group of Pfizer, Inc., and Fort Dodge Animal Health, Overland Park, Kansas, for their subsidies of this book, which will enable it to be within the price range of veterinary students, who are an important part of our audience. Pfizer's and Fort Dodge Animal Health's commitment to supporting in this way the improved usage of antibiotics in animals deserves wide recognition and thanks.

We are grateful to Joan Hamilton for help with some of the keyboarding and to Sue Ann Walker for help with some of the figures. We thank the staff of Iowa State University Press, particularly Judi Brown,

Lynne Bishop, and Gretchen Van Houten, for their support of this book. We also are grateful to Rosemary Sheffield for her editing expertise. John Prescott revised this book while on leave for this purpose from the Ontario Veterinary College. He thanks the College for support of this venture and for support from the Bull Fund. We hope that readers will continue to send comments to John Prescott, so that any future editions can be improved.

John Prescott, Desmond Baggot, Bob Walker

Important Notice and Abbreviations

The indications and dosages of all drugs in this book are the recommendations of the authors and do not always agree with those given on the package inserts prepared by the pharmaceutical manufacturers in different countries. The medications described do not necessarily have the specific approval of national regulatory authorities, including the U.S. Food and Drug Administration, for use in the diseases and dosages for which they are recommended. In addition, while every effort has been made to check the contents of this book, errors may have been missed. The package insert for each drug product should therefore be consulted for use, route of administration, dosage, and (for food animals) withdrawal period, as approved by the reader's national regulatory authorities.

The following abbreviations are used in this book:

MIC = minimum inhibitory concentration
MBC = minimum bactericidal concentration
PO= *per os*, oral administration
IM= intramuscular administration
IV= intravenous administration
SC= subcutaneous administration
q6, q8, q12 hours, etc. = every 6, 8, 12 hours, etc.

The following abbreviations relating to antimicrobial therapy in animals are sometimes used:

SID = single daily administration
BID = twice daily administration (every 12 hours)
TID = three times daily administration (every 8 hours)
QID = four times daily administration (every 6 hours)

A dosage of, for example, "10 mg/kg TID IM" means 10 mg/kg administered every 8 hours intramuscularly.

Antimicrobial Therapy in Veterinary Medicine

THIRD EDITION

1

Antimicrobial Drug Action and Interaction: An Introduction

J. F. PRESCOTT

Antimicrobial drugs exploit differences in structure or biochemical function between host and parasite. Modern chemotherapy is traced to Paul Ehrlich, a pupil of Robert Koch's who devoted his career to discovering agents that possessed selective toxicity so that they might act as "magic bullets" in the fight against infection. The remarkable efficacy of modern antimicrobial drugs still retains a sense of the miraculous. Sulfonamides, the first clinically successful broad-spectrum antibacterial agents, were produced in Germany in 1935.

It was the discovery by Fleming in 1929 of the antibiotic penicillin, a fungal metabolite, and its later development by Ernst Chain and Howard Florey during World War II that led to the antibiotic revolution. An *antibiotic* is a substance that is produced by a microorganism and at low concentrations inhibits or kills other microorganisms. Many other antibiotics were described within a few years of the introduction of penicillin. Their chemical modification has led to the continuing development of increasingly powerful and effective new antimicrobial drugs. Although there are several important non-antibiotic synthetic antibacterial agents, such as the sulfonamides and fluoroquinolones, antibiotics are the most important source of antibacterial agents. The word *antimicrobial* has a broader definition than *antibiotic* and includes any substance of natural, semisynthetic, or synthetic origin that kills or inhibits the growth of a microorganism but causes little or no damage to the host. *Antimicrobial* is often used synonymously with *antibiotic*.

The marked structural and biochemical differences between prokaryotic and eukaryotic cells give antimicrobial agents greater opportunities for selective toxicity against bacteria than against fungi, which are nucleated like mammalian cells, or against viruses, which reproduce using their host's genetic material. Nevertheless, in recent years increasingly effective antifungal and antiviral drugs have been introduced into clinical practice.

Important milestones in the development of antibacterial drugs are shown in Figure 1.1. The therapeutic use of these agents in veterinary medicine has usually followed their use in human medicine because of the enormous costs of development. Some antibacterial drugs have been developed specifically for animal health and production, such as tylosin and tiamulin. Figure 1.1 highlights the relationship between antibiotic use and the development of resistance in many target microorganisms.

Spectrum of Activity of Antimicrobial Drugs

Antimicrobial drugs may be classified in a variety of ways, based on three basic features.

Class of Microorganism

Antiviral and antifungal drugs generally are active against only viruses and fungi, respectively. Antibacterial agents are described as *narrow-spectrum* if they inhibit only bacteria or as *broad-spectrum* if they also inhibit mycoplasmas, rickettsias, and chlamydiae. The spectrum of activity of common antibacterials is shown in Table 1.1.

Antibacterial Activity

Some antibacterial drugs are also considered narrow-spectrum in that they inhibit only Gram-positive or Gram-negative bacteria. Broad-spectrum drugs inhibit both Gram-positive and Gram-negative bacteria. Other agents may be most active against Gram-positive bacteria but will also inhibit some Gram-negatives (Table 1.2). With the greater availability of broad-spectrum antibacterial drugs, these terms are increasingly uncommon.

Bacteriostatic or Bactericidal Activity

Some antibacterial agents inhibit the growth of a bacterium at one concentration, the minimum inhibitory concentration (MIC) (eg, 0.25 µg/ml), but a higher concentration, the minimum bactericidal concentration (MBC), is necessary to kill it (eg, 4.0 µg/ml). An antibacterial agent that exhibits a large dilution difference between inhibitory and cidal effects is considered to be a *bacteriostatic* drug. On the other hand, an antibacterial agent that kills the bacterium at or near the same drug concentration that inhibits its growth is considered to be a *bactericidal* drug. Under certain clinical conditions this distinction is important, but it is not

Human Infectious Disease

Antibacterial Agents

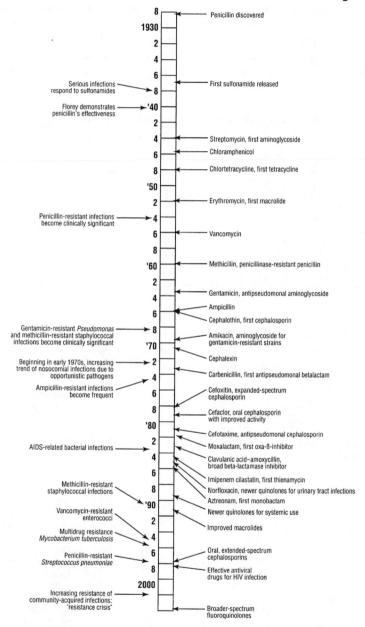

Fig. 1.1. Milestones in human infectious disease and their relationship to development of antibacterial drugs. Modified and reproduced with permission from Kammer (1982).

absolute. In other words, some drugs are often bactericidal (eg, beta-lactams, aminoglycosides) and others are usually bacteriostatic (eg, chloramphenicol, tetracyclines), but this distinction is an approximation, depending on both the drug concentration and the organism involved. Thus, benzyl penicillin is bactericidal at usual concentrations and bacteriostatic at low concentrations. Fluoroquinolones are bactericidal at low

TABLE 1.1. **Spectrum of activity of common antibacterial drugs**

	Class of Microorganism					
	Bacteria	Fungi	Mycoplasmas	Rickettsias	Chlamydiae	Protozoa
Aminoglycosides	+	−	+	−	−	−
Beta-lactams	+	−	−	−	−	−
Chloramphenicol	+	−	+	+	+	−
Fluoroquinolones	+	−	+	+	+	−
Lincosamides	+	−	+	−	−	+
Macrolides	+	−	+	−	+	−
Pleuromutilins	+	−	+	−	+	−
Tetracyclines	+	−	+	+	+	−
Sulfonamides	+	−	+	−	+	+
Trimethoprim	+	−	−	−	−	+

TABLE 1.2. **Antibacterial activity of selected antibiotics**

	Aerobic Bacteria		Anaerobic Bacteria		
Spectrum	Gram +	Gram −	Gram +	Gram −	Examples
Very broad	+	+	+	+	Azlocillin; cefoxitin; chloramphenicol; imipenem; moxalactam; tetracyclines
Intermediately broad	+	+	+	(+)	Carbenicillin; cefoperazone; cefotaxime; ceftriaxone; first- and second-generation cephalosporins
	+	(+)	+	(+)	Ampicillin, amoxycillin
Narrow	−	+	−	−	Aztreonam, mecillinam, cefsulodin, polymyxin
	+	(+)	+	(+)	Penicillin
	(+)	+	−	−	Aminoglycosides, spectinomycin, sulfonamides, trimethoprim
	+	−	+	+	Lincosamides, macrolides, pleuromutilins, spiramycin, vancomycin
	+	−	+	−	Bacitracin
	−	−	+	+	Nitroimidazoles

serum or tissue concentrations to MIC values (1:1), bactericidal at higher ratios, and then bacteriostatic again at very high values.

Mechanisms of Action of Antimicrobial Drugs
Antibacterial Drugs

The diverse sites of action of the antibacterial drugs are summarized in Figure 1.2. Their mechanisms of action fall into four categories: inhibition of cell wall synthesis, damage to cell membrane function, inhibition of nucleic acid synthesis or function, and inhibition of protein synthesis.

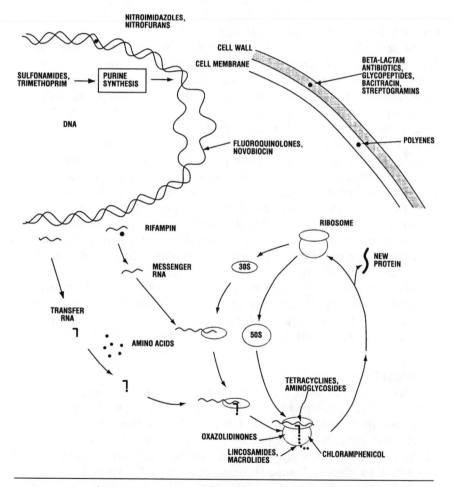

Fig. 1.2. Sites of action of commonly used antibacterial drugs that affect virtually all important processes in a bacterial cell. Modified and reproduced with permission after Aharonowitz and Cohen (1981).

Antibacterial drugs that affect cell wall synthesis (beta-lactam antibiotics, bacitracin, vancomycin) or inhibit protein synthesis (aminoglycosides, chloramphenicol, lincosamides, macrolides, pleuromutilins, tetracyclines) are more numerous and important than those that affect cell membrane function (polymixins) or nucleic acid function (nitroimidazoles, nitrofurans, quinolones, rifampin), although the development of fluoroquinolone antibiotics has been a major recent advance in antimicrobial therapy. Agents that affect intermediate metabolism (sulfonamides, trimethoprim) have greater selective toxicity than those that affect nucleic acid synthesis.

Searching for New Antibacterial Drugs

Most antibacterial drugs in major use are analogs of only six major classes of antibiotics (aminoglycosides, cephalosporins, macrolides, penicillins, quinolones, and tetracyclines). The problem of increasing resistance is leading to increased efforts to find novel antibiotics, particularly narrow-spectrum antibiotics with activity against defined pathogens. The approaches in the search for novel antibiotics include further development of analogs of existing agents; identifying novel targets based on a biotechnological approach, including use of information obtained from bacterial genome sequencing and gene cloning; screening of natural products from plants and microorganisms from unusual ecological niches other than soil; development of antibacterial peptide molecules derived from phagocytic cells of many species; screening for novel antimicrobials using combinatorial chemical libraries; development of synthetic antibacterial drugs with novel activities, such as oxazolidinones; development of new antibiotic classes that were abandoned early in the antibiotic revolution because existing drug classes had similar activities; development of "chimeramycins" by laboratory recombination of genes encoding antibiotics of different classes; and combination of antibacterial drugs with iron-binding chemicals targeting bacterial iron uptake mechanisms.

Antifungal Drugs

Most currently used systemic antifungal drugs damage cell membrane function by binding ergosterols that are unique to the fungal cell membrane (polyenes, azoles) (see Chapter 17). The increase in the number of AIDS patients and of people undergoing organ or bone marrow transplants has resulted in increased numbers of immunosuppressed individuals in many societies. The susceptibility of these people to fungal infections has renewed interest in the discovery and development of new antifungal agents. The focus of antifungal drug development has shifted to cell wall structures unique to fungi (1,3-β-D-glucan synthase inhibitors, chitin synthase inhibitors, mannoprotein binders) (see Chapter 17).

Antiviral Drugs

Antiviral drugs act only during viral replication; newer analogs are targeted at inhibition of absorption or penetration of viruses into the cell or inhibition of their assembly and release (Fig. 18.1). The distinction between deoxyribonucleic acid (DNA) and ribonucleic acid (RNA) viruses is important in antiviral therapy. The AIDS crisis has led to a dramatic increase in discovery and development of new, clinically effective antiviral drugs.

Antibacterial Drug Interactions: Synergism, Antagonism, and Indifference

Knowledge of the different mechanisms of action of antimicrobials provides some ability to predict their interaction when they are used in combination. It was clear from the early days of their use that combinations of antibacterials might give antagonistic rather than additive or synergistic effects. Concerns regarding combinations include the difficulty in defining synergism and antagonism, particularly their method of determination in vitro; the difficulty of predicting the effect of a combination against a particular organism; and the uncertainty of the clinical relevance of in vitro findings. The clinical use of antimicrobial drug combinations is described in Chapter 5. With the availability of broad-spectrum antibacterial drugs, combinations of these drugs are less commonly used, except for specific purposes.

An antibacterial combination is *additive* or *indifferent* if the combined effects of the drugs equal the sum of their independent activities measured separately; *synergistic* if the combined effects are significantly greater than the independent effects; and *antagonistic* if the combined effects are significantly less than their independent effects. Synergism and antagonism are not absolute characteristics. Such interactions are often hard to predict, vary with bacterial species and strains, and may occur only over a narrow range of concentrations or ratios of drug components. Because antimicrobial drugs may interact with each other in many different ways, it is apparent that no single in vitro method will detect all such interactions. Although the techniques to quantify and detect interactions are relatively crude, the observed interactions occur clinically.

The two methods commonly used, the *checkerboard* and the *killing curve* methods, measure two different effects (growth inhibition and killing) and have sometimes shown poor clinical and laboratory correlation. In the absence of simple methods for detecting synergism or antagonism, the following general guidelines may be used.

Synergism of Antibacterial Combinations

Antimicrobial combinations are frequently synergistic if they involve (1) sequential inhibition of successive steps in metabolism (eg, trimethoprim-sulfonamide); (2) sequential inhibition of cell wall synthesis (eg, mecillinam-ampicillin); (3) facilitation of drug entry of one antibiotic by another (eg, beta-lactam–aminoglycoside); (4) inhibition of inactivating enzymes (eg, ampicillin–clavulanic acid); and (5) prevention of emergence of resistant populations (eg, erythromycin-rifampin).

Antagonism of Antibacterial Combinations

To some extent the definition of antagonism as it relates to antibacterial combinations reflects a laboratory artifact. However, there have been clinical situations in which antagonism is clinically important. Antagonism may occur if antibacterial combinations involve (1) inhibition of bactericidal activity such as treatment of meningitis in which a bacteriostatic drug prevents the bactericidal activity of another, (2) competition for drug-binding sites such as macrolide-chloramphenicol combinations (of uncertain clinical significance), (3) inhibition of cell permeability mechanisms such as chloramphenicol-aminoglycoside combinations (of uncertain clinical significance), and (4) induction of beta-lactamases by beta-lactam drugs such as imipenem and cefoxitin combined with older beta-lactam drugs that are beta-lactamase unstable.

The impressive complexity of the interactions of antibiotics, the differences of such effects among bacterial species, and the uncertainty of the applicability of in vitro findings to clinical settings make predicting the effects of some combinations hazardous. For example, the same combination may cause both antagonism and synergism in different strains of the same species. Laboratory determinations are really required but may give conflicting results, depending on the test used. Knowledge of the mechanism of action is probably the best approach to predicting the outcome of the interaction in the absence of other guidelines.

In general, the use of combinations should be avoided, because the toxicity of the antibiotics will be at least additive and may be synergistic, because the ready availability of broad-spectrum bactericidal drugs has made their use largely unnecessary, and because they may be more likely to lead to bacterial superinfection. There are, however, well-established circumstances, discussed in Chapter 5, in which combinations of drugs are more effective and often less toxic than drugs administered alone.

Bibliography

Aharonowitz Y, Cohen G. 1981. The microbiological production of pharmaceuticals. Sci Am 245:141.

Chan EL, Zabransky RJ. 1987. Determination of synergy by two methods with eight antimicrobial combinations against tobramycin-susceptible and tobramycin-resistant strains of *Pseudomonas*. Diagn Microbiol Infect Dis 6:157.

Eliopoulos GM, Moellering RC. 1991. Antimicrobial combinations. In: Lorian V, ed. Antibiotics in Laboratory Medicine. Baltimore: Williams and Wilkins.

Ford CW, et al. 1997. Oxazolidinones: new antibacterial agents. Trends Microbiol 5:196.

Hirsh DC, et al. 1990. Lack of supportive data for use of ampicillin together with trimethoprim-sulfonamide as broad-spectrum antimicrobial treatment of bacterial disease in dogs. J Am Vet Med Assoc 197:594.

Kammer RB. 1982. Milestones in antimicrobial therapy. In: Morin RB, Gorman M, eds. Chemistry and Biology of Beta-lactam Antibiotics. Vol 3. Orlando, FL: Academic Press.

Lehrer RI, et al. 1993. Defensin: antimicrobial and cytotoxic peptides of mammalian cells. Annu Rev Immunol 11:105.

Moellering RC. 1979. Antimicrobial synergism—an elusive concept. J Infect Dis 140:630.

Rahal JJ. 1978. Antibiotic combinations: the clinical relevance of synergy and antagonism. Medicine 57:179.

Ryback MJ, McGrath BJ. 1996. Combination antimicrobial therapy for bacterial infections. Drugs 52:390.

Silen JY, et al. 1998. Screening for novel antimicrobials from encoded combinatorial libraries by using a two-dimensional agar format. Antimicrob Agents Chemother 42:1447.

Williams JD, ed. 1979. Antibiotic Interactions. New York: Academic Press.

2

Antimicrobial Susceptibility Testing and Interpretation of Results

R. D. WALKER

Unlike almost all other chemical therapies administered to animals, which target specific sites within the animal, antimicrobial chemotherapy targets the microorganism causing the infectious disease process. It is the elimination of that microorganism that will resolve the disease. Antimicrobial agents, however, rarely eradicate a pathogen without the assistance of the host's specific and nonspecific defenses. The purpose of antimicrobial chemotherapy is to assist the host's defense mechanisms in eradicating the causative agent. When antimicrobial agents are used, it is important that the right drug be used, at the right concentration, at the right dosing interval, for the right length of time.

In choosing the right agent, several factors must be considered. The pathogens' susceptibility to the agent is first in importance. In conjunction with this are the pharmacokinetic and the pharmacodynamic properties of the drug (Fig. 2.1). Pharmacokinetic properties include the route of administration, the rate of absorption, the rate of distribution, the volume of distribution, the protein binding capacity of the drug, and the route and rate of elimination, all of which influence the frequency of dosing. Pharmacodynamic properties include concentration versus time in the tissue and other body fluids, toxicologic effect, concentration versus time at the site of the infection, and antimicrobial effect at the site of the infection. Pharmacodynamic antimicrobial effects at the site of the infection include minimal inhibitory concentration (MIC), minimal bactericidal concentration (MBC), concentration-dependent killing effect, first exposure effect, post-antibiotic effect (PAE), sub-MIC effect (SM-PAE), and post-antibiotic leucocyte enhancement effect (PALE). Other factors, sometimes of equal

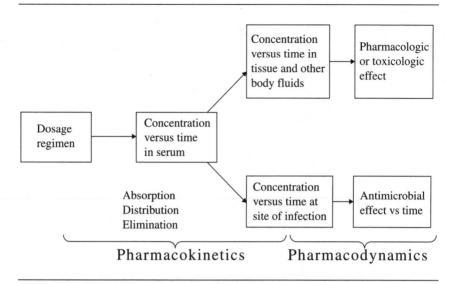

Fig. 2.1. Interaction of pharmacokinetic and pharmacodynamic parameters in antimicrobial chemotherapy. After Craig (1998).

importance, include the cost of the therapy, and the host's immune defenses and renal and hepatic functions.

This chapter describes the various types of in vitro antimicrobial susceptibility tests, how they are performed, and the basis of how a laboratory defines an organism as susceptible or resistant. Chapter 5 discusses considerations involved in choosing an antimicrobial agent and in designing a dosage regimen that maximizes the clinical efficacy of the agent chosen.

Indications for In Vitro Antimicrobial Susceptibility Testing

The target of antimicrobial therapy is the bacterium causing the infection. Different bacterial isolates, even those belonging to the same species, may require different concentrations of drug to inhibit their growth (Table 2.1). In addition, the MIC for a single species may vary within the same animal (Fig. 2.2), and MICs can change over time (Table 2.2). Despite potential variations in a pathogenic bacterium's susceptibility profile, the clinician's experience or knowledge of local susceptibility and resistance patterns of the suspected pathogen can usually guide empirical therapy. Where knowledge of the pathogen's susceptibility profile is either unknown or unpredictable, or if the infection is life threatening and knowledge of the pathogen's susceptibility profile could save the patient's life should the empiric therapy fail, in vitro susceptibility tests should be performed.

TABLE 2.1. **In vitro activity of selected antimicrobial agents against *Pseudomonas aeruginosa* isolated from specimens collected from small animals (SA) and large animals (LA)**

Antimicrobial Agent		Number Tested	MIC (µg/ml)											
			0.03	0.06	0.125	0.25	0.5	1.0	2.0	4.0	8.0	16.0	32.0	≥64.0
Amikacin	SA	149							67	38	14	3		
	LA	28							24	2	2		4	1
Gentamicin	SA	149			6	9	32	47	30	13	7			
	LA	28			3	0	6	15	1	1		1		
Ticarcillin	SA	149									25	70	35	18
	LA	28									1	16	9	1
Enrofloxacin	SA	149	1	2	21	36	57	17	4	2				
	LA	28			1	12	12	3						

Source: Data from Michigan State University, 1989–1999, Walker (unpubl.).

range between isolates

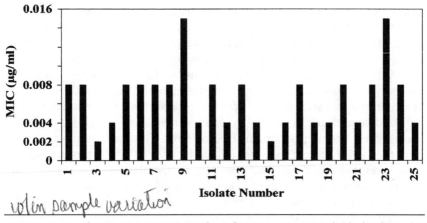

ω[in Dample variation

Fig. 2.2. In vitro activity of enrofloxacin against 25 individual isolates of *E. coli* from a single fecal sample. The MICs ranged from 0.002 μg/ml to 0.016 μg/ml, representing a nearly 10-fold difference between the most susceptible and the least susceptible isolates.

Δ in MIC 90's w/ time

TABLE 2.2. **Changes in MICs of bacterial pathogens from dogs to enrofloxacin**

Organism	Year Tested	Number Tested	MIC$_{50}$	MIC$_{90}$	MIC$_{100}$
Escherichia coli	1991	48		≤0.08	0.16
	1996	78	0.03	0.06	>2.0
Klebsiella pneumoniae	1991	16		≤0.08	≤0.08
	1996	20	0.06	0.125	>2.0
Proteus mirabilis	1991	50		≤0.08	0.16
	1996	38	0.25	0.5	0.5
Staphylococcus intermedius	1991	85		0.16	0.16
	1996	164		0.5	1.0

Source: Modified from Walker and Thornsberry (1998).

   Not all of bacteria isolated from a specimen should be subjected to susceptibility testing. Bacteria that are typically considered to be contaminants or normal flora should not be tested. The reasons for this guideline include the expense associated with unnecessary testing, the possibility that such testing will result in the clinician's treating normal flora, and the potential selection of more expensive or more toxic agents. Susceptibility testing should not be performed on organisms known to be susceptible to inexpensive, nontoxic agents. For example, beta-hemolytic streptococci are universally susceptible to penicillin in vitro and in vivo. They may also be susceptible to gentamicin in vitro. However, when associated with a purulent abscess, they will not be inhibited by gentamicin in vivo, because gentamicin diffuses poorly into abscesses, is inactivated by purulent exudate, and requires an oxidative transport system to penetrate the bacterial membrane, and abscesses are void of oxygen. Thus, results from an in vitro susceptibility test that report that an organism such as *Streptococcus zooepidemicus* is susceptible to gentamicin could be misleading.

Although the results of in vitro antimicrobial susceptibility testing can and have been used successfully to predict clinical responses, the user must keep in mind that such tests are static tests performed under carefully standardized conditions. In the in vivo environment, from which the pathogen was isolated, nothing is standardized or static. Thus, the results generated from the in vitro testing may be nullified by a variety of factors in vivo that are intrinsic to the antimicrobial agent, the host, or the pathogen. Despite this proviso, when tested under standardized conditions, use of antimicrobial agents classified as susceptible by in vitro susceptibility testing has a high probability of predicting a favorable outcome, whereas use of antimicrobial agents classified as resistant predicts a poor clinical response (Craig, 1993).

Susceptibility Testing Methods

Although there are several methods for performing in vitro antimicrobial susceptibility tests, one basic concept is that they use inhibition rather than killing of the bacterium as the end point, with test results being reported qualitatively or quantitatively. Qualitative results are reported as susceptible, intermediate, or resistant, whereas quantitative results are reported as minimal inhibitory concentrations (MICs) in $\mu g/ml$ or mg/l. Testing procedures that generate quantitative results usually also interpret them qualitatively. Methods of performing in vitro susceptibility tests include disk diffusion, agar dilution, broth macrodilution, broth microdilution, and a concentration gradient test (E test®). Of these, the disk diffusion and the broth microdilution tests are the ones most commonly used in veterinary medicine, although the E test® is gaining in popularity. The decision on which test method to use is based on cost, ease of use, and flexibility as it relates to the needs of the laboratory's clientele.

Disk Diffusion Test

The disk diffusion test has been the testing method most widely used in veterinary medicine because of its flexibility in types and number of drugs that can be tested on a daily basis, and its relatively low cost. As the name implies, the disk diffusion test is based on the diffusion of an antimicrobial agent from a disk (commercially prepared and thus standardized, if stored properly) placed on an agar surface of standardized growth medium that has been seeded with approximately 1.0×10^8 colony-forming units (CFU)/ml of a pure culture of the test bacterium. When the disk is applied to the seeded agar surface, a race is initiated between the growth of the bacterium on the agar surface and the diffusion of the drug through the agar. The diffusion of the antimicrobial agent results in a drug concentration gradient. When the concentration of the antimicrobial agent becomes too dilute to inhibit the growth of the bacterium, a zone of inhibition is formed. This zone of inhibition correlates inversely with the MIC of the test organism. In other words, the larger the zone of inhibition, the smaller the concentration of drug required to inhibit the pathogen. The use of too many bacteria in the original inoculum results in smaller zones of inhibition, whereas the use of too few organisms, as is usually the case in plates inoculated directly from clinical samples, results in larger zones of inhibition. The latter circumstance may make some bacteria appear susceptible that might be resistant if tested under the standardized conditions of the test.

The major disadvantage of the disk diffusion test is that results are qualitative. The submitting veterinarian is told by the laboratory that the organism is susceptible but is not told how susceptible. If the clinician knew how susceptible the pathogen was to a particular antibacterial agent, the dose might be adjusted to maximize clinical efficiency or reduce costs. The potential value of quantitative information to the clinician has prompted the development of two variations of the disk diffusion test. The first is a computerized system that calculates the MIC of an antimicrobial agent from the zone of inhibition generated by the disk diffusion tests, and the second is a concentration gradient system. Both systems were developed for use in human medicine but are beginning to be applied in veterinary medicine. The interpretation of the data generated by the computerized system is based on data collected from testing bacterial isolates from humans. This system has recently been tested on bacteria isolated from animals and found to be potentially useful to the veterinary community but would require an extensive database in order to include many important animal pathogens (Hubert et al., 1998).

The concentration gradient strip (E test®) is a modification of the diffusion test that generates quantitative results. The test relies on the diffusion of a continuous concentration gradient of an antimicrobial agent from a plastic strip into an agar medium seeded with a pure culture of the test bacterium. The plastic strip has a defined concentration of a stabilized dried drug on one side, in a continuous gradient from top to bottom, and a continuous MIC interpretive scale on the other. After incubation, the MIC is determined by reading the concentration on the strip where the zone of inhibition intersects the strip. The cost of the E test® prohibits its use for routine testing in the laboratory, but it is valuable for susceptibility testing of yeast or fastidious organisms, such as anaerobic bacteria and certain species of mycoplasma.

Dilution Susceptibility Tests

Quantitative susceptibility testing may be performed using agar dilution, broth macrodilution, or broth microdilution. Of these, agar dilution is the "gold standard" but together with broth macrodilution is too cumbersome for routine use. The broth microdilution test is, however, being used with increasing frequency in veterinary laboratories. This test is performed in microtiter plates, with round or truncated V-bottom wells, using antimicrobial agents of known potency in progressive two-fold dilutions that encompass concentrations similar to those obtained in serum and tissue at recommended doses. The microtiter trays may be prepared using a variety of formats, but each tray usually contains several antimicrobial agents that are tested against a single isolate. The microtiter trays may be prepared in-house or obtained commercially. Those obtained commercially may be purchased as dehydrated trays or as frozen trays. Dehydrated trays generally have a shelf life of 1 to 2 years and may be stored at room temperature, whereas frozen trays have a shelf life of 6 months and must be stored at –10° C or –70° C, depending on the antibacterial agents contained in the tray. Microdilution tests are more expensive than the disk diffusion test and lack the day-to-day flexibility of a disk diffusion test in choice of the antimicrobial agents. This problem of lack of flexibility may be compounded by bulk buying (to reduce cost) and the need to finish using a 2-year supply of plates before introducing a new antibiotic to the panel. To reduce the cost associated with microtiter dilution trays, some laboratories use "breakpoint" trays. These have more antimicrobial agents than the "full range" trays, but each agent has only two or three dilutions, usually one dilution below the susceptible breakpoint, the susceptible breakpoint, and sometimes one dilution above the susceptible breakpoint. Another modification of the breakpoint panel is to use fewer antimicrobial agents but design the panel so that two or three organisms may be tested on it. Results generated by the use of breakpoint panels are thus qualitative and therefore similar to but often more expensive than those generated by a disk diffusion test.

To perform a broth microdilution test, a bacterial suspension is made from an overnight culture or a culture in logarithmic phase of growth and diluted to a turbidity comparable to that of a 0.5 McFarland turbidity standard (approximately 1.0×10^8 CFU/ml). This suspension is further diluted in sterile water, saline, or broth so that ultimately the final concentration of bacteria per well should be 5×10^4 CFU/well. Once inoculated, the trays are stacked two high in a 35° C incubator with ambient air and incubated for 16–20 hours. When reading the trays, the MIC is recorded as the lowest concentration of antimicrobial agent that completely inhibits the growth of the organism, as determined by the unaided eye.

There is considerable variation globally in the methods used for antimicrobial susceptibility testing of animal pathogens, and there is an urgent need to develop international standards for performance and for interpretation of such tests. One such approach that might form the basis for an international standard is the process and standards used by the National Committee for Clinical Laboratory Standards (NCCLS) in the United States. For more complete details on in vitro antimicrobial suscep-tibility testing, including testing of fastidious organisms such as *Haemophilus somnus* or *Actinobacillus pleuropneumoniae*, the reader is referred to NCCLS M31-A document (NCCLS 1999a).

Interpretation of Susceptibility Tests: Determining the Interpretive Criteria

The results generated by in vitro antimicrobial susceptibility tests, whether they are determined by disk diffusion or dilution methodologies, are generally provided to clinicians by designating the tested pathogen as susceptible, intermediate, or resistant. These designations are arrived at by determining in vitro *breakpoints*—those zones of inhibition or MICs at which an organism is considered to be susceptible, intermediate, or resis-tant based on obtainable serum concentrations of the drug and clinical tri-als. In other words, when a laboratory reports that an organism is suscepti-ble, it implies that the recommended dosage of the antimicrobial agent will reach serum or tissue concentrations sufficient to inhibit the bacterium's growth in vivo. Resistant breakpoints represent those concentrations that cannot be achieved using normal dosage. Intermediate breakpoints are those zones of inhibition or MICs that fall between the susceptible and resistant breakpoints; traditionally these have represented a "buffer zone" that prevented resistant organisms from being categorized as susceptible, or vice versa, because of uncontrolled technical problems in the laboratory. However, this category may also represent susceptible organisms for antimicrobial agents with wide pharmacotoxicity margins, which allow the drug to be administered at higher than recommended doses or are concen-trated at the body site where the infection is occurring, such as beta-lactams or fluoroquinolones in the urinary tract. Recently in the United States, the NCCLS Subcommittee on Veterinary Antimicrobial Susceptibility Testing (VAST) established a fourth interpretive criterion. This criterion has been designated as *flexible* and is used with quantitative testing procedures. *Flex-ible* indicates the availability of a U.S. Food and Drug Administration flexi-ble label, which allows the clinician to adjust the dose, within a given range, based on the MIC of the pathogen (NCCLS 1999a).

Interpretation of In Vitro Antimicrobial Susceptibility Test Results

There are a variety of reasons to suspect that in vitro tests cannot always predict the efficacy of an antimicrobial agent in vivo. In vitro tests involve the continuous exposure of a relatively small concentration of bacteria to a constant level of an antimicrobial agent under standardized testing conditions. These conditions differ considerably from those in vivo, where large numbers of bacteria are exposed to fluctuating levels of the drug at wide variations in pH, oxygen tension, and host defenses. Despite these considerable differences, studies in human medicine have demonstrated the clinical value of in vitro susceptibility tests (Gudmundsson and Craig, 1986; McCabe and Treadwell, 1986; Lorian and Burns, 1990; Stratton, 1991; Craig, 1993; Johnson, 1996). In situations in which a bacterium fails to respond to an antibacterial agent, clinicians should ask the following questions: Did the report indicate that the organism was susceptible, with no additional information, or did the report also include an MIC value for each antimicrobial agent? If the results were limited to susceptible, how susceptible was the pathogen? Was the size of the zone of inhibition at the susceptible breakpoint the smallest susceptible zone size? Studies have shown that smaller zones of inhibition have been associated with increased rates of bacteriological failure (Gerber and Craig, 1981; Thornsberry et al., 1982). This contrasts to favorable clinical responses in patients treated with antimicrobial agents that had low MICs (large zones of inhibition) against the pathogens (Craig, 1993). By generating full-range MICs, a laboratory gives clinicians information that may allow them to individualize the therapeutic regimen, especially with regard to dose and dosing frequency. In other words, if the MIC is very low, the dose or frequency of dosing may be decreased, reducing the cost of the antimicrobial therapy. On the other hand, if the MIC is higher, but the organism is still considered susceptible (flexible category), or the drug has a wide pharmacotoxicity margin, a higher dose of a less expensive or less toxic drug may be given. In other words, interpretation of susceptibility depends on knowing the relationship between in vitro–determined susceptibility and factors involved in its relationship to tissue drug concentrations (which depend on factors such as dose and pharmacokinetic and pharmacodynamic properties of the drug or drug class, discussed in Chapter 5). With greater understanding of efficacious use of different classes of antimicrobial agents, with increased costs of some of these agents, and with decreased susceptibility of many bacteria to commonly used antimicrobial agents, the more that can be determined from in vitro susceptibility testing, the greater the chance of using these drugs successfully.

Historically, the interpretive criteria used in veterinary medicine have come from two sources. The first source is the interpretive criteria established by a drug's sponsor. How these were derived depended on the criteria set by the sponsor and were subject to change based on such things as market influences. The second source was from interpretive criteria set by the NCCLS for antimicrobial drugs used in humans. These interpretive criteria were based on population dynamics, using bacterial isolates from humans, pharmacokinetic data generated in humans, and clinical trials conducted in humans. In 1993 the NCCLS established a subcommittee to develop interpretive criteria for bacterial pathogens isolated from animals, the Subcommittee on Veterinary Antimicrobial Susceptibility Testing. This subcommittee is composed of representatives from academia, industry, and regulatory agencies, a mix consistent with the NCCLS tripartite approach in its consensus process. Determining when to interpret a bacterium as susceptible or resistant to an antimicrobial drug involves two phases in the NCCLS process. The first phase is to establish quality control (QC) ranges, using both diffusion and dilution testing, for the QC organism, in order to validate the in vitro testing of the clinical isolates. The second phase is to determine the interpretive criteria.

To evaluate the performance of in vitro susceptibility tests, the limits of acceptable variability in zones of inhibition or MIC ranges are first defined by testing the agent against all appropriate QC strains of bacteria. These strains are from a single source, usually the American Type Culture Collection. In the early part of this phase of development, the agent is tested against the QC organisms at different pHs and at different concentrations of bacteria to determine the influence these variables have on the test results. Broth microdilution test results are compared with agar dilution test results, using different isolates. Once these data have been generated to establish QC limits, the agent is tested in a minimum of 7 different laboratories, using both the disk diffusion and the broth microdilution testing methods on or in a minimum of 3 different lots of media. For the disk diffusion test, 2 lots of disks are evaluated. At least 10 separate tests are performed for each QC organism over 10 days. A control drug of the same class as the test agent that has already had QC guidelines established is run concurrently with the test agent. Once the QC ranges for the QC organisms have been established, (Figs. 2.3 and 2.4), the interpretive criteria can be determined.

The determination of the interpretive criteria involves generating three pieces of data: (1) the population distribution of the bacterial species for which the test agent is being marketed; (2) the pharmacokinetic parameters of the test agent in the target animal species; (3) the results of the clinical trials. In general, the population distribution study is performed on 300–600 recent clinical isolates representing all species of bacteria likely to be tested, using both the disk diffusion and the broth microdilution testing methods. These isolates should represent a wide geographic distribution but may be determined in a single laboratory in accordance with the NCCLS M37-A document (NCCLS 1999b). Interpretation of the data involves generating a scattergram by plotting the zone of inhibition

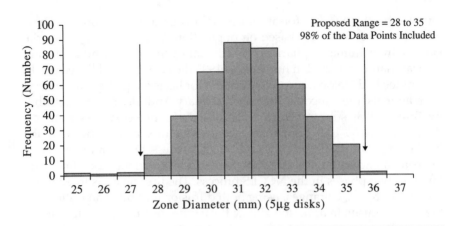

Fig. 2.3. Example of data points generated in a seven-laboratory study designed to define the quality control limits of a new antibacterial agent against a standardized quality control bacterium.

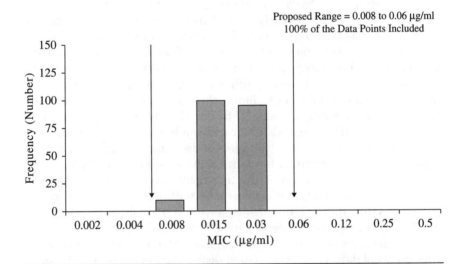

Fig. 2.4. Example of data points generated in a seven-laboratory study designed to define the quality control limits of a new antibacterial agent when tested against a standardized quality control bacterium.

against the MIC for each pathogen and calculating a linear regression line (Fig. 2.5). The selection of breakpoints—susceptible, intermediate, and resistant—is then based on regression line analysis, error rate-bounding, pharmacokinetics, and clinical verification of the breakpoints by clinical and bacteriological response rates.

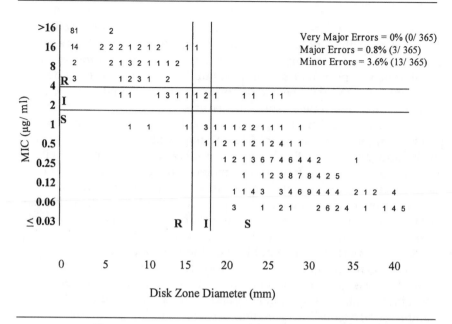

Fig. 2.5. Scattergram comparing MICs and zones of inhibition, which, in conjunction with pharmacokinetic data and results from clinical trials, contribute to the development of interpretive criteria. Numbers refer to number of isolates at each point. *R,* resistant; *I,* intermediate; *S,* susceptible.

Failure of Antimicrobial Susceptibility Tests to Predict Clinical Outcomes

The results of in vitro antimicrobial susceptibility testing of bacteria have the potential to influence decisions on the treatment of individual patients. This is based on the assumption that susceptibility results are predictive of therapeutic efficacy. These assumptions have been validated by several clinical studies in human medicine (Bryan et al., 1983; Gudmundsson and Craig, 1986; Lorian and Burns, 1990; McCabe and Treadwell, 1986; Stratton, 1991), but there is a paucity of similar data in veterinary medicine. Some veterinary clinicians think that in vitro test results are a poor indicator of clinical efficacy. There are several reasons that in vitro susceptibility tests do not always predict clinical outcome. In general, these include errors associated with in vitro testing, errors associated with dosing regimens, and differences between the in vitro environment in which the testing was performed and the in vivo environment in which the drug must be effective.

In Vitro Testing

Several factors may affect the ability of in vitro results to predict clinical efficacy, the most important being the bacterium. Was it the right pathogen? Was it a pure culture? Was it grown under the appropriate conditions at the right concentration? The testing procedure itself may influence the results. For example, bacteria that grow poorly on the artificial medium may appear to be susceptible, but this may be an artifact due to their slow growth rate. The use of appropriate QC should provide protection against improper testing procedures. The interpretive criterion may be misleading. For example, the current NCCLS susceptible breakpoint for ampicillin is 8.0 µg/ml when testing the Enterobacteriaceae and enterococci (NCCLS 1999b). The peak serum concentration of ampicillin, when dosed at 11 mg/kg, is approximately 3.6 µg/ml. The clinical efficacy of ampicillin, as with all beta-lactam antibiotics, is determined by the length of time the serum concentrations exceed the MIC of the pathogen (see Chapter 5). If an organism, such as *Escherichia coli*, isolated from a soft tissue infection, has an MIC of 8.0 µg/ml when tested against ampicillin, it would be reported as susceptible even though the peak serum concentration is much lower than that. The reason for this discrepancy is that the breakpoint was generated from studies involving human isolates, pharmacokinetic values from humans, and human clinical trials. Another example of erroneous interpretation is that a penicillinase-producing (ie, resistant) *Staphylococcus aureus* may be susceptible to concentrations of penicillin G if it is present in the urinary tract, but would not be susceptible if it were present in other tissues. Since the development of the NCCLS-VAST, interpretive criteria for veterinary-specific antimicrobial agents are being generated using animal isolates, pharmacokinetic data collected from the target animal species, and clinical trials conducted in that animal species.

Dosing Regimens

The clinical efficacy of the different classes of antimicrobial agents is dependent on different factors discussed in detail in Chapter 5. For example, the clinical efficacy of the fluoroquinolones is dependent on the concentration of the drug above the MIC of the pathogen in relation to time. Dosage regimens for fluoroquinolones that produce peak serum concentrations that are only 1 to 2 times the MIC of the pathogen contribute to therapeutic failures and the selection of resistant organisms rather than to clinical and microbiological cures, even though the pathogen may have been properly identified and tested and the results indicated that it was susceptible. Errors such as this occur more frequently when qualitative results are reported without quantitative results or when the clinician does not increase the dose to treat susceptible pathogens with higher MICs.

In Vitro versus In Vivo Conditions

In vitro tests must be and are conducted under standardized testing conditions. The pH, the oxygen tension, the temperature, and the concentration and growth rate of the organisms are just a few of the conditions that must be carefully controlled when performing in vitro tests. On the other hand, the in vivo environment in which the selected antimicrobial agent must perform is just the opposite. Nothing is standardized—not the pH, the oxygen tension, the concentration of bacteria, or the ability of the drug to diffuse into or away from the site of the infection. Some antimicrobial agents perform very poorly under the circumstances in which they are used even though the in vitro results indicated that the bacterium would be susceptible. For example, antimicrobial agents that are highly bound to serum proteins diffuse poorly into abscesses. Aminoglycosides, although they are not highly protein bound, are not lipid soluble and therefore do not diffuse in abscesses, are inactivated by purulent exudate and require an oxidative transport to cross a bacterium's cell membrane in order to interact with the ribosome. Purulent exudates are anaerobic, and thus there is no oxygen for an oxygen transport system. The presence of a bacterial biofilm will also impede the effectiveness of an antimicrobial agent. Biofilms form when bacteria are allowed to colonize viable and nonviable tissue or material within the host. Foreign bodies or sequestra provide ideal surfaces for such colonization. Once embedded in these biofilms, the bacteria are out of reach of antimicrobial agents. On the other hand, this does not contribute to why the in vitro testing is not predictive of in vivo results.

Bibliography

Bryan CS, et al. 1983. Analysis of 1,180 episodes of Gram-negative bacteremia in non-university hospitals: the effect of antimicrobial therapy. Rev Infect Dis 5:629–638.

Craig WA. 1993. Qualitative susceptibility versus quantitative MIC tests. Diagn Microbiol Infect Dis 16:231.

Craig WA. 1998. Pharmacokinetic/pharmacodynamic parameters: Rationale for antibacterial dosing of mice and men. Clin Infect Dis 26:1.

Gerber AU, Craig WA. 1981. Worldwide clinical experience with cefoperazone. Drugs 22 (Suppl 1):108.

Gudmundsson S, Craig WA. 1986. Role of antibiotics in endotoxic shock. In: Proctor RA, ed. Clinical Aspects of Endotoxic Shock. Amsterdam: Elsevier.

Hubert SK, et al. 1998. Evaluation of a computerized antimicrobial susceptibility system with bacteria isolated from animals. J Vet Diagn Invest 10:164.

Johnson CC. 1996. In vitro testing: correlation between bacterial susceptibility, body fluid levels, and effectiveness of antibacterial therapy. In: Lorian V, ed. Antibiotics in Laboratory Medicine, 4th ed. Baltimore: Williams and Wilkins.

Lorian V, Burns L. 1990. Predictive value of susceptibility tests for the outcome of antimicrobial therapy. J Antimicrob Chemother 25:175.

McCabe WR, Treadwell TL. 1986. In vitro susceptibility tests: correlations between sensitivity testing and clinical outcome in infected patients. In: Lorian V, ed. Antibiotics in Laboratory Medicine, 2nd ed. Baltimore: Williams and Wilkins.

National Committee on Clinical Laboratory Standards. 1999a. Performance standards for antimicrobial disk and dilution susceptibility tests for bacteria isolated from animals; Approved Standard. NCCLS Document M31-A. Wayne, PA: NCCLS.

National Committee on Clinical Laboratory Standards. 1999b. Development of in vitro susceptibility testing criteria and quality control parameters for veterinary antimicrobial agents; Approved Guidelines. NCCLS Document M37-A. Wayne, PA: NCCLS.

Stratton CW. 1991. In vitro testing: correlation between bacterial susceptibility, body fluid levels, and effectiveness of antibacterial therapy. In: Lorian V, ed. Antibiotics in Laboratory Medicine, 3rd ed. Baltimore: Williams and Wilkins.

Thornsberry C, et al. 1982. Antimicrobial susceptibility tests with cefoxime and correlation with clinical bacteriologic response. Rev Infect Dis 4 (Suppl):S316.

Walker RD, Thornsberry C. 1998. Decrease in antibiotic susceptibility or increase in resistance. J Antimicrob Chemother 41:1.

3 | Antimicrobial Drug Resistance and Its Epidemiology

J. F. PRESCOTT

The use of antibacterial drugs selects for resistant bacteria, and that selection tends to occur in stepwise increments. For reasons that are not fully clear, resistant bacteria have a tendency to acquire multiple resistant mechanisms. Once a bacterium has acquired a resistance mechanism, it tends to retain it. The use of these drugs does not create resistance but rather eliminates the susceptible bacteria in the host and spares the resistant ones. Use of antibacterial drugs thus provides the selection force for the Darwinian process of natural selection. Only the "fittest," resistant bacteria survive antibacterial drugs. Indeed, antibacterial use over the last 50 years has significantly changed the frequency of different types of bacterial infections observed in animals and humans. The potential for mutation by bacteria and for genetic exchange between bacteria, combined with the short generation time of bacteria, can rapidly produce resistant populations, which will be selected by the use of antibacterial drugs, although this selection effect is often bacterial species–specific and is not inevitable. The development of resistance has commonly followed the introduction of new antibacterial drugs (see Fig. 1.1). Increasing resistance to commonly used antibiotics in common Gram-positive aerobic pathogens of medical interest has led to the apparent crisis of antibiotic resistance in human medicine, with important implications for use of certain antibacterial drugs in animals, as described later.

The Meaning of Resistance

The susceptibility of organisms to antimicrobial drugs was discussed in Chapter 2. Resistance in an organism can be defined in two ways. First,

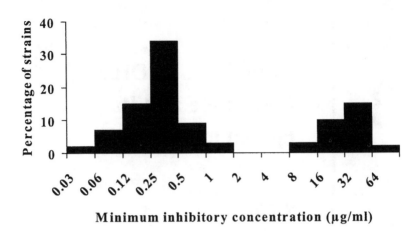

Minimum inhibitory concentration (µg/ml)

Fig. 3.1. Hypothetical minimum inhibitory concentration of an antibiotic against 100 isolates of the same pathogenic species recovered from various infectious processes. This shows the clear difference often observed between a susceptible and a resistant population. Such a clearly bimodal population distribution (rather than a normal distribution) is typical for most (but not all) antibiotics and for most pathogens. Breakpoints in susceptibility tests are designed in part to distinguish these populations. The Fig. also illustrates the jump to resistance that occurs when a susceptible bacterium acquires transferable resistance.

it can be defined in relation to the population as a whole of which the organism is a part. There is often a "break" between the susceptibility in vitro of susceptible and resistant bacteria within a population (Fig. 3.1). Second, resistance can be defined in relation to the mean serum or tissue concentration of an antimicrobial drug administered at the usual dosage by the usual route. This relationship can be used to define a breakpoint for interpretation of in vitro susceptibility data, a value that sometimes also incorporates break values obtained by studying susceptible and resistant bacteria within the population of the particular species being examined (see Chapter 2).

Types and Mechanisms of Resistance

Resistance is classified as either *intrinsic* (constitutive) or *acquired.*

Intrinsic Resistance

Bacteria may be intrinsically or naturally resistant to antibiotics because the organisms lack the cellular mechanisms required for antibiotic action. Among many examples are the inherent resistance of Enterobacteriaceae to vancomycin and of Gram-positive bacteria to polymyxin B. In addition, bacteria that are susceptible in vitro may be resistant in vivo. For example, sometimes Gram-positive bacteria may lose their cell wall and subsequently persist in the body as L forms, which makes them resistant to beta-lactam antibiotics.

Acquired Resistance

Acquired, genetically based resistance can arise because of chromosomal mutation or, more importantly, through the acquisition of transferable genetic material. There are many mechanisms of acquired resistance, including activation of drug efflux pumps and induction of enzymes that degrade the antibacterial agent. Acquired resistance is not a problem in all bacterial species. Gram-positive bacteria, apart from staphylococci, often lack the ability to acquire R plasmids (resistance plasmids), so that their significance as causes of disease in animals and people has, for a number of species, declined considerably since the antibiotic era started. Nevertheless, in recent years acquired resistance among Gram-positive bacteria has become increasingly problematic. In contrast to resistance in a few Gram-positive bacteria, resistance to many antibiotics is serious and important in Enterobacteriaceae and occurs increasingly in a broad range of other Gram-negative pathogens, such as *Bordetella, Haemophilus, Pasteurella,* and *Pseudomonas.* Acquired resistance has been identified in most but not all pathogenic bacterial genera, as well as in the commensal flora. Two factors contribute to the seriousness of the problem once multiresistant organisms develop: they may persist in the host or the environment in the absence of antibiotic selection, and they may act as reservoirs of resistance genes that may spread to other bacteria. Bacteria that are resistant to one antibiotic are likely to become resistant to other antibiotics for reasons that are not well understood but may relate to the presence of mutational defects in DNA mismatch repair mechanisms ("mutator phenotype"), making these strains more prone both to chromosomal mutation and to promiscuous exchange of DNA between species.

CHROMOSOMAL MUTATION TO RESISTANCE

Chromosomal mutations that lead to resistance often produce structural changes in the bacterial cell, whereas transferable resistance tends to code for enzymes that metabolize antibiotics. Mutations that result in antibiotic resistance are spontaneous events involving changes in chromosomal nucleotide sequences uninfluenced by the presence of antibiotics. Chromosomal resistance is generally a gradual, stepwise process, whereas transferable resistance is often high-level all-or-none. The induction in certain bacterial species of stable, heritable derepression of chromosomal beta-lactamases by newer cephalosporin and other newer beta-lactam drugs to produce broad-spectrum, high-level resistance to beta-lactam drugs is an exception to this generalization. The development of chromosomally based resistance can be a major problem. For example, among the fluoroquinolones a series of small increments in resistance as a result of individual nucleotide mutations in different genes can quickly lead to inefficacy of the drug. Among the beta-lactamases, which cause resistance to beta-lactam drugs, minor differences in molecular structure may have dramatic differences in the function of the beta-lactamase enzyme. For example, a mutation producing a single nucleotide change can convert a TEM-1 to a TEM-12 beta-lactamase (see Chapter 6), and a second single nucleotide change can convert this TEM-12 enzyme into a TEM-26 beta-lactamase, with a dramatic increase in resistance to ceftazidime. Mutations are sometimes associated with other cell changes, so that these cells may be at a disadvantage compared with the parent and may therefore be diluted out from the population in the absence of antibiotic selection. Some mutants, however, are as viable as the parents and are therefore inevitably selected by antibiotic use.

Mutations leading to resistance may be dramatic, as in the case of streptomycin, whose minimum inhibitory concentration (MIC) can increase 1,000-fold with a single mutation, or they may be gradual, as in the development of multistep resistance to fluoroquinolones. The variation in mutational events is characteristic for each antibiotic; it occurs at high frequency for streptomycin, nalidixic acid, and rifampin (1 in 10^8 cells), at slightly lower rates for erythromycin, and perhaps never for some agents such as vancomycin and polymyxin B. Antibiotics to which bacteria readily develop chromosomal resistance (erythromycin, rifampin, streptomycin) are therefore often used in combination with other antibiotics, since the chance of two mutations occurring simultaneously in the same bacterium is the product of the chance of each mutation occurring alone. Antibiotic-resistant mutants emerge less frequently in vivo than in vitro because host defenses kill many of them. The development of mutational resistance is said to be favored by underdosing (dose, frequency).

TRANSFERABLE DRUG RESISTANCE

Genetic exchange as a cause of antibacterial drug resistance is of major significance. Transfer of genetic material produces epidemic or infectious resistance, often to several antibiotics at the same time even, although uncommonly, in the absence of antibiotics selecting for resistant organisms. The extrachromosomal DNA responsible for the resistance can reproduce itself within the cell and then spread to other cells by several different mechanisms. Acquisition of transferable resistance genes by a susceptible bacterium is usually associated with a marked increase ("jump") in resistance (see Fig. 3.1).

Bacterial populations have remarkable abilities to share genetic information that will promote their survival in adverse environments. The absence of a nuclear membrane means that genes can move readily between the chromosome and other genetic elements in the cell and from there—through bacteriophages, plasmid- or transposon-mediated conjugation, or simple transformation—to other bacteria in the population. Limiting scientific interest largely to documenting only pathogens' progressive acquisition of resistance may have neglected the progressive acquisition of antimicrobial drug resistance by nonpathogenic members of the normal bacterial flora of animals and people, and may have underestimated the important reservoir of resistance genes that this flora may contain.

Transduction. In transduction, plasmid DNA is incorporated by a bacterial virus and transferred to another bacterium. The best example of phage transduction is transfer of the beta-lactamase gene from resistant to susceptible staphylococci. This mechanism is thought to be relatively unimportant because of the specificity of bacteriophages.

Transformation. Transformation is a critically important method of gene transfer in which naked DNA passes from one cell to another, potentially leading to development of new forms of resistance genes, usually among closely related genera, as a result of joining and crossover of homologous DNA. For example, acquisition of the penicillin-binding protein 2 (PBP2) gene by a *Streptococcus* species from another *Streptococcus* species through transformation can result in crossover of DNA molecules in regions where PBP2 sequences are similar, if a break occurs in the target DNA strand during replication and one DNA strand is joined to the other. The result is the formation of a unique "mosaic" PBP2 gene, which may have reduced affinity for penicillin. Penicillin-resistant streptococci carrying this new gene may then emerge through selection by penicillin because of the bactericidal effect that penicillin has on the bacteria not carrying this gene. Horizontal transfer of DNA between related genera of bacteria and recombination to produce new forms of resistance genes are increasingly recognized as an important source of emergence of resistance. Bacteria in which this process occurs are usually those with a high frequency of natural transformation (eg, some *Streptococcus* spp., *Neisseria* spp.), and transformation is from related genera because of the need for high homology of nucleotide sequences for recombination to occur.

Conjugation. In the common process of gene transfer known as conjugation, a donor bacterium synthesizes a plasmid-mediated sex pilus that attaches to a recipient bacterium in a mating process and transfers copies of plasmid-mediated resistance genes to the recipient. The donor

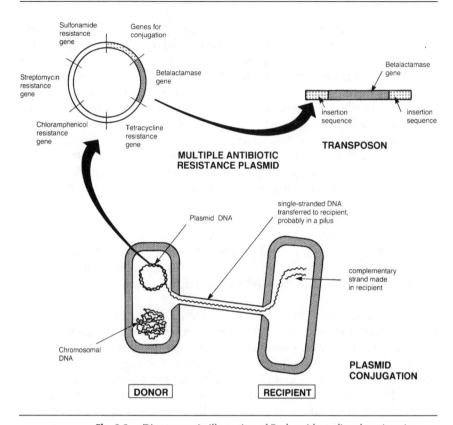

Fig. 3.2. Diagrammatic illustration of R plasmid–mediated conjugation
and transfer of antibiotic resistance genes (bottom), the composition of a
multiple antibiotic R plasmid (upper left), and the composition of a
transposon (upper right). Transposons are a central element in the formation
of R plasmids.

retains copies of the plasmid, and the recipient now becomes a potential
donor (Fig. 3.2). This transfer may occur between bacterial strains of the
same species, within species of the same genus, or even between species
belonging to different families. For example, *Staphylococcus aureus* can
exchange genetic material with *Enterococcus faecalis* or *Escherichia coli.*

The genetic elements responsible for transfer of antibiotic resistance
are the R (resistance) plasmids, or R factors. They are present in bacteria
as extrachromosomal circular DNA, which replicates independently of,
but synchronously with, chromosomal DNA. They are relatively stably
inherited but are not required by the bacterium for its survival. They possess regions with the resistance genes, which may code for resistance to
between 1 and 10 different antibiotics *(multiple antibiotic resistance)* and for

the ability of bacteria to transfer genes by conjugation. Use of any one antibiotic to which the plasmid encodes resistance will select for the maintenance of the entire plasmid. In some cases, however, these plasmids may encode other attributes, such as the ability to colonize or resistance to heavy metals, which may help ensure their maintenance in the absence of antibiotic selection. Some plasmids may not have the genes required for conjugal transfer but can be mobilized to move by using the conjugal apparatus of other, self-transmissible plasmids in the cell.

Transposons. Short sequences of DNA known as transposons ("jumping genes") can transpose from plasmid to plasmid, from plasmid to chromosome, or vice versa. A transposon copy does not remain at the original site. The frequency of transposition is characteristic of the transposon and the bacterial strain. Many transposons (class I) contain an antimicrobial drug-resistance gene flanked by two insertion sequences, which in turn are made of a central sequence with the genes for transposition flanked by short inverted repeats (Figs. 3.2 and 3.3). Other classes are more complex. The key property of all transposable elements is their ability to move and integrate into foreign DNA sequences by nonhomologous ("illegitimate") recombination. Transposons are readily acquired by plasmids and may readily incorporate into chromosomal DNA. Because of transposons, plasmids of very diverse origin possess identical antibiotic-resistance genes. The rapid transfer of transposons between plasmids in a cell and between chromosomes and plasmids, together with the interbacterial transfer of plasmids, can result in the rapid development of antibiotic resistance within bacterial populations. The phenomenon of nonhomologous recombination means that the same transposon may be found in the genome or plasmids of highly unrelated organisms. In addition, certain conjugative transposons may excise from DNA to form a circular transfer form, which, like plasmids, carries the genes needed for conjugation between bacteria.

Integrons. Integrons are a class of mobile genetic element often found on plasmids and are distinct from transposons and insertion sequences. They are associated with antibiotic resistance and other changes in bacteria. An integron is a site-specific recombination system containing an integrase (recombinase) enzyme, a gene-capture (attachment) site, and a captured gene or genes. The captured genes occur as mobile gene cassettes, a unique family of small mobile elements that include only a single antibiotic resistance gene and a specific recombination site. The recombination site confers mobility because it is recognized by site-specific integrases, which catalyze integration of the cassettes at

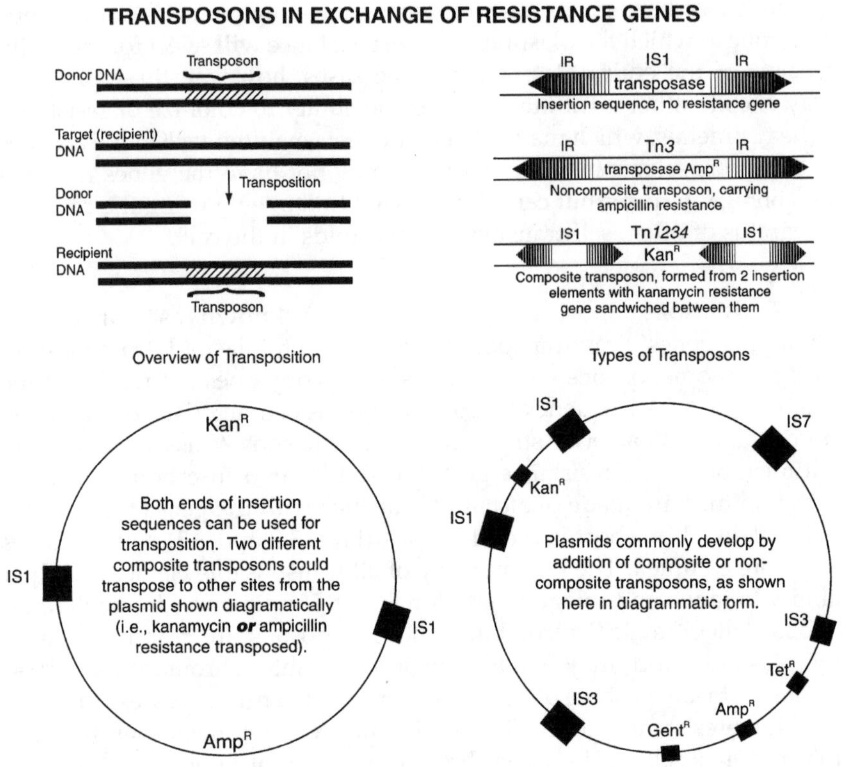

TRANSPOSONS IN EXCHANGE OF RESISTANCE GENES

Fig. 3.3. Diagrammatic illustration of transposons and their role in the development of transferable resistance. *Upper left:* Transposition involves excision of the transposable element and insertion by nonhomologous recombination in another DNA molecule. *Upper right:* The simplest transposon is an insertion element (e.g., IS1) which does not have an antibiotic resistance gene but encodes the transposase necessary for movement; some insertion elements (e.g., Tn3) contain a single resistance gene; composite transposons (e.g., Tn1234) are composed of two insertion elements flanking an antibiotic resistance gene or genes. *Bottom right:* R plasmids commonly develop by addition of composite (e.g., Tn1234) or noncomposite transposons. *Bottom left:* Since both ends of insertion sequences can be used for transposition, two different composite transposons could transpose to other DNA molecules from the plasmid shown.

specific sites within the integron. By this means, integrons containing multiple antibiotic resistance gene cassettes can develop.

The development of resistance plasmids usually follows progressive acquisition of transposons of different types or of integrons. Obviously, mutation can lead to further change in plasmid-mediated resistance genes.

Cross-resistance

Cross-resistance occurs when one organism, becoming resistant to one antibiotic, thereby becomes resistant to another. The classic example is the aminoglycosides, in which chromosomal resistance to a newer drug such as gentamicin is associated with resistance to older drugs such as neomycin. Cross-resistance is common among the macrolides and fluoroquinolones.

Mechanisms of Resistance

Important mechanisms of resistance include (1) enzymatic inactivation or modification of antibiotics; (2) impermeability of the bacterial cell wall or membrane; (3) active expulsion of the drug by the cell efflux pump; and (4) alteration in target receptors. The mechanisms of resistance to individual antimicrobial drugs, which may include combinations of the mechanisms listed, are discussed in the chapters describing these drugs. Although most of the mechanisms listed are specific for individual drugs, nonspecific resistance to a wide range of structurally unrelated antibiotics has been described in several common pathogens associated with mutations leading to overexpression of the multi-antibiotic resistance (Mar) locus, which controls multidrug efflux pumps in bacteria. Mar mutations can be selected by low concentrations of an antimicrobial drug; the clinical importance of Mar mutations leading to broad-spectrum resistance remains, however, to be determined.

Extent of Antibiotic Resistance

A causal relationship has been shown between antimicrobial use and the development of resistance. This selection is bacterial species specific, so that some species have remained highly susceptible for decades while others have rapidly become resistant and hence emerged prominently as pathogens. In veterinary medicine, the tendency has been to focus on the well-documented development of resistance in certain *Salmonella* strains, which cause zoonotic infection, and in other enteric bacteria, especially *Escherichia coli,* in part because the intestine is the major site of antibiotic resistance transfer. Relatively little systematic study has been done on the development of resistance in nonenteric and opportunist pathogens in animals. Antibiotic resistance in opportunist pathogens is a major problem in human hospital practice, but there are few reports of such problems in veterinary hospitals.

Resistance in Intestinal *E. coli*

Extensive study of antimicrobial resistance in intestinal *E. coli* has provided information on the mechanisms and ecology of such resistance

(Hinton et al., 1986). Studies of E. coli isolated from different animal species showed the relationship between the degree of antimicrobial drug use and the extent of resistance (Linton, 1977). Resistance is extensive in animals kept under intensive conditions where antibiotics are in common use (pigs, broiler chickens). Large numbers of these normal intestinal E. coli show resistance, mostly plasmid mediated, in some cases to as many as 10 clinically useful antibiotics. Although resistant isolates are not more virulent than nonresistant strains, some reports note the acquisition of virulence genes (LT-toxin, ST-toxin) by R plasmids.

In England, Smith (1975) recorded the increased resistance of intestinal E. coli of animal origin that occurred over the years as a result of the widespread use of antimicrobial drugs in animals. This was first evident in 1957 when Smith showed that feeding rations containing tetracyclines to pigs and poultry resulted in the recovery from their feces of large numbers of tetracycline-resistant E. coli. The increase in resistance to commonly used antibiotics between 1956 and 1980 was striking. It seems that over the years the tetracycline-resistant E. coli have become increasingly able to compete with sensitive bacteria in the intestine. The linkage of resistance genes on the same plasmid means that the use of any one antibiotic for which resistance was determined by the plasmid promotes continued resistance to all the antibiotics. Withdrawing the use of all antibiotics in a herd may not result in the loss of resistance by E. coli, because such genes, which are on transposons, may be incorporated into the bacterial chromosome and because possession of R plasmids may not be deleterious to bacterial survival in the intestine. In some cases it may even promote colonization.

Transfer of R Plasmids in the Intestine

In a test tube, drug resistance can be transferred rapidly throughout a susceptible bacterial population, but the frequency of transfer in vivo is lower. Within a short time of treatment of an animal with an antibiotic, the commensal E. coli population becomes resistant to that drug. This mainly results from the selection of resistant organisms and only to a lesser extent from the transfer of resistance. In general, conditions in the large bowel do not favor the transfer of resistance plasmids. The persistence of resistant bacteria is related to the persistence of the antibiotic. Thus in a cow treated for mastitis with short-term administration of antibiotics, resistant E. coli do not persist long in the intestine. It is the prolonged use of antibiotics that is more likely to be associated with persistence of resistant organisms even after the drug is no longer administered.

The persistence of R plasmids is generally a function of the bacterial strain, not the plasmids. The majority of R plasmid–containing E. coli are not good intestinal colonizers, but the persistent presence of an antibiotic will select for these organisms even though they may not be good colonizers.

The development of resistance in normal bacterial flora may impair the efficacy of antimicrobial treatment. For example, Devriese and Dutta (1984) showed that chickens colonized experimentally or naturally by an erythromycin-inactivating *Lactobacillus* flora failed to attain therapeutic blood levels after oral administration of the drug when compared with control chickens that did not possess an inactivating flora.

Antimicrobial Resistance in *Salmonella typhimurium*

Antibiotic resistance is a major problem in *Salmonella typhimurium* but not in other *Salmonella* serotypes. Certain phage types of the organism, such as type 29 and DT104, are ready recipients of R plasmids from *E. coli*. These phage types make resistance in *S. typhimurium* a special case with serious effects.

Multiple antibiotic resistance has been reported in *S. typhimurium* of animal origin throughout the world. It is most marked when only calf isolates are examined, since the extensive use of antibiotics in certain types of calf rearing, the tendency of resistant *E. coli* to colonize the intestine of young calves, and the nature of salmonellosis in calves provide intensive pressure for the emergence of antibiotic-resistant *Salmonella*.

From 1960 in Britain there was a progressive increase in infection in calves due to phage type 29 of *S. typhimurium*. Between 1960 and 1965 the type progressively acquired resistance genes, so that by 1965 several strains were resistant to six antimicrobial drugs (Fig. 3.4) (Anderson, 1968). At the same time, the organism started to appear in the human population. In 1965 the majority of this phage type isolated from human infections were drug resistant, and some deaths in humans were reported. The outbreak resulted from the intensive rearing of calves started at about the same time and was associated with the dissemination of the animals throughout Britain from a few sources. The progressive development of resistance by the calf strains appeared to follow the sequence of use of antibiotics on the farm where the disease was thought to have started.

In 1978, multiple-resistant strains of H2-bearing plasmids of *S. typhimurium* phage type 204 (and the closely related type 193) caused many outbreaks of salmonellosis in calves in Britain, and they spread to Europe and to the human population. Possession of these plasmids may enhance the ability of *S. typhimurium* to colonize the intestine of the calf. There have been studies in the United States of human infections caused by antibiotic-resistant *Salmonella* and their relationship to antimicrobial drug use in animals (Sun, 1984; Cohen and Tauxe, 1986; Spika et al., 1987).

More recently, a multiresistant and highly virulent strain of *S. typhimurium*, phage type DT104, has been isolated from cattle, for which it is particularly pathogenic, and from a wide variety of their contacts, including humans. The strain appears to have originated in England but has spread to and become common on most continents. Like phage types 29 and 204, it is unusual in that multiple antibiotic resistance is a characteristic of the clone, but unlike the other two phage types, the genes encoding at least some of the multiple resistance have become chromosomally integrated, probably through the activity of an integron. This organism is an example of the association between therapeutic antibiotic use in animals and the development of resistance in bacteria that can cause serious illness in people.

Hospital-acquired Infections by Resistant Bacteria

Nosocomial infection by multiple-resistant resident bacteria is a major problem in human medicine but has been little studied in veterinary hospitals, although it undoubtedly occurs. Analogy to the ecology of resistance in *E. coli* and *Salmonella* in farm animals is useful. There is a causal relationship between the use of antibiotics in hospitals and the selection of resistant pathogens. Colonization of patients by resistant, opportunist bacteria is hard to prevent because of shared air spaces, environment, utensils, and nursing staff; the presence of bacteria that colonize patients easily; and the use of antibiotics that destroy the normally protective bacterial flora of the patient. In addition, the ability of R plasmids

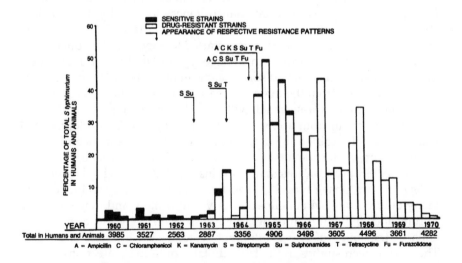

Fig. 3.4. Incidence of *Salmonella typhimurium* phage type 29 as a percentage of total human isolates of this serovar in the United Kingdom in 1960–1970. Based in part on Anderson (1968). Data supplied by and published with permission of the author.

to transfer across bacterial genera is a major cause of the development of resistant bacteria in hospitals.

Antibiotic Resistance in Animal Pathogens and Human Health

The effect of antimicrobial drug resistance in bacteria of animal origin on human health is the subject of prolonged, acrimonious, and ongoing debate. It is the biggest issue currently affecting antimicrobial drug use in animals. In particular, the focus has been on the unrestricted and often widespread use of antimicrobial drugs important in treating human infections for growth promotional and disease prophylactic ("subtherapeutic") purposes in food animals. The recent emergence of vancomycin-resistant enterococci, of multiresistant *S. typhimurium* DT104, and of fluoroquinolone-resistant *Campylobacter* has restimulated discussion of this important issue.

Bacteria from animals may reach the human population by many routes (Fig. 3.5). Drug-resistant bacteria of animal origin, such as *E. coli*,

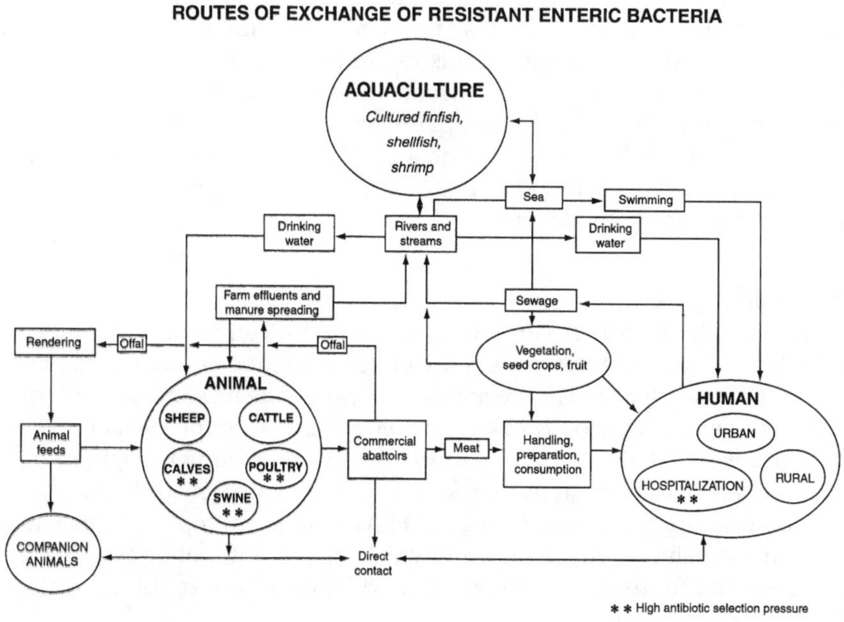

ROUTES OF EXCHANGE OF RESISTANT ENTERIC BACTERIA

** ** High antibiotic selection pressure

Fig. 3.5. Routes of exchange of *E. coli* between animals and humans. Note the areas where antibiotic selection for resistance is most likely. After Linton (1977), modified by R. Irwin; reproduced with permission.

can colonize humans, an effect particularly likely with enteric bacteria. Heavily exposed individuals, such as slaughterhouse workers, food handlers, and farmers feeding antibiotics to animals, have a higher frequency of resistant *E. coli* than the general population. At slaughter, animal carcasses are significantly contaminated by intestinal bacteria. The extent of acquisition by people of bacteria of medical significance which are resistant as a result of the use of growth promotional and disease prophylactic antibiotics is hard and perhaps impossible to quantify, in part since these same resistant bacteria may have become resistant as a result of medical use of the same or related antibiotics. In addition, the scale of acquisition of transmissible resistance genes by human pathogens from animal-derived bacteria has been difficult to quantify. Most antibiotic resistance in human pathogens relates to use of antimicrobial drugs in human medicine rather than in animals, but there is increasing evidence, discussed below, for the contribution to resistance of selected pathogens of growth promotional drugs.

Many pathogenic bacteria from the intestines of animals cause zoonotic infection in humans, including *Salmonella, Campylobacter jejuni, Yersinia enterocolitica,* and certain *E. coli.* Such human infections may be hard to treat because of acquired resistance or may be precipitated by the use of antimicrobial drugs to treat unrelated conditions. Such zoonotic infections caused by resistant organisms are probably a striking example of a more insidious process by which resistant bacteria or resistance genes are acquired among the nonpathogenic microbial flora of people. Antibiotic-resistant bacteria, such as *E. coli* and enterococci, are often acquired in people from food. The extent of this acquisition remains unknown but may be widespread.

The Swann Report

In 1968 the British government established a committee of inquiry under Sir Michael Swann to assess the effect of feeding antibiotics to animals on antimicrobial resistance in human health. The reasons for concern were as follows: (1) the outbreak of antibiotic-resistant type 29 *Salmonella typhimurium* in Britain in calves and its spread to the human population; (2) the experiences with an outbreak of chloramphenicol-resistant *S. typhi* in Central America; (3) the evidence of H. Williams Smith of resistance in *E. coli* in intensively reared pigs and chickens fed antibiotics as growth promoters and for disease prophylaxis; and (4) the discovery of transmissible antibiotic resistance.

The use of antimicrobial drugs in animals results in antibiotic-resistant bacteria reaching the human population; this is well established with *Salmonella* infections. The main argument before the Swann committee was the extent to which R plasmid–containing nonpathogens, such as *E. coli,* reached the human population and remained as reservoirs of R plasmids that could be acquired by human pathogens.

The Swann Report (Joint Committee, 1969) recommended that antibiotics important in human medicine be withdrawn from unrestricted use as growth promoters and disease prophylactics in animals in Britain. Similar measures have since been adopted in Europe and Japan. Swann distinguished between feed and therapeutic antibiotics. The committee recommended the continued use of feed antibiotics if (1) the agents had limited application in human medicine; (2) they did not impair the use of therapeutic antibiotics in humans through cross-resistance; and (3) they reduced the costs of producing the animals. Penicillin and tetracyclines were withdrawn from unrestricted use as growth promoters and could be used only in disease prophylaxis or treatment under veterinary prescription. The committee was especially critical of the use of subtherapeutic levels of antibiotics to animals described as "stressed." The spirit of the Swann report was to restrict the use of therapeutically effective antibiotics as feed additives, while allowing veterinarians their professional right to prescribe.

The findings of the Swann committee have been criticized, especially in the United States. Critics think that the findings were based on too little evidence or on special pleading, such as in the case of a limited range of phage types of *S. typhimurium.* They think that the unproved and, in their view, slender risk of human pathogens acquiring R plasmids from resistant bacteria is outweighed by the economic contribution of antibiotics to agriculture. Nevertheless, there is increasing evidence of the harmful effects for people of antibiotic resistance in *Salmonella,* which likely developed from use of drugs in animals. Food animals are a major source of *Salmonella* infections in humans that are resistant to antimicrobial drugs, and such drug resistance is associated with antimicrobial drug use on the farm.

The Situation in North America

In North America and elsewhere outside Europe, many antibiotics are incorporated in feed, without veterinary prescription, at low levels both to promote growth and to protect against disease (see Chapter 32). Approximately half of all antibiotics produced in North America are said to be used in agriculture, the majority as growth promoters and disease prophylactics in swine. In early investigations of the relationship of agricultural use of antibiotics and resistance in human pathogens, the U.S. Food and Drug Administration (FDA) concluded that antibiotic-resistant and antibiotic-susceptible bacteria of animal origin could be pathogenic to humans and that the use of certain of these drugs might promote animal carriage of *Salmonella* (Report, 1972). The FDA task force required manufacturers to show that their products did not increase the reservoir of *Salmonella* in animals. It proposed that there was sufficient evidence to stop the feeding of subtherapeutic penicillin and chlortetracycline to animals, except under veterinary prescription. This proposal was not accepted. The 1979 report of the U.S. Office of Technology Assessment determined that these drugs should be replaced by others to promote growth, even though this would result in short-term economic loss (Technical Report, 1979). The 1981 Council of Agricultural Science and Technology report suggested that the cost of banning the subtherapeutic use of such drugs would be $3.5 billion annually. The National Academy of Sciences (Committee Report, 1980) was commissioned by the FDA to study definitively the epidemiologic effects on human health of feeding animals subtherapeutic antibiotics to promote growth. The academy's conclusion, which was probably correct at the time, was that such an epidemiologic study was not feasible. Use of discriminating DNA-based techniques have, however, now been used to identify individual strains of resistant bacteria obtained from animals and people (eg, Jensen, 1998; Jensen et al., 1999). More recently, the Institute of Medicine report (1989) concluded that it was unable to find a substantial body of direct evidence of a human health hazard in the use of subtherapeutic penicillin and tetracyclines in animal feeds. Nevertheless, it calculated that the use in animals of these drugs caused an estimated 26 human deaths a year from antibiotic-resistant *Salmonella* infection. The 1995 Office of Technology Assessment report recommended collecting certain relevant new information that would finally resolve the issue of the contribution of use of feed antimicrobials in animals to adverse effects in humans and would lead to decisive action, rather than a further review of the topic that might lead to a further inconclusive report. Finally, the National Research Council (1998) concluded that use of drugs in food animal production was not without some problems and concerns but did not appear to constitute an immediate public health concern. It acknowledged that there were many gaps in knowledge and that additional data might alter this conclusion. It estimated that banning nontherapeutic use of antibiotics in food animals would add $5–$10 a year to the cost of food for each United States' citizen.

Arguments over the unrestricted use of penicillin, sulfonamides, and tetracyclines as growth promoters have ignored the more serious effects of the unrestricted use of such agents as disease prophylactics ("subtherapeutics"), because higher levels of drugs are more likely to promote resistance. Such unrestricted use leads to resistance in bacteria of veterinary importance, including zoonotic pathogens, and may conceivably contribute to resistance in host-specific human pathogens. In addition, however, resistance in host-nonspecific human pathogens, notably enterococci, has been linked to use of growth promoters in animals.

Recent Developments in Use of Antibiotics in Food Animals
FLUOROQUINOLONE USE IN FOOD ANIMALS

A fluoroquinolone drug, sarafloxacin, was licensed in the United States for use for the water-borne treatment of *E. coli* infections in poultry in 1995. This licensing came only after intensive public discussion of the potential of this drug to select for resistant food-borne pathogens. The issue was that fluoroquinolones are the only important new class of antibiotics developed in the decade, and resistance to them develops readily. In Europe, where the drug class has been administered to chickens for years, resistance to fluoro-quinolones has developed in *Campylobacter jejuni* isolated from chickens, the major source of infection for people. Fluoroquinolone resistance develops readily in *C. jejuni*. In response to public concern, the U.S. Center for Veterinary Medicine issued a license for use under veterinary prescription only for the specific purpose of treatment of *E. coli* infections, with no leeway for extra-label use. In addition, a unique active program of monitoring of antimicrobial drug resistance in chicken and other-source *Campylobacter jejuni* and *Salmonella* was instituted as part of the approval process (National Antimicrobial Resistance Monitoring System, Chapter 34). Enrofloxacin has been approved for treating *E. coli* infections in chickens and *Pasteurella multocida* infections in turkeys, and for use in beef cattle for treatment of acute bovine respiratory disease caused by *P. haemolytica*, *P. multocida*, and *Haemophilus somnus*. Fluoroquinolone resistance in *C. jejuni* of poultry origin appears to be emerging in the United States (Smith et al., 1999).

VANCOMYCIN-RESISTANT ENTEROCOCCI: THE TRAGEDY OF AVOPARCIN

Avoparcin is a growth promoter in chickens and pigs that was used extensively in Europe. It was introduced as a growth promoter precisely because it had no use in human medicine. Avoparcin is a glycopeptide in the same class of antibiotic as vancomycin. Because it is of the same class, its use in animals has been associated with the selection of vancomycin resistance in enterococci, organisms found normally in the intestines of people and animals. Although enterococci, such as *Enterococcus faecium*, have traditionally been viewed as nonpathogenic, they have emerged as a major cause of hospital-acquired infection in immunosuppressed human patients treated with broad-spectrum antimicrobial drugs. Enterococci are naturally resistant to many commonly used antibiotics, with the exception of vancomycin, but they readily acquire resistance genes (*vanA, vanB*) that are found on transposable elements. Since vancomycin has been virtually the only antibiotic available for treatment of these infections, the emergence of vancomycin-resistant enterococci (VRE) has become a major problem in hospital-acquired infections. The widespread distribution in Europe but not the United States of VREs in farm and pet animals, in fresh meats, and sewage has been attributed to the extensive use of avoparcin as a growth promoter in Europe, and for this reason avoparcin was withdrawn as a growth promoter in Europe. There is evidence that VREs from animals may colonize people (Jensen, 1998; Jensen et al., 1999; Willems et al., 1999). Paradoxically, VREs have emerged as a significant problem in hospital-acquired infection especially in the United States, a country in which avoparcin is not used in animals. The widespread use of vancomycin in hospitals in the United States to treat pseudomembranous colitis caused by *Clostridium difficile*, as well as inadequate infection control practices, rather than animal use of avoparcin may explain this emergence. A streptogramin derivative, quinipristin-dalfopristin, has recently been approved for treatment of patients with VRE infections. Because enterococci resistant to virginiamycin—another growth promoter used extensively in swine and poultry—are also resistant to this drug, it has also been withdrawn as a growth promoter in the European Union, as it has been in Denmark. Because of the resistance problem in human medicine, antibiotics introduced specifically for growth promotion in animals because they were not at the time used in medicine have now become the core of some new medically useful drugs. The "tragedy" of avoparcin and virginiamycin is that these drugs were used in agriculture precisely because they were not used in medicine. Growth promoters are discussed further in Chapter 32. The trend for a decline in human fecal carriage of vancomycin-resistant enterococci in Europe, which has followed the withdrawal of avoparcin for use in animals, will, if it continues, be an indication of the unsupected scale of movement of resistant bacteria from food animals into the human population (Klare et al., 1999; Pantosti et al., 1999).

THE WORLD HEALTH ORGANIZATION'S RECOMMENDATIONS

A meeting of specialists convened by the World Health Organization in 1998 reiterated an earlier recommendation that the use of any antimicrobial agent for growth promotion in animals be stopped if it is used in human therapeutics or is known to select for cross-resistance to antimicrobials used in human medicine. Other recommendations included improvements in national and international monitoring of antimicrobial resistance in food animals and foods of animal origin, a requirement for veterinary prescription of antibiotics, and recommendations relating to education of users as well as enforcement of policies adopted.

THE FUTURE OF ANTIBIOTICS IN AGRICULTURE

The crisis of resistance in medically important pathogens has led to renewed calls for considerable reductions in antibiotic use in animals, particularly as growth promoters and disease prophylactics, and to the withdrawal of certain classes of these drugs from agricultural use. It is reasonable to withdraw antibiotics from growth promotional and subtherapeutic use if they contribute significantly to resistance in human pathogens. In addition, medically important drugs should be used prudently for therapeutic purposes in animals. The European Union in 1999 banned bacitracin, spiramycin, tylosin, and virginiamycin as growth promoters. Other growth-promoting drugs may follow.

In the United States, the Center for Veterinary Medicine of the Food and Drug Administration is developing a framework for evaluating and assuring human safety of antimicrobial drugs used for food animals. The proposed evaluation will depend on the importance of the antimicrobial drug or drug class in human medicine and on the potential human exposure to resistant bacteria acquired from food-producing animals. Drugs may be categorized into three groups, depending on the value of the drug in human medicine. For example, vancomycin and streptogramin antibiotics might be Category I class, "critical" antimicrobial drugs, whereas Category III drugs might be those such as monensin not used (or unimportant) in human medicine. Subcategories for each of these three groups would depend on the likelihood of human exposure to resistant (usually enteric) pathogens produced by use of these drugs in food animals. For example, high potential for human exposure would be likely to follow use of a drug such as avoparcin for growth promotional purposes, whereas short-term use of a drug for therapeutic purposes would be categorized as giving rise to low potential for human exposure. In addition, the framework proposes obtaining preapproval data showing that the level of resistance transfer from proposed use of drugs is safe, and establishing resistance and monitoring "thresholds" to ensure that approved uses do not result in significant development of resistance in animal-derived bacteria or their transfer to people.

Increasing controls of antibiotic use in agriculture, such as those proposed in the United States, may require considerable changes in the management of food animals under intensive conditions to maintain a high level of production in the face of infectious disease. Swedish experience may be helpful in this regard (Report, 1997).

Control of Antibiotic Resistance

Until recently, the problem of antimicrobial drug resistance has largely been overcome by the development of new antibiotics, but the expense, inefficiency, and self-defeating nature of this approach are focusing interest in the preservation of the efficacy of existing drugs. Since there is a direct relationship between antimicrobial use and the selection of resistance among bacteria generally, the major approach to control of antimicrobial drug resistance is the reduction of use of these drugs. A number of approaches can be taken to limit the development and spread of antimicrobial drug resistance, but there is need to document the value of such approaches. Control of antibiotic resistance, insofar as it is possible, depends on the careful and appropriate use of antibiotics by knowledgeable veterinarians who cooperate with clinical microbiologists and laboratories of excellent standards in adopting measures to control the problem.

Rational Use

Antibiotics should be used only where a bacterial infection is known or suspected to be present. This determination can be either by direct demonstration of the infection (Gram- or Wright-stained smear, polymerase chain reaction (PCR), culture) or from clinical data (eg, at least two of fever, leukocytosis, localized inflammation, components of the Wright-stained sample, radiographic evidence, elevated serum fibrinogen) (Hirsh, 1995). In human medicine, up to 70% of antibiotic use has been estimated to be either unnecessary or inappropriate. No similar assessments have been attempted in veterinary medicine. Antibacterial drugs should be administered at therapeutic doses only for short periods, which for acute infections is usually for 48 hours after clinical cure; prolonged use selects for resistant strains that may persist. Selection of antibiotic resistance is more likely with suboptimal antimicrobial exposure, so full therapeutic dosage should be used. Where possible, narrow-spectrum drugs are preferred over broad-spectrum drugs. Drug combinations may overcome the development of chromosomal mutations to resistance or of plasmid-mediated resistance (eg, clavulanic acid or sulbactam resistance to beta-lactamases). Antibiotics should be used in prophylaxis only where proven effective and usually for not more that 48 hours.

National policies should ensure that antibiotics be available only by prescriptions by veterinarians, who should be responsible for educating users about their proper use. There should, however, be no financial gain made by the provider from prescribing or supplying antibiotics. Antibiotic use should be guided where necessary by use of susceptibility tests, and users should be aware of the errors possible in the performance and interpretation of these tests.

Although antibiotic policies are often a source of conflict, a number of hospitals have developed policies in which antibiotics are divided into those freely available for prescription, those used for special purposes, and those whose use is allowed only after agreement by infectious disease specialists. Such policies have been developed in human medicine in collaboration with hospitals' antimicrobial drug susceptibility testing. To prevent antibiotic resistance from spreading in some human hospitals, strategies of rotating their use have been advocated. For example, one or more antibiotics would not be used for a year or two, and unrelated drugs would be administered instead. The effectiveness of such strategies in their application into veterinary use requires confirmation. Decreased use or withdrawal of certain drugs from human hospitals has been followed sometimes by dramatic reductions in resistance to these and other antibiotics.

Reduction of Spread of Resistance
Hygiene and management approaches should aim to limit the spread of antibiotic resistance, where this is a problem. For example, isolating sick animals prevents transmission of bacteria that may be resistant. Because many diseases are self-limiting, hygienic and management measures to prevent spread of bacteria during infection are important. Approaches other than antibacterial use to control infections, such as vaccines or management methods, should be favored over antibiotics.

Surveillance
Data on the prevalence of antimicrobial drug resistance in veterinary pathogens are generally fragmentary and unbalanced. There have been only varied and limited attempts to monitor drug resistance on national levels but no such attempts internationally. Agreement on standard methods for resistance testing and reporting on a global level are critical (see Chapter 2), although the data resulting from such studies may be difficult to interpret and to use. Resistance data from accredited clinical microbiological laboratories using common, internationally agreed upon and quality-controlled methods and interpretive criteria could be collated and published annually by a designated national organization. National and international surveillance schemes for monitoring resistance might include "sentinel" bacteria isolated from the intestine of healthy animals (eg, for food animals, enterococci, *Salmonella, C. jejuni*) in a systematic sampling process and tested in an internationally agreed upon manner. The total quantity of different types of antibiotics used in a country should be determined and made public on an annual basis by a designated national organization. The availability of data of this type will provide the evidence on which national and international policies for control of antibiotic resistance might be based.

Bibliography

Aarestrup FM, et al. 1998. Surveillance of antimicrobial resistance in bacteria isolated from food animals to antimicrobial growth promoters and related therapeutic agents in Denmark. APMIS 106:606.

Anderson ES. 1968. Drug resistance in *Salmonella typhimurium* and its implications. Br Med J 3:333.

Animal Health Industry. 1998. Antibiotic use in food animals. <www.ahi.org.info.general/antibiotics.htm>.

Bager F, et al. 1997. Avoparcin used as a growth promoter is associated with the occurrence of vancomycin-resistant *Enterococcus faecium* on Danish poultry and pig farms. Prev Vet Med 31:95.

Barton MD. 1998. Does the use of antibiotics in animals affect human health? Aust Vet J 76:177.

Bates J, et al. 1994. Farm animals as a putative reservoir for vancomycin-resistant enterococcal infection in man. J Antimicrob Chemother 34:507.

Bywater RJ, Verschueren C. 1993. Antimicrobials in veterinary medicine: public health and good veterinary practice. Vet Microbiol 35(3–4).

Chiew Y-F, et al. 1998. Can susceptibility to an antimicrobial be restored after halting its use? The case of streptomycin versus Enterobacteriaceae. J Antimicrob Chemother 41:247.

Cohen ML, Tauxe RV. 1986. Drug resistant *Salmonella* in the United States: an epidemiologic perspective. Science 234:964.

Committee on Drug Use in Food Animals. 1998. The use of drugs in food animals: benefits and risks. Washington, DC: National Academy Press.

Committee Report. 1980. The effects on human health of subtherapeutic use of antimicrobials in animal feeds. Washington, DC: National Academy of Sciences.

Council of Agricultural Sciences and Technology. 1981. Report 88, Antibiotics in animal feeds. Ames, IA: Council for Agricultural Science and Technology.

Devriese LA, Dutta GN. 1984. Effects of erythromycin inactivating *Lactobacillus* crop flora on blood levels of erythromycin given orally to chicks. J Vet Pharm Ther 7:49–53.

Endtz HP, et al. 1991. Quinolone resistance in campylobacter isolated from man and poultry following the introduction of fluoroquinolones in veterinary medicine. J Antimicrob Chemother 27:199.

Glynn MK, et al. 1998. Emergence of multidrug-resistant *Salmonella enterica* serotype typhimurium DT104 infections in the United States. N Engl J Med 338:1333.

Hall RM, Collis CM. 1995. Mobile gene cassettes and integrons: capture and spread of genes by site specific recombination. Mol Microbiol 15:593.

Hinton M, et al. 1986. The ecology of drug resistance in enteric bacteria. J Appl Bacteriol (Suppl):77S.

Hirsh DC. 1995. Antimicrobial drugs: a strategy for rational use and ramifications of misuse. Small Anim Med Dig 1:188.

Holmberg SD, et al. 1984. Animal-to-man transmission of antimicrobial-resistant *Salmonella:* investigations of U.S. outbreaks, 1971–1983. Science 225:833.

Institute of Medicine. 1989. Human Health Risks with the Subtherapeutic Use of Penicillin or Tetracyclines in Animals Feed. Washington, DC: National Academy Press.

Jacobs-Reitma WF, et al. 1991. The induction of quinolone resistance in *Campylobacter* bacteria in broilers by quinolone treatment. Lett Appl Microbiol 19:228.

Jensen LB. 1998. Differences in the occurrence of two base pair variants of Tn*1546* from vancomycin-resistant enterococci from humans, pigs, and poultry. Antimicrob Agents Chemother 42:2463.

Jensen LB, et al. 1999. Vancomycin-resistant *Enterococcus faecium* strains with highly similar pulsed-field gel electrophoresis patterns containing similar Tn*1546*-like elements isolated from a hospitalized patient and pigs in Denmark. Antimicrob Agents Chemother 43:724.

Joint Committee on the Use of Antibiotics in Animal Husbandry and Veterinary Medicine (Swann Report). 1969. London: Her Majesty's Stationery Office.

Klare I, et al. 1995. *VanA*-mediated high level glycopeptide resistance in *Enterococcus faecium* from animal husbandry. FEMS Microbiol Lett 125:165.

Klare I, et al. 1999. Decreased incidence of VanA-type vancomycin-resistant enterococci isolated from poultry meat and from fecal samples of humans in the community after discontinuation of avoparcin usage in animal husbandry. Microbial Drug Resis 5:45.

Langlois BE, et al. 1988. Antimicrobial resistance of fecal coliforms from pigs in a herd not exposed to antimicrobial agents for 126 months. Vet Microbiol 18:147.

Linton AH. 1977. Antibiotic resistance: the present situation reviewed. Vet Rec 100:37.

Ministry of Agriculture, Fisheries, and Food. 1998. A review of antimicrobial resistance in the food chain. London: MAFF Publications.

O'Brien T, et al. 1985. Intercontinental spread of a new antibiotic resistance gene on an epidemic plasmid. Science 230:87.

Office of Technology Assessment, U.S. Congress. 1995. Impacts of Antibiotic-Resistant Bacteria. Washington, DC: U.S. Government Printing Office. Available <www.wws.princeton.edu/~ota/>.

Pacer DE, et al. 1989. Prevalence of *Salmonella* and multiple antimicrobial-resistant *Salmonella* in California dairies. J Am Vet Med Assoc 195:59.

Pantosti A, et al. 1999. Decrease of vancomycin-resistant enterococci in poultry meat after avoparcin ban. Lancet 354:741.

Report from the Commission on Antimicrobial Feed Additives. 1997. Antimicrobial Feed Additives. Stockholm: Ministry of Agriculture.

Report to the Commissioner of the Food and Drug Administration by the FDA Task Force. 1972. The Use of Antibiotics in Animal Feeds. Rockville, MD: U.S. Government Printing Office.

Rowe B, et al. 1979. International spread of multiresistant strains of *Salmonella typhimurium* phage types 204 and 193 from Britain to Europe. Vet Rec 105:468.

Sandvang D, et al. 1998. Characterization of integrons and antibiotic resistance genes in Danish multiresistant *Salmonella enterica* Typhimurium DT104. FEMS Microbiol Lett 160:37.

Seoane AS, Levy SB. 1995. Characterization of MarR, the repressor of the multiple antibiotic resistance *(mar)* operon in *Escherichia coli*. J Bact 177:3414.

Smith HW. 1975. Persistence of tetracycline resistance in pig *E. coli*. Nature 258:628.

Smith HW, Lovell MA. 1981. *Escherichia coli* resistant to tetracycline and to other antibiotics in the faeces of U.K. chickens and pigs in 1980. J Hyg 87:477.

Smith KE, et al. 1999. Quinolone-resistant *Campylobacter jejuni* infections in Minnesota, 1992–1998. New Engl J Med 340:1525

Spika JS, et al. 1987. Chloramphenicol-resistant *Salmonella newport* traced through hamburger to dairy farms. N Engl J Med 316:565.

Sun M. 1984. Use of antibiotics in animal feed challenged. Science 226:144.

Technical Report, Office of Technology Assessment. 1979. Drugs in Livestock Feed. Vol 1. Washington, DC: U.S. Government Printing Office.

Thal LA, Zervos MJ. 1999. Occurrence and epidemiology of resistance to virginiamycin and streptogramins. J Antimicrob Chemother 43:171.

Threlfall EJ, et al. 1996. Increasing spectrum of resistance in multiresistant *Salmonella*. Lancet 347:1052.

Timoney JF, Linton AH. 1982. Experimental ecological studies on H2 plasmids in the intestine and feces of the calf. J Appl Bacteriol 52:417.

Van den Bogaard AE, et al. 1997. Vancomycin-resistant enterococci in turkeys and in farmers. N Engl J Med 337:1558.

Wall PG, et al. 1995. Transmission of multiresistant strains of *Salmonella typhimurium* from cattle to man. Vet Rec 136:591.

Willems RJL, et al. 1999. Molecular diversity and evolutionary relationships of Tn*1546*-like elements in enterococci from humans and animals. Antimicrob Agents Chemother 43:483.

Witte W. 1998. Medical consequences of antibiotic use in agriculture. Science 279:996.

Young EJ, et al. 1985. Antibiotic resistance patterns during aminoglycoside restriction. Am J Med Sci 290:223.

4

Principles of Antimicrobial Drug Bioavailability and Disposition

J. D. BAGGOT

In treating microbial infections, it is important that an effective concentration of antimicrobial drug be rapidly attained at the focus of infection and that it be maintained for an adequate duration. The concentration achieved depends on the systemic availability of the drug, which varies with the dosage form (drug preparation) and route of administration, the dosing rate, and the ability of the drug to gain access to the infection site. The chemical nature and physicochemical properties (in particular, lipid solubility and degree of ionization) of the drug influence the extent of absorption (systemic availability), pattern of distribution, and rate of elimination (pharmacokinetic characteristics). The location of the infection can have a major influence on the drug concentration achieved where its action is required, as some sites (eg, central nervous system) are protected by cellular barriers to drug penetration, while others (eg, mammary glands) have a local pH that may favor drug accumulation (systemically administered lipid-soluble organic bases). The urinary tract is unique in that exceedingly high concentrations are achieved in urine, particularly of antimicrobial agents that are mainly eliminated by renal excretion. Microbial susceptibility to the drug concentration achieved at the site of infection is critical in determining the clinical response to therapy (see Chapter 2). Thus, effective antimicrobial therapy depends on a triad of bacterial susceptibility, pharmacokinetic characteristics of the drug, and the dosage regimen. In addition, the competence of host defense mechanisms influences the outcome of therapy.

Routes of Administration

Drugs are administered as prepared dosage forms, such as parenteral preparations for injection, and tablets, capsules, suspensions, or pastes for oral administration. It is highly important that drug preparations be administered only by the route(s) and to the animal species for which their formulation was developed; this information is provided on the label of authorized products. When veterinary preparations of an antimicrobial agent are not available, preparations intended for use in humans could be administered to companion animals. Knowledge of the fate of the drug is important, since dosage must be appropriate for the animal species.

Parenteral therapy should always be used in the treatment of severe infections, and in horses and ruminant species it is generally preferable to oral therapy. Long-acting parenteral preparations should always be administered by IM injection and, apart from procaine penicillin G, are suitable for use only in ruminant species and pigs. Suitable sites of injection are discussed in Chapters 21–30. In mild to moderate infections, oral therapy is preferred in dogs and cats, particularly for antimicrobial agents that are reliably absorbed from the gastrointestinal tract and those for which parenteral preparations cause tissue irritation at the IM site of injection. In the treatment of systemic infections caused by susceptible Gram-negative bacteria, aminoglycosides (such as gentamicin, amikacin) must be administered parenterally (generally IM or SC). Parenteral cephalosporins should be administered by slow IV injection. Certain antimicrobials are approved for administration in the feed or drinking water to pigs or poultry, providing convenience of administration.

Intravenous Administration

The IV injection of a parenteral drug solution ensures that the total dose enters the systemic circulation. The high concentration initially produced in the blood declines rapidly as the drug distributes to other tissues of the body, including the organs of elimination (liver and kidneys). Since passive diffusion is the process by which drug molecules enter cells and penetrate cellular barriers, the chemical nature of a drug, the lipid solubility and degree of ionization of those that are weak organic acids or bases, and the concentration gradient are the factors that determine the concentrations attained in cells, transcellular fluids (eg, cerebrospinal, synovial, ocular), and glandular secretions (eg, milk, saliva, prostatic fluid). After the attainment of pseudodistribution equilibrium, the plasma concentrations decline at a slower rate that is associated entirely with elimination (ie, metabolism and excretion) of the drug. It is on the elimination phase of drug disposition that the half-life of the drug is based (Fig. 4.1).

The IV administration of a parenteral solution assures complete systemic availability of the drug. Intravenous injection provides higher plasma concentrations, which may enhance tissue distribution, but effective plasma concentrations generally persist for a shorter duration than following extravascular drug administration. A shorter dosage interval is

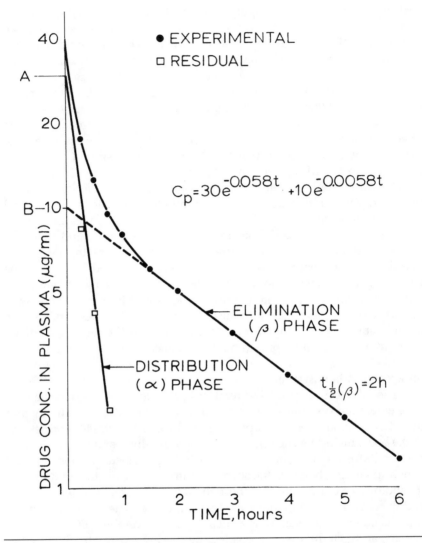

Fig. 4.1. Plasma concentration-time curve for a drug after intravenous injection of a bolus dose. The disposition curve is described by a biexponential equation (inset) and separated into its component phases (distribution and elimination). The half-life of the drug is obtained from the exponent of the elimination phase $\beta = 0.0058$ min^{-1}; t$_{1/2}$ = 0.693/0.0058 = 120 min). Reproduced with permission from Baggot (1977).

required to maintain effective concentrations, and the concentrations achieved will fluctuate to a greater degree. Parenteral solutions contain a drug in salt form dissolved in a vehicle, and the pH reaction of some solutions is far outside the physiologic range. To avoid excessively high initial drug concentrations in the systemic circulation and adverse effects that could be produced by the drug per se or by constituents of the formulation, IV injections should be given slowly. Parenteral solutions (conventional formulation only) that would produce tissue irritation at IM injection sites may be administered IV, but care must be taken to avoid perivascular damage. Pharmacokinetic parameters describing the disposition of a drug are based on the plasma concentration-time data following the IV injection of a single dose.

IV infusion of a parenteral solution containing a fixed concentration of drug is the only method of administration that allows precise control over the rate of drug entry into the systemic circulation and the plasma concentration that will ultimately be attained. Assuming knowledge of the systemic clearance of the drug, this method can be used to achieve and maintain a desired steady-state concentration and avoid fluctuation in concentrations which is a feature of multiple dosing. Whereas the rate of infusion determines the steady-state concentration attained, the time taken to reach steady state is determined solely by the rate of elimination (half-life) of the drug. For practical purposes, it can be predicted that a plasma concentration within 90% of the desired steady-state concentration will be achieved after infusing the drug at a constant rate for a period corresponding to 4 times the half-life. It follows that the use of continuous infusion is most suitable for drugs with short half-lives (<2 hours). Should a change from one steady-state concentration to another be contemplated, infusion at a different rate for a similar length of time (ie, 4 half-lives) will be required to effect the change in steady-state concentration.

Intramuscular and Subcutaneous Injections

Parenteral dosage forms (solutions and suspensions) of most antimicrobial agents can, in general, be administered by IM or SC injection to animals. The composition of the formulation, the concentration of the drug in the preparation, and the total dose to be administered will determine suitability of the dosage form for administration to a particular species. With regard to species, particular attention must be given to the concentration of drug in the preparation, since drug concentration, together with the total dose required, determines the volume to be administered. A volume exceeding 20 ml should not be administered at any one IM injection site. The lateral neck is the preferred site for IM injection in large animals. Although nonirritating parenteral solutions are frequently administered by SC injection in cats, this route of administration is seldom used in horses. Most antimicrobial agents are rapidly and completely absorbed from nonirritating solutions; peak plasma concentrations are reached within 1 hour of giving the injection. Although drug absorption from IM injection sites is generally assumed to be a first-order process, the validity of this assumption is often questionable. Oil-based formulations and unbuffered aqueous solutions or suspensions may cause irritation and produce tissue damage at IM injection sites. Slow and erratic absorption occurs, and systemic availability of the drug is often incomplete.

Absorption from IM and SC injection sites is determined by the formulation of the parenteral preparation, the vascularity of the injection site, and, to a lesser extent, the chemical nature and physicochemical properties of the drug substance. When single doses (10 mg/kg) of amikacin were administered SC to dogs at three different concentrations (50, 100, and 250 mg/ml), the concentration of the solution did not influence the absorption and elimination kinetics of the drug. The bioavailability of gentamicin (50 mg/ml) was not affected by the location of the injection site (Gilman et al., 1987; Wilson et al., 1989). Comparison of the plasma concentration-time curves after IM injection in calves of five different parenteral preparations of ampicillin at similar dose levels (7.7 ± 1.0 mg/kg) shows the marked influence of formulation on the pattern of ampicillin absorption (Nouws et al., 1982) (Fig. 4.2). Only drug preparations that are bioequivalent in the target animal species would be expected to have similar clinical efficacy.

The concentration of drug in a parenteral suspension can influence the plasma concentration profile. For example, when an aqueous suspension of amoxicillin trihydrate was administered IM to horses at the same dose level (10 mg/kg) but at different concentrations (100 and 200 mg/ml), the lower concentration (10%) was better absorbed and produced a more consistent plasma concentration profile. Location of the injection site may also affect the systemic availability and peak plasma concentration of drugs administered as prolonged-release parenteral preparations. This was shown in a study of the influence of injection site location on the plasma concentration-time curves for penicillin G administered as procaine penicillin G to horses (Firth et al., 1986) (Fig. 4.3). The systemic availability and peak plasma concentration of penicillin G were highest following IM injection of the drug product in the neck region (musculus serratus ventralis cervicis). This site was followed, in descending order, by m. biceps, m. pectoralis, and m. gluteus or subcutaneously in the cranial part of the pectoral region. The systemic availability of amoxicillin, administered as amoxicillin trihydrate 20% aqueous suspension, was shown in dairy cows to vary as widely with IM injection site as between IM and SC sites (Rutgers et al., 1980). Based on this study and others in which the conventional formulation of oxytetracycline was

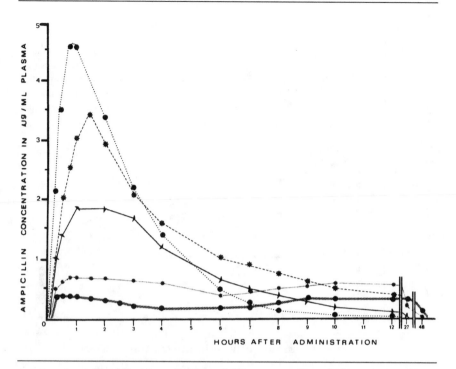

Fig. 4.2. Mean plasma ampicillin concentrations after IM injection of five different parenteral ampicillin formulations at similar dose levels (7.7 ± 1.0 mg/kg) to 5 calves. Reproduced with permission from Nouws et al. (1982).

administered IM at different sites, it can be concluded that the shoulder and neck regions for IM injection are superior to the buttock and to subcutaneous injection in cattle (Nouws and Vree, 1983). Better antimicrobial absorption from the former sites could be attributed to greater access of drug to a larger absorptive surface area with perhaps greater blood flow. Age or body weight of calves influenced the relative systemic availability, based on comparison of area under the curve, of amoxicillin (7 mg/kg) administered IM as amoxicillin trihydrate 10% aqueous suspension (Marshall and Palmer, 1980) (Fig. 4.4). When the same preparation was administered IM to different animal species, the trend was for smaller animals (piglets, dogs, cats) to show an early high peak concentration followed by a rapid decline, whereas larger animals (calves, horses) showed a lower and relatively constant plasma concentration of amoxicillin over at least an 8-hour period.

Prolonged-release preparations are designed to delay absorption and thereby maintain effective drug concentrations for an extended period,

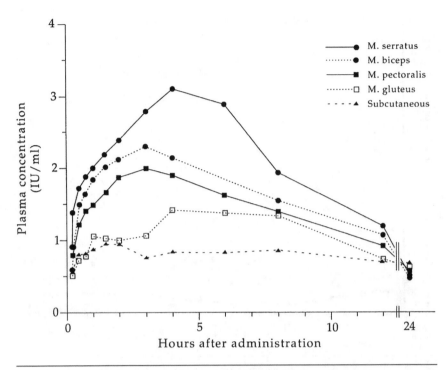

Fig. 4.3. Mean plasma penicillin concentration-time curves after 20,000 IU of procaine penicillin G/kg was administered to 5 horses at five different sites. Reproduced with permission from Firth et al. (1986).

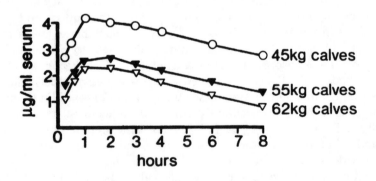

Fig. 4.4. Effect of age and weight on systemic availability of amoxicillin in calves after IM injection of amoxicillin trihydrate aqueous suspension (100 mg/ml) at a dosage of 7 mg/kg body weight. Reproduced with permission from Marshall and Palmer (1980).

which infers several times the elimination half-life of the drug. The aqueous suspension of procaine penicillin G (300,000 IU/ml) probably represents the limit to which decreasing the rate of absorption can be usefully applied to lengthen the dosage interval for penicillin G. A single dose (25,000 IU/kg) of this preparation will maintain effective concentrations against susceptible bacteria for at least 12 hours and generally for 24 hours. An essential feature of prolonged-release preparations is that the rate of drug release be adequate to maintain effective plasma concentrations for the duration of the dosage interval.

A single IM dose (20 mg/kg) of a long-acting preparation of oxytetracycline base in 2-pyrrolidone provided plasma oxytetracycline concentrations greater than 0.5 μg/ml for 48 hours in ruminant calves, cattle, goats, red deer, and fallow deer. Pronounced tissue damage at the injection site was found on examination of excised muscle tissue of pigs slaughtered 1 and 2 weeks after IM administration of a long-acting preparation, whereas the conventional preparation, administered at the same dose level (20 mg/kg), produced little tissue irritation (Xia et al., 1983). Comparison of the pharmacokinetics of three injectable oxytetracycline preparations administered IM in the lateral neck of pigs (20 mg/kg) indicates that 48 hours would be an appropriate dosage interval for either of the long-acting preparations, and 24 hours for the conventional preparation (Banting and Baggot, 1996) (Table 4.1).

Useful methods of evaluating the extent of tissue irritation and rate of resolution at the IM injection site include the use of ultrasonography (Banting and Tranquart, 1991) and determination of the kinetics of plasma creatine kinase (CK) activity (Aktas et al., 1995; Toutain et al., 1995). The use of a tissue-damaging drug preparation in food-producing animals

TABLE 4.1. **Pharmacokinetic parameters describing the absorption and disposition of three oxytetracycline formulations administered intramuscularly (lateral neck) to pigs**

Pharmacokinetic Term	Product A	Product B	Product C
C_{max} (μg/ml)	6.27 ± 1.47	5.77 ± 1.0	4.68 ± 0.61
t_{max} (h)	3.0 (2.0–4.0)	0.5 (0.083–2.0)	0.5 (0.083–2.0)
AUC (μg × h/ml)	79.22 ± 25.02	91.53 ± 20.84	86.64 ± 14.21
MRT (h)	11.48 ± 2.01	25.27 ± 9.22	37.66 ± 15.62
$C_{p(24h)}$ (μg/ml)	0.81 ± 0.34	1.01 ± 0.26	0.97 ± 0.29
$C_{p(48h)}$ (μg/ml)	<LOQ	0.40 ± 0.17	0.50 ± 0.09

Source: Banting and Baggot (1996) with permission.
Note: n = 8; dose = 20 mg/kg body weight. Results are expressed as mean ± standard deviation. LOQ = limit of quantification (0.1 μg/ml). Product A: engemycine 10% in polyvinylpyrrolidone; product B: Oxyter LA 20% in dimethylacetamide; product C: terramycin LA 20% in 2-pyrrolidone and polyvinylpyrrolidone.

must entail a correspondingly long withdrawal period. The withdrawal period for a drug varies with formulation of the dosage form (preparation) and may differ among animal species. Parenteral preparations should be formulated in a manner such that their IM injection does not cause tissue damage with persistence of drug residues at the injection site. Irritating preparations and drugs in oil-based vehicles should *never* be administered to horses. With the notable exception of procaine penicillin G (aqueous suspension), long-acting parenteral preparations currently available are unsuitable for use in the horse.

Since avian and reptilian species appear to have a well-developed renal portal system, first-pass renal excretion may decrease the systemic availability of drugs, such as beta-lactam and aminoglycoside antibiotics, injected IM in the legs of birds or the posterior half of the body of reptiles.

Oral Administration

A wide variety of oral dosage forms are available for use in animals. They include oral solutions, suspensions, pastes, capsules, tablets of various types, and powders. The rate of drug absorption varies with the type of dosage form; oral solutions provide rapid absorption. Dissolution must precede absorption from a solid dosage form and frequently controls the rate of drug absorption. Oral suspensions and pastes generally provide drug for absorption at a rate that is intermediate between solutions and solid dosage forms. Reticular groove closure may enable drug solutions to bypass the rumen, whereas drug suspensions are largely deposited in the rumen. This distinction may be of significance with regard to the clinical efficacy of some anthelmintics. Although the rumen has good absorptive capacity, drug absorption takes place slowly from ruminal fluid (pH 5.5–6.5) because of its large volume and slow onward passage to the abomasum. In monogastric species, gastric emptying is the principal physiologic factor governing the rate of drug absorption. Medication of feed or of drinking water provides a convenient means of antimicrobial administration to pigs and poultry. By contrast, the addition of an antimicrobial agent to the feed is an unreliable method of dosing horses and should not be considered.

The systemic availability, which is the fraction of an oral dose that reaches the systemic circulation unchanged, is of greater clinical importance than the rate of absorption of an antimicrobial agent. Systemic availability is influenced by the stability of an antimicrobial agent in the highly acidic gastric contents (pH 3–4) or its susceptibility to inactivation (by hydrolytic or reductive reaction) by ruminal microorganisms, and by the chemical nature and physicochemical properties of the drug. Since absorption takes place by passive diffusion across the mucosal epithelial barrier, high solubility in lipid is an important property. Having passed through the mucosal barrier, drug molecules are conveyed in hepatic portal venous blood to the liver, the major organ of drug metabolism, prior to reaching the systemic (general) circulation. Presystemic metabolism, referred to as the first-pass effect, can occur in the gut lumen or mucosal epithelium or, most important, in the liver. The first-pass effect decreases the systemic availability of drugs that undergo extensive hepatic metabolism. Presystemic metabolism activates prodrugs of ampicillin, such as pivampicillin and bacampicillin, by hydrolysis of the ester in the intestinal mucosa. Metabolic conversion (N-dealkylation) of enrofloxacin to ciprofloxacin and of difloxacin to sarafloxacin is likely to occur to some extent, but the products formed possess high antimicrobial activity, being drugs in their own right. Presystemic metabolism converts netobimin and febantel (probenzimidazole anthelmintics) to albendazole and fenbendazole, respectively. The low plasma concentrations and lack of clinical efficacy of pyrantel and morantel (tetrahydropyrimidine anthelmintics) against tissue nematodes and larval stages embedded in tissues may be attributed to extensive first-pass hepatic metabolism. Triclabendazole, administered as an oral suspension, appears to be completely converted by hepatic first-pass metabolism to the sulfoxide (active) metabolite, which is subsequently metabolized by the liver to the sulfone (inactive) metabolite.

The systemic availability of aminoglycoside antibiotics, which are polar organic bases, is very low following oral administration, whereas they are rapidly absorbed and completely available systemically when administered by IM or SC injection. It is the absorption process that differs between the gastrointestinal tract and parenteral sites. Passage across the mucosal barrier requires that the drug be at least moderately lipid soluble, whereas absorption from parenteral sites is mainly controlled by capillary blood flow at the absorptive surface.

The presence of food in the stomach or binding to feed constituents decreases the systemic availability of most penicillins, apart from amoxicillin and ampicillin prodrugs, oral cephalosporins, trimethoprim-sulfonamide combinations, and tetracyclines (except doxycycline). The systemic availability of some drugs (eg, doxycycline, erythromycin estolate, ketoconazole) is increased when administered to dogs after feeding. Since the systemic availability of antimicrobial agents administered orally (pastes) or by nasogastric tube (aqueous suspensions) to horses is significantly decreased by feeding prior to dosing, food should be withheld for up to 2 hours after antimicrobial administration. The systemic availability of metronidazole varies widely among individual horses (60–90%) but might not be significantly decreased by feeding prior to oral dosing.

It may be feasible to administer certain antimicrobial agents orally to young foals, calves, and kids, even though these drugs are not suitable for oral use in older and adult herbivorous animals. This is due not only to better absorption but also to the fact that neither the microflora indigenous to the specialized fermentation regions of the gastrointestinal tract nor the hepatic microsomal oxidative reactions have developed. For example, the systemic availability of amoxicillin, administered as a 5% oral suspension of the trihydrate, was 30–50% in 5-to-10-day-old Thoroughbred foals and 5–15% in adult horses. Pivampicillin, a prodrug of ampicillin, has a systemic availability (ampicillin) of 40–53% in foals between 11 days and 4 months of age (Ensink et al., 1994) and 31–36% in adult horses. The systemic availability of cefadroxil (5% oral suspension) decreases from 68% in 1-month-old foals to 14.5% in foals 5 months of age (Duffee et al., 1997). In calves the systemic availability of chloramphenicol, administered as an oral solution, decreases with ruminal development (de Backer and Bogaert, 1983). Ruminal development, which normally occurs during the first 4–8 weeks after birth, is largely influenced by the composition of the diet. In older calves and cattle the ruminal microflora inactivate chloramphenicol by a reductive reaction (Theodorides et al., 1968).

Modified-release ruminal boluses containing certain anthelmintics (eg, ivermectin, oxfendazole, fenbendazole, morantel tartrate) are available for use in cattle. The design of the modified-release bolus determines the pattern of anthelmintic release into ruminal fluid over a prolonged period (generally 90–140 days). The controlled-release ivermectin bolus continuously delivers ivermectin at a constant rate for 135 days, whereas the intermittent-release oxfendazole bolus delivers pulse doses of oxfendazole at 3-week intervals.

Applied Clinical Pharmacokinetics

The chemical nature and related physicochemical properties largely govern the absorption, distribution, and elimination, which refers to biotransformation (metabolism) and excretion, of antimicrobial agents. The majority of antimicrobial agents are weak organic electrolytes, either weak acids or weak bases, while fluoroquinolones, tetracyclines, and rifampin are amphoteric compounds. Lipid solubility and the degree of ionization, which is determined by the pK_a of the drug and the pH of the biologic fluid in question (pH of blood is 7.4), influence the extent of absorption, the pattern of distribution, and the elimination process(es) for antimicrobial agents. Lipid solubility is a requirement for passive diffusion of drugs across cell membranes, and it is the nonionized form of weak organic acids and bases that is lipid soluble.

Since antimicrobial agents, like other drugs, are available as prepared dosage forms, the type and formulation of the dosage form (drug preparation) determine the route of administration, the bioavailability, and the overall rate of elimination of the drug. Because the drug preparation affects pharmacokinetic processes, it influences the dosage regimen for each animal species and the withdrawal period(s) in food-producing animals.

Distribution and Elimination

Following the entry of an antimicrobial agent into the systemic circulation, the free (unbound) fraction is available for distribution to extravascular tissues and for removal from the body by the organs of elimination (liver and kidneys). The extent and pattern of distribution vary between antimicrobial agents of different classes because of differences in their chemical nature. Distribution is determined by blood flow to tissues and the ability of a drug to penetrate (mainly by passive diffusion) cellular barriers. The rate of distribution is largely influenced either by perfusion (lipophilic drugs) or by diffusion (ionized and polar compounds). Extensive (>80%) binding to plasma proteins limits the immediate availability of a drug for extravascular distribution. Accumulation in tissues (pH partition effect) influences the extent of distribution. Selective binding to a tissue component (eg, aminoglycosides in the kidney) may account for only a small fraction of the amount of drug in the body but could produce an adverse, even toxic, effect, or the residue could limit the use of the drug in food-producing animals. Definitive information on the distribution pattern of a drug can be obtained only by measuring levels of the drug in the various organs and tissues of the body, such as kidneys, liver, skeletal muscle, adipose tissue, and skin. Selective binding can reasonably be suspected and should be further investigated when a specific lesion is produced in a tissue.

Whereas some antimicrobial agents are almost entirely eliminated by renal excretion (aminoglycoside, most beta-lactam antibiotics), others are eliminated by hepatic metabolism and, to a lesser extent, by renal or biliary excretion. The extent to which liver damage decreases the rate of elimination of drugs is difficult to assess. However, certain antimicrobial agents (chloramphenicol, erythromycin, metronidazole) inhibit hepatic microsomal enzyme activity, while rifampin induces hepatic microsomal enzymes. The rate of elimination of several therapeutic agents used concurrently with one of these antimicrobials can be affected by the altered microsomal-mediated oxidative reactions. Decreased renal function requires adjustment of aminoglycoside dosage (see Chapter 19). Renal impairment may lead to the accumulation of drug metabolites, although they were formed in the liver or at other sites of biotransformation.

Lipophilic antimicrobial agents readily penetrate cellular barriers, with the exception of the blood-brain barrier. Consequently, these drugs

are well absorbed from the gastrointestinal tract, become widely distributed in body fluids and tissues, and can generally attain effective concentrations at sites of infection. Examples of lipophilic antimicrobial agents
include fluoroquinolones, macrolides and lincosamides, minocycline and
doxycycline, trimethoprim, rifampin, metronidazole, and chloramphenicol. Some of these drugs (erythromycin, clindamycin, doxycycline) are
extensively bound to plasma proteins, which limits their availability for
extravascular distribution. Of the lipophilic antimicrobials, only certain
individual drugs penetrate the blood-brain barrier and attain effective
concentrations in cerebrospinal fluid (eg, metronidazole, chloramphenicol). Lipophilic antimicrobial agents are eliminated mainly by the liver
(metabolism and biliary excretion), while a fraction of most of these drugs
(with the notable exception of doxycycline) is excreted unchanged (and as
metabolites) in the urine. The more rapidly a drug is metabolized, the
smaller the fraction of dose that is excreted unchanged (eg, trimethoprim)
(Table 4.2). The metabolic pathways—various hepatic microsomal oxidative reactions and glucuronide conjugation—are determined by the functional groups present in the drug molecule. Apart from some fluoroquinolones, rifampin, and metronidazole, the metabolites of lipophilic
antimicrobials are inactive. Enrofloxacin is converted to ciprofloxacin,
difloxacin to sarafloxacin, and pefloxacin to norfloxacin by N-dealkylation
(oxidative reaction). The half-lives of individual lipophilic antimicrobials
may differ within a species and among animal species. For example, the
half-lives of various fluoroquinolones in the dog are ciprofloxacin,
2.2 hours; enrofloxacin, 3.4 hours; norfloxacin, 3.6 hours; difloxacin,
8.2 hours; and marbofloxacin, 12.4 hours. The half-lives of metronidazole
in various species are cattle, 2.8 hours; horse, 3.9 hours; dog, 4.5 hours;
chicken, 4.2 hours; and the half-lives of chloramphenicol are horse,
0.9 hours; dog, 4.2 hours; cat, 5.1 hours; chicken, 5.2 hours.

The pharmacokinetic properties of different antibacterial drug classes
and their members, and factors affecting these properties, are discussed
extensively under the description of each drug.

TABLE 4.2.   **Half-life and urinary excretion of trimethoprim**

Species	Half-life (h)	Fraction of Dose Excreted Unchanged (%)
Goat	0.7	2
Cow	1.25	3
Pig	2.0	16
Horse	3.2	10
Dog	4.6	20
Human	10.6	69 ± 17

Pharmacokinetic Parameters

Drug disposition is the term used to describe the simultaneous effects of distribution and elimination—that is, the processes that occur subsequent to the absorption of a drug into the systemic circulation. The major pharmacokinetic parameters that describe the disposition of a drug are the systemic (body) clearance (Cl_B), which measures the ability of the body to eliminate the drug, and the volume of distribution (V_d), which denotes the apparent space in the body available to contain the drug. The *half-life* ($t_{1/2}$) expresses the overall rate of drug elimination; it is only when the dose is administered intravenously that the "true" (elimination) half-life of a drug can be determined. When a drug preparation is administered orally or by a nonvascular parenteral route (eg, IM or SC), the *systemic availability* (F), that fraction of the dose that reaches the systemic circulation unchanged, is an important parameter. Since the absorption process influences the rate of drug elimination, the value obtained for half-life is "apparent"; it will vary with route of administration and formulation of the dosage form (drug preparation). *Bioavailability,* which refers to both the rate and extent of drug absorption, provides a more complete description of the absorption process. The rate and pattern of absorption assume importance when a drug is administered as a prolonged-release (long-acting) preparation.

BIOAVAILABILITY

Bioavailability is defined as the rate and extent to which a drug enters the systemic circulation unchanged. It is influenced not only by the factors that determine drug absorption but also by formulation of the dosage form and the route of administration. Complete systemic availability (extent of absorption) can be assumed only when a drug is administered intravenously.

An estimation of the rate of drug absorption can be obtained from the peak (maximum) plasma concentration (C_{max}) and the time at which the peak concentration is attained (t_{max}), based on a plot of the plasma concentration-time data. However, the blood sampling times determine how well the peak is defined; t_{max} often lies between measured plasma concentrations. Both C_{max} and t_{max} may be influenced by the rate of drug elimination, and C_{max} is also affected by the extent of absorption. The parameter C_{max}/AUC, which can be calculated and is expressed in units of reciprocal time (h^{-1}), is an additional term that may be used to indicate the rate of drug absorption. Even though an absorption rate constant (and half-life) can be calculated, the generally small number of data points on which it is based makes it an inaccurate measurement of drug absorption.

The usual technique for estimating systemic availability (F), extent of absorption, employs the method of corresponding areas:

$$F = \frac{AUC_{PO}}{AUC_{IV}} \times \frac{dose_{IV}}{dose_{PO}}$$

where AUC is the total area under the plasma concentration-time curve relating to the route of drug administration (IV and PO, IM, or SC). The application of this technique involves the assumption that clearance of the drug is not changed by the route of administration. Following the administration of a single dose by any route, the total area under the curve can be estimated by the linear trapezoidal rule, from zero time to the last measured plasma drug concentration, with extrapolation to infinite time, assuming log-linear decline (Fig. 4.5). The accuracy of this method for estimating the total area under the curve (AUC) depends on the number of plasma concentration-time data points from the time of drug adminis-

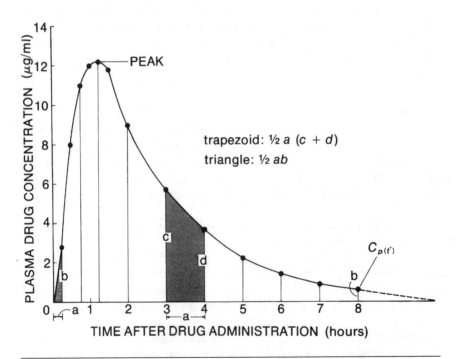

Fig. 4.5. Usual form of the plasma drug concentration profile that follows oral administration or nonvascular (IM, SC) injection of a conventional form of a drug. AUC may be calculated by the trapezoidal rule. Reproduced with permission from Baggot (1977).

tration (zero time) to the last measured plasma concentration and on the relative area under the extrapolated portion of the curve, which should be less than 10% of the total area. When comparison is made of the AUC for an oral dosage form with that for an intravenous preparation of the drug, the absolute bioavailability (systemic availability) is obtained, whereas comparison of the AUCs for two oral dosage forms (test and reference) estimates the relative bioavailability. The latter comparison is used in bioequivalence assessment. In bioavailability studies a crossover design, with an appropriate washout period between the phases of the study, should be used whenever feasible.

The systemic availability of orally administered antimicrobial drugs is often incomplete (<100%). This may be due to poor absorption, degradation in the stomach or rumen, or presystemic metabolism (first-pass effect). Incomplete systemic availability can often be compensated for by administering a higher oral dose. The time of feeding relative to oral dosing may affect the systemic availability (oral bioavailability) of an antimicrobial agent, as discussed earlier. For example, the oral bioavailability of enrofloxacin, trimethoprim, and sulfadiazine is high (>80%) in pigs and is not influenced by the intake of feed. In contrast, the presence of feed in the gastrointestinal tract markedly decreases the oral bioavailability of spiramycin (from 60% to 24%) and lincomycin (from 73% to 41%) (Nielsen, 1997). The systemic availability of rifampin (5 mg/kg) was 26% when the drug was administered to horses 1 hour after feeding, compared with 68% when given 1 hour before feeding (Fig. 4.6). Because of species differences in digestive physiology and in anatomical arrangement of the gastrointestinal tract, the systemic availability and rate of absorption of drugs administered orally differ widely between ruminant and monogastric species.

Parenteral preparations administered by IM injection often vary in systemic availability, while the rate of absorption differs between conventional (immediate-release) and long-acting (prolonged-release) dosage forms. Incomplete systemic availability of parenteral preparations could be attributed either to partial precipitation of the drug at the injection site or to tissue irritation caused by the drug per se, the vehicle, or the pH of the preparation. By decreasing the rate of drug absorption, long-acting preparations provide a prolonged duration of effective plasma concentrations and allow the use of a longer dosage interval. For example, the dosage interval for procaine penicillin G is 12 hours in horses, and 24 hours in pigs and cattle; the dosage interval for the long-acting parenteral formulation of oxytetracycline is 48 hours in pigs, cattle, and goats. Repeated dosage with prolonged-release preparations produces less fluctuation in plasma concentrations than the degree of fluctuation produced by conventional preparations. It is usual to determine the

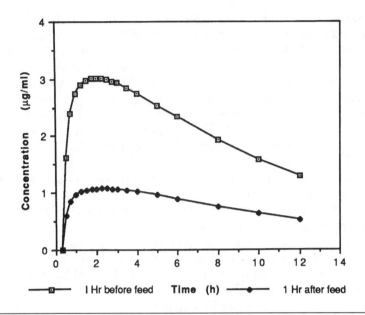

Fig. 4.6. Mean plasma rifampin concentration-curves in horses (n = 5) after oral administration of the drug (5 mg/kg) 1 hour before or 1 hour after feeding.

relative bioavailability of a prolonged-release preparation by comparing area under the curve with AUC for a conventional preparation administered by the same route to the same animals (crossover design). The mean residence times should be compared. The plasma concentration-time curve, plotted on arithmetic coordinates, shows the pattern of drug absorption and the duration of effective plasma concentrations. It is on the latter, rather than the apparent half-life, that the dosage interval is based.

The systemic availability of a drug can be estimated by comparing the cumulative urinary excretion of the unchanged (parent) drug after extravascular administration with the amount excreted unchanged after IV administration. Using this approach, the systemic availability of oxytetracycline was determined in pigs following the IM injection (biceps femoris) of single doses (20 mg/kg) of a conventional (OTC-C) and a long-acting (OTC-LA) preparation (Fig. 4.7). Both preparations provided more than 95% systemic availability of the antibiotic (Xia et al., 1983). Cumulative urinary excretion was used to compare the systemic availability of sulfamethazine administered as three oral dosage forms to yearling cattle (Bevill et al., 1977). The results obtained (Table 4.3) indicate that the oral solution (107 mg/kg) and oral rapid-release bolus (27.8 g of sulfamethazine; similar dose level as for oral solution) provide relatively

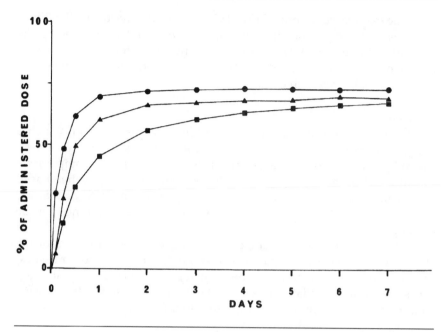

Fig. 4.7. Cumulative urinary excretion of oxytetracycline in pigs after IV injection of conventional OTC preparations (●, n = 3) and IM injection of conventional (▲, n = 4) and a long-acting OTC preparation (■, n = 6). Reproduced with permission from Xia et al. (1983).

TABLE 4.3. **Systemic availability of three oral dosage forms of sulfamethazine in cattle**

Dosage Form	Systemic Availability (%)
Solution	80.8
Rapid-release bolus	63.2
Sustained-release bolus	32.0

effective availability of the drug for absorption from the rumen, whereas the sustained-release bolus (67.5 g of sulfamethazine) is a less satisfactory dosage form. This method is an alternative to comparing area under the plasma concentration-time curves, but it is cumbersome to apply because the total volume of urine voided during the excretion period for the drug (at least 6 half-lives) must be measured. In addition, the stability of the drug in urine during the collection period and storage of the samples must be assured. Use of cumulative urinary excretion data to compare the systemic availability of different dosage forms of a drug administered by the same extravascular route (PO or IM)—that is, relative bioavailability—assumes that the ratio of the total amount excreted unchanged to the amount absorbed remains constant. It is always preferable to base estimation of the rate of drug absorption on plasma concentration data rather than on urinary excretion data.

CLEARANCE

Clearance indicates the volume of blood or plasma from which a drug (or marker substance for an elimination process) would have to be cleared per unit of time to account for its elimination. For comparative purposes, clearance is expressed in units of ml/min × kg. When based on plasma drug concentrations, clearance can assume values that are not "physiologic"; conversion from plasma to blood clearance can be accomplished.

The systemic (body) clearance of a drug represents the sum of the clearances by the various organs (liver, kidneys, "other" organs or tissues) that contribute to elimination of the drug. It can be calculated by dividing the systemically available dose by the total area under the plasma concentration-time curve (from time zero to infinity):

$$Cl_B = \frac{F \times dose}{AUC}$$

where F is the fraction of the dose that enters the systemic circulation unchanged and AUC is the total area under the curve. By definition, the systemic clearance of a drug is the product of the volume of distribution, calculated by the area method, and the overall elimination rate constant:

$$Cl_B = V_{d(area)} \times \beta$$

When an intravenous dosage form of the drug is not available, F cannot be determined; in this situation the term Cl_B/F should be used.

The concept of clearance is extremely useful in clinical pharmacokinetics, since the systemic clearance of most therapeutic (including antimicrobial) agents is constant over the clinically useful range of plasma concentrations. This is because the overall elimination of most drugs obeys first-order kinetics, whereby a constant fraction is eliminated per unit of time (eg, 50% is eliminated each half-life). Systemic clearance is probably the most important pharmacokinetic parameter to consider in defining a drug dosage regimen and is required for calculating dosing rate adjustment that may be necessitated by functional impairment of an organ of elimination. When multiple doses are administered at a constant dosage

TABLE 4.4. **Disposition kinetics of antimicrobial agents in dogs**

Drug	Half-life (h)	$V_{d(area)}$ (ml/kg)	Cl_B (ml/min × kg)
Penicillin G	0.50	156	3.60
Ampicillin	0.80	270	3.90
Ticarcillin	0.95	340	4.30
Cephalexin	1.71	402	2.70
Cefazolin	0.80	700	10.40
Cefotaxime	0.73	480	7.50
Ceftizoxime	1.07	300	3.25
Ceftazidime	0.82	220	3.15
Ceftriaxone	0.85	240	3.26
Gentamicin	1.25	335	3.10
Amikacin	1.10	245	2.61
Kanamycin	0.97	255	3.05
Norfloxacin	3.56	1,770	5.53
Enrofloxacin	3.35	2,454	8.56
Marbofloxacin	12.40	1,900	1.66
Difloxacin	8.20	3,640	5.10
Trimethoprim	4.63	1,849	4.77
Sulfadiazine	5.63	422	0.92
Sulfadimethoxine	13.20	410	0.36
Sulfisoxazole	4.50	300	0.77
Chloramphenicol	4.20	1,770	4.87
Thiamphenicol	1.75	765	5.20
Metronidazole	4.50	948	2.50
Erythromycin	1.72	2,700	18.2
Clindamycin	3.25	1,400	5.25
Oxytetracycline	6.02	2,096	4.03
Doxycycline	6.99	1,010	1.72
Minocycline	6.93	1,952	3.55

interval, systemic clearance relates the average steady-state plasma concentration to the dosing rate of the drug. Systemic or individual organ clearance, depending on the elimination processes for a drug, may be the pharmacokinetic parameter of choice in applying the allometric technique to interspecies scaling of drug elimination.

As an example of one species, values of pharmacokinetic parameters describing the disposition of some antimicrobial agents are presented for dogs (Table 4.4).

VOLUME OF DISTRIBUTION

The volume of distribution, which relates the amount of drug in the body to the concentration in the plasma, provides an estimation of the extent of distribution of a drug. It quantifies the apparent space, in both the systemic circulation and the tissues of distribution, available to contain the drug, but it does not reveal the pattern of distribution. The distribution pattern of a drug can be described only by measuring the level (amount) of drug in the various organs and tissues of the body.

The volume of distribution can be calculated (area method) from the equation:

$$V_{d(area)} = \frac{dose}{AUC \times \beta}$$

where AUC is the total area under the plasma concentration-time curve and β is the overall elimination rate constant of the drug, obtained from the linear terminal (elimination) phase of the semilogarithmic disposition curve (see Fig. 4.1). This implies that the drug was administered as an IV bolus dose. When the drug is administered orally (PO) or by a nonvascular parenteral route (IM, SC), correction must be made for systemic availability (F), and the apparent first-order elimination rate constant (k_d) must be substituted for β.

Drugs that are predominantly ionized in plasma or are relatively polar (penicillins, cephalosporins, aminoglycosides) have volumes of distribution in the range of 150 to 300 ml/kg; this infers only that their distribution is limited in extent. Lipophilic antimicrobial agents (macrolides, lincosamides, chloramphenicol, trimethoprim, fluoroquinolones) have volumes of distribution that are generally between 1 and 3 l/kg. The volumes of distribution of moderately lipid-soluble antimicrobials (eg, metronidazole, rifampin, sulfonamides) are intermediate (400–800 ml/kg). The tetracyclines differ in lipid solubility, and their volumes of distribution vary accordingly.

Species variations in the volume of distribution of a drug can be largely attributed to differences in body composition (Table 4.5), in particular to anatomical features of the gastrointestinal tract, while differences in plasma protein binding may contribute. The greatest variation is found between ruminant and monogastric species, mainly for lipophilic organic bases.

Since volume of distribution, serving as a proportional factor, relates the plasma concentration to the amount of drug in the body, knowledge of this parameter is required for calculating the dose (mg/kg) that would provide a desired plasma drug concentration:

$$Dose_{IV} = C_{p(ther)} \times V_{d(area)}$$

Drug administration by the oral or a nonvascular parenteral route may require upward adjustment of the dose to compensate for incomplete systemic availability of the drug. No provision can be made for variation in the rate of drug absorption.

Volume of distribution has useful applications, but it is a parameter (volume term) that must be properly interpreted. Although $V_{d(area)}$ may be determined following drug administration by any route, it varies with

TABLE 4.5. Body composition of various species (% live weight)

Organ/Tissue	Horse	Dog	Goat	Cow	Human
Blood	8.6	—	—	4.7	7.9
Brain	0.21	0.51	0.29	0.06	2.0
Heart	0.66	0.82	0.48	0.37	0.47
Lung	0.89	0.89	0.88	0.71	1.4
Liver	1.3	2.32	1.95	1.22	2.6
Spleen	1.11	0.26	0.25	0.16	0.26
Kidney	0.36	0.61	0.35	0.24	0.44
Gastrointestinal tract	5.8	3.9	6.4	3.8	1.7
Gastrointestinal contents	12.7	0.72	13.9	18.4	1.4
Skin	7.4	9.3	9.2	8.3	3.7
Muscle	40.1	54.5	45.5	38.5	40.0
Bone	14.6	8.7	6.3	12.7	14.0
Tendon	1.7	—	—	—	2.0
Adipose	5.1	—	—	18.9	18.1
Body weight (kg)	308	16	39	620	70
Source	a	b	b	c	d

Sources: a, Webb and Weaver (1979); b, Neff-Davis et al. (1975); c, Matthews et al. (1975); d, International Commission on Radiological Protection (1975).

change in the elimination rate constant for a drug, even when the distribution space has remained unchanged. The volume of distribution at steady state, $V_{d(ss)}$, is not subject to this disadvantage but can be determined only when the drug is administered as an IV bolus dose. The volume of distribution at steady state can be calculated by the use of areas (Benet and Galeazzi, 1979):

$$V_{d(ss)} = \frac{\text{dose}_{IV} \times \text{AUMC}}{(\text{AUC})^2}$$

where AUC is the total area under the curve (zero moment) and AUMC is the area under the first moment of the plasma concentration-time curve, that is, the area under the curve of the product of time and plasma concentration $(t \times C_p)$ over the time span zero to infinity. This noncompartmental method of calculating V_d does not require the application of a compartmental pharmacokinetic model or mathematical description of the disposition curve. The volume of distribution at steady state represents the volume in which a drug would appear to be distributed during steady state if the drug existed throughout that volume at the same concentration as in the plasma.

The volume of distribution at steady state is somewhat smaller than that calculated by the area method. For trimethoprim in dogs, $V_{d(ss)}$ is 1675 ml/kg and $V_{d(area)}$ is 1849 ml/kg, and for sulfadiazine in dogs, $V_{d(ss)}$ is 392 ml/kg and $V_{d(area)}$ is 422 ml/kg. When interpreting the influence of disease or physiologic state on the disposition kinetics of a drug, the systemic clearance (Cl_B) and $V_{d(ss)}$, rather than $V_{d(area)}$, are the pharmacokinetic parameters that should be used. Neither volume of distribution term allows one to predict drug concentrations that are attained in tissues or at infection sites.

HALF-LIFE

The half-life of a drug expresses the time required for the plasma concentration, as well as the amount in the body, to decrease by 50% through the process of elimination. Half-life ($t_{1/2}$) measures the rate of decline in plasma drug concentrations during the elimination phase of the disposition curve and is calculated from the expression:

$$t_{1/2} = \frac{0.693}{\beta}$$

where β is the overall elimination rate constant of the drug; 0.693 is ln 2. The half-lives of antimicrobial agents are independent of the dose administered (at least within the recommended dose range), since their overall elimination obeys first-order kinetics. The characteristic of first-order elimination is that the time required for a given concentration to decrease by a certain percentage (eg, 50% each half-life) is independent of the concentration.

Half-life is the pharmacokinetic parameter that is used to compare the rate of elimination of drugs in different species (Table 4.6). Even though the relative contribution of hepatic metabolism or renal excretion to antimicrobial elimination may differ among species, this approach is useful for comparative purposes. The half-lives of antimicrobials (and pharmacologic agents) that are mainly eliminated by hepatic metabolism can vary widely among species. Apart from oxytetracycline, which undergoes enterohepatic circulation, variation among mammalian species in the half-lives of antimicrobials that are eliminated by renal excretion is not of clinical significance. For comparative purposes the half-life of gentamicin is about 1 hour in guinea pigs and rabbits; 1.1–1.4 hours in dogs and cats; 1.4–1.8 hours in cattle, sheep, and goats; 1.9 hours in pigs; 2–3 hours in horses and human beings; about 3 hours in llamas and camels; 2.5–3.5 hours in chickens and turkeys; 12 hours in channel catfish *(Ictalurus punctatus)* at 22 ± 2° C; and an average of 51 hours in reptiles.

Compared with the half-lives of antimicrobials in mammalian (and avian) species, those in poikilothermic species (fish and reptiles) are prolonged, which is consistent with their much lower metabolic turnover rate (Calder, 1984) (see Chapters 29 and 30). The half-life of an antimicrobial agent in fish is influenced by the temperature of the water in which the fish are acclimatized (Table 4.7). The overall rate of antimicrobial elimination

TABLE 4.6. **Average half-lives of antimicrobial agents in various species**

Drug	Process(es) of Elimination	Half-life (h) Cattle	Horses	Dogs	Humans
Trimethoprim	M + E(r)	1.25	3.2	4.6	10.6
Sulfadiazine	M + E(r)	2.5	3.6	5.6	9.9
Sulfamethoxazole	M + E(r)	2.3	4.8	—	10.1
Sulfamethazine	M + E(r)	8.2	9.8	16.8	—
Sulfadimethoxine	M + E(r)	12.5	11.3	13.2	40
Sulfadoxine	M + E(r)	10.8	14.2	—	150
Norfloxacin	M + E(r)	2.4	6.4	3.6	5.0
Enrofloxacin	M + E(r)	1.7	5.0	3.4	—
Chloramphenicol	M + E(r)	3.6	0.9	4.2	4.6
Metronidazole	M + E(r)	2.8	3.9	4.5	8.5
Tinidazole	M + E(r)	2.4	5.2	4.4	14.0
Erythromycin	E(h) + M	3.2	1.0	1.7	1.6
Oxytetracycline	E(r ± h)	4.0	9.6	6.0	9.2
Penicillin G	E(r)	0.7	0.9	0.5	1.0
Ampicillin	E(r)	0.95	1.2	0.8	1.3
Cefazolin	E(r)	—	0.65	0.8	1.8
Ceftriaxone	E(r)	—	1.62	0.85	7.3[a]
Gentamicin	E(r)	1.8	2.2–2.8	1.25	2.75
Amikacin	E(r)	—	1.7	1.1	2.3

Note: M, metabolism; E, excretion; r, renal; h, hepatic.
[a]Eliminated by the liver (biliary excretion) in human beings.

TABLE 4.7. **The half-lives of various antimicrobial agents in fish**

Antimicrobial Agent	Species	Acclimatization Temperature (°C)	$t_{1/2}$ (h)
Trimethoprim	Carp	10	40.7
	(*Cyprinus carpio* L.)	24	20.0
Sulfadiazine	Carp	10	47.0
	(*Cyprinus carpio* L.)	24	33.0
Oxytetracycline	Rainbow trout	12	89.5
	(*Salmo gairdneri*)		
	African catfish	25	80.3
	(*Clarias gariepinus*)		
Florfenicol	Atlantic salmon	10.8 ± 1.5	12.2
	(*Salmo salar*)	(seawater)	
Enrofloxacin	Fingerling rainbow trout	15	27.4
	(*Oncorhynchus mykiss*)		
Enrofloxacin (5 mg/kg, IM)	Red pacu	25	28.9
	(*Colossoma brachypomum*)		
Gentamicin	Channel catfish	22	12.0
	(*Ictalurus punctatus*)		
Sulfadimidine	Carp	10	50.3
	(*Cyprinus carpio* L.)	20	25.6
	Rainbow trout	10	20.6
	(*Salmo gairdneri*)	20	14.7

increases (ie, half-life decreases) with increase in water temperatures. The average half-life of trimethoprim, administered IV as trimethoprim-sulfadiazine combination, in carp (*Cyprinus carpio* L.) is 40.7 hours at 10° C and 20 hours at 24° C (Nouws et al., 1993); in cattle, 1.25 hours; in horses, 3.2 hours; in dogs, 4.6 hours; and in human beings, 10.6 hours. Sulfadiazine half-life similarly differs widely: carp, 47 hours at 10° C and 33 hours at 24° C; cattle, 2.5 hours; horses, 3.6 hours; dogs, 5.6 hours; and human beings, 9.9 hours. The prolonged half-lives of lipid-soluble antimicrobials in fish could be attributed to a greater contribution made by enterohepatic circulation. The half-life of oxytetracycline in African catfish *(Clarias gariepinus)* is 80.3 hours at 25° C and in rainbow trout *(Salmo gairdneri)* is 89.5 hours at 12° C (Grondel et al., 1989), whereas half-lives in domestic animals range from 3.4 to 9.6 hours. When developing antimicrobial products for use in farmed fish, studies of the relationship between pharmacokinetics of the drugs and ambient (water) temperature should be performed (see Chapter 30). Furthermore the quantitative susceptibility (MIC) of bacterial pathogens isolated from poikilothermic animals may be temperature dependent.

Half-life is the parameter on which selection of the dosage interval for a drug is based. The rate at which a drug administered by constant infusion or as multiple doses at a fixed interval (eg, approximately equal to the half-life) approaches a steady-state concentration is determined solely by the half-life of the drug; a duration of 4 times the half-life is required to attain an average plasma concentration during the dosage interval within 90% of the eventual steady-state concentration. A drug that selectively binds to tissues or is sequestered in a body compartment may have more than one half-life in any species. The relevance of the half-life chosen depends on the proposed application. The half-life based on the decline in plasma concentrations of clinical interest is relevant to dosage interval selection. That based on the gradual decline in subinhibitory plasma concentrations in the case of an antimicrobial agent may find application in predicting the withdrawal period for the drug in a food-producing species. The half-life of gentamicin (10 mg/kg, IV) in sheep based on the clinically relevant (β) elimination phase is 1.75 hours, whereas that based on the prolonged terminal (γ) phase is 88.9 hours (Brown et al., 1986). For drugs that show linear pharmacokinetic behavior (antimicrobial agents), dissimilar values of clearance based on single dose and average steady-state plasma concentrations (multiple dosing) provide definitive evidence of the presence of a "deep" peripheral compartment (Browne et al., 1990). Requirements of the study design are that the duration of blood sampling be prolonged and the sensitivity of the analytical method be sufficiently high to detect the presence of a deep peripheral compartment; the plasma concentration-time data is analyzed according to a three-compartment open model.

MEAN RESIDENCE TIME

The mean residence time (MRT) represents the average time the molecules of a drug reside in the body after the administration of a single dose. This parameter is the statistical moment analogy to half-life and may vary with the route of administration. The calculation of MRT is based on total areas under the plasma concentration curves, which are estimated by numerical integration using the trapezoidal rule (from time zero to the last measured plasma concentration) with extrapolation to infinite time:

$$MRT = \frac{AUMC}{AUC}$$

where AUC is area under the curve (zero moment) and AUMC is area under the (first) moment curve obtained from the product of plasma concentration and time *versus* time from time zero to infinity. The areas under the extrapolated portion of the curves are estimated as follows: for AUC,

$$\frac{C_{p(last)}}{\beta}$$

and for AUMC,

$$\frac{t^* \times C_{p(last)}}{\beta} + \frac{C_{p(last)}}{\beta^2}$$

where β is the overall elimination rate constant of the drug and t^* is the time of the last measured plasma drug concentration ($C_{p(last)}$). The elimination rate constant, β, is obtained by least squares regression analysis of the terminal 4 to 6 data points. It is desirable that the areas under the extrapolated portion of the curves be less than 10% of the total AUC and less than 20% of total AUMC.

Values of mean residence time and other pharmacokinetic parameters obtained for metronidazole in horses are presented (Table 4.8).

The advantage of using noncompartmental methods for calculating pharmacokinetic parameters, such as mean residence time (MRT), systemic clearance (Cl_B), volume of distribution ($V_{d(area)}$) and systemic availability (F), is that they can be applied to any route of administration and do not require the selection of a compartmental model. The only assumption made is that the absorption and disposition of the drug obey

TABLE 4.8. **Bioavailability, absorption, and disposition kinetics of metronidazole after administration of single IV and oral doses to quarter horse mares**

	Pharmacokinetic Terms and Units	Mean ± SD
Intravenous		
$V_{d(area)}$	(ml/kg)	661 ± 44
$V_{d(ss)}$	(ml/kg)	651 ± 45
Cl_B	(ml/kg × h)	115 ± 10.8
$t_{1/2}$	(h)	4.04 ± 0.45
MRT_{IV}	(h)	6.02 ± 0.91
Oral		
Lag time	(h)	0.3 (0–0.88)[a]
t_{max}	(h)	1.5 (0.75–4.0)[a]
C_{max}	(μg/ml)	21.2 ± 3.1
$t_{1/2(d)}$	(h)	6.0 ± 2.94
MRT_{PO}	(h)	9.4 ± 4.32
F	(%)	74.5 ± 13.0
		72.7 (58.4–91.5)[a]

Source: Baggot et al. (1988) with permission.
Note: n = 6; IV dose = 10 mg/kg; oral dose = 20 mg/kg.
[a]Median (range).

first-order (linear) pharmacokinetics. After intravenous administration of a bolus dose of drug, the volume of distribution at steady state is given by

$$V_{d(ss)} = Cl_B \times MRT_{IV}$$

CHANGES IN DRUG DISPOSITION

Certain physiologic conditions (neonatal period, pregnancy), prolonged fasting (48 hours or longer), disease states (fever, dehydration, chronic liver disease, renal function impairment), or pharmacokinetic-based drug interactions may alter the disposition of drugs. Assessment of changes in the disposition of a drug should include a comparison of the plasma concentration-time curves in healthy and affected animals and of the following pharmacokinetic parameters: systemic clearance, volume of distribution at steady state and as calculated by the area method, and the half-life of the drug.

The time course of a drug in the body depends upon both the volume of distribution and the systemic clearance, while half-life reflects the relationship between these two parameters:

$$t_{1/2} = \frac{0.693 \times V_{d(area)}}{Cl_B}$$

It follows that an alteration in either or both of the basic parameters, V_d and Cl_B, may result in a change in the half-life, which is a derived parameter. Because of the variables on which the half-life depends, it cannot be used as the sole pharmacokinetic parameter to interpret the underlying changes associated with altered disposition of a drug.

Changes in volume of distribution may occur in disease or physiologic states where membrane permeability is altered (fever), extracellular fluid volume is changed (dehydration, neonatal period), or drug binding to plasma proteins is decreased (hypoproteinemia, uremia, competitive drug displacement). In studies of the effect of *E. coli* endotoxin–induced fever in dogs and etiocholanolone-stimulated fever in human beings on the serum concentrations of gentamicin, it was shown that serum gentamicin concentrations were lower during the febrile state, while the renal clearance (gentamicin is eliminated entirely by glomerular filtration) and the half-life of the drug were not significantly changed (Pennington et al., 1975). The lower serum concentrations could be attributed to increased extravascular distribution, although not of sufficient extent to significantly increase the half-life, of the aminoglycoside. Penicillin G distributes more widely in febrile than in normal animals (Fig. 4.8). Even though infectious diseases have in common the presence of fever, the alterations produced in drug disposition will vary with the pathophysiology of the disease. When corresponding changes occur in volume of distribution and clearance of a drug, the half-life remains unchanged (Abdullah and Baggot, 1984, 1986). Corresponding significant increases in both the volume of distribution and systemic clearance of trimethoprim administered in combination with sulfadimethoxine or sulfamethoxazole occurred in febrile pneumonic pigs compared with healthy pigs; the half-life of trimethoprim remained unchanged. The disposition kinetics of neither sulfonamide was altered in the disease state (Mengelers et al., 1995). In the presence of an experimentally induced *E. coli* infection in pigs, the systemic clearance of enrofloxacin was significantly decreased while the volume of distribution remained unchanged. This resulted in an approximately 2.5-fold increase in the half-life of enrofloxacin (Zeng and Fung, 1997).

Changes in systemic clearance may occur when glomerular filtration is decreased (renal function impairment) or hepatic microsomal metabolic activity is altered. Alteration of blood flow to the organ of elimination may affect the clearance of antimicrobials. Halothane anesthesia, for example, significantly decreased the clearance of gentamicin, resulting in significantly higher plasma concentrations at 8 hours after IV administration of the drug (Smith et al., 1988).

Chloramphenicol, metronidazole, and erythromycin inhibit hepatic microsomal enzymes, whereas rifampin and various lipid-soluble drugs (eg, phenobarbital) and xenobiotics induce hepatic microsomal enzymes. Prolonged fasting (>48 hours), which is accompanied by hyperbilirubinemia, appears to decrease hepatic microsomal metabolic activity and

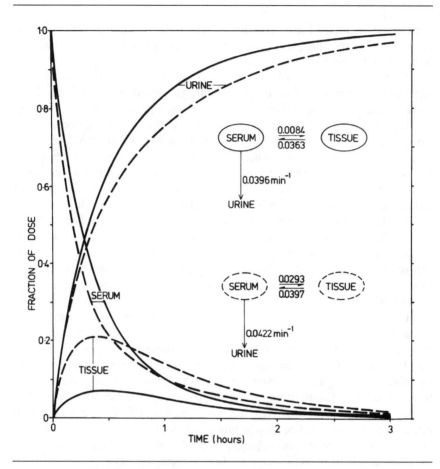

Fig. 4.8. Analog-computer-generated curves showing penicillin G levels (as fraction of IV dose) in the central and peripheral compartments of the two-compartment open model and the cumulative amount excreted in the urine as a function of time. The curves are based on the first-order rate constants associated with the model, which was used to describe the disposition kinetics of the drug in normal (solid line) and febrile (dashed line) dogs. Reproduced with permission from Baggot (1980).

thereby the rate of oxidative reactions and glucuronide synthesis. Although chronic liver disease or altered hepatic function can change the disposition of drugs that undergo extensive hepatic metabolism, indicator tests that would quantify the affected elimination process are not available for clinical application.

There is limited information regarding the influence of disease states, including gastrointestinal disease, on drug absorption. Decreased cardiac output (a feature of congestive heart failure) and, as a consequence, altered blood flow to the intestinal tract may influence the rate but probably not the extent of absorption (systemic availability). Combined IV and oral dose studies (ie, determination of absolute bioavailability) are required to differentiate between altered absorption and disposition processes.

DOSAGE REGIMEN

Factors that affect drug dosage regimens are discussed in Chapter 5. A dosage regimen entails the administration of a series of maintenance doses at a constant dosage interval. Additional features relating to clinical efficacy of the drug selected are the dosage form, which determines the route of administration, and the duration of therapy. The dosing rate and duration of therapy should be appropriate to treat the infection. It is because bacterial susceptibility can be determined in vitro and values of the pharmacokinetic parameters describing bioavailability and disposition are known that dosing rates for antimicrobial agents can be calculated. The minimum effective plasma/serum concentration used in calculating the usual dosing rate for an antimicrobial is based on the MIC for the majority of pathogenic microorganisms that are susceptible to the drug. Variation in the degree of infection and in drug concentrations attained at various sites of infection is partly catered for by the range of doses that is recommended for use in an animal. With the notable exception of penicillins, the maximum dose that can safely be administered does not generally exceed 5 times the dose that would provide minimum effective plasma concentrations. It is usual to estimate the dose that would provide safe and effective plasma concentrations for an 8-hour or 12-hour dosage interval, depending on the (apparent) half-life of the antimicrobial agent.

The dosing rate of a drug can be defined as the systemically available dose (F × dose) divided by the dosage interval (τ):

$$\text{Dosing rate} = \frac{F \times \text{dose}}{\text{Dosage interval}}$$

$$= C_{p(avg)} \times Cl_B$$

where $C_{p(avg)}$ is the average plasma concentration of the drug at steady state, and Cl_B is the clearance of the drug. This relationship can be applied only to drugs that show linear pharmacokinetic behavior—that is, absorption and elimination are first-order processes—and to those for which concentrations exceeding MIC throughout the dosage interval are required. Assuming knowledge of the systemic availability and the clearance of a drug, the average plasma concentration at steady state that would be achieved by applying a fixed dosing rate can be predicted:

$$C_{p(avg)} = \frac{F \times dose}{Cl_B \times \tau}$$

The longer the dosage interval (τ) relative to the half-life of the drug, the greater will be the degree of fluctuation in plasma concentrations at steady state. Selecting a dosage interval similar to the (apparent) half-life of the drug will minimize fluctuation in plasma concentrations; fluctuation will be nonexistent when the drug is administered by IV infusion.

When a drug is administered by IV infusion, the clearance of the drug determines the rate of infusion (R_o) that would be required to produce a desired steady-state (plateau) concentration:

$$R_o = C_{ss} \times Cl_B$$

The steady-state plasma concentration achieved by continuous infusion or the average plasma concentration at steady state produced by multiple dosing at a constant dosage interval depends on the clearance of the drug. The time required to attain steady state depends solely upon the half-life of the drug. After infusion of the drug solution for a period corresponding to 4 times the half-life, the plasma concentration will be within 90% of the eventual steady-state concentration. Steady-state can be attained either gradually by continuous infusion or multiple dosing or promptly by administering a loading dose. The size of the loading dose that would provide a desired plasma concentration can be calculated:

$$Loading\ dose = C_{p(avg)} \times V_{d(area)}$$

Alternatively, the loading dose can be based on the fraction of drug eliminated during the dosage interval and can be related to the maintenance dose of the dosage regimen. This approach is generally applied to antimicrobial agents that produce a bacteriostatic effect and have half-lives between 8 and 24 hours (eg, conventional dosage forms of sulfonamides and tetracyclines).

Development of Antimicrobial Preparations

Blood concentration profiles generated at the low and high ends of the approved dose range, coupled with MIC data for commonly isolated bacterial pathogens, provide a basis for selection of the appropriate dose to use for the particular disease, organ system affected, and causative pathogenic microorganism. The dose range may be defined by a clinically confirmed dose at the lower end and target species safety (including consideration of human food safety for food-producing animals) at the upper end of the dose range (Martinez and Berson, 1998).

Pharmacokinetic-pharmacodynamic (PK-PD) relationships have been well described for many antimicrobials and provide the basis for development of veterinary drug product labels that bear a range of doses. In terms of PK-PD relationship, antimicrobial agents may be assigned to one of three general categories (Craig, 1993), as discussed in Chapter 5.

Time-dependent Bactericidal Action. The category of time-dependent bactericidal action contains antimicrobial agents (eg, beta-lactam antibiotics) that produce a time-dependent bactericidal effect on susceptible bacteria (see Figure 5.2). The overall effectiveness of therapy with these drugs is largely influenced by the aggregate time over which effective plasma concentrations (>MIC for pathogenic microorganisms) are maintained. The peak height determines the rate of penetration of a beta-lactam antibiotic to accessible sites of infection. The clinical effectiveness of dosage regimens that maintain plasma concentrations above the MIC for most of the dosage interval could be attributed to the combination of time-dependent bacterial killing (principal activity) and the postantibiotic sub-MIC effect (minor contribution) beta-lactams exert on susceptible Gram-positive bacteria.

Concentration-dependent Bactericidal Action. The category of concentration-dependent bactericidal action contains antimicrobial agents (eg, aminoglycosides and fluoroquinolones) that produce a concentration-dependent bactericidal effect (see Fig. 5.2). The clinical effectiveness of aminoglycosides and fluoroquinolones is influenced both by the height of the peak plasma concentration relative to the MIC (C_{max}:MIC ratio) and by the area under the plasma concentration-time curve that is above the MIC during the dosage interval. The area under the inhibitory plasma concentration-time curve (AUIC = AUC/MIC) indicates the degree of exposure of a microorganism to the drug. This parameter may be more closely related to the success of treatment with an aminoglycoside, whereas the C_{max}:MIC ratio is important for fluoroquinolones. The maximum activity of fluoroquinolones appears to be achieved when the C_{max}:MIC ratio is in the range 5–10:1. Aminoglycosides and fluoroquinolones induce a postantibiotic sub-MIC effect on most species of Gram-negative aerobic bacteria, which is probably due to their inhibition of protein and DNA synthesis. Because of its variable duration, generally 1–6 hours, this effect is not taken into account when calculating dosage regimens.

Bacteriostatic Antimicrobial Action. The category of bacteriostatic antimicrobial action contains antimicrobial agents (eg, tetracyclines, chloramphenicol, sulfonamides, macrolides, lincosamides) that produce a predominantly bacteriostatic effect. For these agents it is essential that plasma concentrations be maintained above the MIC throughout the dosage interval. The success of therapy also depends upon the participation of host defense mechanisms.

The bioavailability of a drug varies with the formulation of the dosage form and the route of administration. It is a most important pharmacokinetic parameter in developing a dose range label for an antimicrobial preparation. Bioequivalence assessment of generic formulations is based on the estimation of relative bioavailability and the confidence interval for the parameters that measure the rate and extent of absorption of the drug.

Passage into Milk

The bovine udder is richly supplied with blood mainly through the external pudendal arteries and supplemented by a subsidiary supply, cranially through the subcutaneous abdominal artery and caudally via the perineal artery. The ratio of the volume of blood circulating through the mammary gland to volume of milk produced has been estimated to be 670:1, at a moderate level of milk production. This provides ample opportunity for the unbound fraction of lipid-soluble drugs to passively diffuse from the systemic circulation into milk. The passage of antimicrobial agents into milk shows the influence of chemical nature, degree of ionization and lipid solubility, and extent of plasma protein binding on the equilibrium concentration attained across a cellular barrier. The validity of using the milk-to-plasma equilibrium concentration ratio for predictive purposes is highly dependent on the experimental design applied in obtaining the results. Steady state can be achieved either by infusing the drug intravenously for a period exceeding 4 times the half-life or by administering a loading dose followed by maintenance doses, each one-half the loading dose, at intervals equal to the half-life of the drug. After attaining equilibrium, blood and milk samples should be collected at regular (30-minute) intervals, and drug concentration should be determined in ultrafiltrates of plasma and milk.

The majority of antimicrobial agents cross the blood-milk barrier, which is a somewhat restrictive functional rather than anatomical barrier, by passive diffusion. Both nonpolar lipid-soluble compounds and polar substances that possess sufficient lipid solubility passively diffuse through the predominantly lipoidal barrier. The rate of transfer is directly proportional to the concentration gradient across the barrier and the lipid solubility of the drug. The equilibrium concentration ratio of total (non-ionized plus ionized) drug is determined by the degree of ionization in blood and milk, the charge on the ionized moiety, and the extent of binding to plasma proteins and milk macromolecules. It has been shown that only the lipid-soluble, nonionized moiety of a weak organic acid or base that is free (not bound to protein) in the plasma can penetrate cell membranes, enter the milk, and diffuse into transcellular fluids. The milk-to-plasma equilibrium concentration ratio ($R_{m/p}$) can often be predicted (Rasmussen, 1966):

For an acid,

$$R_{milk/plasma} = \frac{1 + 10^{(pH_m - pK_a)}}{1 + 10^{(pH_p - pK_a)}}$$

or for a base,

$$R_{milk/plasma} = \frac{1 + 10^{(pK_a - pH_m)}}{1 + 10^{(pK_a - pH_p)}}$$

where pH_m and pH_p are the pH reactions of milk and plasma, respectively, and pK_a is the negative logarithm of the acidic dissociation constant of an organic acid or base. In normal lactating cows (milk pH range 6.5–6.8), weak organic acids attain milk ultrafiltrate–to–plasma ultrafiltrate concentration ratios less than or equal to 1; organic bases, excluding aminoglycosides and spectinomycin (which are polar), attain equilibrium concentration ratios greater than 1 (Table 4.9). Some lipophilic bases concentrate (ion-trapping effect) in milk; these drugs have an advantage over other antimicrobial agents in the systemic treatment of mastitis. The significance of this favored distribution decreases with increasing pH of milk, particularly for macrolides (Table 4.10), and is largely influenced by the susceptibility of the pathogenic microorganisms causing mastitis. The higher pH of mastitic milk (6.9–7.2) does not interfere with antibacterial activity of macrolides and aminoglycosides, whereas their activity would be decreased in a more acidic environment. Lipid solubility appears to be the principal factor that governs the passage of tetracyclines (amphoteric compounds) into milk and the equilibrium concentration ratios attained. Even though doxycycline is 85–90% bound to plasma proteins and oxytetracycline is only 20% bound, the equilibrium concentration ratio of doxycycline is 1.53 whereas that of

TABLE 4.9. Comparison of calculated and experimentally obtained milk:plasma concentration ratios for antimicrobial agents under equilibrium conditions

Drug	Lipid Solubility	pK_a	Milk pH	Concentration Ratio (milk ultrafiltrate: plasma ultrafiltrate) Theoretical	Experimental
Acids					
Penicillin G	Low	2.7	6.8	0.25	0.13–0.26
Cloxacillin	Low	2.7	6.8	0.25	0.25–0.30
Ampicillin	Low	2.7, 7.2	6.8		0.24–0.30
Cephaloridine	Low	3.4	6.8	0.25	0.24–0.28
Cephaloglycin	Low	4.9	6.8	0.25	0.33
Sulfadimethoxine	Moderate	6.0	6.6	0.20	0.23
Sulfadiazine	Moderate	6.4	6.6	0.23	0.21
Sulfamethazine	Moderate	7.4	6.6	0.58	0.59
Bases					
Tylosin	High	7.1	6.8	2.00	3.5
Lincomycin	High	7.6	6.8	2.83	3.1
Spiramycin	High	8.2	6.8	3.57	4.6
Erythromycin	Very high	8.8	6.8	3.87	8.7
Trimethoprim	High	7.3	6.8	2.32	2.9
Aminoglycosides	Low	7.8[a]	6.8	3.13	0.5
Spectinomycin	Low	8.8	6.8	3.87	0.6
Polymyxin B	Very low	10.0	6.8	3.97	0.3
Amphoteric					
Oxytetracycline	Moderate	—	6.5–6.8	—	0.75
Doxycycline	Moderate/ high	—	6.5–6.8	—	1.53
Rifampin[b]	Moderate/ high	7.9	6.8	0.82	0.90–1.28

[a]The pK_a value given for aminoglycosides is unconfirmed.
[b]Theoretical concentration ratio for rifampin is based on its behavior as an organic acid (pK_a 7.9).

oxytetracycline is 0.75 at milk pH within the range 6.5–6.8. Tetracyclines exert their greatest activity at an acidic pH close to their isoelectric point (5.5 for all tetracyclines apart from minocycline, whose isoelectric point is 6.0). This implies that their antimicrobial activity would be less in mastitic milk (pH 6.9–7.2).

The principal differences in mammary gland physiology are in the relative volume of milk produced by various species and in the composition of the milk, particularly the fat (triglycerides) and protein (casein) content.

TABLE 4.10. Comparison of the fraction of dose recovered in normal and mastitic milk for antibiotics administered intramuscularly to cows

Drug	pK$_a$	Percentage Nonionized in Plasma	Percentage of Dose Recovered in Milk	
			Normal	Mastitic
Acids				
Penicillin G	2.7	0.002	0.001	0.001
Cloxacillin	2.7	0.002	0.001	0.001
Ampicillin	2.7, 7.2		0.08	0.10
Amoxicillin	2.7, 7.2		0.06	0.15
Bases				
Tylosin	7.2	66.67	2.60	1.40
Spiramycin	8.2	13.68	6.80	2.40
Erythromycin	8.8	3.85	3.80	2.20
Spectinomycin[a]	8.8	3.85	0.04	0.08
Gentamicin[a]	7.8	28.47	0.006	0.01
Polymyxin	10.0	0.25	0.001	0.001
Amphoteric				
Oxytetracycline	—	—	0.07	0.08
Doxycycline	—	—	0.15	0.15

[a]Polar drug with low solubility in lipid.

Bibliography

Abdullah AS, Baggot JD. 1984. Influence of *Escherichia coli* endotoxin-induced fever on pharmacokinetics of imidocarb in dogs and goats. Am J Vet Res 45:2645.

Abdullah AS, Baggot JD. 1986. Influence of induced disease states on the disposition kinetics of imidocarb in goats. J Vet Pharm Ther 9:192.

Aktas M, et al. 1995. Disposition of creatine kinase activity in dog plasma following intravenous and intramuscular injection of skeletal muscle homogenates. J Vet Pharm Ther 18:1.

Baggot JD. 1977. Principles of Drug Disposition in Domestic Animals: The Basis of Veterinary Clinical Pharmacology. Philadelphia: WB Saunders.

Baggot JD. 1980. Distribution of antimicrobial agents in normal and diseased animals. J Am Vet Med Assoc 176:1085.

Baggot JD, et al. 1988. Clinical pharmacokinetics of metronidazole in horses. J Vet Pharm Ther 11:417.

Banting A de L, Baggot JD. 1996. Comparison of the pharmacokinetics and local tolerance of three injectable oxytetracycline formulations in pigs. J Vet Pharm Ther 19:50.

Banting A de L, Tranquart F. 1991. Echography as a tool in clinical pharmacology. Acta Vet Scand, Suppl 87:215.

Benet LZ, Galeazzi RL. 1979. Noncompartmental determination of the steady-state volume of distribution. J Pharm Sci 68:1071.

Bevill RF, et al. 1977. Disposition of sulfonamides in food-producing animals. IV: Pharmacokinetics of sulfamethazine in cattle following administration of an intravenous dose and three oral dosage forms. J Pharm Sci 66:619.

Brown SA, et al. 1986. Dose-dependent pharmacokinetics of gentamicin in sheep. Am J Vet Res 47:789.

Browne TR, et al. 1990. New pharmacokinetic methods. III: Two simple tests for "deep pool effect." J Clin Pharm 30:680.

Calder WA. 1984. Size, Function and Life History. Cambridge: Harvard University Press.

Craig W. 1993. Pharmacodynamics of antimicrobial agents as a basis for determining dosage regimens. Eur J Clin Microb Infect Dis 1 (Suppl):6.

de Backer P, Bogaert MG. 1983. Drug bioavailability in the developing ruminant. In: Ruckebusch Y, et al., eds. Veterinary Pharmacology and Toxicology. Lancaster, England: MTP Press.

Duffee NE, et al. 1997. The pharmacokinetics of cefadroxil over a range of oral doses and animal ages in the foal. J Vet Pharm Ther 20:427.

Ensink JM, et al. 1994. Oral bioavailability of pivampicillin in foals at different ages. Vet Q 16:S113.

Firth EC, et al. 1986. Effect of the injection site on the pharmacokinetics of procaine penicillin G in horses. Am J Vet Res 47:2380.

Gilman JM, et al. 1987. Plasma concentration of gentamicin after intramuscular or subcutaneous administration to horses. J Vet Pharm Ther 10:101.

Grondel JL, et al. 1989. Comparative pharmacokinetics of oxytetracycline in rainbow trout (Salmo gairdneri) and African catfish (Clarias gariepinus). J Vet Pharm Ther 12:157.

International Commission on Radiological Protection. 1975. Report of the Task Group on Reference Man, 1st ed. Oxford: Pergamon.

Marshall AB, Palmer GH. 1980. Injection sites and drug bioavailability. In: Van Miert ASJPAM, et al., eds. Trends in Veterinary Pharmacology and Toxicology. Amsterdam: Elsevier.

Martinez MN, Berson MR. 1998. Bioavailability/bioequivalence assessments. In: Hardee GE, Baggot JD, eds. Development and Formulation of Veterinary Dosage Forms, 2nd ed. New York: Marcel Dekker.

Matthews CA, et al. 1975. External form and internal anatomy of Holsteins and Jerseys. J Dairy Sci 58:1453.

Mengelers MJB, et al. 1995. Pharmacokinetics of sulfadimethoxine and sulfamethoxazole in combination with trimethoprim after intravenous administration to healthy and pneumonic pigs. J Vet Pharm Ther 18:243.

Metzler CM. 1989. Bioavailability/bioequivalence: study design and statistical issues. J Clin Pharm 29:289.

Neff-Davis C, et al. 1975. Comparative body composition of the dog and goat. Am J Vet Res 36:309.

Nielsen P. 1997. The influence of feed on the oral bioavailability of antibiotics/chemotherapeutics in pigs. J Vet Pharm Ther 20 (Suppl 1):30.

Nouws JFM, Vree TB. 1983. Effect of injection site on the bioavailability of an oxytetracycline formulation in ruminant calves. Vet Q 5:165.

Nouws JFM, et al. 1982. Comparative plasma ampicillin levels and bioavailability of five parenteral ampicillin formulations in ruminant calves. Vet Q 4:62.

Nouws JFM, et al. 1993. Pharmacokinetics of sulphadiazine and trimethoprim in carp (Cyprinus carpio L.) acclimated at two different temperatures. J Vet Pharm Ther 16:110.

Pennington JE, et al. 1975. Gentamicin sulfate pharmacokinetics: lower levels of gentamicin in blood during fever. J Infect Dis 132:270.

Rasmussen F. 1966. Studies on the Mammary Excretion and Absorption of Drugs. Copenhagen: Carl Fr. Mortensen.

Rutgers LJE, et al. 1980. Effect of the injection site on the bioavailability of amoxycillin trihydrate in dairy cows. J Vet Pharm Ther 3:125.

Smith CM, et al. 1988. Effects of halothane anesthesia on the clearance of gentamicin sulfate in horses. Am J Vet Res 49:19.

Theodorides VJ, et al. 1968. Serum concentrations of chloramphenicol after intraruminal and intraabomasal administration in sheep. Am J Vet Res 29:643.

Toutain P-L, et al. 1995. A non-invasive and quantitative method for the study of tissue injury caused by intramuscular injection of drugs in horses. J Vet Pharm Ther 18:226.

Vree TB, et al. 1985. Pharmacokinetics of sulfonamides in animals. In: Vree TB, Hekster YA, eds. Pharmacokinetics of Sulfonamides Revisited, Antibiot Chemother 34:130. Basel: Karger.

Webb AI, Weaver BMQ. 1979. Body composition of the horse. Equine Vet J 11:39.

Wilson RC, et al. 1989. Bioavailability of gentamicin in dogs after intramuscular or subcutaneous injections. Am J Vet Res 50:1748.

Xia W, et al. 1983. Comparison of pharmacokinetic parameters for two oxytetracycline preparations in pigs. J Vet Pharm Ther 6:113.

Zeng Z, Fung K. 1997. Effects of experimentally induced *Escherichia coli* infection on the pharmacokinetics of enrofloxacin in pigs. J Vet Pharm Ther 20 (Suppl 1):39.

5 | Principles of Antimicrobial Drug Selection and Use

J. F. PRESCOTT and R. D. WALKER

The aim of antimicrobial therapy is to rapidly produce and then to maintain an effective concentration of drug at the site of infection for sufficient time to allow host-specific and nonspecific defenses to eradicate the pathogen so that the host can return unharmed to normal function.

Antimicrobial therapy involves a calculated risk that selective toxicity of the drug for the microorganism will occur before any toxic effect on the host. A requirement of all drug therapy is that it be rational. The increasing choice of a wide array of highly effective antimicrobial drugs, with dosage based on pharmacokinetic analysis of drug disposition and with selection based on clinical microbiological data, means that most forms of drug therapy in animals can be rational.

The considerations affecting the choice of an antimicrobial drug are illustrated in Figure 5.1.

Risks Associated with Antimicrobial Treatment

Antimicrobial agents can have a wide variety of damaging effects, including the following: (1) direct host toxicity; (2) adverse interactions with other drugs; (3) interference with the protective effect of normal host microflora or disturbance of the metabolic function of microbial flora in the digestive tract of herbivores; (4) selection or promotion of antimicrobial resistance; (5) tissue necrosis at injection sites; (6) production of residues in animal products for human consumption; (7) impairment of the host's immune or defense mechanisms; and (8) damage to fetal or neonatal tissues.

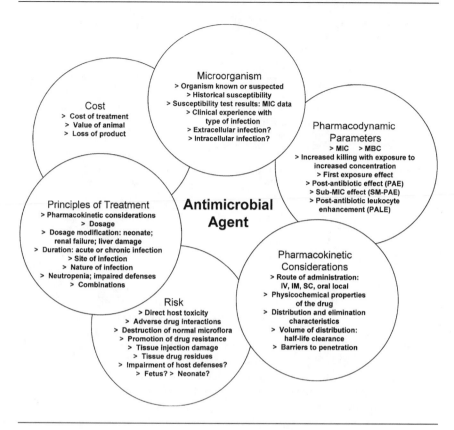

Fig. 5.1.   Some considerations in selection and use of antimicrobial drugs.

Direct Host Toxicity

Direct host toxicity is the most important factor limiting drug dosage. The selective toxicity of antimicrobials is variable. Some agents, such as beta-lactams, are generally very safe, whereas others, such as the aminoglycosides, are potentially toxic. Antimicrobial drugs can damage the function of many organs or tissues, particularly the kidneys (eg, aminoglycosides, amphotericin B), nervous system (eg, aminoglycosides, polymyxins), liver (eg, tetracyclines, chloramphenicol), heart (eg, aminoglycosides, monensin, tetracyclines), immune system (eg, penicillin G), hematopoietic system (eg, chloramphenicol), and joint cartilage (eg, fluoroquinolones). The toxicity of antibiotics with a narrow margin of safety can be minimized by using the lowest effective doses and the shortest duration of treatment or by substituting equally effective but less toxic agents.

TABLE 5.1. **Adverse in vivo effects of drug interactions between antibiotics and other agents**

Antimicrobial Drug	Interacting Drug	Adverse Effect
Aminoglycoside	Cephaloridine, cephalothin, polymyxins, furosemide	Nephrotoxicity
	Polymyxins, curare-like drugs, anesthetics	Neuromuscular blockade
Amphotericin B	Aminoglycosides	Nephrotoxicity
Chloramphenicol	Dicoumarol, barbiturates	Prolonged anesthesia, anticoagulation
Griseofulvin	Dicoumarol, barbiturates	Reduced anticoagulant effect
Lincomycin	Kaolin-pectate	Decreased lincomycin absorption
Monensin	Tiamulin	Neurotoxicity
Polymyxins	Aminoglycosides	Nephrotoxicity, neuromuscular blockade
Rifampin	Theophylline	Enhanced theophylline clearance
Sulfonamides	Oral anticoagulants	Prolonged anticoagulant effect
Tetracyclines	Barbiturates	Anesthetic potentiation
	Oral iron, calcium, magnesium	Decreased tetracycline absorption

Drug Interactions Involving Antimicrobial Agents

Adverse drug interactions can occur in many ways, both in vitro and in vivo, and should be anticipated. These interactions can affect intestinal absorption, enhance or slow liver metabolism, interfere with kidney excretion, or result in competition for receptors or plasma proteins. Examples are shown in Table 5.1.

Absorption from the intestine may be affected nonspecifically by food or through pH, fat, or ionic chelating effects (ie, divalent cations). The influence of food on oral absorption of some antibiotics is summarized in Table 22.5. Liver microsomal enzyme induction by drugs such as rifampin and to a lesser extent griseofulvin may enhance the metabolism and decrease the activity of other drugs, whereas inhibition of microsomal enzymes can reduce the metabolism and increase the activity of other drugs. Notable examples are described in sections on individual drugs. In the kidney, the pH of the urine may, depending on the pK_a of the drug, affect the excretion and absorption of weak acids and weak bases. Many acidic drugs such as penicillins and sulfonamides are secreted actively in the proximal tubules and may interact with other drugs that are similarly excreted. For example, probenecid was used for many years to reduce kidney excretion and to prolong the activity of penicillin.

DRUG INCOMPATIBILITIES

Antimicrobials may be physicochemically incompatible with other agents in vitro. In general, drugs should not be mixed in the same syringe;

chemical inactivation may have occurred even if a visible precipitate is not present. Agents should not generally be mixed in the same saline for IV administration. Normal saline is compatible with most antimicrobial drugs, but benzyl penicillin G and sodium ampicillin are incompatible with dextrose saline, and tetracyclines are incompatible with any solution containing calcium or magnesium.

Antibiotics and the Immune System

Antimicrobial drugs may enhance or suppress host defenses. It is an intriguing thought that some antibiotics may cause some of their beneficial effects through immunomodulation. The complexity of the interactions of antimicrobial drugs with bacteria and phagocytic cells and the use of widely different methods of study in vitro make firm conclusions difficult. Microorganisms that have been damaged by antimicrobial drugs are more susceptible to killing by phagocytes, an effect that may be balanced against any direct deleterious effect on the host's phagocytic cell activity. Beta-lactam drugs have little effect on phagocyte cell function, but tetracyclines consistently reduce phagocytosis, chemiluminescence, and chemotactic activity. Aminoglycosides often inhibit phagocytosis. Some cephalosporins and fluoroquinolones may enhance chemiluminescence. Azithromycin is dramatically concentrated inside phagocytic cells. These findings are often regarded as largely of theoretical interest, with possible clinical application in immunosuppressed or neutropenic patients. Though not guaranteeing efficacy, the ability of some antibiotics to penetrate and to concentrate within cells, particularly phagocytic cells, is an important consideration in the treatment of intracellular bacterial infections.

Factors Determining Choice of Antibiotic

Rational therapy demands an accurate diagnosis. Such a diagnosis may be made clinically but requires bacteriologic investigation in cases of nonspecific infection. Samples for bacteriologic culture should be collected from the actual site of infection before administration of an antimicrobial drug. A Gram stain may provide insight as to the etiological agent, but in many cases it is necessary to identify the pathogen and determine its susceptibility profile. Because of the delay in receiving the outcome of laboratory tests, empirical antibiotic treatment is usually started before results are available; efforts should nevertheless be made to obtain a firm diagnosis.

Empirical antibiotic treatment requires the following: (1) making a diagnosis of microbial infection; (2) taking laboratory samples where possible; (3) making a presumptive microbiologic diagnosis clinically or on the basis of direct examination of stained material; (4) determining the need for antimicrobial treatment; and (5) starting appropriate treatment. The selection of an antimicrobial agent depends on (1) knowledge of the potential susceptibility of the suspected pathogen(s); (2) knowledge of factors that affect drug concentration at the site of infection; (3) knowledge of drug toxicity and factors that enhance it; (4) the cost of treatment; and (5) considerations of regulations about drug use, including drug withdrawal times where applicable.

Bacterial Susceptibility

Antimicrobial susceptibility of some bacterial pathogens, notably many Gram-positive bacteria, is predictable (Chapter 2), but this is not the case for Gram-negative genera that readily acquire resistance (Chapter 3). Every veterinary practice should have access to laboratories in which antimicrobial susceptibility can be determined quickly and reliably.

Laboratory results may be misleading for several reasons, including failure to isolate the causative agent (such as inappropriate sample collection or anaerobes), misinterpretation of the significance of normal flora, and mishandling of specimens or swabs in transit to the laboratory. Other reasons for the failure of some tests to predict susceptibility were discussed in Chapter 2.

Choice of Antimicrobial Drugs

The ideal drug is one to which the organism is most susceptible and one that achieves effective concentration at the site of infection without damaging the host. MIC data may be more useful than results of disk-diffusion susceptibility tests because MIC data define more precisely the degree of susceptibility and consequently the drug dosage; the apparently increased precision of such laboratory-derived data is, however, potentially misleading.

Microbicidal drugs are required (1) in serious life-threatening infections; (2) when host defenses are impaired; (3) in infections of vital tissues such as meninges, endocardium, and bones where host defenses are also not fully functional; and (4) in immunodeficient or immunosuppressed animals. In other cases bacteriostatic agents may be equally useful.

Where appropriate, a narrow-spectrum drug may be more appropriate than a broad-spectrum antibacterial because the narrow-spectrum drug interferes less with the normal microbial flora. In this regard, pharmacokinetic considerations are also relevant. For example, drugs excreted via the bile will disturb the intestinal flora more than those excreted via the kidneys. Drug combinations should be considered in seriously ill patients with severe infections when results of bacteriologic tests are not available. The availability of a dosage form of the antimicrobial drug of choice that is suitable for administration to the particular species of animal is another factor influencing the final choice of antimicrobial drug.

Principles of Antimicrobial Treatment

To some extent, drug dosage can be tailored to the susceptibility of the organism, the site of infection, and the pharmacokinetic and pharmacodynamic properties of the selected antimicrobial agent. However, it should be recognized that in vitro susceptibility data are laboratory derived and the standardized conditions under which the susceptibility data were generated does not exist at the site of infection. It is also important to recognize that pharmacokinetic data represent mean data obtained from different animals and that the immune status of the host, as well as its physiological and psychological status, can influence the therapeutic outcome.

Factors involved in tailoring a dosing regimen include, among other things, the susceptibility of the pathogen in terms of MICs, the concentration of the antimicrobial agent at the site of infection in active form (pharmacokinetic properties of the drug), and the pharmacodynamic properties of the antimicrobial agent (see Figure 2.1). Pharmacokinetic properties correlating with efficacy are shown in Table 5.2. Initially, the pharmacodynamic properties of clinical interest were MICs and MBCs (minimal bactericidal concentrations). However, more recent studies have demonstrated that other bacterial pathogen–antimicrobial agent interactions may influence dosing strategies and therapeutic outcome. These other pharmacodynamic properties include concentration-dependent killing, first-exposure effect, post-antibiotic effect (PAE), sub-MIC post-antibiotic effect (SM-PAE), and post-antibiotic leukocyte enhancement effect (PALE).

TABLE 5.2. **Pharmacokinetic parameters correlating with efficacy of selected antimicrobial drug classes**

Drug Class	Pharmacokinetic Parameter	Optimal Dosing Regimen
Beta-lactams	Time above MIC	Serum concentration continuously above MIC
Aminoglycosides	Peak concentration	Peak serum > 8–10 times MIC
Vancomycin	Area under the curve (AUC)	High serum concentration; may not need to be > MIC throughout dosing interval
Fluoroquinolones	AUC; peak concentration	Peak serum > 10–12 times MIC or 24-hour AUC/MIC > 125
Macrolides	Time above MIC, MBC	High serum concentration; > MIC through dosing interval
Lincosamides	Time above MIC	High serum concentration; > MIC through dosing interval

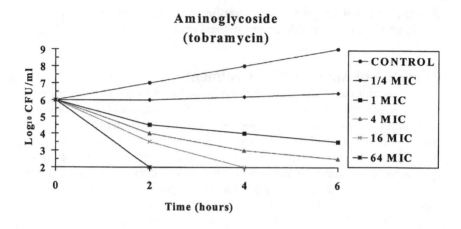

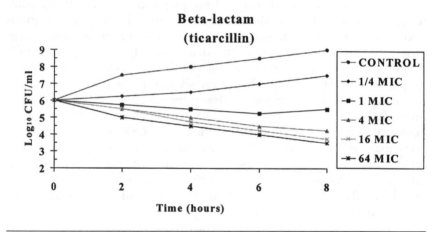

Fig. 5.2. Example of concentration-dependent killing by an aminoglycoside (tobramycin). This effect contrasts with the killing by beta-lactams, which depends on the presence of drug concentration above the MIC (time-dependent killing) but is otherwise independent of drug concentration. Reproduced with permission from Craig and Ebert (1991).

Concentration-dependent killing is dependent on class of antimicrobial agent. This is best illustrated in Figure 5.2. For an aminoglycoside, such as tobramycin, as the concentration of the antimicrobial agent increases above the MIC of the pathogen *Pseudomonas aeruginosa*, the number of viable organisms decreases dramatically. On the other hand, for a beta-lactam drug, such as ticarcillin, the number of viable organisms decreases as concentration of ticarcillin increases from 0.25 of the MIC to

4 times the MIC. However, there is very little decrease in viable organisms as the concentration of ticarcillin continues to increase to 64 times the MIC. Thus, as the concentration of an aminoglycoside increases above the MIC of the pathogen, there is increased killing of the pathogen, which contrasts markedly with the action of a beta-lactam drug. The first-exposure effect refers to the effect the antimicrobial agent has on a bacterial pathogen at the time of the initial therapy. Ideally, initial exposure will destroy most of the invading organisms. However, for bacteria that survive there is often a time in which they will be unaffected by a repeat exposure to the drug. This down-regulation of susceptibility and the length of its duration are dependent on the antimicrobial agent and its mechanism of action. For example, antimicrobial agents that interfere with protein synthesis will have little effect against bacteria whose protein-synthesizing capabilities have not been restored to normal function.

The PAE refers to the persistent suppression of bacterial growth following the removal of an antimicrobial agent. While this was initially recognized in vitro it has been shown, by the use of animal models, to occur in vivo. The length of the PAE is dependent on the microorganism, the class of antimicrobial agent, the concentration of drug to which the bacteria are exposed, and the duration of the exposure. For example, this effect has been observed for all antibacterial drugs that have activity against Gram-positive bacteria in vitro and in vivo with the exception of beta-hemolytic streptococci. These organisms do not show a PAE when exposed to beta-lactams in vivo. It has been suggested that this may be due to their slow growth rate in vivo. In contrast to their action on the Gram-positive bacteria, the beta-lactams produce no or very short PAEs against Gram-negative bacteria either in vitro or in vivo, with the possible exceptions of the carbapenems against *P. aeruginosa*. On the other hand, antimicrobial agents that inhibit DNA (eg, fluoroquinolones) or protein synthesis (eg, aminoglycosides) have prolonged PAEs against Gram-negative bacteria. There are multiple mechanisms that may contribute to an antimicrobial agent exhibiting a PAE on a bacterial pathogen. These post-antibiotic effects are also dependent on class of antimicrobial agent. For example, for the beta-lactams the PAE may be associated with the length of time it takes to synthesize new penicillin-binding proteins, whereas for the aminoglycosides it may be the length of time required for the antimicrobial agent to diffuse from the ribosomes and for protein synthesis to resume. This latter effect may contribute to the SM-PAE. In other words, in vivo, where there is a slow removal of the drug from the site of infection, subinhibitory concentration may continue to inhibit DNA and protein synthesis, depending on the drug's mechanism of action. The PALE describes a bacterium's increased susceptibility to phagocytosis and intracellular killing following exposure to an antimicrobial agent. The

PALE has been shown to increase PAEs both in vitro and in vivo, with those drugs that produce the longest PAEs also exhibiting the greatest PALEs.

Although all the factors listed above determine optimal dosage, the factor that most frequently limits dosage is toxicity to the host. The upper level of the recommended dosage should not be exceeded, because this is often determined by toxicity. Sometimes, however, a drug's antibacterial effects may be limiting and may determine the upper level of dosage. For example, as discussed above, the killing rate of penicillin G (and other beta-lactam drugs) has an optimal concentration, whereas that of the aminoglycosides or fluoroquinolones is proportional to drug concentration. Penicillin G is virtually nontoxic in nonallergenic patients, but its dosage is limited by its antibacterial action, whereas the dosage of aminoglycoside is limited not by antibacterial effects but rather by the drug's toxicity to the host.

Recommended dosing intervals should be followed. With the exception of the penicillins and aminoglycosides, the interval for IV-administered drugs required to maintain therapeutic plasma concentrations should not usually exceed twice their elimination half-life. Because elimination half-life is based on IV dosing, however, administering appropriate formulations by other routes can be a highly effective way to lengthen the interval between doses, since absorption may be delayed. For example, a single dose of procaine penicillin G administered IM can maintain effective drug levels for 12–24 hours because of slow absorption, even though in all species the elimination half-life of penicillin G is less than 1 hour. The detrimental effects of not following dose interval recommendations were observed by Waltner-Toews et al. (1986), who reported that calves treated with chloramphenicol once daily were 4 times more likely to die of pneumonia than calves treated twice daily.

One way to increase the concentration of a drug at the site of infection is to administer an IV bolus injection slowly, because tissue penetration is a function of peak serum concentration.

Dosages may have to be modified in neonates and in animals with impaired liver or kidney function (see Chapter 19).

Duration of Treatment

Although it is axiomatic that a drug must be present at an adequate concentration for an adequate time at the site of infection, the variables affecting length of treatment have not been defined. Responses of different types of infections to antimicrobial drugs vary, and clinical experience with many infections is important in assessing response to treatment. For acute infections, it will be clear within 2 days whether or not therapy is clinically effective. If no response is seen by that time, both the diagnosis and the treatment should be reconsidered. Treatment of acute infections should be continued for at least 2 days after clinical and microbiologic resolution of infection. For serious acute infections, treatment should last 7–10 days. For chronic infections, particularly intracellular infections, treatment will be considerably longer and may involve months (see Chapter 19). Some uncomplicated infections, such as cystitis in human females, have been successfully treated with single doses of antibiotics, but the efficacy of single-dose treatments in animals must be established in appropriate infections before this approach is recommended.

Adjunctive Treatment

Adjunctive treatments to antimicrobial therapy are essential in promoting healing. They include debriding necrotic tissues, removing pus, draining abscesses, removing foreign bodies, correcting acid base and fluid balance successfully, and providing rest and nursing. It is virtually impossible to treat infection associated with a foreign body without removing the foreign body.

Other Considerations

Other considerations in antimicrobial therapy include cost of the drug and convenience of administration. In food-producing animals, one must know the likelihood of drug residues remaining in tissues or in milk, and therefore the required withdrawal times of agents. Labeled directions for drug products for food-animal use must be followed or intelligently interpreted. The danger of selection of resistant bacteria by antibiotic use is another important consideration.

EXTRALABEL DRUG USE

Antimicrobial drugs are licensed in many countries only for use for particular purposes at specific dosage, as shown on the manufacturer's product label. Because of the high costs of obtaining approval, many drugs are not approved or may be approved only for narrowly specified purposes at dosages that, in food animals at least, may be based more on the potential for drug residues or economics of treatment than on optimal clinical efficacy. In the United States, the Food and Drug Administration's Center for Veterinary Medicine, besides having a "professional flexible labeling" approach, has a discretionary "extralabel" policy (with notable exceptions; see Chapter 34). This means that veterinarians who use drugs in ways not in accord with label directions, but with certain other specifications, will not be prosecuted so long as no illegal tissue residues occur in edible products. The specifications include the need for a careful diagnosis within the context of a valid veterinarian-client-patient relationship, a determination that there are no alternative drugs or that dosage is inappropriate, identification of treated animals, and extended drug withdrawal to ensure no tissue residues. The increasing availability of simple in-house tests for drug residues (see Chapter 33) has aided extralabel drug use. For non-food-producing animals, the position is generally that veterinarians may use any legally obtainable antimicrobial drug to treat disease, subject only to subsequent scientific justification before courts of law or professional ethics groups, should this use need to be defended.

CORTICOSTEROID USE

The benefits of using corticosteroids with antimicrobial drugs in the treatment of acute bacterial infections are both controversial and poorly investigated. Clear guidelines are not available. Corticosteroids have many effects on nonspecific and specific host defenses: suppressing inflammation, impairing phagocytosis, delaying healing, reducing fever, and impairing the immune response. Use of corticosteroids in the treatment of infections would therefore generally be expected to have deleterious effects and should be avoided. In the virtual absence of experimental or clinical data supporting their concurrent use, however, certain circumstances may justify their short-term use: (1) in severe, life-threatening septicemia or endotoxemia, with septic shock; (2) in extensive, severe, acute local infections to prevent lysosomal enzyme release from neutrophils and resulting tissue destruction; (3) in the treatment of meningitis to control cerebral edema and to control inflammation due to release of inflammatory mediators induced by beta-lactam antibiotics. Short-acting steroids should probably not be used for more than 3–5 days.

RAPID ATTAINMENT OF HIGH TISSUE CONCENTRATIONS OF DRUGS

In acute bacterial infections, especially when using bacteriostatic drugs, it may be useful to administer a *priming (loading) dose* to establish therapeutic drug levels rapidly, usually by giving a high dose by IV injection.

LOCAL ADMINISTRATION OF ANTIMICROBIAL DRUGS

Antimicrobial drugs are administered locally in the treatment of a wide variety of infections, including endometritis; skin, outer ear, and wound infections; mastitis; osteomyelitis; and occasionally bronchopneumonia (by endotracheal or aerosol administration). Local administration usually achieves significantly higher and more persistent drug concentrations than systemic administration, so that local treatments may be administered less frequently than systemic treatments. The principles of drug selection and use are those described for systemic antimicrobial drugs, with the caution that the drug vehicle and the drug must not provoke tissue inflammation. For endometritis, local treatment may not penetrate important sites, such as the oviducts or cervix, in contrast to systemic treatment. In the cow and the mare, intrauterine treatment of the involuted uterus is often with 1 g of antibiotic dissolved in 100–250 ml sterile saline administered daily for 3–5 days, depending on severity and chronicity of infection. Acute, severe endometritis requires systemically administered antibiotics, which may be supplemented by local treatments. Endotracheal administration of antibiotics, particularly aminoglycosides, results in high, persistent drug concentrations in the tracheobronchial tree and, while not generally recommended, may have a place in treatment of tracheobronchial infections that respond poorly to systemic treatment, as, for example, in kennel cough in dogs. Aerosol administration of antimicrobial drugs is rarely used but may have a place in the treatment of severe infections of the bronchial tract that are unresponsive to other treatments, including severe viral respiratory infections (see Chapter 18). Antimicrobial-impregnated polymethyl methacrylate for the treatment of osteomyelitis may maintain effective local concentrations of drug for several weeks. Gentamicin-impregnated collagen sponges have also been used successfully in the local treatment of septic arthritis in animals.

Antimicrobial Drug Combinations

From the earliest days of antibiotic use, it was known that combinations of drugs sometimes had dramatic synergistic effects where individual agents had failed. A classic example was in the treatment of enterococcal endocarditis with a combination of penicillin G and streptomycin. On the other hand, early studies of the use of combinations to treat certain types of meningitis showed that antagonism between drugs might have fatal results. The importance of antagonism is greatest in patients whose, or at sites where, immune defenses are poor, such as in meningitis, endocarditis, or chronic osteomyelitis, particularly where combination of a bacteriostatic drug with a bactericidal drug prevents the required killing activity of the bactericidal drug. Mechanisms of synergism and antagonism are discussed in Chapter 1.

There are four indications for the use of antimicrobial combinations. Bactericidal combinations are effective in serious infections where host defenses are impaired. Two or more agents may be administered to treat polymicrobial infections (intra-abdominal infections, aspiration pneumonia, female genital tract infections), as well as to prevent emergence of chromosomal resistance. Enzymatic destruction of one drug may be overcome by using a combination. Finally, combined therapy may decrease drug toxicity and provide broad-spectrum coverage in severe but undefined infections. Examples of clinically effective combinations are shown in Table 5.3. Combinations should be used only where their

TABLE 5.3.   **Clinically useful antimicrobial drug combinations in veterinary medicine**

Indication	Drug Combination	Comment
Bovine *Staphylococcus aureus* mastitis	Penicillin-streptomycin Ampicillin–clavulanic acid	Synergistic combination
Rhodococcus equi pneumonia of foals	Erythromycin-rifampin	Synergistic combination
Brucella canis in dogs	Minocycline-streptomycin	Synergistic combination
Peritonitis after intestinal spillage	Gentamicin-clindamycin Cefuroxime-metronidazole	Broad-spectrum antibacterial activity
Coliform meningitis	Trimethoprim-sulfamethoxazole	Synergistic; good CSF penetration
Cryptococcal meningitis	Amphotericin-flucytosine	Synergistic; decreased toxicity
Severe undiagnosed infection	Amoxycillin-gentamicin Cefoxitin-clindamycin	Broad-spectrum, often synergistic combination

efficacy is established. The increasing availability of highly active, broad-spectrum bactericidal drugs may reduce the need for combination therapy.

Combined antimicrobial treatment also has disadvantages. For example, a bacteriostatic drug may neutralize bactericidal effects where these effects are required. Combinations may have additive or synergistic toxicity. They may produce superinfection after destroying normal microbial flora and may have possible adverse pharmacokinetic interactions in vivo. When combination therapy is used, it should be done so in such a way as to maximize the synergistic effect. For example, in using an aminoglycoside-beta-lactam combination, the aminoglycoside should be administered once a day for its concentration-dependent killing effect, whereas the beta-lactam should be administered so as to maintain continuous serum concentrations above the MIC of the organism.

Failure of Antimicrobial Therapy

Treatment failure has many causes. The antibiotic selected may be inappropriate because of misdiagnosis, inactivity at the site of infection, failure to culture infections, inaccurate results of laboratory tests (see Chapter 2), resistance of pathogens, intracellular location of bacteria, metabolic state of the pathogen, or errors in sampling. These factors are more likely to cause failure than inadequate dosage or the use of drugs of low bioavailability, although the latter factors may also be important.

When failure occurs, diagnosis must be reassessed and samples collected for laboratory analysis. Patient factors such as the persistence of foreign bodies, neoplasia, and impairment of host defenses are important to consider. It is important also to ensure that persons medicating their own animals comply with dosing instructions.

TABLE 5.4. **Examples of antimicrobial prophylaxis in veterinary medicine**

Disease/Purpose	Drug	Duration	Comment
Feedlot pneumonia of calves	Tetracycline, penicillin G	1–3 doses	Treat upon arrival at feedlot
Dry-cow therapy	Many	Single dose	
Leptospiral abortion in cows	Streptomycin	Single dose	Removes carriers
Swine erysipelas	Penicillin, long-acting	Single dose	Treat pigs at risk
Atrophic rhinitis in pigs	Tetracycline	First weeks of life	
Strangles in horses	Penicillin, long-acting	1–3 doses	Treat horses at risk
Pulpy kidney infection in lambs	Tetracycline	Period at risk	

Prophylactic Use of Antibiotics

Prophylactic administration of antimicrobial drugs has made a remarkable contribution in controlling infectious disease. Its potential disadvantages are toxicity, the encouragement of drug resistance, residues in edible animal products, and cost.

Successful use of prophylactic antimicrobial drugs is based on several principles. Medication should be directed against a specific pathogen or disease condition, and it is most effective against bacteria that do not readily develop resistance. The duration of prophylaxis should be as short as possible, and prophylaxis should be used only where its efficacy is clearly established. Finally, the dosage must be the same as that used therapeutically. Examples of well-established prophylactic use of antimicrobial drugs are shown in Table 5.4.

In certain well-described circumstances, the use of prophylactic antibiotics in veterinary medicine may be deleterious. For example, the routine use of neomycin pessaries to prevent postparturient metritis in cows has adversely affected subsequent fertility. Concurrent infusion of gentamicin in inseminated mares may reduce ability to conceive. Oral administration of tetracyclines via drinking water to feedlot calves has been associated with increased mortality (Martin et al., 1982). More studies are needed to determine the value of prophylactic antibiotics in different usage in veterinary medicine.

Antibiotics are often administered prophylactically when young animals (pigs, calves) are moved from breeding to growing areas, because disturbances in microbial flora and physiology and the presence of previously unencountered pathogens can spark outbreaks of infectious disease. Because of the disadvantages, the use of antimicrobial drugs for such purposes should be replaced by preventive husbandry practices. The use of antibiotics as growth promoters and disease prophylactics is discussed in Chapter 32.

A similar type of prophylactic drug use in herds is "preemptive medication," exemplified by dry-cow therapy. Such drug use is based on knowledge that disease is present in the population and will continue to affect individuals in the population. Preemptive medication of the herd or individuals reduces shedding of pathogens.

The concept of herd medication is to treat the whole group at risk rather than individuals. Typical examples are (1) giving drugs at prophylactic concentrations to prevent swine dysentery; (2) using "blitz" therapy with intramammary penicillin G to eradicate *Streptococcus agalactiae* infection from a cow herd; and (3) ensuring specified disease-free pigs by the medicated-early-weaning system. Herd medication is employed extensively in veterinary medicine.

PROPHYLACTIC DRUGS IN SURGERY

The principles upon which drugs are used prophylactically to prevent surgical infections are based on extensive studies in human medicine, since there have been few or no randomized trials in veterinary surgery on which to base recommendations.

The key concepts are that antimicrobial drugs are highly effective and necessary in preventing certain postoperative infections and should be used in surgical procedures associated with high risk, where infection rates associated with a particular procedure exceed about 5%. These procedures therefore include cardiovascular, intestinal tract, emergency cesarean, and numerous orthopedic procedures; neurosurgical operations; and procedures requiring prolonged surgery (>4 hours). Antimicrobial prophylaxis is contraindicated for clean surgical procedures not associated with significant infection rates, because of the danger of adverse reactions following antimicrobial use, the selection of resistant bacteria, and the unnecessary cost. For maximum effect, antibiotics should be at the site of infection at the time of bacterial contamination. One dose of antibiotic is therefore given IV immediately before surgery. The duration of prophylaxis is controversial, but most studies have found that administration after the first 24 hours provides no additional protection, although a few suggest prophylaxis for 48–72 hours. For example, Klein and Firth (1988) found that 4 days of antibiotic prophylaxis of umbilical hernia repair operations in calves gave significantly lower wound infection rates than 1 day of prophylaxis. The drugs of choice will vary with hospital and site of operation. Current human surgical protocols suggest cefazolin or cefamandole for cardiovascular or orthopedic surgery and cefoxitin (with or without gentamicin and metronidazole) for abdominal surgery associated with intestinal perforation. There is a need for trials on the value of antimicrobial prophylaxis of infections in veterinary surgery, with recommendations concerning drugs of choice and dosage.

Drug Withdrawal

Most countries require that antimicrobial drugs not be present in foods for human consumption, and they specify the time during which animals cannot be slaughtered and milk cannot be sold after antibiotic treatment. These withdrawal periods are specified for different agents (see Chapter 33) and extra-label drug use (see Chapter 34).

Targeted Drug Delivery

Therapeutic efficacy of antimicrobial drugs in vivo may be reduced by their inability to reach the site of infection in adequate amounts. Considerable effort has been devoted to finding ways to target drugs to the appropriate site. One approach has been to encapsulate drugs in liposomes (microscopic, closed lipid vesicles). After IV injection, liposomes are taken up by cells of the reticuloendothelial system. One notable example is liposomal incorporation of amphotericin B (see Chapter 17), which markedly reduces the toxicity of the drug and thereby increases its efficacy. The directed targeting of liposomally entrapped drugs—for example, with monoclonal antibodies to target cell surface structures—is under active investigation.

Bibliography

Barza M, Cuchural G. 1985. General principles of antibiotic tissue penetration. J Antimicrob Chemother 15A:59.

Craig WA, Ebert SC. 1991. Killing and regrowth of bacteria in vitro: a review. Scand J Infect Dis Suppl 74:63.

Hirsbrunner G, Steiner A. 1998. Treatment of infectious arthritis of the radiocarpal joint of cattle with genatamicin-impregnated sponges. Vet Rec 142:399.

Kaiser AB. 1986. Antimicrobial prophylaxis in surgery. N Engl J Med 315:1129.

Klein WR, Firth EC. 1988. Infection rates in contaminated surgical procedures: a comparison of prophylactic treatment for one day or four days. Vet Rec 123:564.

Krainock RJ. 1991. Prolonged milk residue in two cows after subcutaneous injections of penicillin at an extra-label dose. J Am Vet Med Assoc 198:862.

Martin SW, et al. 1982. Factors associated with mortality and treatment costs in feedlot calves: the Bruce County beef project, years 1978, 1979, 1980. Can J Comp Med 46:341.

Paape MJ, et al. 1991. Pharmacologic enhancement or suppression of phagocytosis by bovine neutrophils. Am J Vet Res 52:363.

Riviere JE, et al. 1988. Pharmacokinetic estimation for therapeutic dosage regimens (PETDR)—a software program designed to determine intravenous drug dosage regimens for veterinary applications. J Vet Pharmacol Ther 11:390.

Strom B, Linde-Forsberg C. 1993. Effects of ampicillin and trimethoprim-sulfamethox-azole on the vaginal bacterial flora of bitches. Am J Vet Res 54:891.

Townsend GC, Scheld WM. 1996. The use of corticosteroids in the management of bacterial meningitis in adults. J Antimicrob Chemother 37:1051.

Trostle SS, et al. 1996. Use of antimicrobial-impregnated polymethyl methacrylate beads for treatment of chronic, refractory septic arthritis and osteomyelitis of the digit in a bull. J Am Vet Med Assoc 208:404.

Waltner-Toews D, et al. 1986. Calf-related drug use on Holstein dairy farms in southwestern Ontario. Can Vet J 27:17.

6 Beta-lactam Antibiotics: Penam Penicillins

J. F. PRESCOTT

Introduction to Beta-lactam Antibiotics

Alexander Fleming's observation in 1928 that colonies of staphylococci were lysed on a plate contaminated with a *Penicillium* mold was the discovery that led to the development of antibiotics. In 1940, Chain and Florey and their associates were the first to produce sufficient quantities of penicillin from cultures of *Penicillium notatum*. Almost a decade later, penicillin G became widely available for clinical use. In its clinical application, this antibiotic was found to have limitations, which included relative instability in gastric acid, susceptibility to inactivation by beta-lactamase (penicillinases), and relative inactivity against clinically important Gram-negative bacteria. This inactivity against Gram-negative rods was subsequently found to result from (1) inability of the antibiotic to penetrate the Gram-negative cell wall, (2) lack of available binding sites (penicillin-binding proteins); or (3) enzymatic inactivation. Intensive research led to the isolation of the active moiety, 6-aminopenicillanic acid, in the penicillin molecule. This moiety, which consists of a thiazolidine ring (A) attached to a beta-lactam ring (B) that carries a secondary amino group (R–NH–), is essential for antibacterial activity (Fig. 6.1). Isolation of the active moiety has resulted in the design and development of semisynthetic penicillins that overcome some but not all of the limitations associated with penicillin G.

The development of the cephalosporin family, which shares the beta-lactam ring with penicillins (Fig. 6.2), led to a remarkable array of drugs with varying ability to penetrate different Gram-negative bacterial species and to resist several beta-lactamase enzymes (see Chapter 7). Other naturally occurring beta-lactam antibiotics have subsequently been described that lack the bicyclic ring of the classic beta-lactam penicillins and

105

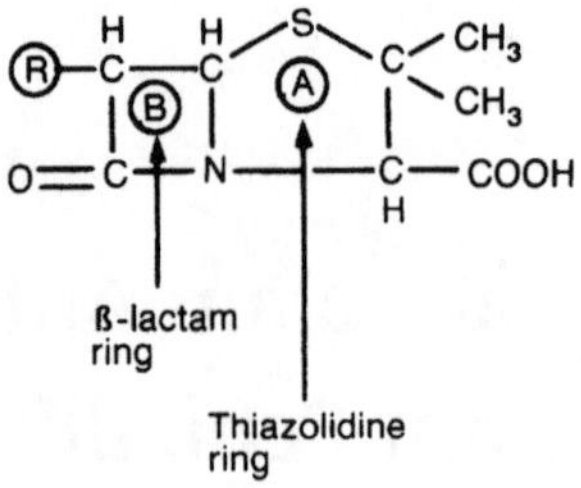

Fig. 6.1. Structural formula of penicillin.

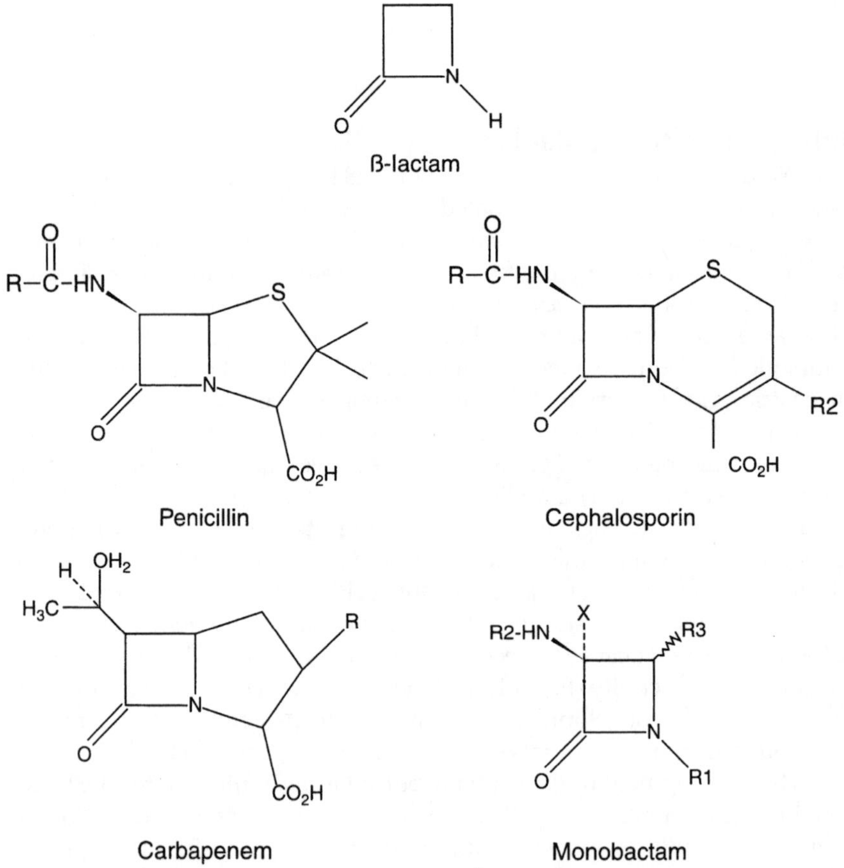

Fig. 6.2. Core structures of naturally occurring beta-lactams.

cephalosporins. Many have potent antibacterial activity and are highly inhibitory to beta-lactamase enzymes. Some, such as the carbapenems, oxacephems, penems, and monobactams, have potent antibacterial activity, whereas others, such as the oxapenam clavulanic acid, have no antibacterial activity of their own but possess potent beta-lactamase inhibitory activity (see Chapter 8). These latter drugs are combined with older beta-lactams to increase their range of antibacterial activity. Beta-lactam antibiotics are in widespread use because of their selectivity, versatility, and low toxicity.

Chemistry

The penicillins, cephalosporins, carbapenems, monobactams, and penems are referred to as beta-lactam antibiotics. Rupture of the beta-lactam ring, which is brought about enzymatically by bacterial beta-lactamases, results in loss of antibacterial activity. Hypersensitivity reactions appear to be associated with the active moieties of the beta-lactam drugs, and because these drugs are of similar structure, caution should be exercised when administering cephalosporins to penicillin-sensitive animals. Substitutions can be made on the beta-lactam ring for specific purposes, such as (1) increasing resistance to beta-lactamases of clinically important families or species of bacteria; (2) enhancing activity against selected pathogens; or (3) ensuring favorable pharmacokinetic properties. Semisynthetic beta-lactam drugs have in some cases thus been designed for specific purposes.

Mechanism of Action

Beta-lactam antibiotics prevent the bacterial cell wall from forming by interfering with the final stage of peptidoglycan synthesis. They inhibit the activity of the transpeptidase and other peptidoglycan-active enzymes that are called penicillin-binding proteins (PBPs) (transpeptidases, carboxypeptidases), which catalyze cross-linkage of the glycopeptide polymer units that form the cell wall. The drugs exert a bactericidal action but cause lysis only of growing cells, that is, cells that are undergoing active cell wall synthesis. The exact mechanism of lysis is unknown.

Variation in the activity of different beta-lactams results, in part, from differences in affinity of the PBPs for the drugs. The difference in susceptibility between Gram-positive and Gram-negative bacteria depends on differences in receptor sites (PBPs), on the relative amount of peptidoglycan present (Gram-positive bacteria possess far more), on the ability of the drugs to penetrate the outer cell membrane of Gram-negative bacteria, and on resistance to the different types of beta-lactamase enzymes produced by the bacteria. These differences are summarized in Figures 6.3 and 6.4.

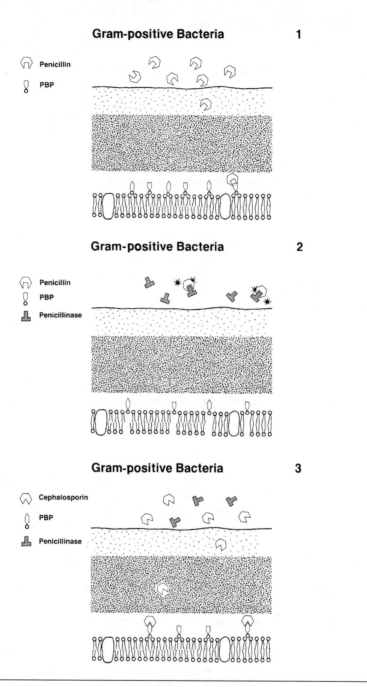

Gram-positive Bacteria 1

Penicillin

PBP

Gram-positive Bacteria 2

Penicillin

PBP

Penicillinase

Gram-positive Bacteria 3

Cephalosporin

PBP

Penicillinase

Fig. 6.3. Summary of action and resistance to beta-lactam drugs: Gram-positive bacteria. *1,* Susceptible bacterium; *2,* exogenous beta-lactamase-producing bacterium, eg *Staphylococcus aureus; 3,* penicillinase-producing bacterium susceptible to cephalosporin. Modified from a figure by R. D. Walker.

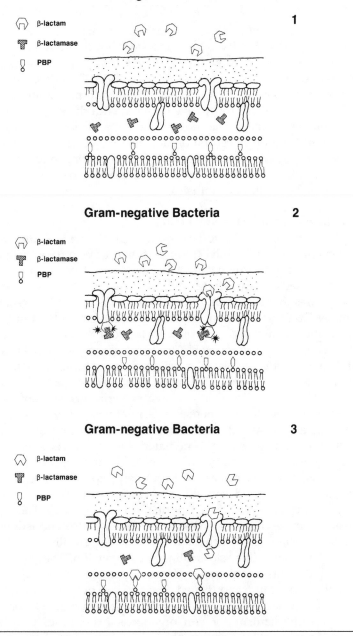

Fig. 6.4. Summary of action and resistance to beta-lactam drugs: Gram-negative bacteria. *1,* Bacterium constitutively resistant to penetration by beta-lactam; *2,* penetration by beta-lactam but destruction by periplasmic beta-lactamase; *3,* susceptible Gram-negative bacterium. Modified from a figure by R. D. Walker.

Beta-lactam antibiotics are bactericidal drugs with slower kill rates than those exhibited by aminoglycosides or fluoroquinolones. Killing activity starts after a lag period. Against Gram-positive bacteria, all beta-lactams exhibit an in vitro postantibiotic effect. This does not carry over for the streptococci in vivo. The beta-lactams do not exhibit a postantibiotic effect against Gram-negative bacteria, with the possible exception of carbapenems against *Pseudomonas*. Optimal antibacterial efficacy is time-dependent and not concentration-dependent (see Chapter 5) and requires that serum concentrations exceed MIC of the pathogen for essentially the entire dosing interval, so that these drugs are best administered frequently or by continuous infusion.

Resistance to Beta-lactam Antibiotics

In Gram-positive bacteria, especially *Staphylococcus aureus*, resistance to penicillin G is mainly through the production of beta-lactamase enzymes that break the beta-lactam ring of most penicillins. *Staphylococcus aureus* secretes beta-lactamase enzymes extracellularly as inducible exoenzymes that are plasmid mediated (see Fig. 6.3). Inherent resistance of many Gram-negative bacteria to penicillin G results from low permeability of the Gram-negative cell wall, lack of PBPs, and a wide variety of beta-lactamase enzymes (see Fig. 6.4). Most Gram-negative bacteria inherently express low levels of species-specific, chromosomally mediated beta-lactamase enzymes within the periplasmic space that sometimes contribute to resistance. These enzymes hydrolyze susceptible cephalosporins more rapidly than penicillin G, but they hydrolyze ampicillin, carbenicillin, and beta-lactamase–resistant penicillins poorly.

Production of plasmid-mediated beta-lactamases is widespread among common Gram-negative primary and opportunist bacterial pathogens. The enzymes are constitutively expressed, are present in the periplasmic space, and cause high-level resistance. The majority are penicillinases rather than cephalosporinases (see Fig. 6.4). The most widespread are those classified on the basis of their hydrolytic activity as TEM-type beta-lactamases, which readily hydrolyze penicillin G and ampicillin rather than methicillin, cloxacillin, or carbenicillin. The less widespread OXA-type beta-lactamases hydrolyze penicillinase-stable penicillins (oxacillin, cloxacillin, and related drugs). More details on beta-lactamases are given in Chapter 8. Beta-lactamases probably evolved from PBPs as a protective mechanism for soil organisms exposed to beta-lactams in nature, in which they are thought to be widespread through their production by molds. Because of spread of transferable resistance, beta-lactamase production by pathogens is now widespread.

A major advance has been the discovery of broad-spectrum beta-lactamase-inhibitory drugs (eg, clavulanic acid, sulbactam, tazobactam).

These drugs have weak antibacterial activity but show extraordinary synergism when administered with penicillin G, ampicillin, or amoxicillin, because of the irreversible binding of the beta-lactamase enzymes of resistant bacteria. Other beta-lactamase inhibitors, such as cefotaxime and carbapenems, have potent antibacterial activity in their own right (see Chapter 8).

Bibliography

Bush K. 1988. Recent developments in beta-lactamase research and their implications for the future. Rev Infect Dis 10:681.

Craig WA, Ebert SC. 1992. Continuous infusion of β-lactam antibiotics. Antimicrob Agents Chemother 36:2577.

Juteau J-M, et al. 1991. Molecular distribution of ROB-1 beta-lactamase in *Actinobacillus pleuropneumoniae*. Antimicrob Agents Chemother 35:1397.

Livrelli VO, et al. 1988. Generic determinant of the ROB-1 beta-lactamase in bovine and porcine *Pasteurella* strains. Antimicrob Agents Chemother 32:1282.

Palzkill T. 1998. β-Lactamases are changing their activity spectrums. ASM News 64:90.

Soriano F, et al. 1996. Correlation of pharmacodynamic parameters of five β-lactam antibiotics with therapeutic efficacies in an animal model. Antimicrob Agents Chemother 40:2686.

Penam Penicillins
General Considerations

The acidic radical (R) attached to the amino group of 6-aminopenicillanic acid (see Fig. 6.1) determines the susceptibility of the resulting penicillin to hydrolytic degradation or enzymatic inactivation by bacterial beta-lactamase and determines the antibacterial activity of the molecule. Both these factors influence the clinical effectiveness of penicillins, which is also determined by the concentration attained at the site of infection. The nature of the acidic radical has little influence on the rate of elimination of penicillins, but it determines the extent of plasma albumin binding and, to a lesser degree, membrane-penetrating ability. The 6-aminopenicillanic acid moiety and the structure of the acid radicals of some penicillins are shown in Figure 6.5.

Penam penicillins are readily distinguished on the basis of antimicrobial activity into six groups ("generations" that largely correspond to their time of introduction into clinical use) (Table 6.1): benzyl penicillin and its long-acting parenteral forms; orally absorbed penicillins similar to benzyl penicillin; staphylococcal penicillinase-resistant isoxazolyl penicillins; extended-spectrum, or broad-spectrum, penicillins; antipseudomonal penicillins; and beta-lactamase-resistant penicillins.

Since the 1940s, the progressive development of penicillins for clinical use has resulted in derivatives with activity similar to that of benzyl penicillin but which could be administered orally and/or were resistant

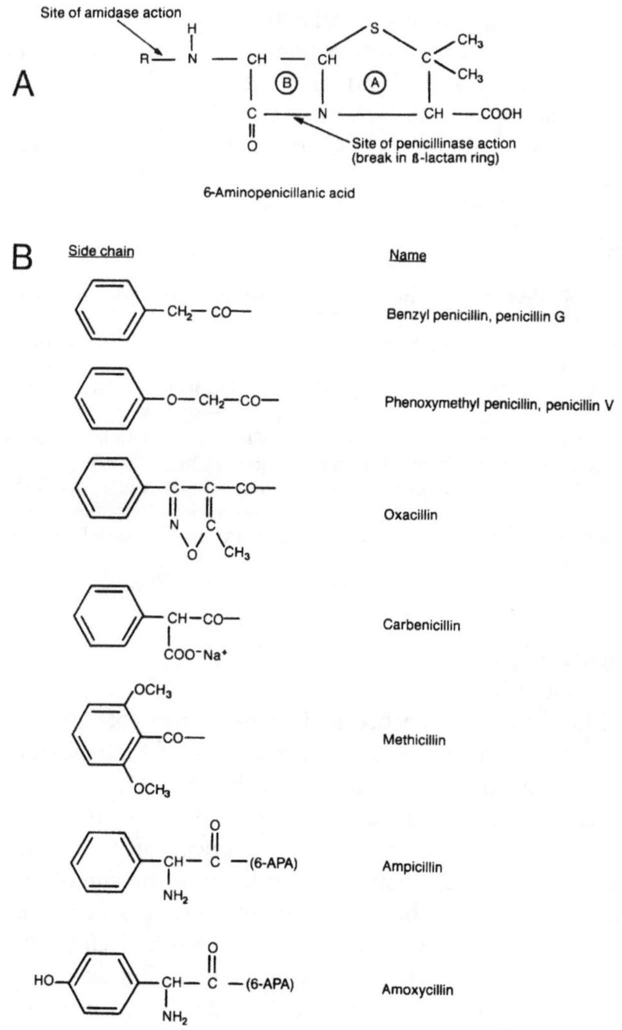

Fig. 6.5. Structural formulas of some penicillins. *A*, Basic structure of penicillin G; *B*, structures that can be substituted at the R to produce a new penicillin.

to *Staphylococcus aureus* beta-lactamase (penicillinase). Subsequently, orally administered penicillins with a broader spectrum of activity, which involved greater Gram-negative antibacterial activity, and penicillins active against *Pseudomonas aeruginosa* were developed. Despite considerable effort, however, with the exception of temocillin, extended-spectrum

TABLE 6.1. Classification of the six groups of penam penicillins
(6-aminopenicillanic acid derivatives)

Group	Important Derivatives	Antimicrobial Advantage
1. Benzyl penicillins	Procaine, benzathine (long-acting forms)	Gram-positive bacteria
2. Orally absorbed penicillins similar to benzyl penicillins	Phenoxymethyl penicillin	Gram-positive bacteria
3. Antistaphylococcal isoxazolyl penicillins	Cloxacillin, dicloxacillin, oxacillin, methicillin, nafcillin	Activity against *Staphylococcus aureus*
4. Extended-spectrum (broad-spectrum) penicillins	Aminobenzylpenicillins (ampicillin, hetacillin, pivampicillin, amoxicillin); amidopenicillins (mecillinam)	Broader spectrum than benzyl penicillins but beta-lactamase sensitive
5. Antipseudomonal penicillins	Ureidopenicillins (azlocillin, mezlocillin, piperacillin); carboxypenicillins (carbenicillin, ticarcillin)	*Pseudomonas aeruginosa* activity, reduced Gram-positive
6. Beta-lactamase–resistant penicillins	Temocillin	Beta-lactamase resistance

penicillins are susceptible to beta-lactamase-producing Gram-negative bacteria. For this reason the use of penicillins against common Gram-negative bacteria is limited in favor of more recently introduced cephalosporin beta-lactams (see Chapter 7) or combination with beta-lactamase inhibitors (see Chapter 8).

Mechanism of Action

The targets of all beta-lactam drugs are the penicillin-binding proteins (PBPs) found on the outside of the cytoplasmic membrane and involved in synthesizing and remodeling the cell wall. As described, susceptibility of a bacterium to a penicillin depends on a combination of affinity for the PBP, ability to penetrate the cell wall, and ability to resist beta-lactamase enzymes (Figs. 6.3 and 6.4). Usually 4–7 PBPs are present in bacteria and are the targets for penicillins. The bactericidal effect in Gram-negative bacteria results from osmotically induced lysis of cells weakened by loss of their peptidoglycan layer, although the exact mechanism has not been elucidated. In Gram-positive bacteria, which have considerably greater quantities of peptidoglycan in their cell walls than Gram-negative bacteria, an effect of beta-lactams is not only to prevent the final peptidoglycan cross-linking, which gives peptidoglycan its strength, but also to release lipoteichoic acid, causing a suicide response by degradation of peptidoglycan by autolysins (endogenous endopeptidase, carboxypeptidase PBPs).

For some Gram-positive cocci, exposure to beta-lactam antibiotics above an optimal killing concentration results in a reduction of killing, which can be considerable (the Eagle effect, or paradoxical effect). Its basis appears to be interference of growth by penicillin binding to PBPs other than the major target PBP. Since beta-lactams are effective only against growing bacteria that are actively synthesizing cell walls, failure of the bacteria to grow results in failure to be killed. The Eagle effect is an important concept, given that there may be a tendency to overdose with beta-lactam antibiotics because they are generally so safe.

Antimicrobial Activity

Benzyl penicillin and orally administered benzyl penicillins (phenoxymethyl penicillin; Table 6.2) have outstanding activity against many Gram-positive bacteria, notably beta-hemolytic streptococci, nonresistant staphylococci, *Actinomyces* spp., *Bacillus* spp., *Clostridium* spp., *Corynebacterium* spp., and *Erysipelothrix rhusiopathiae*. Susceptible Gram-negative species include some *Bacteroides* spp., some *Fusobacterium* spp., and a variety of Gram-negative aerobic bacteria such as *Haemophilus* spp., and many *Pasteurella* spp. Enterobacteriaceae, *Bacteroides fragilis*, most *Campylobacter* spp., *Nocardia* spp., and *Pseudomonas* spp. are resistant. Penicillinase-resistant, antistaphylococcal isoxazolyl penicillins (cloxacillin, dicloxacillin, methicillin, nafcillin, oxacillin) have activity similar to but slightly less than that of benzyl penicillin, with the exception that they are active against penicillinase-producing *Staphylococcus aureus* (see Table 6.2). Extended-spectrum penicillins (aminobenzylpenicillins such as ampicillin and its esters, and amoxicillin) retain the activity of benzyl penicillin against Gram-positive bacteria but have increased activity against Gram-negative bacteria, including *Escherichia coli, Proteus* spp., and *Salmonella* spp. They are, however, ineffective against *Pseudomonas aeruginosa* and are inactivated by beta-lactamases. Mecillinam, another member of the extended penicillin group, differs from aminobenzylpenicillins in its lower activity against Gram-positive bacteria but considerably greater activity against Gram-negative bacteria, including a broad spectrum of the Enterobacteriaceae; however, it is still inactivated by many beta-lactamases. Penicillins (carboxypenicillins, ureidopenicillins) active against *P. aeruginosa* (carbenicillin, azlocillin, mezlocillin, piperacillin) are effective against both Gram-positive and Gram-negative bacteria, including *P. aeruginosa* (see Table 6.2).

Resistance to Penam Penicillins

Most resistance results from production of a beta-lactamase enzyme, although modification of PBPs with reduced drug affinity or reduced bacterial permeability are additional and sometimes concurrent mechanisms of intrinsic or acquired resistance to penam penicillins. Beta-lactamases are discussed in Chapter 8. Resistance because of exogenously produced

TABLE 6.2. Activity (usual MIC, μg/ml) of penicillins against bacteria of human origin

Organisms	Narrow-spectrum Penicillins		Penicillinase-stable Penicillins		Broad-spectrum Penicillins	
	Penicillin G	Penicillin V	Methicillin	Cloxacillin	Ampicillin	Carbenicillin
Staphylococcus aureus						
Beta-lactamase⁻	0.02	0.05	1.25	0.1	0.05	1.25
Beta-lactamase⁺	R	R	2.5	0.25	R	25
Streptococcus agalactiae	0.005	0.01	0.2	0.06	0.02	0.2
Beta-hemolytic streptococci	0.005	0.01	0.2	0.04	0.02	0.2
S. faecalis	3	6	≥25	≥25	1.5	50
Clostridium perfringens	0.05	0.1	1	0.5	0.05	0.5
Escherichia coli	50	125	R	R	5	5
Proteus mirabilis	5	50	250	R	5	2.5
Proteus, indole⁺	R	R	R	R	1.25	5
Klebsiella pneumoniae	250	R	R	R	250	250
Enterobacter spp.	R	R	R	R	250	12.5
Pseudomonas aeruginosa	R	R	R	R	R	50

Source: Garrod et al. (1981) with permission.
Note: R, resistant. Any MIC ≥ is resistant.

beta-lactamase is now widespread in *S. aureus*, particularly in clinical isolates, as a result of bacteriophage- or plasmid-mediated resistance. Among Gram-negative bacteria, plasmids encoding beta-lactamases have also become widespread and are the cause of extensive acquired resistance. Modification of PBPs is recognized to be increasingly important as another mechanism of resistance to penam penicillins. The most important example in human medicine is methicillin (oxacillin) resistance in *S. aureus* (MRSA) but resistance because of this mechanism has not been well documented in animal pathogens.

Pharmacokinetic Properties

The penicillins are organic acids that are generally available as the sodium or potassium salt of the free acid. In dry, crystalline form, penicillins are stable but lose their activity rapidly when dissolved. Apart from the isoxazolyl penicillins (cloxacillin, dicloxacillin, oxacillin) and penicillin V, acid hydrolysis limits the systemic availability of most penicillins from oral preparations. The penicillins (pK_a 2.7) are predominantly ionized in plasma, have relatively small apparent volumes of distribution (0.2–0.3 l/kg), and have short half-lives (0.5–1.2 hours) in all species of domestic animals. After absorption, they are widely distributed in the extracellular fluids of the body, but they cross biologic membranes poorly because they are ionized and poorly lipid soluble. Concentration in milk, for example, is about one-fifth that of serum. Entry across biologic membranes or through the blood-brain or blood-cerebrospinal fluid barrier is enhanced by inflammation, so that inhibitory drug concentrations may be attained at these sites, which are normally inaccessible to penicillin.

Penicillins are eliminated almost entirely by the kidneys, which results in very high levels in the urine; nafcillin is an exception, in that it is excreted mainly in bile. Renal excretion mechanisms include glomerular filtration and tubular secretion. The latter is subject to competitive inhibition by other organic acids, such as probenecid. Impaired renal function delays excretion of the penicillins, but the wide margin of safety of this class of drug offsets the absolute need to adjust dosage.

Drug Interactions

Penicillins are usually synergistic with the aminoglycosides against many bacteria, which are susceptible to each drug alone, because they enhance penetration of the aminoglycoside. Such synergism may occur with penicillinase-producing *S. aureus*. Penicillins are synergistic against these organisms with drugs that bind beta-lactamase enzymes, such as cloxacillin, clavulanic acid, sulbactam, tazobactam, and some cephalosporins. Aminobenzylpenicillins and ureidopenicillins are increasingly combined with beta-lactamase inhibitors (see Chapter 8).

Toxicity and Adverse Effects

Penicillins and beta-lactam antibiotics generally are remarkably free of toxic effects even at doses grossly in excess of those recommended. The major adverse effects are acute anaphylaxis and collapse; milder hypersensitivity reactions (urticaria, fever, angioneurotic edema) are more common. All penicillins are cross-sensitizing and cross-reacting, but cross-reactions occur in only about 5–8% of human patients treated with cephalosporins. Anaphylactic reactions are less common after oral administration than after parenteral administration. Penicillins must not be used in animals known to be sensitive. Less common adverse reactions include hemolytic anemia and thrombocytopenia.

Dosage Considerations

Beta-lactams produce killing and lysis of bacteria at concentrations above MIC. Post-antibiotic effects are observed only for staphylococci in vivo, so that dosage requires that drug concentrations exceed MIC for most of the dosage interval. Excessive drug concentrations may be counterproductive because of the Eagle effect described earlier, in which sometimes dramatic reduction of killing occurs in the presence of high, supra-MIC concentrations of the beta-lactam antibiotic.

Clinical Usage

Penicillins are important antibacterial drugs in the treatment of infections in animals (see Table 6.1). The often exquisite susceptibility of Gram-positive bacteria, such as the beta-hemolytic streptococci, means that benzyl penicillin is often a drug of choice for these infections, because of its high potency and low toxicity. Antistaphylococcal penicillins are in widespread use in the prevention and treatment of staphylococcal mastitis in cows. The extended-spectrum penicillins, particularly aminobenzylpenicillins, have lost much of their potency against Gram-negative bacteria over the decades but have been revitalized by their combination with beta-lactamase inhibitors (see Chapter 8). The antipseudomonal penicillins remain important for this activity but are rivaled by antipseudomonal cephalosporins.

Group 1, Benzyl Penicillin and Long-acting Parenteral Forms

Sodium benzyl penicillin G is available as the benzyl, the procaine benzyl, and the tribenzyl ethylenediamine (benzathine) forms. Frequent dosing of benzyl penicillin is required because of the drug's rapid excretion, so that long-acting, delayed-absorption forms (procaine, benzathine) have been developed, with procaine penicillin being the most extensively used because dosing frequency is usually q24 hours. The principle behind the use of procaine and benzathine penicillin is that both forms delay absorption from the injection site. Thus, although the elimination half-life is the same, the absorption half-life is much longer, reducing the need for frequent dosing. Delayed absorption also means a lower peak concentration.

Antimicrobial Activity

The activity of penicillin G was originally defined in units. Crystalline sodium penicillin G contains approximately 1,600 units/mg (1 unit = 0.6 µg; 1 million units of penicillin = 600 mg, or 0.6 g). Most semisynthetic penicillins are prescribed by weight (mg/kg) rather than units.

Good Susceptibility (MIC ≤0.12 µg/ml) is shown by many aerobic Gram-positive bacteria, including all beta-hemolytic streptococci (such as *Streptococcus agalactiae, S. canis, S. zooepidemicus, S. dysgalactiae, S. suis, S. uberis, Bacillus anthracis, Actinomyces* spp., most corynebacteria (including *C. pseudotuberculosis, C. renale), Erysipelothrix rhusiopathiae,* and most *Listeria monocytogenes* (Table 6.2). Susceptible anaerobes include *Clostridium* spp., most *Fusobacterium* spp., and some *Bacteroides.* Susceptible Gram-negative aerobes include *Haemophilus somnus.*

Variable Susceptibility is shown by *Staphylococcus aureus* and other staphylococci, although in the absence of resistance, staphylococci are highly susceptible.

Moderate Susceptibility (MIC 0.25–2 µg/ml), which may sometimes vary because of acquired resistance, is shown by *Actinobacillus* spp., *Borrelia* spp., *Brucella* spp., *Haemophilus* spp., *Leptospira* spp., *Moraxella* spp., *Pasteurella* spp., *Proteus* spp., *Taylorella equigenitalis,* and *Serpulina* spp.

Resistance (MIC ≥4 µg/ml) is shown by Enterobacteriaceae (other than some *Proteus* spp.), *Bacteroides fragilis, Bordetella* spp., most *Campylobacter* spp., and *Nocardia* spp.

Antibiotic Resistance

Despite extensive use of penicillin in veterinary medicine for many years, most Gram-positive bacteria remain susceptible to the drug. *Staphylococcus aureus* is an exception. The beta-lactamase enzymes of *S. aureus* are mainly active against penicillin G, ampicillin, and carbenicillin but hydrolyze penicillinase-stable penicillins (methicillin, cloxacillin) and cephalosporins poorly. Resistance in usually susceptible Gram-negative bacteria such as *Haemophilus* and *Pasteurella* is the result of R plasmid–mediated production of beta-lactamases, but this is rarer.

Pharmacokinetic Properties

Pharmacokinetic properties of the benzyl penicillins were discussed earlier in this chapter under Penam Penicillins: Pharmacokinetic Properties. Acid hydrolysis in the stomach limits the systemic availability of benzyl penicillin administered orally.

Drug Interactions

Penicillin G is synergistic with the aminoglycosides against many Gram-positive bacteria, except those showing high-level aminoglycoside resistance. Such synergism may be seen even with penicillinase-producing *Staphylococcus aureus*. Penicillin is synergistic against these organisms with drugs that bind beta-lactamase enzymes (see Chapter 8). Penicillin G has been combined with streptomycin for use in animals, but there is little clinical evidence supporting the clinical value of the combination (Whittem and Hanlon, 1997). For this reason, because streptomycin is associated with tissue residues, the combination is no longer available in some countries, including the United States. In addition, there are significant differences in pharmacokinetic properties among different combined preparations (Groen et al., 1996).

Toxicities and Adverse Effects

The parent benzyl penicillin and its numerous derivatives are relatively safe drugs; toxic effects were described under Penam Penicillins: General Considerations. Many of the acute toxicities reported in animals are the result of the toxic effects of the potassium or procaine with which penicillin is combined in the dosage form. To avoid cardiac arrest, care should be taken with the rate at which potassium penicillin G is injected IV; administration of the sodium salt is safer. Procaine penicillin G should never be given IV. In high doses given IM, the procaine form may cause nervous excitement (incoordination, ataxia, excitability) and death, particularly in horses (Nielsen et al., 1988). It should not be administered to horses within 2 weeks before a race, so as to avoid procaine-positive drug test results. Procaine penicillin should be stored in the refrigerator and not used past expiration dates; repeated use of the same injection site should be avoided, especially in horses. Severe, immune-mediated hemolytic anemia with icterus has been reported in horses (Blue et al., 1987).

Administration and Dosage

Recommended dosages for penam penicillins are shown in Table 6.3. Because of the relative lack of toxicity of penicillins, their dosage can be tailored, to some extent, to the susceptibility of the infecting bacteria more than with any other class of antibiotic. The effectiveness of penicillin therapy is related to the time that tissue concentration exceeds the MIC of the

TABLE 6.3. **Usual dosages of penam penicillins in animals**

Drug	Route	Dose (IU/kg or mg/kg)	Interval (h)	Comment
Penicillin G, sodium aqueous	IM, IV	15,000–20,000 IU/kg	6–8	
Procaine penicillin G	IM	25,000 IU/kg	24	Every 12 hours for serious infections
Benzathine penicillin	IM	40,000 IU/kg	72	Highly susceptible bacteria only; little use
Penicillin V	Oral	10 mg/kg	6–8	Erratic absorption; amoxicillin preferred
Cloxacillin, dicloxacillin, methicillin, oxacillin	Oral	15–25 mg/kg	6–8	Monogastrates only; avoid ingesta
Ampicillin sodium	IM, IV	10–20 mg/kg	6–8	
Ampicillin (hetacillin)	Oral	10–20 mg/kg	8	Monogastrates only; avoid ingesta
Amoxicillin	Oral	10–20 mg/kg	8–12	Monogastrates only
Amoxicillin	IM (SC)	10 mg/kg	12	
Amoxicillin, long-acting	IM	15 mg/kg	48	Very susceptible bacteria only
Amoxicillin trihydrate	IM	10–20 mg/kg	12	
Pivampicillin	Oral	25 mg/kg	12	Monogastrates only
Carbenicillin, indanyl sodium	Oral	33 mg/kg	6–8	Urinary tract only
Carbenicillin	IM, IV	33 mg/kg	6–8	
Piperacillin	IV (IM)	50 mg/kg	8	May be used with tazobactam
Ticarcillin	IV (IM, SC)	25–40 mg/kg	8	Often used with clavulanic acid

pathogen. Because of the short half-lives of penicillins, preparations that provide rapid absorption must be administered at short intervals (q6 hours). Low systemic availability from oral forms must be compensated for by increasing the size of the dose.

Penicillin G is available as a potassium or sodium salt that can be administered parenterally as freshly prepared solutions. Procaine penicillin G is a special form developed to prolong absorption from the IM injection site. A single dose of 25,000 IU/kg provides effective serum concentrations against susceptible bacteria for at least 12 hours and generally for up to 24 hours in all species of domestic animals. For moderately susceptible bacteria, high doses of procaine penicillin given once daily may be useful; an example is administration of 45,000 IU/kg in the once-daily treatment of bovine *Pasteurella haemolytica* pneumonia, but more clinical data is needed on the efficacy of such high dosing, since the Eagle effect may reduce the efficacy of the drug. Oral potassium penicillin G has been

TABLE 6.4. **Applications of penicillin G (or penicillin V) in clinical infections in animals**

Species	Primary Applications	Secondary Applications
Cattle, sheep, goats	Anthrax, clostridial and corynebacterial infections, *Arcanobacterium pyogenes*, streptococcal mastitis, listeriosis	Actinobacillosis, anaerobic infections, possibly infectious keratoconjunctivitis, leptospirosis
Swine	Streptococcal and clostridial infections, erysipelas, *A. pyogenes*, *A. suis*	Glasser's disease, pasteurellosis, anaerobic infections
Horses	Streptococcal and clostridial infections	Actinobacillosis, anaerobic infections
Dogs, cats	Streptococcal and clostridial infections	Cat bite abscess, anaerobic infections, leptospirosis

used to treat canine urinary tract infections caused by *E. coli* or *Proteus mirabilis*. The response is due to the high concentrations of penicillin that are attained in urine.

Benzathine penicillin is a long-acting, slow-release formulation of penicillin G administered every 72 hours. Serum concentrations are usually so low that it can, at best, be recommended only for extremely susceptible bacteria and is best avoided.

Clinical Applications

The general clinical applications of penicillin G are shown in Table 6.4. Penicillin G is the drug of choice in treating infections caused by Gram-positive bacteria such as streptococci, corynebacteria, *Erysipelothrix*, clostridia, and perhaps *Listeria*, as well as some Gram-negative bacteria such as *Haemophilus somnus*, *Pasteurella*, and many anaerobes. In addition, it is a drug of choice in treating the spirochetal agent of Lyme disease, *Borrelia burgdorferi*. The advantages of penicillin G are its potent bactericidal activity against susceptible bacteria and its wide margin of safety; dosage can be tailored to the susceptibility of the pathogen by selecting the form of drug to be administered. Disadvantages are its activity against only actively growing bacteria, its narrow spectrum, the widespread resistance in *Staphylococcus aureus* and Gram-negative bacteria, and the drug's failure to cross biological membranes well, except in acute inflammation.

CATTLE, SHEEP, AND GOATS

Penicillin G is the most commonly used antibiotic for food animals. It is probable that it was initially licensed at an inappropriately low dosage. Parenterally administered penicillin G is the drug of choice for the treatment of disease caused by susceptible bacteria, including anthrax, clostridial infections, *Corynebacterium renale* infection, *Haemophilus somnus* infection, pneumonic pasteurellosis caused by sensitive *Pasteurella,* and infections caused by non-spore-forming anaerobes such as *Fusobacterium necrophorum* and *Porphyromonas asaccharolytica.* Penicillin G's poor activity against slowly multiplying bacteria and its relative inability to penetrate biologic membranes may explain its often disappointing effect in treating *Arcanobacterium pyogenes,* actinomycosis, or chronic *Staphylococcus aureus* mastitis. For most conditions that are penicillin responsive, a dosage of 20,000–25,000 IU/kg once daily is adequate for procaine penicillin G.

Listeriosis has been successfully treated with a daily dose of 44,000 IU/kg of procaine penicillin administered for 7–14 days (Rebhun and deLaHunta, 1982), but ampicillin is preferred. Penicillin G is effective against acute leptospirosis, although again, ampicillin is probably preferable. Procaine penicillin G (300,000–600,000 IU in 1–2 ml) administered subconjunctivally has been used extensively in the treatment of *Moraxella bovis* keratoconjunctivitis because this maintains therapeutic concentrations for up to 36 hours. One controlled study did not, however, confirm the value of this treatment (Allen et al., 1995).

Pneumonic pasteurellosis has been treated successfully with daily intramuscular or subcutaneous injections of 45,000 IU/kg of procaine penicillin (Hjerpe, 1976). Resistance among *Pasteurella haemolytica,* however, is increasing, and further increases in dose are not justified. Serious, acute mastitis caused by streptococci or susceptible *S. aureus* can be treated by IM procaine penicillin 20,000–25,000 IU/kg, q12 or q24 hours depending on severity, as a probably useful adjunct to frequent stripping of the infected quarter. Penicillin is more commonly administered intramammarily, often combined with streptomycin, and has given excellent results in the treatment of streptococcal infections during lactation, but only modest results against *S. aureus.* Penicillin G in fixed combination with streptomycin has been used successfully against severe *Dermatophilus* infection, but this combination is no longer available in many countries.

SWINE

Penicillin is the parenteral drug of choice in preventing and treating erysipelas, and streptococcal, clostridial, and corynebacterial infections. For acute erysipelas and streptococcal infections, procaine penicillin is preferred, but benzathine penicillin is used in prophylaxis. *Streptococcus suis* meningitis may be treated successfully with daily injections of procaine penicillin given early in the disease. Attempts to eradicate *S. suis* infection by treating farrowing sows with benzathine penicillin have yielded variable results. Oral administration of procaine penicillin significantly reduced the incidence of spontaneous *S. suis* meningitis in pigs, a surprising effect in view of the low tissue concentrations achieved (McKellar et al., 1987). Penicillin-streptomycin combination (25 mg/kg) administered for 1, 3, or 5 days removed the kidney carrier state in swine infected with *Leptospira pomona* (Allt and Bolin, 1996).

HORSES

Penicillin G is used against beta-hemolytic streptococci in neonatal foals for *Streptococcus zooepidemicus* polyarthritis and meningitis and in adult animals for infections of wounds, lower respiratory and urinary tracts, and the uterus, where it may be given by parenteral administration and local infusion. It is the drug of choice in strangles, when treatment is required. Penicillin is the preferred antibiotic in tetanus. Injection of procaine penicillin G in the neck or biceps gave higher serum concentrations than injection in the gluteal muscle or SC (Firth et al., 1986). Penicillin should not be administered orally to horses, because of its poor absorption and the digestive disturbances it may cause.

DOGS AND CATS

Penicillin G is a drug of choice for streptococcal and clostridial infections, for actinomycosis, and for infections caused by susceptible Gram-negative bacteria such as *Pasteurella multocida*. Because of penicillin G's activity against anaerobic bacteria, it is particularly suitable in the treatment of periodontal disease, tooth abscesses, wound infections, and perhaps pyometra. However, amoxicillin (and to a lesser extent ampicillin) is preferred for all these uses. Unlike penicillin G, which is erratically absorbed in dogs and cats after oral administration and which therefore is administered parenterally, amoxicillin is well absorbed following oral administration, which increases tissue concentrations and decreases the amount of drug remaining in the gut to cause intestinal disturbance. Because of the very high urinary concentrations attained after administration of penicillin G and amoxicillin by any route, either drug may be used in the treatment of canine urinary tract infections caused by *Staphylococcus aureus* (even penicillinase-producing), streptococci, *E. coli*, and *Proteus mirabilis*.

POULTRY

Penicillin is used by oral administration in the prevention and treatment of necrotic enteritis, ulcerative enteritis, and intestinal spirochetosis and, in combination with streptomycin, in treating erysipelas in turkeys.

Bibliography

Allen LJ, et al. 1995. Effect of penicillin or penicillin and dexamethasome in cattle with infectious bovine keratoconjunctivitis. J Am Vet Med Assoc 206:1200.

Allt DP, Bolin CA. 1996. Preliminary evaluation of antimicrobial agents for treatment of *Leptospira interrogans* serovar *pomona* infection in hamsters and swine. Am J Vet Res 57:59.

Blue JT, et al. 1987. Immune-mediated hemolytic anemia induced by penicillin in horses. Cornell Vet 77:263.

Divers TJ. 1996. Penicillin therapy in bovine practice. Compend Contin Educ Pract Vet 18:703.

Firth EC, et al. 1986. Effect of the injection site on the pharmacokinetics of procaine penicillin in horses. Am J Vet Res 47:2380.

Garrod LP, et al. 1981. Antibiotics and Chemotherapy, 5th ed. New York: Churchill Livingstone.

Groen K, et al. 1996. Bioequivalence study in calves of three commercial penicillin/dihydrostreptomycin fixed combination products for intramuscular injection. J Vet Pharm Ther 19:370.

Hjerpe CA. 1976. Practical and theoretical considerations concerning treatment of bacterial pneumonia in feedlot cattle, with special reference to antibiotic therapy. Proc Am Assoc Bovine Pract, pp97–140.

Ling GV, et al. 1980. Urine concentrations of five penicillins following oral administration to normal adult dogs. Am J Vet Res 41:1123.

McKellar QA, et al. 1987. Penicillin therapy of spontaneous streptococcal meningitis in pigs. Vet Rec 121:347.

Nielsen IL, et al. 1988. Adverse reaction to procaine penicillin G in horses. Aust Vet J 65:181.

Papich MG, et al. 1994. Disposition of penicillin G after administration of benzathine penicillin G, or a combination of benzathine penicillin G and procaine penicillin. Am J Vet Res 55:825.

Rebhun WC, deLaHunta A. 1982. Diagnosis and treatment of bovine listeriosis. J Am Vet Med Assoc 180:395.

Watson ADJ, et al. 1987. Systemic availability of penicillin V from six oral preparations in dogs. J Vet Pharm Ther 10:180.

Whittem T, Hanlon D. 1997. Dihydrostreptomycin or streptomycin in combination with penicillin G in dairy cattle therapeutics: a review and re-analysis of published data. Part 1: Clinical pharmacology. N Z Vet J 45:178.

Group 2, Orally Absorbed Penicillins

Phenoxymethyl penicillin (penicillin V) resists stomach acid hydrolysis and is therefore administered orally. It has a spectrum of activity similar to that of benzyl penicillin and is therefore used for the same purposes in monogastrates. Oral administration of penicillin V is used in the effective prophylaxis and treatment of *Streptococcus suis* meningitis in swine.

Group 3, Antistaphylococcal Isoxazolyl Penicillins: Cloxacillin, Dicloxacillin, Methicillin, Nafcillin, and Oxacillin

The antistaphylococcal penicillins are resistant to *Staphylococcus aureus* penicillinase and are used mainly in the treatment or prevention of bovine staphylococcal mastitis. The isoxazolyl penicillins (cloxacillin, oxacillin) are acid stable and may be given orally to monogastric animals, for example, in the treatment of staphylococcal skin infections in dogs.

Penicillinase production in *S. aureus* may be detected by the use of nitrocefin-impregnated paper disks.

All of these penicillins are resistant to *S. aureus* penicillinase, although activity against other penicillin-sensitive bacteria is less than that of penicillin G. Activity of the different drugs is similar in vivo. Resistance to methicillin in bovine *S. aureus* isolates is rare. Figures purporting to show extensive resistance probably reflect inappropriate test conditions or drug inactivity, as methicillin deteriorates readily in storage. Methicillin-resistant (heteroresistant) *S. aureus* may be overlooked. Although no single method is ideal, methicillin-resistant *S. aureus* are best detected using oxacillin disks, with *S. aureus* grown 18–24 hours at 30° C or 35° C. Heteroresistant *S. aureus* are often multiply resistant (to other beta-lactams, aminoglycosides, macrolides, tetracyclines) but susceptible to rifampin, quinolones, and trimethoprim-sulfamethoxazole.

Activity of these penicillins against streptococci-causing mastitis in cows is good. Cure rates approximate those for penicillin-streptomycin combinations. While apparent clinical cure of *S. aureus* mastitis is usual, bacteriologic cure is often disappointing. There may be no benefit to IM as well as intramammary administration of dicloxacillin, since serum drug concentrations achieved were negligible (Pyorala et al., 1994). Daigneault and George (1990) established the value of high topical doses (375 mg) of benzathine cloxacillin in the treatment of experimental *Moraxella bovis* keratoconjunctivitis applied twice at 3-day intervals.

In dogs, IV use of nafcillin during surgery to prevent staphylococcal infection has been associated with the development of acute renal failure within 2–4 days of surgery, probably as a result of direct renal damage by the drug (Pascoe et al., 1996). Studies of the pharmacokinetics of dicloxacillin in dogs suggest that IM administration (25 mg/kg, q8 hours) is more reliable than oral administration in achieving serum concentrations of drug consistently greater than or equal to MIC of penicillinase-producing *S. aureus* (Dimitrova et al., 1998).

Bibliography

Daigneault J, George LW. 1990. Topically applied cloxacillin for treatment of experimentally induced bovine keratoconjunctivitis. Am J Vet Res 51:376.

Dimitrova DJ. 1996. Pharmacokinetics of dicloxacillin sodium following intravenous and intramuscular administration to domestic cats. J Vet Pharm Ther 19:405.

Dimitrova DJ, et al. 1998. Dicloxacillin pharmacokinetics in dogs after intravenous, intramuscular, and oral administration. J Vet Pharm Ther 21:414.

Pascoe PJ, et al. 1996. Case-control study of the association between intraoperative administration of nafcillin and acute postoperative development of azotemia. J Am Vet Med Assoc 208:1043.

Pyorala P, et al. 1994. Pharmacokinetics and tissue irritation of sodium dicloxacillin in lactating cows after intravenous and intramuscular injection. J Vet Pharm Ther 17:157.

Ziv G, et al. 1983. Concentrations of methicillin in blood, normal milk, and mastitic milk of cows after intramuscular injection of methicillin and tamethicillin. J Vet Pharm Ther 6:41.

Group 4, Extended-spectrum Penicillins: Aminobenzylpenicillins

Aminobenzylpenicillins (ampicillin, amoxicillin, and the related esters bacampicillin, hetacillin, pivampicillin, and talampicillin) have similar antimicrobial activity, but amoxicillin and possibly pivampicillin have the advantage of achieving higher tissue concentrations because of better absorption from the intestine. The broad-spectrum aminobenzylpenicillins are slightly less active than penicillin G against Gram-positive and anaerobic bacteria and also are susceptible to staphylococcal penicillinase. These broad-spectrum drugs have considerably greater activity against Gram-negative bacteria such as *E. coli, Proteus mirabilis,* and *Salmonella.* Nevertheless, acquired resistance has considerably reduced the effectiveness of these drugs. An exciting development has been their combination with beta-lactamase–inhibiting drugs, which increases their effectiveness considerably (see Chapter 8) and with which these drugs should generally be combined.

Antimicrobial Activity

Good Susceptibility (MIC ≤1): As for benzyl penicillin group but includes *Borrelia* spp. and *Leptospira* spp., which are highly susceptible, as well as *Actinobacillus* spp., *Haemophilus* spp., *Moraxella* spp., and *Pasteurella* spp. (Tables 6.2 and 6.5).

Moderate Susceptibility (MIC 2–4 µg/ml): As for benzyl penicillin but also *Campylobacter* spp., enterococci, and *Rhodococcus equi.* Variable moderate activity (because of acquired resistance) against *E. coli, Proteus mirabilis,* and *Salmonella.* Acquired resistance in Enterobacteriaceae is widespread.

Resistance (MIC >4 µg/ml, approximately): Bacteroides fragilis, Bordetella bronchiseptica, *Citrobacter* spp., *Enterobacter* spp., *Klebsiella* spp., other *Proteus* spp., *Pseudomonas aeruginosa, Serratia* spp., and *Yersinia enterocolitica.*

Antimicrobial Resistance

Plasmid-mediated acquired resistance is common in Gram-negative bacteria and is often multiple, such as that in most enterotoxigenic *E. coli* and *Salmonella typhimurium.* Many *E. coli* that cause bovine mastitis are resistant. Aminobenzylpenicillins are susceptible to *Staphylococcus aureus* beta-lactamase (see Tables 6.2 and 6.5).

TABLE 6.5. In vitro activity (μg/ml) of new penicillins against various medically important opportunist bacteria

Organism	Ampicillin		Mecillinam		Ticarcillin		Azlocillin		Piperacillin	
	MIC_{50}	MIC_{90}	MIC_{50}	MIC_{90}	MIC_{50}	MIC_{90}	MIC_{50}	MIC_{90}	MIC_{50}	MIC_{90}
Streptococcus agalactiae	0.06	0.12	2	8	2	4	0.25	1	0.25	1
Escherichia coli	4	128	1	4	16	128	8	128	8	128
Klebsiella pneumoniae	128	128	2	128	128	128	32	128	8	128
Citrobacter diversus	4	128	0.5	4	16	128	4	8	4	4
Enterobacter cloacae	128	128	2	32	8	128	4	32	4	32
Proteus mirabilis	1	4	4	16	0.5	16	0.5	16	0.5	16
Pseudomonas aeruginosa	128	128	128	128	16	128	4	128	4	128
Bacteroides spp.[a]	1	32	2	16	4	32	2	8	2	4

Source: Modified from Prince and Neu (1983) with permission.
[a] Other than *B. fragilis.*

Pharmacokinetic Properties

The basic pharmacokinetic properties of penicillins were described under Penam Penicillins: General Considerations. Both ampicillin and amoxicillin are relatively stable in acid. In dogs, the systemic availability of amoxicillin (60–70%) is about twice that of ampicillin (20–40%), so that peak blood concentrations are often twice or more than those that occur after the same dose of ampicillin. The absorption of amoxicillin is unaffected by feeding, unlike absorption of ampicillin. Hetacillin and pivampicillin are esters of ampicillin developed to increase systemic availability, but it is questionable whether this occurs in dogs. Pivampicillin has significantly better bioavailability in horses than amoxicillin after oral administration (Ensink et al., 1992). Ampicillin is available as a sodium salt that can be administered parenterally in a freshly prepared solution. The trihydrate salts are less soluble and therefore poorly absorbed from the intestine but form aqueous suspensions that can be injected either IM or SC. These preparations produce low peak concentrations in the serum, but they extend the dosing interval to 12 hours. Long-acting preparations of ampicillin trihydrate, which produce therapeutic serum concentrations for 48 hours, have been introduced. The lower peak plasma concentrations, however, may decrease penetration of the antibiotic to sites of infection.

Drug Interactions

Aminobenzylpenicillins are commonly synergistic with aminoglycosides against Gram-positive bacteria and often also against Gram-negative bacteria, but only if the latter are not resistant to both drugs. The broad-spectrum beta-lactamase inhibitors clavulanic acid and sulbactam show remarkable synergism with aminobenzylpenicillins against beta-lactamase-producing bacteria (see Chapter 8).

Toxicities and Adverse Effects

Toxic effects are similar to those described under Penam Penicillins: General Considerations. One hazard with broad-spectrum penicillins is the potential to disturb the normal intestinal flora. In dogs and cats, the effect may be less marked with amoxicillin, which is better absorbed. Ampicillin should not be administered to small rodents (guinea pigs, hamsters, gerbils) or to rabbits, because it may produce clostridial colitis (*Clostridium difficile* or, in rabbits, *C. spiroforme*). Administration of pivampicillin in horses was associated with less loose feces or diarrhea than observed in horses given trimethoprim-sulfadiazine (Ensink et al., 1996b). Moderate diarrhea has been described in calves after several days' treatment with oral ampicillin, which appears to result from malabsorption caused by a direct effect on intestinal mucosa.

Administration and Dosage

Recommended dosages are shown in Table 6.3. The soluble sodium salts can be administered parenterally and orally, but the poorly soluble trihydrate form should only be administered IM. Reconstituted aqueous sodium salts are unstable after more than a few hours. Because of their short half-lives, preparations that are rapidly absorbed should be administered every 6 hours to maintain serum drug concentrations over 1 µg/ml for a significant length of time. Amoxicillin is preferred for oral administration because it is better absorbed than ampicillin, and its absorption is unaffected by feeding. Another advantage of oral amoxicillin over ampicillin is that it can be given twice daily to small animals. Long-acting preparations of amoxicillin are available, but it is doubtful whether they maintain therapeutic serum concentrations for the 48-hour recommended dosing interval.

Clinical Applications

The aminobenzylpenicillins are bactericidal, relatively nontoxic drugs with a broader spectrum of activity than penicillin G and are better distributed in the body. Even with these advantages, relatively high doses are required to treat infections caused by Gram-negative bacteria. The relatively high prevalence of acquired resistance has limited their place. Amoxicillin is the best penicillin for the treatment of urinary tract infections and enteric infections caused by susceptible organisms and has similar activity to penicillin G in the treatment of anaerobic infections. Although amoxicillin offers pharmacokinetic advantages over ampicillin, it has some of the same difficulty as ampicillin in attaining concentration in tissues approximating those necessary for susceptible Gram-negative bacteria.

The main clinical applications are similar to those shown in Table 6.4. Amoxicillin is a drug of choice in the treatment of leptospirosis. Ampicillin is preferred to penicillin to treat listeriosis.

In cattle, sheep, and goats, oral ampicillin has been used to treat *E. coli* and *Salmonella* infections, but acquired resistance limits their effectiveness for this purpose. Ampicillin is effective against bovine respiratory disease but seems to offer no advantage over penicillin G. Ampicillin has been used intramammarily in the treatment of coliform mastitis, but resistance largely limits its use. Long-acting amoxicillin administered twice IM at 15 mg/kg q48 hours was effective in removing the *Leptospira hardjo* kidney carrier state from the majority of experimentally infected cattle (Smith et al., 1997).

Indications in horses for ampicillin or amoxicillin are few, since they offer little advantage over benzyl penicillins, largely because of acquired resistance in Gram-negative bacteria. One indication is in the treatment of

Rhodococcus equi, but drugs should be administered IM at 11–15 mg/kg q6 hours. Oral administration of amoxicillin (or preferably pivampicillin) is appropriate for infections in foals caused by organisms with good susceptibility but cannot be recommended for adult horses.

Ampicillin or amoxicillin is used in the treatment of canine urinary tract infections, because over 90% of *Staphylococcus aureus,* streptococci, and *Proteus mirabilis,* nearly 90% of *E. coli,* and 65% of *Klebsiella* are regarded as susceptible to urinary concentrations of the drug. Nevertheless, treatment results in one study were not conspicuously better than those obtained with penicillin G (Ling and Gilmore, 1977). The combination of clavulanic acid–amoxicillin is preferred for these purposes. Clinical trials in cats showed once-daily dosing with a 50-mg tablet of amoxicillin to be as effective as twice-daily dosing (Keefe, 1978b). Field trial comparison in cats of 50-mg amoxicillin twice daily versus 50-mg hetacillin twice daily showed a significant advantage for amoxicillin (Keefe, 1978a). Amoxicillin, metronidazole, and omeprazole have been used to produce bacteriologic cure in the treatment of *Helicobacter* gastritis in cats, but the organism could still be detected by polymerase chain reaction (PCR) (Perkins et al., 1996). Unfortunately, PCR does not distinguish between viable and nonviable organisms. Amoxicillin produced clinical cure of *Borrelia burgdorferi* infection in the majority of treated dogs, but the organism was not eradicated (Straubinger et al., 1997).

In poultry, ampicillin is sometimes administered orally for the prevention or treatment of *E. coli* or *S. aureus* septicemia or of salmonellosis.

Bibliography

Agerso H, et al. 1998. Water medication of a swine herd with amoxycillin. J Vet Pharm Ther 21:199.

Baggot JD, et al. 1990. Oral dosage of penicillin V in adult horses and foals. Equine Vet J 22:290.

Ensink JM, et al. 1992. Bioavailability of oral penicillins in the horse: a comparison of pivampicillin and amoxicillin. J Vet Pharm Ther 15:221.

Ensink JM, et al. 1996a. Oral bioavailability and in vitro stability of pivampicillin, bacampicillin, talampicillin, and ampicillin in horses. Am J Vet Res 57:1021.

Ensink JM, et al. 1996b. Side effects of oral antimicrobial agents in the horse: a comparison of pivampicillin and trimethoprim/sulphadiazine. Vet Rec 138:253.

Keefe TJ. 1978a. Clinical efficacy of amoxicillin oral suspension. Feline Pract 8:33.

Keefe TJ. 1978b. Result of a clinical study to determine frequency of dosage for amoxycillin trihydrate in cats. Vet Med Small Anim Clin 73:447.

Kueng G, Wanner M. 1994. Bioavailability of different forms of amoxycillin administered orally to dogs. Vet Rec 135:552.

Ling GV, Gilmore CJ. 1977. Penicillin G or ampicillin for oral treatment of canine urinary tract infections. J Am Vet Med Assoc 171:358.

Nouws JFM, et al. 1986. Age difference in pharmacokinetics of an amoxicillin trihydrate–15% formulation administered intramuscularly to ruminants. Vet Q 8:339.

Perkins SE, et al. 1996. Use of PCR and culture to detect *Helicobacter pylori* in naturally infected cats following triple antimicrobial therapy. Antimicrob Agents Chemother 40:1486.

Prince AS, Neu HC. 1983. New penicillins and their use in pediatric practice. Pediatr Clin North Am 32:3–16.

Smith CR, et al. 1997. Amoxycillin as an alternative to dihydrostreptomycin sulphate for treating cattle infected with *Leptospira borgpetersenii* serovar *hardjo*. Aust Vet J 75:818.

Straubinger RK, et al. 1997. Persistence of *Borrelia burgdorferi* in experimentally infected dogs after antibiotic treatment. J Clin Microbiol 35:111.

Group 4, Extended-spectrum Penicillins: Amidopenicillins

Mecillinam (amidinopenicillin) is active against a broader range of Enterobacteriaceae than ampicillin, being highly active against *Citrobacter* spp., *Enterobacter* spp., *E. coli*, *Klebsiella pneumoniae*, *Proteus* spp., and *Yersinia* spp. Mecillinam has little activity against Gram-positive bacteria and none against *Pseudomonas aeruginosa* (see Table 6.5). It has high affinity only for PBP2, the enzyme mediating cylindric growth in Gram-negative rods. Mecillinam is synergistic with many beta-lactamase-inhibiting drugs. It is inactivated by many beta-lactamases. Its efficacy against some beta-lactamase-producing bacteria is due to its rapid penetration of cells as well as its low affinity for some of their degradative enzymes.

In calves, Soback et al. (1986) suggested that dosage of 16 mg/kg every 5 hours would maintain drug concentrations sufficient to inhibit 90% of *E. coli*, *Pasteurella multocida*, and *Salmonella* spp.

Mecillinam may have potential for use in veterinary medicine for infections caused by susceptible Enterobacteriaceae.

Bibliography

Soback S, et al. 1986. Clinical pharmacology of mecillinam in calves. J Vet Pharm Ther 9:385.

Group 5, Antipseudomonal Penicillins: Carboxypenicillins and Ureidopenicillins

Carbenicillin was the first carboxypenicillin with good activity against *Pseudomonas aeruginosa* and *Proteus* (see Table 6.2) but has now been largely replaced by the more active carboxypenicillin and by the ureidopenicillins ticarcillin, azlocillin, and piperacillin. It is administered IV. Two esters of carbenicillin (carindacillin, carfecillin) are available for oral administration for urinary tract infections caused by *Proteus* or *P. aeruginosa*. Ticarcillin has a similar spectrum of activity to that of carbenicillin. It is active against most *E. coli* and *Proteus* spp. and more active than carbenicillin against *P. aeruginosa* (see Table 6.5). Most *Klebsiella*, *Citrobacter*, and *Serratia* and all *Enterobacter* enterococci are resistant. Ticarcillin is generally reserved for *P. aeruginosa* infections but is less active than azlocillin or piperacillin. It is administered IV.

Because of the expense of carbenicillin and ticarcillin, the high dosages required, the usually IV administration, and the general lack of clinical application, it is unlikely that carbenicillin and ticarcillin will be used for parenteral treatment of *Pseudomonas* or other infections in animals. These drugs have potential use in the local treatment of *P. aeruginosa* infections caused by otherwise resistant bacteria, such as otitis externa in dogs, bovine mastitis, metritis in mares, and, possibly, otherwise resistant urinary tract infections. Ticarcillin is licensed in the United States for the treatment of uterine infections in mares caused by beta-hemolytic streptococci (6g in 250–500 ml by intrauterine infusion at estrus once daily for 3 days). For this purpose, ticarcillin would have no advantage over benzyl penicillin and should be reserved for infections caused by *P. aeruginosa* and other susceptible Gram-negative bacteria. Spensley et al. (1986) found that diluting the drug in large volumes (250 ml) gave higher endometrial concentrations after intrauterine administration than did smaller volumes (60 ml). Ticarcillin was administered IV to a foal (110 mg/kg, QID) in the effective treatment of bacterial arthritis (Sweeney and Markel, 1984). A parenteral (IM) dosage suggested for dogs is 25–40 mg/kg q6–8 hours; IV-administered drug should be given every 4–6 hours. Ticarcillin (IV, 15–25 mg/kg q8 hours) has been used successfully, combined with topical administration, in the treatment of otitis externa in dogs caused by otherwise resistant *P. aeruginosa* (Nuttall, 1998). Because of the danger of *P. aeruginosa*'s developing resistance, these agents are probably best used in conjunction with a broad-spectrum aminoglycoside or with beta-lactamase inhibitors.

The expanded spectrum of activity of the antipseudomonal ureidopenicillins (azlocillin, mezlocillin, piperacillin) results from their interaction with PBPs other than those that bind aminopenicillins, their increased penetration of Gram-negative bacteria, and their resistance to some species-specific chromosomal beta-lactamases. Ureidopenicillins bind PBP3, septal murein synthetase. They have increased activity against Gram-negative bacteria relative to activities of carboxy- or aminobenzylpenicillins, notably against *Klebsiella* and *Pseudomonas aeruginosa* (see Tables 6.2 and 6.5) and increased activity against *Bacteroides fragilis*.

Mezlocillin is more active than azlocillin against Enterobacteriaceae, although resistance is not infrequent, because the bacteria are susceptible to common beta-lactamases (see Table 6.5). Most *Enterobacter* and *Serratia* are resistant. Piperacillin combines the spectra of mezlocillin and azlocillin and is more active than both. It inhibits over 95% of *P. aeruginosa* and many Enterobacteriaceae and is active against many anaerobes, including many *Bacteroides fragilis*. Piperacillin is the most active broad-spectrum penicillin but is also susceptible to some common beta-lactamases as well as to the penicillinase of *Staphylococcus aureus*. Ureidopenicillins may be combined with beta-lactamase inhibitors (eg, piperacillin with tazobactam; see Chapter 8) or with aminoglycosides. There is incomplete cross-resistance among ureidopenicillins and carboxypenicillins.

Ureidopenicillins are administered IV, although azlocillin may be administered by (painful) IM injection. Expense limits their application. Clinical applications are probably limited to treatment of *P. aeruginosa* infections and, combined with an aminoglycoside or beta-lactamase inhibitor, to serious infections caused by Gram-negative bacteria in immunocompromised hosts.

Bibliography

Nuttall TJ. 1998. Use of ticarcillin in the management of canine otitis externa complicated by *Pseudomonas aeruginosa*. J Small Anim Pract 39:165.

Spensley MS, et al. 1986. Pharmacokinetics and endometrial tissue concentrations of ticarcillin given to the horse by intravenous and intrauterine routes. Am J Vet Res 47:2587.

Sweeney CR, Markel MD. 1984. Ticarcillin therapy in a foal with septic arthritis. Mod Vet Pract 65:841.

Tilmant L, et al. 1985. Pharmacokinetics of ticarcillin in the dog. Am J Vet Res 46:479.

Group 6, Beta-lactamase-resistant Penicillins: Temocillin

Temocillin is ticarcillin modified by the addition of a 6α-methoxy group to increase resistance to beta-lactamase. Temocillin's high activity against Enterobacteriaceae is at the expense of resistance of *Pseudomonas*, *Bacteroides fragilis*, and Gram-positive bacteria. More than 90% of Enterobacteriaceae are inhibited at MIC ≤8 μg/ml. The drug is stable to expanded-spectrum, plasmid-mediated beta-lactamases that inactivate third-generation cephalosporins. Temocillin has a long half-life (4.5 hours) in humans, allowing for once-daily dosage. Temocillin has many potential applications, but its use, like that of the antipseudomonal penicillins, is limited by expense and the need for IV administration.

7

Beta-lactam Antibiotics: Cephalosporins and Cephamycins

J. F. PRESCOTT

General Considerations

In cephalosporins, the beta-lactam ring is attached to a 6-membered dihydrothiazine ring with the effect that the cephalosporin nucleus is inherently more resistant to beta-lactamases than is the penicillin nucleus (Fig. 7.1). The 7-aminocephalosporanic acid molecule also provides more sites than the aminopenicillanic acid molecule for manipulation in the production of semisynthetic drugs. Changes at position 7 (R_1) alter beta-lactamase stability and antibacterial properties particularly, whereas changes at position 3 (R_2) tend to alter metabolic stability and pharmacokinetic properties. True cephalosporins contain the common 7-aminocephalosporanic acid of *Cephalosporium acremonium*, whereas cephamycins are derived from *Streptomyces* species (cefotetan, cefoxitin) or are synthetic derivatives produced by substituting oxygen for sulfur (latamoxef).

Cephalosporins in general have the advantages of beta-lactamase stability, good activity against target proteins (PBPs), and good ability to penetrate bacterial cell walls. Although they may be active against a wide range of organisms, such activities are not uniform and produce often subtle differences among the different molecules. Pharmacokinetically they are generally similar and have typical beta-lactam properties, usually requiring parenteral injection, having short (1–2 hour) half-lives, and being excreted usually through the kidneys in the urine. They are bactericidal, are relatively nontoxic, and can be used in many penicillin-sensitive individuals.

Classification

Cephalosporins have a wide range of antibacterial activity but show considerable diversity in their antibacterial properties. One approach to

134

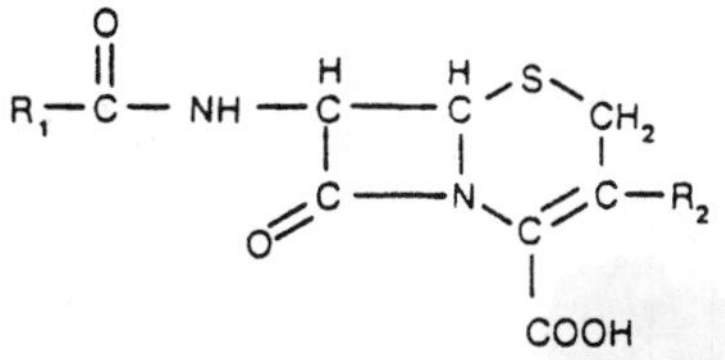

Fig. 7.1. Structural formula of the cephalosporin nucleus.

TABLE 7.1. **Classification of cephalosporins into groups (and generations) based on route of administration and antibacterial activity**

Group	Characteristics	Examples
1 (first generation)	Parenteral; resistant to staphylococcal beta-lactamase; sensitive to enterobacterial beta-lactamase; moderately active	Cephacetrile, cephaloridine, cephalothin, cephapirin, cephazolin
2 (first generation)	Oral; resistant to staphylococcal beta-lactamase; moderately resistant to some enterobacterial beta-lactamases; moderately active	Cefaclor, cefadroxil, cephadrine, cephalexin
3 (second generation)	Parenteral; resistant to many beta-lactamases; moderately active	Cefotetan, cefoxitin, cefuroxime, cefamandole
4 (third generation)	Parenteral; resistant to many beta-lactamases; highly active	Cefotaxime, ceftiofur, ceftriaxone, latamoxef
5 (third generation)	Oral; resistant to many beta-lactamases; highly active	Cefetamet, cefixime
6 (third generation)	Parenteral; resistant to many beta-lactamases; active against *Pseudomonas aeruginosa*	Cefoperazone, cefsulodin, ceftazidime
7 (fourth generation)	Parenteral; resistant to staphylococcal, enterobacterial, and pseudomonal beta-lactamases; highly active	Cefepime, cefpirome

Note: Classification is that of Wise (1997). By convention, cephalosporins discovered before 1975 are spelled with *ph* and after 1975 with *f*.

classification has been chronological or historical, with the different cephalosporins introduced since 1975 being described somewhat arbitrarily as generations (Tables 7.1 and 7.2). This has implied that each of the generations introduced has added another general level of advantage over the previous generation rather than adding some advantage(s) at the expense of another or others (Williams, 1987). Differences within the generations often appear subtle but are important. Cephalosporins were originally introduced (first generation) for the treatment of penicillinase-resistant staphylococcal infections, with the advantage that these drugs also had a spectrum of activity against Gram-negatives similar to that of

TABLE 7.2. **Antibacterial activity (MIC$_{90}$, µg/ml) of cephalosporins**

Organism	First Generation		Second Generation		Third Generation	
	Cephalothin	Cefadroxil	Cefuroxime	Cefoxitin	Cefotaxime	Moxalactam
Staphylococcus aureus	0.5	2	1	4	2	6
S. aureus, penicillinase[a]	0.5	4	1	4	2	4
S. pyogenes	0.12	0.5	0.03	0.5	0.06	0.6
Escherichia coli	8	16	4	4	0.1	0.2
Klebsiella spp.	4	16	4	4	0.1	0.1
Enterobacter spp.	R[a]	R[a]	8	R[a]	0.1-R[a]	0.15
Proteus mirabilis	4	16	4	4	0.06	0.1
Proteus, indole[a]	R[a]	R[a]	8	8	0.2-2	0.05
Salmonella spp.	2	8	4	4	0.5	0.05
Pseudomonas aeruginosa	R[a]	R[a]	R[a]	R[a]	16-R[a]	16-R[a]
Bacteroides fragilis	32	—	8-64	4-32	0.25	0.8

Source: Garrod et al. (1981) with permission.

Note: Many species show wide strain variation and considerable inoculum effect.

[a] >32 µg/ml.

the extended-spectrum aminobenzylpenicillins. Alterations of the side chains on the 7-aminocephalosporanic acid nucleus and the discovery of the cephamycins led to increasing stability to the beta-lactamases of Gram-negative bacteria, including those of *Bacteroides fragilis* and *Pseudomonas aeruginosa*. This increase in stability is usually at the expense of decreasing activity against Gram-positive bacteria and gives pharmacokinetic differences. Because of the inadequacies of classification as generations, an expanded classification has been developed on the basis of antimicrobial activity, including beta-lactamase stability and pharmacological properties (Williams, 1987, developed by Wise, 1997; see Table 7.1). This classification will be followed here.

The "generations" are broadly characterized as follows.

- First generation: primarily Gram-positive antibacterial activity, administered parenterally (IV, IM, SC) or in some cases orally
- Second generation: Gram-positive and Gram-negative antibacterial activity, administered by all routes
- Third generation: decreased Gram-positive but increased Gram-negative antibacterial activity, administered parenterally and in a very few cases orally
- Fourth generation: increased Gram-positive and Gram-negative antibacterial activity, administered by all routes

Antimicrobial Activity

The mechanism of action of the cephalosporins is that of beta-lactam antibiotics (see Chapter 6). For susceptibility testing, cephalothin is the class drug for groups 1 and 2, first-generation, cephalosporins. For groups 3–7, second- to fourth-generation cephalosporins, there is no class representative. For susceptibility testing of Enterobacteriaceae, cefotaxime can usually substitute for ceftazidime, ceftizoxime, and ceftriaxone (and vice versa) and cefamandole for cefonicid and cefuroxime (and vice versa). For *Pseudomonas aeruginosa*, cefoperazone will substitute for ceftazidime (and vice versa) and cefotaxime for ceftriaxone and latamoxef (and vice versa).

Cephalosporins are usually active against beta-hemolytic streptococci and against beta-lactamase–producing staphylococci, but not against staphylococci resistant to methicillin (oxacillin). Most enterococci are resistant. Among Enterobacteriaceae, in the absence of acquired resistance, *Escherichia coli* and *Salmonella* are susceptible, as are some *Proteus* and *Klebsiella* species. Fourth-generation, group 7, cephalosporins are effective against Enterobacteriaceae and other Gram-negative bacteria resistant to earlier generations of cephalosporins because of acquired beta-lactamase–based resistance. Susceptibility among common Gram-negative aerobic species such as *Haemophilus* and *Pasteurella*, including beta-lactamase producers, is usual. Only third-generation antipseudomonal (group 6) and fourth-generation (group 7) cephalosporins are effective against *P. aeruginosa*. Mycobacteria are resistant. Against non-spore-forming anaerobic bacteria, activity is variable and resembles that of aminobenzylpenicillins. Cefoxitin is notably resistant to beta-lactamase-producing anaerobes, including *Bacteroides fragilis*.

Resistance to Cephalosporins

The three basic mechanisms of resistance to cephalosporins result from reduced permeability, enzymatic inactivation, or absence of specific penicillin-binding proteins. Constitutive and acquired resistance caused by periplasmic beta-lactamases active against the different cephalosporins forms a central basis of the classification of these drugs (see Table 7.1).

Shortly after the development of second- and some third-generation agents, it was recognized that certain Gram-negative pathogens (*Citrobacter, Enterobacter, Providencia, Pseudomonas,* and *Serratia* spp.) might develop resistance to newer cephalosporins, which emerged rapidly during therapy. These organisms possessed inducible, chromosomally mediated group 1 beta-lactamases, which only slowly inactivated the newer cephalosporins, so that these bacteria were usually killed by these agents. Resistance was associated with stable mutation to derepression and high-level production of these enzymes. Most of the third-generation cephalosporins can select for such stably derepressed mutants. Resistance has emerged in perhaps 15% of human patients infected with these relatively unusual genera. Derepressed beta-lactamase-producing organisms are resistant to all cephalosporins (other than fourth-generation), to monobactams, and to penicillins. Such resistance, which appears to involve the extracellular expression of beta-lactamases through efflux pumps, has to some extent limited the use of these valuable antibiotics. Outbreaks of nosocomial infection with these resistant organisms have occurred in hospitals. This mechanism is the major cause of resistance to newer cephalosporins and has been noted particularly with ceftazidime. Some mutants with altered outer membrane permeability and with drug efflux pump activity may show cross-resistance with aminoglycosides, chloramphenicol, fluoroquinolones, tetracyclines, and trimethoprim. Plasmid-mediated acquired resistance to newer cephalosporins has also been described (Payne et al., 1991).

Pharmacokinetic Properties

The basic pharmacokinetic and drug disposition characteristics of cephalosporins are typical of beta-lactams (see Chapter 6), with an elimination half-life of 1–2 hours. Some drugs, however, such as cefotetan and ceftriaxone have significantly longer half-lives. Group 2 (second-generation) and 5 (third-generation) oral cephalosporins are well absorbed after oral administration, which may be enhanced by formulations as prodrugs, which are metabolized to active compounds in the body. Some fourth-generation cephalosporins can be administered orally to monogastrates. Clearance is through the kidney in most cases, although drugs with high molecular weight and protein binding, such as cefoperazone, are largely excreted in the bile.

Drug Interactions

Cephalosporins are synergistic with aminoglycosides, with which they are sometimes combined in the treatment of infections in neutropenic patients in human medicine.

Toxicity and Adverse Effects

Cephalosporins are among the safest antimicrobial drugs. They have the safety associated with penicillins, although individual drugs may have specific adverse effects. For example, hypoprothrombinemia and platelet abnormalities causing bleeding disorders have been noted with some newer cephalosporins. The broad spectrum of antibacterial activity of second- to fourth-generation drugs may cause overgrowth ("superinfection") of the patients by inherently resistant bacteria that no longer have to compete with susceptible members of the microbial flora. The emergence of multiresistant enterococci as nosocomial infections in human hospital intensive care units is an example of this effect. Gastrointestinal disturbances are therefore also among adverse effects, particularly with drugs excreted through the bile. Human patients allergic to penicillin are sometimes (5–8%) also allergic to cephalosporins. Many second- and third-generation drugs are painful on injection and are usually therefore administered IV, but orally administered third-generation (group 5) cephalosporins are now available.

Dosage Considerations

As with all beta-lactams, the aim of treatment is to maintain serum and tissue concentrations of drug at $\geq$MIC for the majority or all of the dosing intervals.

Clinical Usage

Cephalosporins are an important class of antimicrobial agents with widespread potential use. First-generation cephalosporins have a spectrum of activity and clinical use similar to that of extended-spectrum aminobenzylpenicillins, with the addition of resistance to staphylococcal beta-lactamase. First-generation oral cephalosporins are therefore used in the treatment of canine *Staphylococcus intermedius* skin infections and urinary tract infections, as well as bovine *S. aureus* and streptococcal mastitis. Second- and some third-generation (groups 3 and 4) parenteral cephalosporins are used to treat infections caused by bacteria resistant to first-generation drugs. For example, ceftiofur, which has antimicrobial characteristics between those of second- and third-generation cephalosporins, is used in animals to treat systemic infections caused by Gram-negative aerobes, including *E. coli, Pasteurella,* and *Salmonella* infections. Cefoxitin has a special place in the treatment of mixed aerobic-anaerobic infections. The antipseudomonal, group 6, cephalosporins are used exclusively in the treatment of *Pseudomonas aeruginosa* infections. Other third-generation (group 5) and the fourth-generation cephalosporins are usually (but not always) reserved in human medicine for the treatment of hospital-based bacterial infections resistant to earlier cephalosporins or alternative antimicrobial drugs. The broad-spectrum and bactericidal activity (at concentrations ≥ 4 MIC) may be drawbacks of newer cephalosporins, since they are associated with the selection of resistant bacterial superinfection and gastrointestinal disturbance.

Bibliography

Adu A, Armour CL. 1995. Drug utilization review (DUR) of the third generation cephalosporins. Drugs 50:423.

Caprile KA. 1988. The cephalosporin antimicrobial agents: a comprehensive review. J Vet Pharmacol Ther 11:1.

Garrod LP, et al. 1981. Antibiotic and Chemotherapy, 5th ed. New York: Churchill Livingstone.

Glauser M, Francioli P. 1997. Fourth-generation cephalosporins in severe infections. Clin Microbiol Infect 3 (Suppl 1).

Papich MG. 1987. The beta-lactam antibiotics: clinical pharmacology and recent developments. Compend Contin Educ Pract Vet 9:68.

Payne DJ, et al. 1991. Transferable resistance to extended-spectrum beta-lactams: a major threat or minor inconvenience? J Antimicrob Chemother 27:255.

Phillips I, Shannon K. 1989. Class I beta-lactamases: induction and derepression. Drugs 37:402.

Williams JD. 1987. Classification of cephalosporins. Drugs 34 (Suppl 2):15.

Wise R. 1997. β-lactams: cephalosporins. In: O'Grady F, et al., eds. Antibiotic and Chemotherapy. New York: Churchill Livingstone.

Group 1, First-generation Cephalosporins: Cephacetrile, Cephapirin, Cephaloridine, Cefazolin, Cephradine, Cephalothin

First-generation, group 1, parenteral cephalosporins share the characteristics of the oral first-generation cephalosporins of high activity against Gram-positive bacteria, including beta-lactamase-producing *Staphylococcus aureus;* moderate activity against certain nontransferable, beta-lactamase-producing, Gram-negative Enterobacteriaceae and fastidious Gram-negatives; and no activity against *Enterobacter* spp., *Pseudomonas aeruginosa,* and *Serratia* spp., among others. For susceptibility testing, cephalothin is the class drug, but cefazolin may also be tested since it is more active against Gram-negative bacteria. Activity is shown for selected bacteria in Tables 7.2 and 7.3.

Acquired resistance is common in Gram-negative but rare in Gram-positive bacteria. Methicillin-resistant *S. aureus* is resistant to all beta-lactam drugs, including cephalosporins.

TABLE 7.3. **Activity (µg/ml) of cephalothin against selected bacteria**

Organism	MIC_{50}	MIC_{90}
Gram-positive aerobes		
Arcanobacterium pyogenes	0.5	4
Bacillus anthracis	0.25	0.5
Corynebacterium pseudotuberculosis	≤1	≤1
Erysipelothrix rhusiopathiae	0.25	0.5
Listeria monocytogenes	2	4
Nocardia asteroides	64	128
Rhodococcus equi	>128	>128
Staphylococcus aureus	0.5	0.8
Streptococcus agalactiae	≤0.12	0.5
S. uberis	0.5	2
Gram-positive anaerobes		
Actinomyces spp.	0.06	0.12
Clostridium perfringens	0.5	1
C. septicum	≤0.12	≤0.12
Clostridium spp.	0.5	1
Gram-negative aerobes		
Actinobacillus spp.	≤1	16
A. pleuropneumoniae	≤1	
Bordetella avium	≤1	≤1
B. bronchiseptica	16	64
Brucella canis	8	16
Campylobacter jejuni	≥512	≥512
E. coli	8	64
Klebsiella pneumoniae	4	>64
Leptospira sp.	1	8
Pasteurella haemolytica	1	8
P. multocida		
Cattle	1	8
Pigs	≤1	≤1
Pseudomonas aeruginosa	>64	>64
Salmonella sp.	2	8
Gram-negative anaerobes		
Bacteroides fragilis	>32	>32
Bacteroides spp.	16	>32
Fusobacterium spp.	0.5	≥1
F. necrophorum	0.06	0.5
Porphyromonas asaccharolytica	1	16

Pharmacokinetic Properties

IM or SC injection of first-generation cephalosporins results in rapid absorption with high bioavailability. There is widespread distribution in extracellular fluids in the body but poor penetration across biological membranes (including into the udder) and physiological barriers (such as the cerebrospinal fluid). Cephalothin and cephapirin are metabolized into the less active desacetyl derivatives. The majority of drug is rapidly eliminated in the urine, and tubular secretion (but not glomerular filtration) can be inhibited by probenecid to reduce clearance from the body. The specific mechanism of renal excretion varies with the agent. Half-life is less than 1 hour.

Toxicities and Side Effects

Pain on IM injection of cephalothin means that this drug is little used. Non-dose-related hypersensitivity, fever, skin rash, and eosinophilia occur uncommonly. At very high doses, nephrotoxicity caused by acute tubular necrosis may occur. Because of this, cephaloridine is no longer available for clinical use.

Administration and Dosage

Recommended dosage is shown in Table 7.4. Because of the margin of safety, a range of dosage can be used depending on the MIC of susceptible bacteria.

Clinical Applications

Clinical applications of parenteral first-generation cephalosporins have become fewer with the development of beta-lactamase-stable cephalosporins. Applications are as described for oral cephalosporins below, which are used extensively in small animal medicine. These drugs have been used extensively in prophylaxis of surgical wound infections in human patients and are used for this purpose in dogs and cats. Cefazolin

TABLE 7.4. **Parenteral dosage (IV, IM, SC) of group 1 parenteral cephalosporins**

Species	Drug	Dose (mg/kg)	Interval (h)	Comments
Dogs, cats	Cephradine	22	6–8	
	Cephalothin	20–40	6–8	IV only (painful IM)
	Cefazolin	15–30	12	IM, IV
Horse	Cephapirin	20	8	Highly susceptible, eg, *Staphylococcus aureus*
	Cefazolin	15–20	8	
	Cephalexin	10	8–12	
Cattle, sheep	Cefazolin	15–20	12	Poor penetration into the udder
	Cephapirin	10	8–12	As cefazolin

has been suggested for administration (20 mg/kg IV) at the time of surgery, repeated SC 6 hours later (Rosin et al., 1993). In dogs and cats, parenteral first-generation drugs might be used to establish high tissue levels rapidly before using an oral cephalosporin. In horses, an important indication would be parenteral treatment of *Staphylococcus aureus* infections. In the absence of susceptibility testing, their use in treating infections caused by Gram-negative Enterobacteriaceae is not generally recommended, since activity is unpredictable (as is the case also for aminobenzylpenicillins). In cattle, these cephalosporins are in widespread use in treatment and prevention (dry-cow therapy) of mastitis caused by the Gram-positive cocci, as alternatives to pirlimycin, cloxacillin, and penicillin-novobiocin combination. Administration is by the intramammary route.

Bibliography

Gagnon H, et al. 1994. Single-dose pharmacokinetics of cefazolin in bovine synovial fluid after intravenous regional injection. J Vet Pharmacol Ther 17:31.

Henry MM, et al. 1992. Pharmacokinetics of cephadrine in neonatal foals after single oral dosing. Equine Vet J 24:242.

Marcellin-Little DJ, et al. 1996. Pharmacokinetic model for cefazolin distribution during total hip arthroplasty in dogs. Am J Vet Res 57:720.

Petersen SW, Rosin E. 1995. Cephalothin and cefazolin in vitro antibacterial activity and pharmacokinetics in dogs. Vet Surg 24:347.

Prades M, et al. 1988. Pharmacokinetics of sodium cephapirin in lactating dairy cows. Am J Vet Res 49:1888.

Rosin E, et al. 1993. Cefazolin antibacterial activity and concentrations in serum and the surgical wound in dogs. Am J Vet Res 54:1317.

Silley P, et al. 1988. Pharmacokinetics of cephalexin in dogs and cats after oral, subcutaneous, and intramuscular administration. Vet Rec 122:15.

Soback S, et al. 1987. Clinical pharmacology of cefazolin in calves. J Vet Med 34A:25.

Group 2, Oral First-generation Cephalosporins: Cefadroxil, Cephradine, Cephalexin, and Cephaloglycin

First-generation, group 2, oral cephalosporins share the characteristics of the group 1 parenteral cephalosporins in high activity against Gram-positive bacteria, including beta-lactamase-producing *Staphylococcus aureus;* moderate activity against certain nontransferable, beta-lactamase-producing, Gram-negative Enterobacteriaceae and fastidious Gram-negatives; and no activity against *Enterobacter* spp., *P. aeruginosa*, and *Serratia* spp., among others (see Tables 7.2 and 7.4).

Antimicrobial Activity

Antimicrobial activity of oral cephalosporins is similar to that of aminopenicillins with the addition of resistance to the beta-lactamase of *S. aureus.*

Good Susceptibility (MIC ≤8 μg/ml) is shown by many Gram-positive bacteria, including *S. aureus*, streptococci (not enterococci), *Actinomyces* spp., *Bacillus* spp., *Corynebacterium* spp., *Erysipelothrix rhusiopathiae*, and most *Listeria monocytogenes* (see Table 7.2). Susceptible anaerobes include some *Bacteroides*, most *Clostridium* spp., and most *Fusobacterium* spp. Susceptible aerobes include fastidious organisms such as *Bordetella avium*, *Haemophilus* spp., and *Pasteurella* spp.

Variable Susceptibility, due to acquired resistance, is shown by *E. coli*, *Klebsiella* spp., *Proteus* spp., and *Salmonella* spp.

Moderate Susceptibility (MIC 16 μg/ml): Actinobacillus spp., *Brucella* spp., and some *Bacteroides* spp.

Resistance (MIC ≥32 μg/ml): Acinetobacter spp., *Bacteroides fragilis*, *Bordetella bronchiseptica, Campylobacter* spp., *Citrobacter* spp., *Enterobacter* spp., *Nocardia* spp., *Enterococcus faecalis, Pseudomonas aeruginosa, Rhodococcus equi, Serratia* spp., and *Yersinia* spp.

Antibiotic Resistance

Acquired resistance occurs in Gram-negative bacteria and is particularly important in Enterobacteriaceae.

Pharmacokinetic Properties

Oral cephalosporins have pharmacokinetic properties similar to those of penicillin V and the aminobenzylpenicillins. Generally cephalosporins are rapidly and largely absorbed after oral administration in monogastrates; these drugs are unaffected by the presence of food (except for cephradine). Relatively wide distribution occurs in extracellular fluids, but penetration across biological membranes is poor. Inflammation enhances passage across barriers. Half-lives are short, usually less than 1 hour, although cefadroxil has a longer half-life in dogs. Cephalosporins are largely excreted unchanged in urine. Plasma protein binding is low. Absorption in horses and ruminants is poor and highly erratic.

Drug Interactions

Oral cephalosporins are potentially synergistic with aminoglycosides, although indications for such combinations would be unusual.

Toxicities and Side Effects

Cephalosporins are among the safest of antimicrobial drugs. Allergic reactions, including acute anaphylactic hypersensitivity, are rare. In

TABLE 7.5. **Recommended oral dosage of oral cephalosporins in animals**

Species	Drug	Dose (mg/kg)	Interval (h)	Comments
Dogs, cats	Cefadroxil	22	12	Range 15–30 mg/kg
	Others	10–15	8	
Calves	Cefadroxil	25	12	
(preruminants)	Cefaclor	3.5	12	
	Cephadrine	7	12	
Horses	Cefadroxil	20–40	8	Foals only

humans, the majority of allergic reactions are not cross-reactive with penicillin. A small proportion of human patients may develop eosinophilia, rash, and drug fever. Vomiting and diarrhea may occur in a small proportion of monogastrates given oral cephalosporins.

Administration and Dosage

Recommended dosage is shown in Table 7.5. Oral cephalosporins should be administered to monogastrates 3 times daily, although cefadroxil may be administered twice daily at the higher dose. Oral cephalosporins should not be used in herbivores.

Clinical Applications

Oral cephalosporins have applications similar to those of penicillinase-resistant penicillins and aminobenzylpenicillins in monogastrate animals, so that they are widely used in small animal medicine. The cephalosporins are thus potentially useful in a variety of nonspecific infections caused by staphylococci, streptococci, Enterobacteriaceae, and some anaerobic bacteria. Long-term use (30 days) in the treatment of chronic *Staphylococcus aureus* pyodermas in dogs is one useful application. Prophylactic use on 2 consecutive days a week prevented recurrence of German Shepherd recurrent furunculosis (Bell, 1995). Cephalexin has been described as the drug of choice for *Klebsiella pneumoniae* urinary tract infections (Ling and Ruby, 1983), although a fluoroquinolone is now a better choice. Apart from skin and urinary tract infections caused by susceptible organisms, other applications include the treatment of abscesses and wound infections caused by susceptible organisms in dogs and cats.

Bibliography

Angarano DW, MacDonald JM. 1989. Efficacy of cefadroxil in the treatment of bacterial dermatitis in dogs. J Am Vet Med Assoc 194:57.

Bell A. 1995. Prophylaxis of German Shepherd recurrent furunculosis (German Shepherd dog pyoderma) using cephalexin pulse therapy. Aust Vet Pract 25:30.

Campbell BG, Rosin E. 1998. Effect of food on absorption of cefadroxil and cephalexin in dogs. J Vet Pharmacol Ther 21:418.

Duffee NE, et al. 1997. The pharmacokinetics of cefadroxil over a range of oral doses and animal ages in the foal. J Vet Pharmacol Ther 20:427.

Frank LA, Kunkle GA. 1993. Comparison of the efficacy of cefadroxil and generic and proprietary cephalexin in the treatment of pyoderma in dogs. J Am Vet Med Assoc 203:530.

Ling GV, Ruby AL. 1983. Cephalexin for oral treatment of canine urinary tract infection caused by *Klebsiella pneumoniae*. J Am Vet Med Assoc 182:1346.

Silley P, et al. 1988. Pharmacokinetics of cephalexin in dogs and cats after oral, subcutaneous, and intramuscular administration. Vet Rec 122:15.

Soback S, et al. 1987. Clinical pharmacology of five oral cephalosporins in calves. Res Vet Sci 43:166.

Thornton JR, Martin PJ. 1997. Pharmacokinetics of cephalexin in cats after oral administration of the antibiotic in tablet and paste preparations. Aust Vet J 75:439.

Whittem T, Slacek B. 1996. Contrast between the pharmacokinetics of two formulations of cephalexin after intramuscular administration in cattle. N Z Vet J 44:145.

Group 3, Second-generation Parenteral Cephalosporins: Cefaclor, Cefoxitin, Cefotetan, Cefuroxime, and Cefamandole

Second-generation, group 3, parenteral cephalosporins have a wide spectrum of antibacterial activity largely because of their stability to a broad range of beta-lactamases. They are moderately active against Gram-positive bacteria. Cephamycins (cefotetan, cefoxitin) are products of *Streptomyces* rather than of *Cephalosporium* species and differ from cephalosporins in the presence of a methoxy group in the 7 position of the cephalosporin nucleus. Cephamycins are very stable to beta-lactamases, including those of *Bacteroides fragilis* but, like other second-generation drugs, are not active against *Pseudomonas aeruginosa*.

Antimicrobial Activity

Cefoxitin is resistant to most bacterial beta-lactamases, although it penetrates Gram-negative bacteria relatively poorly. Antimicrobial activity is slightly broader and greater than that of cefazolin and other first-generation cephalosporins for Gram-negative bacteria and includes *Enterobacter* spp. and *Serratia* spp. Activity against Gram-positive bacteria is slightly less. Cefoxitin is stable to the beta-lactamase of *Bacteroides fragilis* and has good activity against this and other *Bacteroides, Porphyromonas,* and *Prevotella* spp. *Pseudomonas aeruginosa,* enterococci, and some Enterobacteriaceae are resistant (Tables 7.2 and 7.6). Of the 7-methoxy cephalosporins, cefotetan has the greatest activity against Gram-negative bacteria, but *P. aeruginosa* is resistant. A proportion of *Citrobacter, Enterobacter,* and *Serratia* species are resistant. Activity against anaerobes is similar to that of cefoxitin, but a proportion of *B. fragilis* are resistant. Cefmetazole has a spectrum of activity similar to that of cefoxitin but is more active against Enterobacteriaceae.

TABLE 7.6. **Susceptibility of human medical opportunist pathogens to selected beta-lactam antibiotics**

Organism	Susceptibility (%)							
	Ampicillin	Carbenicillin	Cefamandole	Cefoxitin	Cephalothin	Latamoxef	Oxacillin
Enterobacter aerogenes	27	73	73	0	0	100	0
E. agglomerans	20	30	90	40	40	90	0
Escherichia coli	65	68	90	98	75	100	0
Klebsiella pneumoniae	2	10	98	90	90	100	0
Proteus mirabilis	85	85	94	97	88	100	0
P. rettgeri	46	69	92	85	0	100	0
Pseudomonas aeruginosa	—	72	—	—	—	53	0
Serratia spp.	7	63	19	70	0	96	0
Staphylococcus aureus	—	—	99	97	97	92	94

Source: Modified from Perryman et al. (1983) with permission.

Resistance

Stable derepression of inducible beta-lactamases in certain Gram-negative pathogens is an important mechanism of resistance. Cefoxitin is a powerful beta-lactamase inducer and can therefore antagonize the effects of other beta-lactams. Transferable, broad-spectrum plasmid-mediated resistance to beta-lactamase-stable cephalosporins has increasingly been described.

Pharmacokinetic Properties

Pharmacokinetic properties and toxicities are similar to those of first-generation parenteral cephalosporins. With one exception, they are not absorbed following oral administration. Excretion, which can be delayed by probenecid, is largely renal. Half-lives in cattle and horses are about 1 hour. The 3-hour half-life of cefotetan in humans allows twice-daily dosing. Cefuroxime axetil is an ester of cefuroxime that is hydrolyzed in the intestinal mucosa and liver to yield active drug, producing good bioavailability after oral administration.

Toxicities and Adverse Effects

Second-generation cephalosporins cause pain on IM injection and may cause thrombophlebitis when administered IV. One of six mares administered cefoxitin IM developed acute laminitis (Brown et al., 1986). Cefoxitin may cause hypoprothrombinemia and a tendency to bleed in human patients. Cefamandole in humans produces alcohol intolerance by blocking liver acetaldehyde dehydrogenase and may cause a coagulopathy associated with hypoprothrombinemia, which is reversible by vitamin K. For this latter reason, cefamandole is rarely if ever used in human medicine. Use in animals has been too limited to describe toxicities, but the broad antibacterial activity of second-generation cephalosporins may lead to gastrointestinal disturbances and superinfection by resistant microorganisms, including yeasts. This has been particularly marked with cefuroxime axetil administered orally to human patients.

Administration and Dosage

Administration is usually IV because of pain associated with IM dosage. Dosage in animals, which in some cases is empirical, is shown in Table 7.7. Cefuroxime axetil is administered orally in monogastrates.

Clinical Applications

Clinical applications in animals are limited by the expense of these drugs but may be similar to those identified in human medicine where cefoxitin is valued particularly for its broad activity against anaerobes,

TABLE 7.7. **Dosage of group 3 and 4 parenteral cephalosporins**

Species	Drug	Dose (mg/kg)	Interval (h)
Dogs, cats	Cefotaxime IM	20–40	8
	Cefotaxime SC	20–40	12
	Cefoperazone IV, IM	20–25	6–8
	Cefoxitin IV, IM, SC	15–30	6–8
	Ceftiofur IM	2.2	24
	Ceftizoxime IV, IM	25–40	8–12
	Ceftriaxone IV, IM	25	12–24
	Cefuroxime axetil PO	10–15	8–12
	Cefuroxime IV	10–15	8–12
Cattle	Ceftiofur IM	1–2.2	24
	Cefquinome IM	1	24
Goats	Cefotaxime IV, IM	20–40	12
Horses	Cefotaxime IV	20–30	6–8
	Cefoxitin IV, IM	20	8
	Ceftiofur IM	2.2	12–24
	Ceftriaxone IV, IM	25	12 (not adults?)
Swine	Ceftiofur IM	2.2	24

Note: Many dosages listed here are empirical.

especially *Bacteroides fragilis*, as well as against Enterobacteriaceae. Indications are thus treatment of severe mixed infections with anaerobes (aspiration pneumonia, severe bite infections, gangrene, peritonitis, pleuritis) and prophylaxis in colonic surgery or ruptured intestine. Cefuroxime is available and effective for short-lasting dry-cow therapy. Cefuroxime axetil is used by the oral route in human medicine for the treatment of otitis media and upper respiratory infections caused by susceptible bacteria. The widespread use of cephalosporins for this purpose may have been largely responsible for the extensive emergence of penicillin resistance in *Streptococcus pneumoniae*, an important human pathogen, in recent years.

Bibliography

Brown MP, et al. 1986. Pharmacokinetics and body fluid and endometrial concentrations of cefoxitin in mares. Am J Vet Res 47:1734.

Caprile KA. 1988. The cephalosporin antimicrobial agents: a comprehensive review. J Vet Pharmacol Ther 11:1.

Garrod LP, et al. 1981. Antibiotics and Chemotherapy, 5th ed. New York: Churchill Livingstone.

Perry CM, Brogden RN. 1996. Cefuroxime axetil: a review of its antibacterial activity, pharmacokinetic properties, and therapeutic efficacy. Drugs 52:125.

Perryman F, et al. 1983. In vitro activity of moxalactam against pathogenic bacteria and its comparison with other antibiotics. Chemotherapy 29:37.

Petersen SW, Rosin E. 1993. In vitro antibacterial activity of cefoxitin and pharmacokinetics in dogs. Am J Vet Res 54:1496.

Soback S. 1988. Pharmacokinetics of single doses of cefoxitin given by the intravenous and intramuscular routes to unweaned calves. J Vet Pharmacol Ther 11:155.

Group 4, Third-generation Parenteral Cephalosporins: Cefmenoxime, Cefotaxime, Cefquinome, Ceftizoxime, Ceftriaxone, Ceftiofur, and Latamoxef

Third-generation, group 4, parenteral cephalosporins are distinguished by their high antibacterial activity and their broad resistance to beta-lactamases; they have particularly good activity against most Enterobacteriaceae. Exceptions include *Enterobacter* and *Serratia*. Streptococci are highly susceptible, staphylococci are moderately susceptible, and enterococci are resistant. Latamoxef (moxalactam) is an oxacephem with an oxygen atom replacing the sulfur at the C-1 position of the cephalosporin nucleus. Its wide anti-Enterobacteriaceae activity is similar to that of others in the group, but latamoxef is more active against *Bacteroides fragilis, Citrobacter* spp., and *Enterobacter* spp. and less active against *Staphylococcus aureus* (Tables 7.6 and 7.8). Some *Pseudomonas aeruginosa* are resistant.

Good Susceptibility (MIC ≤2 μg/ml): Highly active against streptococci, including *Streptococcus suis* (not enterococci). Good activity against many other Gram-positive bacteria (benzyl penicillin sensitive) (see Tables 7.2, 7.6, and 7.8). Among Gram-negative bacteria, *E. coli, Klebsiella* spp., *Proteus* spp., and *Salmonella* spp. are susceptible. Fastidious Gram-negative bacteria (*Actinobacillus* spp., *Haemophilus* spp., *Pasteurella* spp.), including beta-lactamase producers, are all highly susceptible. *Clostridium* spp. and *Fusobacterium* spp. are susceptible, but *Bacteroides* spp. are often resistant.

Moderately Susceptible (MIC 4 μg/ml): *Staphylococcus aureus;* some *Citrobacter* spp., *Enterobacter* spp., some *Pseudomonas aeruginosa,* and *Serratia* spp. (see Table 7.6).

TABLE 7.8. Susceptibility (MIC$_{90}$, μg/ml) of selected animal pathogens to ceftiofur

Organism	MIC$_{90}$	Organism	MIC$_{90}$
Gram-positive aerobes			
Staphylococcus aureus	1	*S. equi*	≤0.004
S. hyicus	1	*S. suis*	0.12
Streptococcus dysgalactiae	≤0.004	*S. uberis*	0.03
Gram-negative aerobes			
Actinobacillus pleuropneumoniae	≤0.008	*Pasteurella haemolytica*	≤0.016
Escherichia coli	0.5	*P. multocida*	≤0.004
Haemophilus somnus	≤0.004	*Salmonella* spp.	1
Moraxella bovis	0.25		
Anaerobic bacteria			
Bacteroides fragilis	≥16	*Fusobacterium necrophorum*	≤0.06
Bacteroides spp.	4	*Peptostreptococcus anaerobius*	0.12

Sources: Data from Salmon et al. (1996); Samitz et al. (1996); Shryock et al. (1998).

Resistance (MIC ≥8 μg/ml): Acinetobacter spp., *Bordetella* spp., some *Enterobacter* spp. and *Serratia* spp., some *Pseudomonas aeruginosa,* enterococci, and methicillin-resistant *Staphylococcus aureus.*

Antibiotic Resistance

Stable derepression of inducible beta-lactamases in certain Gram-negative pathogens is an important mechanism of resistance. Transferable, broad-spectrum plasmid-mediated resistance to beta-lactamase-stable cephalosporins has increasingly been described. Both are threats to the continued use of these cephalosporins.

Pharmacokinetic Properties

Third-generation, group 4, parenteral cephalosporins are not absorbed after oral administration but are rapidly and well absorbed after IM or SC administration, giving peak serum levels in 0.5–1 hour. Although data are often lacking, the half-life is about 1 hour following IV infection. In cattle, the half-life of ceftiofur is about 2.5 hours. By contrast, the half-lives for many of these cephalosporins are 1–2 hours for humans, with the marked exception of ceftriaxone, which, because of extensive protein-binding, has a half-life of 8 hours, giving it the potential for once-daily dosing. Half-life of latamoxef in humans is about 2 hours. Distribution into tissues in extracellular fluid is widespread, but passage across membranes or physiological barriers is poor. Meningeal inflammation significantly enhances otherwise poor CSF penetration so that, because of exceptional antibacterial activity, these cephalosporins are drugs of choice for bacterial meningitis caused by Enterobacteriaceae. Cefotaxime is metabolized in the body to the less active desacetyl-cefotaxime. Excretion is largely through the urinary tract, with cefotaxime being excreted through tubular mechanisms and the others through glomerular filtration. Probenecid administration delays tubular excretion. Biliary elimination also occurs, notably for ceftriaxone and latamoxef. These drugs should therefore be avoided in species with expanded large intestines. Ceftriaxone has a long elimination half-life, giving this drug the advantage of twice-daily dosing.

Drug Interactions

Group 4 cephalosporins are synergistic with aminoglycosides, with which they often need to be combined in the treatment of febrile illness in neutropenic human patients.

Toxicities and Side Effects

Toxicities and side effects are similar to those described for cephalosporins of groups 1–3, but the nephrotoxic potential is low. Cefmenoxime in humans produces alcohol intolerance by blocking liver acetaldehyde dehydrogenase and a coagulopathy associated with hypoprothrombinemia, which is reversible by vitamin K. Clinically important bleeding disorders caused by hypoprothrombinemia or disorders of platelet function are more common with latamoxef than with any other cephalosporin in human patients (about 20%), so that this drug is not generally recommended for clinical use. Vitamin K prophylaxis is suggested if the drug is used. Because of the broad antibacterial activity of these cephalosporins, gastrointestinal disturbances and superinfection by resistant microorganisms, including yeasts, might be anticipated. In human medicine, there is a strong association between group 4 and 6 cephalosporin use and *Clostridium difficile* diarrhea. In horses, IM administration has been occasionally associated with gastrointestinal disturbance, including severe colitis. Gastrointestinal disturbances were noted in 4 of 6 mares administered ceftriaxone IV (Gardner and Aucoin, 1994), probably because of its biliary excretion, so this drug should be used cautiously if at all in horses. Cutaneous drug reaction to ceftiofur, characterized by hair loss and pruritus, has been described in a cow (Tyler et al., 1998).

Administration and Dosage

Recommended IM dosages, which in some cases are empirical, are shown in Table 7.7. To some extent, dosage can be tailored to the susceptibility of the organism, with the aim to maintain drug concentrations at $\geq$MIC throughout the majority of the dosing interval. For example, dosage of ceftiofur for highly susceptible organisms associated with lower respiratory disease is usually 1.1–2.2 mg/kg q24 hours, but for *E. coli* infections caused by susceptible organisms the dose might be as high as 2.2–4.4 mg/kg q12 hours. Ceftriaxone has the advantage that dosage is twice daily, whereas dosage of other group 4 cephalosporins (other than ceftiofur) is usually q8 hours; q12-hour administration of cefotaxime was found to be as effective as q8-hour administration in the treatment of mild to moderate, non-CNS infections in people (Brogden and Spencer, 1997).

Clinical Applications

Because of expense, the availability of cheaper alternatives, and the potential to select for resistant bacteria, third-generation group 4 cephalosporins should be reserved for serious, probably life-threatening infections caused by Gram-negative bacteria, especially Enterobacteriaceae. These cephalosporins are drugs of choice in meningitis caused by *E. coli* or *Klebsiella* spp. They are recommended, in combination with an aminoglycoside, in severe infections caused by multiply resistant bacteria in compromised hosts, such as neutropenic hosts. These drugs have potential application in septicemia, serious bone and joint infections, some lower respiratory tract infections, intra-abdominal infections caused by Enterobacteriaceae, and some soft-tissue infections where cheaper alternative drugs are not available. There is increasing interest in their value in treating systemic complications of human salmonellosis (bacteremia, meningitis, osteomyelitis). The poor activity of some of these cephalosporins against Gram-negative anaerobes is a drawback; ceftiofur, however, has good activity against anaerobes.

CATTLE, SHEEP, AND GOATS

Ceftiofur is used extensively for the treatment of acute, undifferentiated bovine pneumonia with the advantage of a low recommended dose (1.1–2.2 mg/kg q24 hours) and zero drug withdrawal time. Treatment is for 3–5 days and has proved as effective as treatment with sulbactam-ampicillin or potentiated sulfonamides for this purpose (Schumann and Janzen, 1991; Jim et al., 1992). Nebulization may improve efficacy (Sustronck et al., 1995) but may be difficult to achieve in the field. A single needleless IM sustained-release implant of 250 mg drug was as effective in treating calves with respiratory disease as IM injection of 250 mg daily for 3 days (Kesler and Bechtol, 1999). Dosage IM of 3 mg/kg q12 hours was inadequate for the parenteral treatment of mastitis caused by *E. coli*, and dosage IM of 2.2 mg/kg q24 hours failed to remove *Streptococcus agalactiae* infections, since udder distribution is poor because of ceftiofur's high plasma protein binding (Erskine et al., 1995, 1996). Dosage at 1 mg/kg IM was effective in the treatment of foot rot in feedlot cattle (Morck et al., 1998). Cefquinome is used in treatment of bovine respiratory disease and, by intramammary administration, in the treatment of coliform and other bacterial mastitis.

HORSES

Ceftiofur is suitable for use in horses in treating bacterial infections caused by susceptible bacteria (Table 7.8). At 2.2 mg/kg IM q24 hours, it was shown to be as effective as ampicillin in the treatment of respiratory infections in adult horses (Folz et al., 1992). Doses up to 11 mg/kg per day for 30 days were well tolerated (Mahrt, 1992). Intramuscular rather than oral administration is a drawback. The drug has potential application for treatment of septicemia in foals, perhaps combined with an aminoglycoside. It has been used successfully to treat pleuritis and peritonitis caused by susceptible organisms. Cefotaxime has been used effectively in the treatment of neonatal septicemia and meningitis caused by *Acinetobacter* spp., *Enterobacter* spp., and *Pseudomonas aeruginosa* (Morris et al., 1987). Ceftriaxone may be particularly suitable for the treatment of meningitis in foals because it crosses the healthy blood–cerebrospinal fluid barrier. A dosage suggested for Gram-negative bacterial meningitis was 25 mg/kg q12 hours (Ringger et al., 1998). This drug should, however, be used with caution in adult horses because of its hepatic excretion.

SWINE

Ceftiofur is available for use in swine in the treatment of respiratory or systemic infections caused by susceptible bacteria such as *Pasteurella multocida* and beta-lactamase-producing *Actinobacillus* spp. It may also have application for IM administration in the treatment of neonatal colibacillosis.

DOGS AND CATS

Ceftiofur and other group 4 cephalosporins might be useful in the treatment of urinary tract infections caused by otherwise resistant bacteria.

POULTRY

Ceftiofur is administered IM to poults for the control of *E. coli* infections.

Bibliography

Atef M, et al. 1990. Pharmacokinetic profile of cefotaxime in goats. Res Vet Sci 49:34.

Brogden RN, Spencer CM. 1997. Cefotaxime. Drugs 53:483.

Brown SA, et al. 1995. Plasma and urine disposition and dose proportionality of ceftiofur and metabolites in dogs after subcutaneous administration of ceftiofur sodium. J Vet Pharmacol Ther 18:363.

Cervantes CC, et al. 1993. Pharmacokinetics and concentrations of ceftiofur sodium in body fluids and endometrium after repeated intramuscular injections in mares. Am J Vet Res 54:573.

Erskine RJ, et al. 1995. Ceftiofur distribution in serum and milk from clinically normal cows and cows with experimental *Escherichia coli*–induced mastitis. Am J Vet Res 56:481.

Erskine RJ, et al. 1996. Intramuscular administration of ceftiofur sodium versus intramammary infusion of penicillin/novobiocin for treatment of *Streptococcus agalactiae* mastitis in dairy cows. J Am Vet Med Assoc 208:258.

Folz SD, et al. 1992. Treatment of respiratory infections in horses with ceftiofur sodium. Equine Vet J 24:300.

Gardner SY, Aucoin DP. 1994. Pharmacokinetics of ceftriaxone in mares. J Vet Pharmacol Ther 17:155.

Jim GK, et al. 1992. A comparison of trimethoprim-sulfadoxine and ceftiofur sodium for the treatment of respiratory disease in feedlot calves. Can Vet J 33:245.

Kesler DJ, Bechtol DT. 1999. Efficacy of sustained release needle-less ceftiofur sodium implants in treating calves with bovine respiratory disease. J Vet Med 46B:25.

Mahrt CR. 1992. Safety of ceftiofur sodium administered intramuscularly in horses. Am J Vet Res 53:2201.

McElroy D, et al. 1986. Pharmacokinetics of cefotaxime in the domestic cat. Am J Vet Res 47:86.

Meyer JC, et al. 1992. Pharmacokinetics of ceftiofur sodium in neonatal foals after intramuscular injection. Equine Vet J 24:485.

Morck DW, et al. 1998. Comparison of ceftiofur sodium and oxytetracycline for treatment of acute interdigital phlegmon (foot rot) in feedlot cattle. J Am Vet Med Assoc 212:254.

Morris DD, et al. 1987. Therapy in two cases of neonatal foal septicemia and meningitis with cefotaxime sodium. Equine Vet J 19:151.

Peeryman F, et al. 1983. In vitro activity of moxalactam against pathogenic bacteria and its comparison with other antibiotics. Chemotherapy 29:37.

Ringger NC, et al. 1998. Pharmacokinetics of ceftriaxone in neonatal foals. Equine Vet J 30:163.

Salmon SA, et al. 1996. In vitro activity of ceftiofur and its primary metabolite, desfuroylceftiofur, against organisms of veterinary importance. J Vet Diagn Invest 8:332.

Samitz EM, et al. 1996. In vitro susceptibilities of selected obligate anaerobic bacteria obtained from bovine and equine sources to ceftiofur. J Vet Diagn Invest 8:121.

Schumann FJ, Janzen ED. 1991. Comparison of ceftiofur sodium and sulbactam-ampicillin in the treatment of bovine respiratory disease. Wien Tieraertzl Monatsschr 78:185.

Shryock TR, et al. 1998. Antimicrobial susceptibility of Moraxella bovis. Vet Microbiol 61:305.

Soback S. 1989. Pharmacokinetics of single-dose administration of moxalactam in unweaned calves. Am J Vet Res 50:498.

Soback S, Ziv G. 1988. Pharmacokinetics and bioavailability of ceftriaxone administered intravenously and intramuscularly to calves. Am J Vet Res 49:535.

Soback S, et al. 1989. Pharmacokinetics of ceftiofur administered intravenously and intramuscularly to lactating cows. Isr J Vet Med 45:119.

Sustronck B, et al. 1995. Evaluation of the nebulization of sodium ceftiofur in the treatment of experimental Pasteurella haemolytica bronchopneumonia in calves. Res Vet Sci 59:267.

Tell L, et al. 1998. Pharmacokinetics of ceftiofur sodium in exotic and domestic avian species. J Vet Pharmacol Ther 21:85.

Tyler JW, et al. 1998. Probable ceftiofur-induced cutaneous drug reaction in a cow. Can Vet J 39:296.

Group 5, Third-generation Oral Cephalosporins: Cefetamet and Cefixime

Third-generation, group 5, oral cephalosporins are highly active cephalosporins resistant to many beta-lactamases and available for oral administration. Cefixime is structurally related to cefotaxime and ceftizoxime and shares their antibacterial activity. Cefetamet pivoxil is a prodrug hydrolyzed to the active cefetamet and largely shares the antibacterial spectrum of cefixime and group 4 parenteral cephalosporins.

Among Gram-positive aerobes, third-generation oral cephalosporins are largely inactive against Staphylococcus aureus, active against pyogenic streptococci, and inactive against enterococci. They have broad activity against Enterobacteriaceae, which may exclude Citrobacter and Enterobacter. Pseudomonas are resistant. Among human pathogens, they are active against beta-lactamase-producing Haemophilus spp. but inactive against penicillin-resistant Streptococcus pneumoniae. Bacteroides fragilis is resistant. Activity against animal bacterial pathogens has not been significantly assessed.

Absorption of cefetamet occurs well after oral administration and indeed is increased by food, but otherwise its pharmacokinetic properties are typical of those of beta-lactams generally. Adverse effects relate mainly to gastrointestinal disturbance (diarrhea, nausea, vomiting), which occurs in about 10% of human patients. Dosage recommended for cefetamet in children is 20 mg/kg q12 hours. Cefetamet is used in the treatment of upper respiratory and urinary tract infections in people.

Cefixime's long elimination half-life allows once-daily administration in people. It is used in people for the same purposes as cefetamet, but its use as an orally administered "follow-up" to a group 4 parenteral cephalosporin has also been advocated. Adverse effects are largely limited to gastrointestinal disturbance. Dosage recommendations in children are 8 mg/kg q24 hours or 4 mg/kg q12 hours. A suggested dosage for dogs is in the same range (Lavy et al., 1995) and for preruminant calves 10 mg/kg q24 hours (Ziv et al., 1995).

Bibliography

Bryson HM, Brogden RN. 1993. Cefetamet pivoxil. Drugs 45:589.
Lavy E, et al. 1995. Clinical pharmacologic aspects of cefixime in dogs. Am J Vet Res 56:633.
Markham A, Brogden RN. 1995. Cefixime. Drugs 49:1007.
Ziv G, et al. 1995. Clinical pharmacology of cefixime in unweaned calves. J Vet Pharmacol Ther 18:94.

Group 6, Antipseudomonal Parenteral Cephalosporins: Cefoperazone, Cefsulodin, and Ceftazidime

Antipseudomonal, group 6, parenteral cephalosporins are distinguished by the high activity against *Pseudomonas aeruginosa*. Cefsulodin has otherwise a very narrow spectrum of activity. Ceftazidime and cefoperazone have a spectrum of activity almost identical to group 4 cephalosporins but with approximately 10 and 3 times greater activity against *P. aeruginosa*, respectively. Resistance to ceftazidime is rare in *P. aeruginosa*. The group 6 drugs are otherwise slightly less active than group 4 drugs against most organisms. Antipseudomonal cephalosporins are synergistic with aminoglycosides, with which they are often combined in the treatment of *P. aeruginosa* infections in neutropenic human patients. Resistance, through mutation to stable derepression of chromosomally mediated beta-lactamases, in *Enterobacter, Citrobacter, Serratia*, and other genera of the Enterobacteriaceae, or through plasmids has been described.

Pharmacokinetic properties are similar to those described for other parenteral cephalosporins. One exception is the largely hepatic elimination of cefoperazone, which therefore tends to be relatively often associated with gastrointestinal disturbance in humans. Thus, this drug is contraindicated in horses and other herbivores with an expanded large bowel. Cefoperazone, but not ceftazidime, elimination in urine is reduced by

TABLE 7.9. Empirical IM dosage of group 6 antipseudomonal parenteral cephalosporins

Species	Drug	Dose (mg/kg)	Interval (h)
Dogs, cats	Cefoperazone	30	6–8
	Ceftazidime	25–50	8–12
Cattle	Cefoperazone	30	6–8
	Ceftazidime	20–40	12–24
Horses (caution)	Cefoperazone	30	6–8
	Ceftazidime	25–50	8–12

probenecid. There has been little study of the pharmacokinetic properties in animals. In calves, half-life is about 2 hours (Soback and Ziv, 1989a, 1989b).

Toxicities and side effects are the same as for other cephalosporins generally. Cefoperazone is likely contraindicated in those herbivore species with an expanded large bowel. Empirical dosage is shown in Table 7.9.

These drugs are largely reserved in human medicine for *P. aeruginosa* and other Gram-negative septicemias in neutropenic human patients, in which efficacy is considerably enhanced by combination with an aminoglycoside. Cephalosporins have slow bactericidal activity relative to aminoglycosides.

Cefoperazone is used by the intramammary route as a broad-spectrum antibiotic for the treatment of bovine mastitis (Wilson et al., 1986). The advantage claimed is that a single infusion of 250 mg in an oil base gives milk concentrations of ≥MIC of common pathogens for up to 48 hours but, because of systemic absorption, milk concentrations are very low by the fifth milking, which reduces the discard loss of milk. The drug may have particular advantage in the treatment of coliform mastitis. The rapid development of resistance during therapy in bacteria possessing inducible, chromosomal cephalosporinases must be anticipated but has not yet been documented in veterinary medicine.

Bibliography

Rains CP, et al. 1995. Ceftazidime. Drugs 49:577.

Rice LB, et al. 1990. Outbreak of ceftazidime resistance caused by extended-spectrum beta-lactamases at a Massachusetts chronic-case facility. Antimicrob Agents Chemother 34:2193.

Soback S, Ziv G. 1989a. Pharmacokinetics of ceftazidime given alone and in combination with probenecid to unweaned calves. Am J Vet Res 50:1566.

Soback S, Ziv G. 1989b. Pharmacokinetics of single doses of cefoperazone given by the intravenous and intramuscular routes to unweaned calves. Res Vet Sci 47:158.

Wilson CD, et al. 1986. Field trials with cefoperazone in the treatment of bovine clinical mastitis. Vet Rec 118:17.

Group 7, Fourth-generation Parenteral Cephalosporins: Cefepime, Cefpirome

The fourth-generation, group 7, parenteral cephalosporins have high activity against Enterobacteriaceae, moderate activity against *Pseudomonas aeruginosa*, and enhanced activity against staphylococci. They are stable to hydrolysis by many plasmid- or chromosomally mediated beta-lactamases and are poor inducers of group 1 beta-lactamases. They have recently been introduced into human medicine.

Antimicrobial Activity

Cefepime is an enhanced-potency, extended-spectrum cephalosporin, the zwitterionic nature of which gives it rapid ability to penetrate through the porins of Gram-negative bacteria to the cell membrane. Both cefepime and cefpirome have higher affinity for essential PBPs and greater resistance to hydrolysis by beta-lactamases than other cephalosporins. In particular, they are resistant to, and a poor inducer of, group 1 beta-lactamases. There are no reports of activity against specific animal pathogens, however.

Good Susceptibility (MIC ≤8 µg/ml): Methicillin-susceptible *Staphyloccus* spp.; *Streptococcus* spp.; Enterobacteriaceae, including *Citrobacter* spp., *Enterobacter* spp., *E. coli,* and *Serratia* resistant to group 4 cephalosporins; *Pseudomonas aeruginosa,* including isolates resistant to group 6 cephalosporins; beta-lactamase-producing *Haemophilus* spp.; *Clostridium perfringens,* and *Peptostreptococcus* spp. (Table 7.10).

Resistance (MIC ≥32 µg/ml): *Enterococcus* spp., *Listeria monocytogenes,* *Bacteroides* spp., and *Clostridium difficile.*

Pharmacokinetic Properties

Pharmacokinetic properties of these parenterally administered cephalosporins are typical of those of other parenteral cephalosporins generally. Most drug is excreted through the urine.

TABLE 7.10. **Antimicrobial activity (MIC_{90}, µg/ml) of cefepime and cefpirome**

Organism	Cefepime	Cefpirome
Staphylococcus aureus (methicillin-sensitive)	2	0.5
Streptococcus agalactiae	0.12	0.06
Enterococcus faecalis	16	4
Escherichia coli	0.12	0.12
Proteus mirabilis	0.06	0.06
Pseudomonas aeruginosa	4	8
Acinetobacter spp.	8	4

Drug Interactions

Combination of cefepime with aztreonam is synergistic against *P. aeruginosa* with derepressed cephalosporinases, since aztreonam protects cefepime against these enzymes in the extracellular environment (Lister et al., 1998).

Toxicities and Adverse Effects

Toxicities and adverse effects in people are those of cephalosporins generally, with the major effect being gastrointestinal disturbance. Treatment was withdrawn in about 5% of patients treated with cefpirome and 1–3% of patients treated with cefepime because of adverse effects. Gastrointestinal effects must be anticipated if these drugs are used in animals.

Administration and Dosage

These drugs are administered IV or IM twice daily to human patients; dosage can to some extent be tailored to the nature and severity of the infection. In horses, a dosage recommendation was 2.2 mg/kg q8 hours (Guglick et al., 1998). This is a very low dosage based on extrapolation from the empirical dose of 50 mg/kg q8 hours in children.

Clinical Applications

Fourth-generation cephalosporins are used in human medicine in the treatment of nosocomial or community-acquired lower respiratory disease, bacterial meningitis, urinary tract infections, and uncomplicated skin or skin-related infections. They have shown no advantage in clinical trials comparing them to cefotaxime or ceftazidime in treatment of infections in people. These drugs are valuable extended-spectrum cephalosporins for the treatment of serious infections in people. As such, it is unlikely that they will have much application in animals in the near future.

Bibliography

Barradell LB, Bryson HM. 1994. Cefepime. Drugs 47:471.
Guglick MA, et al. 1998. Pharmacokinetics of cefepime and comparison with those of ceftiofur in horses. Am J Vet Res 59:458.
Lister PD, et al. 1998. Cefepime-aztreonam: a unique double β-lactam combination for *Pseudomonas aeruginosa*. Antimicrob Agents Chemother 42:1610.
Sanders CC. 1993. Cefepime: the next generation? Clin Infect Dis 17:369.
Wiseman LR, Lamb HM. 1997. Cefpirome. Drugs 54:117.

8

Other Beta-lactam Antibiotics: Beta-lactamase Inhibitors, Carbapenems, and Monobactams

J. F. PRESCOTT

The continuing development of beta-lactam antibiotics by changes of atoms within the basic beta-lactam ring or its attachment to the thiazolidine ring has produced compounds with significantly different activity from penam penicillins and the cephalosporins and cephamycins. Carbapenem and monobactam class antibiotics (see Fig. 6.2) have been introduced into human medicine, but none have been approved for use in veterinary medicine. By contrast, some beta-lactamase inhibitors (clavulanic acid, sulbactam) have been successfully introduced into veterinary medicine in combination with aminobenzylpenicillins, producing broad-spectrum antibacterial drugs that overcome the limitations that some of the acquired resistance had placed on the older extended-spectrum penicillins.

Beta-lactamase Inhibitors: Clavulanic Acid, Sulbactam, and Tazobactam
Introduction
Beta-lactamase production is a major factor in constitutive or acquired resistance of bacteria to beta-lactam antibiotics. The clinical importance of beta-lactamases has been associated particularly with the rapid ability of plasmid-mediated resistance to spread through bacterial populations. Such resistance has considerably reduced the value of what were once important drugs, such as amoxicillin. Three beta-lactamase inhibitors—clavulanic acid, sulbactam, and tazobactam—have considerably enhanced the activity of penicillins against bacteria with acquired plasmid-mediated resistance (Fig. 8.1). Although possessing weak antibacterial activity on their own, their irreversible binding to susceptible

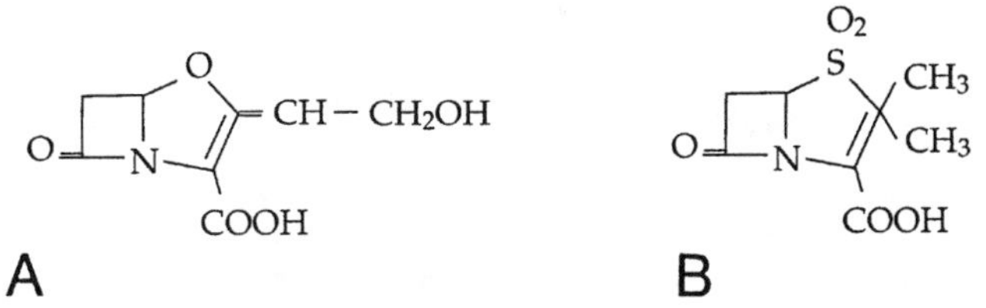

Fig. 8.1. Structural formulas of clavulanic acid *(A)* and sulbactam *(B)*.

beta-lactamases allows the active beta-lactam antibiotic, with which they are combined, to bind to the penicillin-binding proteins (PBPs), resulting in lysis of the bacterial pathogen (Table 8.1). Antibiotics combined for clinical use with clavulanic acid or sulbactam, which both have a similar spectrum of beta-lactamase-inhibiting activities, have included amoxicillin, ampicillin, and ticarcillin. Clavulanic acid and sulbactam are synergistic with a number of penicillins and cephalosporins that are readily hydrolyzed by plasmid-mediated beta-lactamases, including benzyl- and aminobenzylpenicillins and third-generation cephalosporins. Introduction of clavulanic acid and sulbactam has been a significant advance in antimicrobial therapy of infections in animals. The beta-lactamase inhibitors should be used with caution in herbivores with expanded large intestines because of potential for disrupting normal flora, resulting in diarrheic illness.

Beta-lactamases: Classification

Beta-lactamases are enzymes that degrade beta-lactam drugs by opening the beta-lactam ring (see Fig. 6.5A). The beta-lactamases of clinically important pathogens have been studied in exquisite detail and shown to consist of a wide variety of related proteins, with more than 200 unique beta-lactamases described. They may be chromosomally mediated (inducible or constitutive) or plasmid-mediated. Beta-lactamases of Gram-positive bacteria may be exported extracellularly, whereas beta-lactamases of Gram-negative bacteria are found in the periplasmic space but may be found extracellularly when the bacterium lyses (see Figs. 6.3 and 6.4).

Classification is now usually based on a combination of molecular characterization (nucleotide, amino acid sequence) and functional characterization (substrate, inhibition profile) (see Table 8.1) (Bush et al., 1995). Bush groups are identified according to substrate hydrolysis profiles (eg, benzyl penicillin, cephaloridine, ceftazidime, cefotaxime, aztreonam, imipenem) and according to inhibition by clavulanic acid and EDTA.

TABLE 8.1. Classification of bacterial beta-lactamases

Bush Group	Preferred Substrates	Inhibition by Clavulanate	Inhibition by EDTA	Representative Enzymes	Molecular Class
1	Cephalosporins	–	–	AmpC, chromosomal cephalosporinases from Gram-negatives	C
2a	Penicillins	+	–	Gram-positive penicillinases	A
2b	Penicillins, cephalosporins	+	–	TEM-1, TEM-2, SHV-1	A
2be	Penicillins, narrow- and broad-spectrum cephalosporinases, monobactams	+	–	TEM-3 ... TEM-26, SHV-2 ... SHV-6	A
2c	Penicillins, cloxacillin	+	–	PSE-1, PSE-3, PSE-4	A
2d	Penicillins, cloxacillin	+	–	OXA-1 ... OXA-11	D
2e	Cephalosporins	+	–	Proteus vulgaris–inducible cephalosporinase	?
3	Most beta-lactams, including carbapenems	–	+	Xanthomonas maltophilia L1	B
4	Penicillins	–	?	Berkholderia cepacia penicillinase	?

Source: After Bush et al. (1995).

Hydrolysis is normalized in relation to hydrolysis rates for benzyl penicillin or cephaloridine. Although there is general correlation with molecular-based typing approaches, a functional approach to classification is preferred because very fine differences in molecular character may cause dramatic differences in function. For example, a mutation producing a single nucleotide change can convert a TEM-1 to a TEM-12 beta-lactamase, and a second single nucleotide change can convert this TEM-12 enzyme into a TEM-26 beta-lactamase, with marked effects on hydrolysis of ceftazidime.

The genes for beta-lactamases are found in the chromosome or on plasmids and may be moved from these sites by transposons. Transfer of some of these genes has been widespread within and among species, genera, and families. The evolution of beta-lactamases has occurred at a dramatic rate among bacteria, probably in response to selection by the extensive use of beta-lactam antibiotics, especially those with an increasing spectrum of activity. Plasmid-mediated beta-lactamases are centrally important in beta-lactamase resistance. For example, plasmid-mediated TEM-1 beta-lactamase, which encodes ampicillin resistance, has become widespread in *E. coli* that is being isolated from animals and from people from around the world, and it is now found in many other Enterobacteriaceae. More recently, plasmid-mediated extended-spectrum beta-lactamases (Bush group 2be) have emerged among *Klebsiella* spp. and other Enterobacteriaceae, some of which are not susceptible to beta-lactamase inhibitors. All Gram-negative bacteria produce beta-lactamases, usually Bush group 1, from genes located on their chromosomes. In some genera (eg, *Acinetobacter, Citrobacter, Enterobacter, Serratia*), they are inducible, producing high concentrations of enzyme that overwhelm local concentrations of beta-lactamase inhibitors. In some cases, therefore, mutants with derepressed inducible beta-lactamases have emerged among the genera listed that are resistant to the beta-lactams that previously were effective against them. Bush group 3 beta-lactamases are metalloenzymes that hydrolyze most beta-lactams and resist beta-lactamase inhibitors. Although not widespread, genes for these enzymes have been identified on plasmids among opportunist bacteria isolated from human patients.

Beta-lactamase Inhibitors

The concept behind the use of beta-lactamase inhibitors is that they exhibit little antibacterial activity in their own right, but they have a high affinity for beta-lactamases and can be administered with a beta-lactam that would be highly active against the pathogen if it were not for its beta-lactamases. In other words, the inhibitors (clavulanic acid, sulbactam, tazobactam) have high substrate specificity for a wide variety of beta-lactamases. Their binding to these enzymes is irreversible, thus allowing

TABLE 8.2. Activity (MIC$_{90}$, µg/ml) of amoxicillin and ampicillin with or without clavulanic acid and sulbactam, respectively

Organism	Amoxicillin	Amoxicillin-clavulanate	Ampicillin	Ampicillin-sulbactam
Gram-positive aerobes				
Staphylococcus aureus	64	8	16	1
Gram-negative aerobes				
Enterobacter spp.	>128	>128	>128	>128
Escherichia coli	>128	8	>128	8
Klebsiella spp.	>128	1	>128	8
Proteus spp.	>128	>128	>128	8
Pseudomonas aeruginosa	>128	>128	>128	>128
Salmonella spp.	>16	<1		
Gram-positive anaerobes				
Clostridium spp.	>256	16	0.3	16
Gram-negative anaerobes				
Bacteroides fragilis	256	4	32	0.5
Bacteroides spp.	32	1	0.5	1
Fusobacterium spp.	16	4	16	8

the active beta-lactam (amoxicillin, piperacillin, etc) to kill the organism since beta-lactamase is effectively absent. The efficacy of these inhibitors is shown in Table 8.2.

Bibliography

Amyes SG, Miles RS. 1998. Extended-spectrum β-lactamases: the role of inhibitors in therapy. J Antimicrob Chemother 42:415.

Bush K, et al. 1995. A functional classification scheme for β-lactamases and its correlation with molecular structure. Antimicrob Agents Chemother 39:1211.

Girard AE, et al. 1987. Activity of beta-lactamase inhibitor sulbactam plus ampicillin against animal isolates of *Pasteurella, Haemophilus, Staphylococcus*. Am J Vet Res 48:1677.

Ho JL. 1991. Beta-lactamase inhibition: therapeutic implications in infectious diseases. Rev Infect Dis 13:S723.

Livermore DM. 1995. β-lactamases in laboratory and clinical resistance. Clin Microbiol Rev 8:557.

Petrosino J, et al. 1998. β-lactamases: protein evolution in real time. Trends Microbiol 6:323.

Clavulanic Acid

Clavulanic acid is a synthetic compound, the bicyclic nucleus of which has similarities to a penicillin, apart from the oxygen in place of the sulfur and a missing acylamino side chain at position 6. It has good affinity for the majority of plasmid-mediated beta-lactamases (see Table 8.1) and all chromosomally mediated penicillinases, but little for chromosomal cephalosporinases. This latter group of enzymes, however, usually

TABLE 8.3. Activity (MIC$_{90}$, µg/ml) of amoxicillin-clavulanic acid against selected veterinary pathogens

Organism	MIC$_{90}$	Organism	MIC$_{90}$
Gram-positive cocci			
Staphylococcus aureus	0.6	Streptococcus agalactiae	≤0.08
S. intermedius	0.16	S. dysgalactiae	≤0.08
		S. suis	≤0.08
Gram-positive rods			
Arcanobacterium pyogenes	0.16	Listeria monocytogenes	0.16
Gram-negative aerobes			
Actinobacillus pleuropneumoniae	0.32	P. multocida	0.32
Escherichia coli	8	Proteus mirabilis	0.5
Haemophilus somnus	0.06	Pseudomonas spp.	≥32
Moraxella bovis	0.04	Salmonella	2.5
Pasteurella haemolytica	0.12		
Anaerobic bacteria			
Bacteroides fragilis	0.5	Fusobacterium spp.	≥32
Clostridium perfringens	0.5	Porphyromonas asaccharolytica	1.0

Source: C Hoare, Smith Kline Beecham (unpubl. obs.) with permission.

hydrolyze amoxicillin and ticarcillin, with which clavulanic acid is combined, poorly. Clavulanic acid is combined with amoxicillin in the ratio of 2:1 and with ticarcillin in the ratio of 15:1. The combinations are usually bactericidal at one or two dilutions below the MIC of amoxicillin or ticarcillin used alone.

CLAVULANIC ACID–AMOXICILLIN

Amoxicillin–clavulanic acid has a spectrum of activity similar to that of a first- or second-generation cephalosporin.

Good Susceptibility (MIC ≤8/4 µg/ml; for S. aureus, ≤4/2) is shown with several bacteria and excellent susceptibility of Gram-positive bacteria, including beta-lactamase-producing *S. aureus*. Fastidious Gram-negative bacteria (*Actinobacillus* spp., *Bordetella* spp., *Haemophilus* spp., *Pasteurella* spp.) are susceptible, including strains resistant to amoxicillin. Enterobacteriaceae such as *Escherichia coli, Klebsiella* spp., *Proteus* spp., and *Salmonella* spp. are usually susceptible; most anaerobes, including *Bacteroides fragilis*, are susceptible (Table 8.3).

Variable Susceptibility is found in some *E. coli* and *Klebsiella* spp.

Resistance (MIC ≥32/16 µg/ml) is shown among *Citrobacter* spp., *Enterobacter* spp., *Pseudomonas aeruginosa, Serratia* spp., and methicillin-resistant *Staphylococcus aureus*.

Antibiotic Resistance. Clavulanic acid may induce beta-lactamases in susceptible *Providencia* and *Enterobacter*. Emergence of resistance to clavulanic acid has not, however, been reported as a clinical problem in bacteria isolated from animals. Among human clinical bacterial isolates, a variety of resistance mechanisms have emerged. These include overproduction of resistant cephalosporinases that do not bind to clavulanic acid (see Table 8.1), hyperproduction of TEM beta-lactamases, reduced antibiotic uptake, and production of inhibitor-resistant beta-lactamases derived from TEM-1.

Pharmacokinetic Properties. Clavulanic acid is well absorbed after oral administration and has pharmacokinetic properties similar to amoxicillin. Tissue distribution in extracellular fluids is widespread, but penetration into milk and into uninflamed cerebrospinal fluid is relatively poor. Half-life is about 75 minutes. The drug is largely eliminated by renal excretion (unchanged in the urine).

Toxicity and Side Effects. The combination is well tolerated. The major side effect reported in about 10% of human patients has been gastrointestinal effects of nausea, vomiting, and diarrhea, after oral administration. This is associated with a direct effect on gastrointestinal motility of the clavulanic acid component, so recommended oral doses should not be exceeded. Mild gastrointestinal upset has been reported in dogs and cats. Other side effects are those of penicillins generally. The combination should not be used in penicillin- or cephalosporin-sensitive animals. The drug should not be administered orally to herbivores or by injection to horses. It should also not be used in rabbits, guinea pigs, hamsters, or gerbils.

Administration and Dosage. Recommended dosage is shown in Table 8.4. The recommendations by the manufacturers for once-daily dos-

TABLE 8.4. **Suggested dosage of penicillins potentiated by clavulanic acid, sulbactam, or tazobactam**

Drug	Species	Route	Dose (mg/kg)	Interval (h)
Clavulanate-amoxicillin	Dogs, cats	PO	12.5–20	8–12
		SC	10	8
	Cattle	IM	7	12–24
	Preruminant	PO	5–10	12
	Sheep	IM	8.75	12–24
Clavulanate-ticarcillin	Dogs, cats	IV	40–50	6–8
	Horses	IV	50	6
Sulbactam-ampicillin	Cattle	IM	10	24
Piperacillin-tazobactam	Dogs, cats	IV	4	6

ing of parenterally administered drug in food animals represents under-dosing, with twice-daily or more frequent administration taking advantage of the time-dependent pharmacodynamic requirement for efficacy of beta-lactam drugs. Clinical trials comparing dosage in food animals might confirm this deduction.

Clavulanic acid is highly moisture sensitive, so precautions must be taken to ensure dryness during storage.

Clinical Applications. Clavulanic acid–amoxicillin is a valuable addition as an orally administered antibiotic in monogastrates. It extends the range of amoxicillin against beta-lactamase-producing common opportunist pathogens, including fastidious organisms, Enterobacteriaceae, and anaerobic bacteria. It is not effective against *Pseudomonas aeruginosa*. Some *E. coli*, *Proteus*, and *Klebsiella* are susceptible only to urinary concentrations of the combination, so the combination can be recommended for empirical treatment of urinary tract infections in dogs and cats. Activity against anaerobes is a particularly useful attribute.

The drug should not be administered orally to herbivores or by injection to horses, rabbits, guinea pigs, hamsters, or gerbils.

The combination is a valuable addition as a parenterally (IM) administered drug in food-producing animals, particularly for lower respiratory tract infections of cattle and pigs caused by beta-lactamase-producing *Actinobacillus*, *Haemophilus*, and particularly *Pasteurella*. Its potential in the treatment of *E. coli* diarrhea and of salmonellosis needs to be explored in clinical trials.

Cattle, Sheep, and Goats. Clavulanic acid–amoxicillin has been introduced for use in cattle. Potential use includes the treatment of lower respiratory tract infections, particularly of soft tissue infections, including anaerobic infections, plus possibly neonatal calf diarrhea caused by *E. coli* and *Salmonella*. The drug cannot be recommended for parenteral treatment of mastitis but is used for intramammary administration. In sheep, the combination can be recommended in the treatment of pasteurellosis (Gilmour et al., 1990). There are few published data on pharmacokinetic behavior of the drug in ruminants, but the dosing rate recommended by the manufacturer (see Table 8.4) appears low. There may therefore be advantage to at least twice-daily injection of the recommended dose.

Swine. The combination has potential application in the treatment of a variety of infections in swine caused by plasmid-mediated beta-lactamase-producing bacteria, possibly including neonatal diarrheal *E. coli* (Webster, 1990). Clinical trials of the value of this drug for different purposes are needed.

Dogs and Cats. Clavulanic acid–amoxicillin has many applications in dogs and cats, with the advantage of twice-daily oral administration for medication by owners. Among other applications are skin and soft tissue infections caused by *Staphylococcus aureus* and infections following bite wounds that involve mixed bacteria, including anaerobes; upper and lower respiratory tract infections; anal sacculitis; gingivitis; and urinary tract infections involving common opportunist bacteria *(S. aureus, E. coli, Proteus, Klebsiella)*. Apart from urinary tract infections, the drug is not recommended for serious infections caused by *S. aureus, E. coli, Proteus,* or *Klebsiella,* since tissue concentrations may not exceed the MIC for some strains for a sufficient part of the dosing interval. Interestingly, however, doubling the dose was not associated with increased cure in the treatment of canine pyoderma (Lloyd et al., 1997). The drug was less effective than a fluoroquinolone, marbofloxacin, in treating urinary tract infections in dogs (Cotard et al., 1995). The drug may have particular value in peritonitis associated with intestinal content spillage, because of its activity against enteric bacteria, including anaerobes.

Bibliography

Bywater RJ, et al. 1985. Efficacy of clavulanate-potentiated amoxycillin in experimental and clinical skin infections. Vet Rec 116:177.

Cotard JP, et al. 1995. Comparative study of marbofloxacin and amoxicillin–clavulanic acid in the treatment of urinary tract infections in dogs. J Small Anim Pract 36:349.

Gilmour NJL, et al. 1990. Treatment of experimental pasteurellosis in lambs with clavulanic acid and amoxicillin. Vet Rec 126:311.

Indivieri MC, Hirsh DC. 1985. Clavulanic acid–potentiated activity of amoxicillin against *Bacteroides fragilis.* Am J Vet Res 46:2207.

Jones RL, et al. 1994. Clinical observations on the use of oral amoxycillin/clavulanate in the treatment of gingivitis in dogs and cats and anal sacculitis in dogs. Br Vet J 150:385.

Lloyd DH, et al. 1997. Treatment of canine pyoderma with co-amoxyclav: a comparison of two dose rates. Vet Rec 141:439.

Senior DF, et al. 1985. Amoxycillin and clavulanic acid combination in the treatment of experimentally induced bacterial cystitis in cats. Res Vet Sci 39:42.

Webster CJ. 1990. Parenteral amoxycillin-clavulanate in the treatment of diarrhea in young pigs. Vet Rec 126:263

CLAVULANIC ACID–TICARCILLIN

Clavulanic acid–ticarcillin is available as a parenteral (usually IV) drug for use in human medicine. It offers the advantage over clavulanic acid–amoxicillin of the greater activity of ticarcillin against *Enterobacter* and *Pseudomonas aeruginosa.* The combination has good activity against the majority of ticarcillin-resistant Enterobacteriaceae, *Staphylococcus aureus,* anaerobes (including *Bacteroides fragilis*), and many *Pseudomonas aeruginosa.* However, the MIC_{90} of bacterial isolates from disease processes, especially *Enterobacter, Escherichia coli,* and *Klebsiella,* is on the high end of the susceptibility range (MIC ≤16 µg/ml) or in the moderately susceptible range (MIC 32–64 µg/ml) (Sparks et al., 1988). No potentiating activity occurs with the combination for *Enterobacter, P. aeruginosa,* and *Serratia,* and results of treatment of human clinical infections caused by these organisms have sometimes been disappointing, possibly because of induction of beta-lactamases by the clavulanate component. The combination has the disadvantage in animals of requiring frequent (8-hour) IV dosage (see Table 8.4), although a 12-hour dosing interval may be used in neonatal foals. In human medicine, it may have application in the empirical treatment of serious infections in immunocompromised patients, when combined with an aminoglycoside. Applications of clavulanic acid–ticarcillin in veterinary medicine appear to be few.

Bibliography

Garg RC, et al. 1987. Serum levels and pharmacokinetics of ticarcillin and clavulanic acid in dogs following parenteral administration of timentin. J Vet Pharmacol Ther 10:324.

Sanders C, Cavalieri SJ. 1990. Relevant breakpoints for ticarcillin–clavulanic acid should be set primarily with data from ticarcillin-resistant strains. J Clin Microbiol 28:830.

Sparks SE, et al. 1988. In vitro susceptibility of bacteria to a ticarcillin–clavulanic acid combination. Am J Vet Res 49:2038.

Sweeney RW, et al. 1988. Pharmacokinetics of intravenously and intramuscularly administered ticarcillin and clavulanic acid in foals. Am J Vet Res 49:23.

Wilson WD, et al. 1991. Pharmacokinetics and bioavailability of ticarcillin and clavulanate in foals after intravenous and intramuscular administration. J Vet Pharmacol Ther 14:78.

Sulbactam

Sulbactam (penicillinic acid sulfone) is a synthetic derivative of 6-aminopenicillanic acid. It is poorly absorbed orally, but a double ester linkage of sulbactam with ampicillin has been developed to produce the prodrug sultamicillin, which is well absorbed orally and releases the two drugs in the intestinal wall. Sulbactam has no antibacterial activity by itself but irreversibly binds the same groups of beta-lactamases as clavulanic acid, though sulbactam's affinity is several times lower. It also binds beta-lactamases of *Citrobacter, Enterobacter, Proteus,* and *Serratia* that clavulanic acid does not. The same level of inhibition as clavulanic acid can, however, be achieved by increasing the concentration of sulbactam (2:1) for clinical use. It is combined with ampicillin in part because of pharmacokinetic similarities but has also been combined with cefoperazone.

SULBACTAM-AMPICILLIN

Antibacterial activity of sulbactam-ampicillin is slightly broader but is marginally lower than that of clavulanic acid–amoxicillin (see Tables 8.1 and 8.2). Sulbactam-ampicillin's lower affinity for beta-lactamases may limit its activity against some potent beta-lactamase-producing bacteria (Gisby and Beale, 1988).

Pharmacokinetic properties are similar to those of amoxicillin–clavulanic acid, but sulbactam is poorly absorbed orally. It is available for use in human medicine as the orally absorbed prodrug sultamicillin. The combination is well absorbed after IM injection, distributes well into tissues in the extracellular space, and penetrates cerebrospinal fluid through inflamed meninges. Penetration into milk is modest. Elimination is largely in the urine. The half-life is about 1 hour.

The combination used for parenteral injection is well tolerated, and the side effects are those of penicillins generally, without the diarrhea that may occur with the orally administered clavulanic acid–amoxicillin. Intramuscular injection may be painful. The combination should not be used in herbivores with expanded large intestines (horses, rabbits, hamsters, guinea pigs), although adverse effects were not observed in foals (Hoffman et al., 1992).

Clinical Applications. Sulbactam-ampicillin restores and extends the antibacterial activity of ampicillin to include common bacteria that have acquired beta-lactamases. Sulbactam-ampicillin has been introduced into food animal medicine for the treatment of bovine respiratory disease for its activity against *Pasteurella* (including beta-lactamase-producing strains), *Haemophilus somnus, Arcanobacterium pyogenes,* and opportunist bacteria, including *E. coli.* The efficacy and superiority of the combination to ampicillin alone has been demonstrated in experimental and field studies (Bentley and Cummins, 1987; Grimshaw et al., 1987a; Gifford et al., 1988). It was as efficacious as ceftiofur in the treatment of bovine respiratory disease in one study (Schumann and Janzen, 1991). Its advantage over ampicillin in the parenteral treatment of undifferentiated diarrhea in neonatal calves has been demonstrated (Grimshaw et al., 1987b). Once-daily dosage in cattle, though clinically effective, appears to represent underdosing based on pharmacokinetic and pharmacodynamic considerations, and there may be advantage to more frequent dosing. The combination might be useful, given at high dosage, for *E. coli* meningitis in calves. This combination may also see extralabel use for diseases such as salmonellosis; however, there have been no clinical trials reporting its use for diseases other than undifferentiated bovine respiratory disease and enteric colibacillosis. Others of the many potential clinical applications are described for cattle under benzyl penicillin and clavulanic acid–amoxicillin, with the combination clearly having the advantage over benzyl penicillin for many applications. Suggested dosing is shown in Table 8.4.

Bibliography

Bentley OE, Cummins JM. 1987. Efficacy of sulbactam, a beta-lactamase inhibitor, combined with ampicillin in the therapy of ampicillin-resistant pneumonic pasteurellosis in feedlot calves. Can Vet J 28:591.

Gifford GA, et al. 1988. Clinical and pathological evaluation of sulbactam/ampicillin for treatment of experimental bovine pneumonic pasteurellosis. Can Vet J 29:142.

Gisby J, Beale AS. 1988. Comparative efficacies of amoxicillin–clavulanic acid and ampicillin-sulbactam against experimental *Bacteroides fragilis–Escherichia coli* mixed infections. Antimicrob Agents Chemother 32:1830.

Grimshaw WTR, et al. 1987a. The efficacy of sulbactam-ampicillin in the therapy of respiratory disease associated with ampicillin resistant *Pasteurella* species in housed cattle. Vet Rec 121:393.

Grimshaw WTR, et al. 1987b. Efficacy of sulbactam-ampicillin in the treatment of neonatal calf diarrhea. Vet Rec 121:162.

Hoffman AM, et al. 1992. Evaluation of sulbactam plus ampicillin for treatment of experimentally induced *Klebsiella pneumoniae* lung infection in foals. Am J Vet Res 53:1059.

Schumann FJ, Janzen ED. 1991. Comparison of ceftiofur sodium and sulbactam-ampicillin in the treatment of bovine respiratory disease. Wien Tieraertzl Monatsschr 78:185.

Tazobactam

Tazobactam is a beta-lactamase inhibitor with activity similar to but broader than that of clavulanic acid and sulbactam. For example, it resists hydrolysis by Bush group 1 and group 3 beta-lactamases in addition to beta-lactamases inhibited by clavulanic acid (see Table 8.1). Unlike clavulanic acid, it is only a poor to moderate inducer of beta-lactamases. Combined with piperacillin in an 8:1 ratio (piperacillin: tazobactam), it has considerably enhanced the activity of this group 5 (antipseudomonal) penicillin against beta-lactamase-producing bacteria generally.

The combination possesses broad-spectrum activity against many Enterobacteriaceae and other Gram-negative bacteria. Minor exceptions include *Enterobacter* spp. and *Xanthomonas maltophilia*. Activity against anaerobic bacteria such as *Bacteroides fragilis,* including cefoxitin-resistant *B. fragilis,* is an important feature of the combination. It is active against a wide range of Gram-positive bacteria. Pharmacokinetic properties are typical of beta-lactam drugs generally.

Indications in humans medicine are generally those where third-generation cephalosporins are indicated, with an emphasis on the additional beneficial effects of this combination against anaerobic bacteria. It rivals imipenem in breadth of antibacterial activity. The drug is, therefore, used in treatment of intra-abdominal infections (where mixed aerobic-anaerobic infections are likely to be present) and other polymicrobial infections. It is as effective for this purpose as clindamycin-gentamicin combination or as imipenem. It is also used in the treatment of fever in neutropenic patients (in combination with an aminoglycoside). Its advantage over ticarcillin–clavulanate combination in the treatment of human community-acquired lower respiratory infection has been convincingly demonstrated. Although indications for use in animals of this broad-spectrum drug are few, empirical dosage is suggested in Table 8.4.

Bibliography

Bryson HM, Brogden RN. 1994. Piperacillin/tazobactam. Drugs 47:506.
Sanders EW, Sanders CC. 1996. Piperacillin/tazobactam: a critical review of the evolving clinical literature. Clin Infect Dis 22:107.

Carbapenems: Imipenem-Cilastatin, Meropenem, and Biapenem

Carbapenems (see Fig. 6.2) are derivatives of *Streptomyces* spp. that differ from penam penicillins by the substitution of a CH_2 group for the sulfur in the five-membered ring attached to the beta-lactam ring. They have the widest activity of any antibiotic, except possibly trovafloxacin, being highly active against a wide variety of Gram-positive and Gram-negative bacteria and resistant to many beta-lactamases. *N*-Formimidoyl thienamycin (imipenem) is stable to bacterial beta-lactamases other than the Bush group 3 beta-lactamases. Its hydrolysis by a dihydropeptidase in the kidney is overcome by 1:1 combination with cilastatin, a dihydropeptidase inhibitor. Other semisynthetic carbapenems—meropenem and biapenem—have activity similar to that of imipenem but resist degradation by the renal dihydropeptidase.

Antibacterial Activity

Carbapenems are active against almost all clinically important aerobic or anaerobic Gram-positive or Gram-negative cocci or rods. Individual species may be resistant. They offer the advantages of broad antimicrobial activity and, in contrast to third- and fourth-generation cephalosporins, resistance to Bush groups 1 and 2 beta-lactamases. Biapenem and meropenem are slightly less active than imipenem against Gram-positive bacteria but equivalent or slightly more active against Gram-negative aerobes.

Good Susceptibility (MIC ≤4 µg/ml) is shown by most pathogenic bacteria, which includes most Gram-positive bacteria; imipenem is highly active against Gram-positive cocci (including most enterococci), similar to that of benzyl penicillin. *Mycobacterium avium-intracellulare, Nocardia* spp., and *Brucella* spp. are susceptible. Carbapenems are highly active against anaerobic bacteria, including *Bacteroides fragilis.* These drugs are the most active of the beta-lactam antibiotics against Gram-negative bacteria. Their activity includes beta-lactamase-producing fastidious organisms; Enterobacteriaceae, including beta-lactamase-producing isolates, and most *Pseudomonas aeruginosa.* They are slightly less active against *Proteus* spp. than against other enteric organisms.

Resistance (MIC ≥16 µg/ml) is shown by methicillin-resistant *Staphylococcus aureus*, *Burkholderia cepacia*, and some *Enterobacter* spp., *Aeromonas* spp., *Pseudomonas aeruginosa*, *Xanthomonas maltophilia*, and *Enterococcus faecium*.

Antibiotic Resistance

Resistance during therapy with imipenem has been commonly reported in *Pseudomonas aeruginosa* and attributed to alterations in outer-membrane proteins, which reduce permeability; many of these isolates are susceptible to meropenem. Resistance through metalloenzyme carbapenemases occurs in some isolates from the species listed under Antibacterial Activity: Resistance, above. Stably derepressed high-level beta-lactamase-producing mutants of *Citrobacter* spp., *Enterobacter* spp., and *Serratia* spp. may be more susceptible to carbapenems than to third- and fourth-generation cephalosporins.

Pharmacokinetic Properties

These carbapenems are not absorbed after oral administration, although orally administered carbapenems are being developed. Following IV administration, they are widely distributed to extracellular fluid throughout the body and reach therapeutic concentrations in most tissues in humans. There is poor penetration into cerebrospinal fluid even with inflamed meninges. They have the low volume of distribution that is typical of beta-lactam drugs. Imipenem is almost exclusively eliminated through the kidneys, being metabolized in renal tubules by a dihydropeptidase enzyme. Addition of cilastatin prevents this metabolism. This increases the elimination half-life and allows the drug to be excreted in large amounts in active form into urine. Half-life of these carbapenems is about 1 hour. Pharmacokinetic studies have not addressed the distribution of this drug in animals of veterinary importance.

Toxicity and Side Effects

The most common side effects in human patients have been gastrointestinal disturbance (nausea, vomiting, diarrhea) in about 4% of patients and hypersensitivity reactions (rash) in about 3% of patients, and, for imipenem, seizures in about 0.5% of patients have been associated with high doses, renal failure, or underlying neurological abnormalities. Liver enzymes may rise transiently during treatment. Meropenem use in people is associated with a lower incidence of gastrointestinal disturbance than imipenem and does not cause seizures.

Drug Interactions

Carbapenems may be synergistic with aminoglycosides against *Pseudomonas aeruginosa*. Rapid emergence of resistance in *P. aeruginosa* (about 20%) during treatment with imipenem suggests that it should be combined with an aminoglycoside for infections with this organism, although the combination may not prevent the emergence of resistance.

Administration and Dosage

Imipenem is administered IV (over 20–30 minutes) or by deep IM injection q8 hours. Dosage in dogs and cats, for which it is used occasionally, is empirical, in the range 5–10 mg/kg q8 hours. Meropenem is administered IV; an empiric dosage is 5–10 mg/kg q8 hours.

Clinical Applications

These extraordinary antimicrobial drugs are used in human medicine in the treatment of hospital-acquired infections caused by multiply resistant Gram-negative bacteria or by mixed aerobic and anaerobic infections, particularly including infections in immunocompromised patients. Purposes for which they are used successfully in human patients include a variety of serious infections: intra-abdominal infections (less effective than piperacillin-tazobactam but equivalent to clindamycin-tobramycin or cefotaxime-metronidazole); severe lower respiratory tract infections (as or more effective than third-generation cephalosporin-amikacin treatment); septicemia (equivalent to ceftazidime-amikacin in febrile neutropenic patients); life-threatening soft tissue infections and osteomyelitis. Imipenem is not recommended for the treatment of bacterial meningitis or of *Pseudomonas aeruginosa* infection. Meropenem is as effective as cefotaxime or ceftriaxone in treatment of bacterial meningitis in people.

Carbapenems should be reserved for the treatment of infections caused by cephalosporin-resistant Enterobacteriaceae and for empirical treatment of febrile illness in neutropenic patients (see Chapter 19). They would likely be used only rarely in veterinary medicine. The potential for emergence of *P. aeruginosa* resistant to imipenem suggests that administration of imipenem with an aminoglycoside would be prudent. The growing tendency of small animal intensive care units, reported anecdotally, to use imipenem as a first-line antibacterial drug in seriously ill animals with undiagnosed infection is likely to result in progressive development of resistant nosocomial infections in these settings. The problem with the use of these drugs is that they have such broad-spectrum bactericidal action that bacterial superinfections with resistant bacteria are likely, leading to contamination of the environment with such naturally resistant bacteria.

Bibliography

Balfour JA, et al. 1996. Imipenem/cilastatin. Drugs 51:99.
Jaccard C, et al. 1998. Prospective randomized comparison of imipenem-cilastatin and piperacillin-tazobactam in nosocomial pneumonia or peritonitis. Antimicrob Agents Chemother 42:2966.

Orsini JA, Perkons S. 1994. New beta-lactam antibiotics in critical care medicine. Compend Contin Educ Pract Vet 16:183.

Rasmussen BA, Bush K. 1997. Carbapenem-hydrolyzing β-lactamases. Antimicrob Agents Chemother 41:223.

Wiseman LR, et al. 1995. Meropenem. Drugs 50:73.

Monobactams: Aztreonam

Monobactams possess the simple beta-lactam ring without the attached thiazolidine ring (see Fig. 6.2). Aztreonam was the first monobactam introduced into human medicine. Other monobactams such as tigemonam, which can be administered orally, are in clinical trials in human medicine. Aztreonam is a synthetic analog of an antibiotic isolated from a *Streptomyces* species. It binds mainly to PBP3, disrupting cell wall synthesis, and is stable to most beta-lactamases. Comments below are largely confined to aztreonam.

Antibacterial Activity

Good Susceptibility (MIC ≤8 µg/ml) is limited by PBP3 binding to almost all Gram-negative aerobic bacteria, particularly fastidious organisms (*Haemophilus* spp., *Pasteurella* spp.) and Enterobacteriaceae. The susceptibility of *Pseudomonas aeruginosa* is variable.

Resistance (MIC ≥32 µg/ml) is shown in Gram-positive bacteria and anaerobic bacteria. Other *Pseudomonas* spp., *Burkholderia cepacia, Citrobacter* spp., and *Enterobacter* spp. are often resistant because they are susceptible to extended-spectrum (Bush group 2be) beta-lactamases.

Antibiotic Resistance

Aztreonam is hydrolyzed by extended-spectrum beta-lactamase producers but is resistant to Bush group 1 cephalosporinases.

Pharmacokinetic Properties

Aztreonam is not absorbed after oral administration. It is rapidly absorbed after IM injection in human patients and distributes widely in extracellular fluid throughout the body. Penetration into the cerebrospinal fluid of human patients with meningitis has achieved concentrations that should eliminate infections with Enterobacteriaceae. Half-life is about 1.6 hours in people; elimination is mainly renal.

Toxicity and Side Effects

Toxicity is similar to that of benzyl penicillin, with no apparent cross-allergy in human patients allergic to penicillins or cephalosporins. These drugs do not cause the gastrointestinal disturbances associated with carbapenems and other broad-spectrum beta-lactam antibiotics. Their inactivity against Gram-positive bacteria may lead to superinfection with yeasts and with Gram-positive aerobes, including *Enterococcus* spp. and *Staphylococcus aureus*.

Drug Interactions

Aztreonam is often synergistic with aminoglycosides, including aminoglycoside-resistant Gram-negative bacteria and *Pseudomonas aeruginosa*. This may have little advantage, since aztreonam is often used clinically as a substitute for an aminoglycoside. Aztreonam may have advantage combined with beta-lactams susceptible to Bush group 1 cephalosporinases, since it is poorly inactivated by these enzymes.

Administration and Dosage

Aztreonam is administered IV (over 3–5 minutes) or IM. An empirical dose in animals is 30–50 mg/kg q8 hours.

Clinical Applications

The narrow spectrum of aztreonam precludes its use in human medicine for empirical treatment of infections, except possibly for urinary tract infections. Its potential lies in the possibility to substitute for the more toxic aminoglycosides in combination therapy—for example, with clindamycin or metronidazole in serious, mixed anaerobic infections or with erythromycin in mixed infections where Gram-positive bacteria may be present. Aztreonam is used on its own in a wide variety of infections involving Gram-negative bacteria (urinary tract, lower respiratory tract, septicemia) with success as a relatively nontoxic drug in human medicine, including in seriously ill, immunocompromised patients infected with multiply resistant Gram-negative aerobes. Its place in veterinary medicine appears to be slight but might include treatment of meningitis in neonatal animals.

Bibliography

Chin N-X, Neu HC. 1988. Tigemonam, an oral monobactam. Antimicrob Agents Chemother 32:84.
Lister PD, et al. 1998. Cefepime-aztreonam: a unique double β-lactam combination for *Pseudomonas aeruginosa*. Antimicrob Agents Chemother 42:1610.
Neu HC, ed. 1990. Aztreonam's role in the treatment of gram-negative infection. Am J Med 88 (Suppl):3C.
Rubinstein E, Isturiz R. 1991. Aztreonam: the expanding clinical profile. Rev Infect Dis 13:S581.

Tribactams

Tribactams have a tricyclic structure related to that of carbapenems. Sanfetrinem cilexetil is the prodrug of sanfetrinem and is administered orally in people. It has high stability to many beta-lactamases and a broad spectrum of activity similar to that of carbapenems.

9 | Peptide Antibiotics: Polymyxins, Glycopeptides, Streptogramins, and Bacitracin

J. F. PRESCOTT

Polymyxins, glycopeptides, streptogramins, and bacitracin are peptide antibiotics with a variety of actions against bacteria. Because of their systemic toxicity, the clinical development of polymyxins and bacitracin has not been pursued since their discovery early in the antibiotic era. In contrast, glycopeptides and streptogramins continue to be of interest, particularly in human medicine, because of their activity against Gram-positive bacteria, including multiresistant enterococci.

Polymyxins

Polymyxins are antibiotic products of *Bacillus polymyxa*. When first described in the 1940s, they were of great interest for their activity against *Pseudomonas aeruginosa*. Their use against this organism has been replaced by less toxic drugs, but there is still interest in their use in chemically inactivating the endotoxin of Gram-negative bacteria. They are used now for local rather than parenteral applications.

Chemistry

Polymyxins are basic cyclic decapeptides. Colistin is polymyxin E and is chemically related to polymyxin B. Colistin is available as the sulfate for oral administration and as the less toxic sulfomethate (colistimethate sodium) for parenteral use. Polymyxin B is available as the sulfate for both purposes; 1 µg = 10 units polymyxin B. They are stable, highly water-soluble drugs.

TABLE 9.1. Activity (MIC$_{90}$, µg/ml) of polymyxin B and colistin against selected Gram-negative aerobes

Organism	Polymyxin B	Colistin
Actinobacillus sp.	0.5	≤4
A. pleuropneumoniae	—	1
Bordetella bronchiseptica	0.5	0.12
Brucella canis	100	16–32
Campylobacter jejuni	32	8
Escherichia coli	1	8–16
Haemophilus somnus	2	≤0.1
Klebsiella pneumoniae	1	4–8
Pasteurella multocida	4	—
Proteus spp.	128	>128
Pseudomonas aeruginosa	8	8
Salmonella spp.	128	—
Serratia spp.	20	—
Taylorella equigenitalis	2	0.5

Mechanism of Action

Polymyxins are cationic, surface-active agents that disrupt the structure of cell membrane phospholipids and increase cell permeability by a detergent-like action. This binding is competitive with calcium and magnesium. Polymyxins disorganize the outer membrane of Gram-negative bacteria by binding lipopolysaccharides (LPSs, endotoxins) through direct interaction with the anionic lipid A region.

Antimicrobial Activity

Polymyxin and colistin are similarly rapidly bactericidal and highly active against many species of Gram-negative organisms, such as *Escherichia coli, Salmonella,* and *Pseudomonas aeruginosa,* but not against *Proteus, Serratia,* or *Providencia* (Table 9.1). Gram-positive bacteria are resistant. Activity against *P. aeruginosa* is reduced in vivo by the presence of physiologic concentrations of calcium. Susceptible bacteria have MIC 1–4 µg/ml.

Coccidioides immitis is inhibited by clinically achievable drug concentrations (5–10 µg/ml), as is *Prototheca zopfii.*

Resistance

Acquired resistance is rare but occurs among *Pseudomonas aeruginosa* as a result of decreased bacterial permeability. There is complete cross-resistance among polymyxins.

Pharmacokinetic Properties

The polymyxins are not absorbed from the gastrointestinal tract. Systemic therapy therefore requires that a parenteral preparation (either polymyxin B sulfate or colistimethate sodium) be injected, preferably IM. After absorption from the injection site, polymyxins bind moderately to plasma proteins, diffuse poorly through biologic membranes, and attain low concentrations in transcellular fluids and in milk. Binding to mammalian cell membranes is a significant feature of distribution of polymyxins and underlies their accumulation in long-term dosing. They are slowly excreted unchanged by glomerular filtration in the urine. High concentrations of these drugs accumulate in patients with renal insufficiency. The polymyxins are highly nephrotoxic, causing damage to the renal tubular epithelial cells. For systemic use, colistin sulfomethate causes less pain at the injection site and less renal toxicity than polymyxin B, but polymyxin B has greater local activity. Methane sulfonate derivatives show better tissue distribution than the bases but are less active and lack the ability to inactivate endotoxin.

Drug Interactions

Polymyxins are synergistic with a variety of antimicrobial drugs through their disorganizing effects on the outer and cytoplasmic membranes. Synergism with sulfonamides and trimethoprim against a variety of Enterobacteriaceae, including otherwise resistant *Proteus* species and *Pseudomonas aeruginosa,* is recognized. Chelating agents such as ethylenediaminetetraacetic acid (EDTA) and cationic detergents such as chlorhexidine act synergistically against *P. aeruginosa* and are often used in the topical treatment of local infections caused by this organism.

Toxicity and Adverse Effects

Polymyxins are well tolerated after oral or local administration, but systemic use causes nephrotoxic, neurotoxic, and neuromuscular blocking effects. Colistin is less toxic than polymyxin B.

In humans, reversible peripheral neuropathy, with paresthesia, numbness around the mouth, blurring of vision, and weakness occur in about 7% of treated patients; neuromuscular blockade causing respiratory insufficiency occurs in about 2% of patients, particularly in those treated with high doses. Evidence of renal damage is found in about 20% of patients, so that renal function should be monitored in all treated patients. Toxicity may be potentiated by other nephrotoxic agents.

Calves treated with 5 mg/kg IM polymyxin B showed lethargy and apathy 2–4 hours after injection, and a small proportion developed transient ataxia. A dose of 5 mg/kg of polymyxin B or its sulfomethate was highly nephrotoxic, but 2.5 mg/kg had minimal effects. Colistin is less toxic. In sheep, 1 of 3 ewes died of respiratory failure within 2 hours of an IM dose of 10 mg/kg of polymyxin B (Ziv, 1981).

Administration and Dosage

Because of toxicity and the availability of less toxic and more efficacious alternatives, the drug should not be used parenterally in animals. An exception may be in the treatment of endotoxemia—for example, in horses. When administered parenterally, an appropriate IM dose of polymyxin B is 2.5 mg/kg at 12-hour intervals; the drug should not be given IV. The usual parenteral dose of colistimethate is 3 mg/kg administered IM at 12-hour intervals. Polymyxin B sulfate, 2.5 mg/kg IM at 12-hour intervals, may be administered to cows with severe coliform mastitis. For treatment of enteric infections, an oral dose of 5 mg/kg q12 hours has been recommended.

Clinical Applications

The advantages of polymyxins are that resistance rarely develops in susceptible Gram-negative bacteria (except some *Pseudomonas aeruginosa*), and they inactivate endotoxin. These benefits are offset by parenteral toxicity and the widespread availability of alternate, more efficacious, and less toxic drugs, so that polymyxins have a marginal place in antimicrobial therapy. The drugs should not be administered parenterally for more than 5 days unless kidney function is closely monitored. They should not be administered IV, nor should they be given in daily doses exceeding 5 mg/kg. Tissue penetration of polymyxins is poor and is associated with extensive cell membrane binding and inactivation.

The major potential applications of polymyxins are in the oral treatment of *E. coli* and *Salmonella* diarrheas, in the local or possibly the parenteral treatment of coliform mastitis, and in the local treatment of *P. aeruginosa*, such as otitis externa and superficial eye infections.

Infections of the skin, mucous membranes, eye, and ear caused by polymyxin B–sensitive microorganisms respond to local applications of the antibiotic as an ointment or in solution. To widen the range of antimicrobial activity, neomycin and bacitracin are combined with polymyxin B in some topical preparations. These combinations are most useful topically in treating local infections such as chronic otitis externa in dogs.

CATTLE

Polymyxins are useful for the treatment of colibacillosis and salmonellosis in calves. Orally administered colistin or polymyxin B may be a preferred drug in the treatment of *E. coli* diarrhea in calves. In salmonellosis, polymyxin B may be administered both orally and parenterally, possibly in combination with trimethoprim-sulfonamides because of the synergistic interactions. The drug must not be administered parenterally for more than 5 days, in doses not exceeding 5 mg/kg per day.

The potential of polymixins to inactivate endotoxin may be of use in the treatment of coliform mastitis, although this is largely a theoretical rather than field-demonstrated consideration. An IM dose of 5.0 mg/kg of polymyxin B should give milk concentrations exceeding 2 μg/ml for 4 hours, which is sufficient to eliminate the more susceptible coliforms. The fully protonized drugs, but not the methane sulfonate derivatives, can neutralize endotoxin of both sensitive and resistant coliforms. Such a protective effect is, however, seen only in the early stages of coliform mastitis, experimentally within 2–4 hours of infusion of endotoxin (Ziv, 1981). Since about 100 μg of polymyxin B inactivates only 0.2 μg of endotoxin, and endotoxin concentrations may reach 10 μg/ml in coliform mastitis, even intramammary doses are inadequate to remove all the endotoxin.

Polymyxin might be useful in *Prototheca* mastitis, but its use for this purpose has not been well documented.

SWINE

Polymyxins may be drugs of choice in the oral treatment of neonatal colibacillosis.

HORSES

Polymyxins are sometimes used locally to treat superficial infections of the eyes or uterus caused by otherwise resistant *Klebsiella* spp. or *Pseudomonas aeruginosa*. Polymixin B sulfate has been recommended at a low dose for the treatment of endotoxemia in horses early in the course of the disease (0.6 mg/kg, IV, q24 hours). Higher doses may produce transient signs of neurotoxicity. Renal function should be monitored if the drug is used systemically. Its use for this purpose has been based on experimental rather than clinical studies.

DOGS AND CATS

Polymyxins are sometimes used in the local treatment of superficial infections of the eyes, otitis externa, and other skin infections caused by susceptible Gram-negative bacteria. They are preferred for local *Pseudomonas* infections and may be combined with chlorhexidine or EDTA for synergistic effect.

Bibliography

Durando MM, et al. 1994. Effects of polymyxin B and *Salmonella typhimurium* antiserum on horses given endotoxin intravenously. Am J Vet Res 55:921.

Hasselman G, Ludvigsen JB. 1980. The effect of oral colistin on scouring in newborn piglets artificially infected with *E. coli*. Int Pig Vet Soc p171.

Pyorala S, et al. 1994. Efficacy of two therapy regimens for treatment of experimentally induced *Escherichia coli* mastitis in cows. J Dairy Sci 77:453.

Vaara M, Vaara T. 1983. Polycations sensitize enteric bacteria to antibiotics. Antimicrob Agents Chemother 24:107.

Yeary RA. 1975. Systemic toxic effects of chemotherapeutic agents in domestic animals. Vet Clin North Am 5:51.

Ziv G. 1981. Clinical pharmacology of polymyxins. J Am Vet Med Assoc 179:711.

Glycopeptides: Vancomycin, Teicoplanin, and Avoparcin

Vancomycin, teicoplanin, and avoparcin are glycopeptide antibiotics with activity against Gram-positive bacteria and particularly Gram-positive cocci. The drugs inhibit synthesis of cell wall peptidoglycan by forming bonds with the D-alanyl-D-alanine terminal of muramyl dipeptide. Vancomycin has limited use in veterinary medicine because of cost and the need for continuous IV infusion. The recently introduced teicoplanin (which has slightly better activity, can be administered IM, and has a remarkably long half-life) shows considerable potential for the use of glycopeptides in treating infections in animals. Avoparcin has, until recently, been used extensively as a growth promoter for chickens and pigs in Europe. It has been withdrawn for use because of its tendency to select for vancomycin-resistant enterococci in these species, which may then be a source of infection of immunosuppressed and thus high-risk human patients.

Vancomycin

Chemistry

Vancomycin is a high-molecular-weight glycopeptide, a fermentation product of *Streptomyces orientalis*. It is available as the stable and highly soluble hydrochloride.

Antimicrobial Activity

Vancomycin is bactericidal to most Gram-positive aerobic cocci and bacilli; most Gram-positive aerobes and anaerobes are susceptible, but the majority of Gram-negative bacteria are resistant. Organisms with MIC $\leq$2–4 µg/ml are regarded as susceptible, those with 8–16 µg/ml as intermediate, and those with $\geq$32 µg/ml as resistant (Table 9.2).

Resistance

Antibiotic resistance is generally uncommon but occurs with some frequency in *Enterococcus* spp., especially *E. faecium*, in which it has been extensively characterized. The *VanA* gene encodes resistance to all gly-

TABLE 9.2. **Activity (MIC$_{90}$, µg/ml) of vancomycin against selected bacteria**

Organism	MIC$_{90}$	Organism	MIC$_{90}$
Actinomyces spp.	8	*Listeria monocytogenes*	$\leq$1
Arcanobacterium pyogenes	1	*Nocardia*	256
Clostridium difficile	1	*Rhodococcus equi*	0.25
C. perfringens	1	*Staphylococcus aureus*	2
C. septicum	2	Beta-hemolytic streptocci	2
Enteroccus spp.	4		

copeptides and is associated with a plasmid-mediated transposable element Tn1546, which changes the D-alanyl-D-alanine part of the pentapeptide side chain of N-acetylmuramic acid to D-alanyl-D-lactate, preventing glycopeptide binding and thus evading inhibition of cell wall synthesis. VanB resistance affects vancomycin but not teicoplanin, is chromosomal in origin, and not usually transferable, but it acts in a similar manner to VanA. VanC resistance is a nontransferable lower-level resistance observed in *E. gallinarum*. Cross-resistance may occur within drugs of the glycopeptide class but not with other drug classes. Semisynthetic glycopeptides are being developed to overcome the problem of VanA and VanB resistance.

Pharmacokinetic Properties

Vancomycin is poorly absorbed after oral administration. Penetration into tissues is adequate but relatively poor, although the drug enters cerebrospinal fluid when the meninges are inflamed. The half-life in humans is about 6 hours; in dogs, 2 hours; and in horses, nearly 3 hours. Most of the IV-administered drug is excreted through the kidneys (glomerular filtration), with a small proportion excreted in bile. Vancomycin hydrochloride causes marked tissue damage, so it is administered only by IV infusion over a 30-minute period. Alteration of dosage is required for patients with renal impairment. Plasma concentrations can be monitored with dose intervals adjusted to give trough concentrations approximating the MIC of susceptible organisms.

Drug Interactions

Vancomycin is synergistic with aminoglycosides against Gram-positive cocci. It appears to be synergistic in vivo with rifampin against *Staphylococcus aureus*.

Toxicity and Adverse Effects

Vancomycin is highly irritant to tissues on injection and must be administered IV in dilute form. Rapid IV injection produces a histamine-like reaction in humans (red-neck syndrome). The drug is ototoxic in humans, particularly in patients treated with large doses or in patients with renal insufficiency, but more recently the purer forms of the drug as well as the lower doses have been associated with a low risk of ototoxicity. The drug is also potentially nephrotoxic, an adverse effect compounded by high doses and concurrent use of nephrotoxic drugs. There is no information on toxicity in domestic animals.

Administration and Dosage

Dosage recommendations are largely empirical. For parenteral administration, dosages have been recommended. These are 20 mg/kg IV at 12-hour intervals diluted in at least 200 ml of 5% dextrose. For treating intestinal disease, 5–10 mg/kg PO every 12 hours has been recommended. In dogs, Zaghlol and Brown (1988) recommended a parenteral dosage of 15 mg/kg q6 hours and in horses Orsini et al. (1992) recommended 4.3–7.5 mg/kg given as a 1-hour IV infusion q8 hours.

Clinical Applications

There are few indications for the use of vancomycin in animals, particularly since this is a "last resort" drug in human medicine. In humans, its primary use is to treat infections caused by multiresistant Gram-positive bacteria that cannot be treated with other drugs. It may also be used to treat patients allergic to penicillins and cephalosporins. It is the drug of choice in people for the oral treatment of *Clostridium difficile* colitis because of its activity and narrow, bactericidal spectrum. It might be suitable for similar use in animals, for example, in the oral treatment of *C. perfringens* enteritis, *C. spiroforme* enteritis in rabbits, or *C. difficile* in hamsters and other species, including horses. Bacitracin might be a less expensive alternative, although it is not effective against *C. difficile*. It is the drug of choice in the treatment of *Rhodococcus equi* infections in people, in which it may be synergistic with imipenem or rifampin. It might be suitable for use in foals infected with erythromycin- and rifampin-resistant *R. equi*, but such a use must be regarded as a treatment of last resort, in view of the "last resort" nature of this drug in human medicine.

Bibliography

Boss SM, et al. 1994. Use of vancomycin hydrochloride for treatment of *Clostridium difficile* enteritis in Syrian hamsters. Lab Anim Med 44:31.

Jackson MW, et al. 1994. Administration of vancomycin for treatment of ascending bacterial cholangiohepatitis in a cat. J Am Vet Med Assoc 204:602.

Nordmann P, et al. 1992. Therapy of *Rhodococcus equi* disseminated infections in nude mice. Antimicrob Agents Chemother 36:1244.

Orsini JA, et al. 1992. Vancomycin kinetics in plasma and synovial fluid following intravenous administration in horses. J Vet Pharmacol Ther 15:351.

Zaghlol HA, Brown SA. 1988. Single- and multiple-dose pharmacokinetics of intravenously administered vancomycin in dogs. Am J Vet Res 49:1637.

Teicoplanin

Teicoplanin has a molecular structure similar to that of vancomycin and is also a derivative of an actinomycete. It is a complex of five closely related antibiotics.

Teicoplanin has activity similar to and slightly greater than that of vancomycin, being restricted also in activity to Gram-positive bacteria. It has excellent activity against *Staphylococcus aureus* (including methicillin-resistant strains) and against streptococci (in which it is more active than vancomycin), *Listeria monocytogenes*, *Clostridium difficile*, *C. perfringens*, and other Gram-positive bacteria. *Enterococcus faecalis* are somewhat less sensitive than other cocci. *Nocardia* are resistant. Susceptible organisms are those with MIC ≤ 4 µg/ml. Teicoplanin is usually bactericidal to organisms with MIC ≤ 16 µg/ml. Activity in vitro is more affected by test conditions than the activity of vancomycin.

As with vancomycin, development of resistance to teicoplanin is uncommon, and these drugs have been regarded as resistance-resistant. Nevertheless, VanA resistance (causing cross-resistance to teicoplanin) occurs in enterococci, and resistance may develop in coagulase-negative staphylococci, either as a result of selection of mutants with progressive increases in MIC occurring in bacteria during treatment or, less commonly, by plasmid-mediated mechanisms.

Teicoplanin is not absorbed after oral administration. Absorption after IM injection is excellent, and the drug distributes widely into tissues in extracellular fluid. The half-life is remarkably prolonged in humans, between 45 and 70 hours after IV injection, but no pharmacokinetic studies have been done in animals. Penetration into cerebrospinal fluid is poor because of high molecular weight and poor lipid solubility. Elimination is almost entirely renal.

Teicoplanin is synergistic with aminoglycosides against some Gram-positive cocci, including penicillin-tolerant enterococci, is indifferent or additive with rifampin, and may be synergistic with imipenem against Gram-positive cocci.

In humans, teicoplanin is usually well tolerated. Adverse effects reported, in order of frequency, include hypersensitivity skin reactions (rash, pruritus, urticaria), pain (IM) or phlebitis (IV) at injection sites, and rarely nephrotoxicity or ototoxicity (usually in patients also receiving aminoglycosides). Teicoplanin, unlike vancomycin, can be administered by rapid IV injection. No information on toxicity in domestic animals is available.

No information is available on dosage for veterinary use. In humans, dosage is usually 6 mg/kg as a loading dose (IV), followed by once-daily dosage of 3–6 mg/kg; the higher dose may be more effective in most infections. Optimal dosage remains to be determined for use in humans since there is evidence that doses higher than those recommended may sometimes be required.

Teicoplanin is used in human medicine for the treatment of serious infections caused by Gram-positive bacteria where a bactericidal drug is needed, where there is resistance to alternative drugs, or where synergism with an aminoglycoside for broad-spectrum or enhanced activity is required. Uses include septicemia, endocarditis, bone and joint infections, and cystitis caused by multiresistant enterococci. It offers the advantage over vancomycin of less frequent dosing as well as reduced potential for ototoxicity or nephrotoxicity. A particular use has been in catheter-associated infections in neutropenic patients, with the focus on staphylococcal infections. However, the selection for resistant bacteria has been a significant problem. Activity of teicoplanin in vivo may not be as good as that in vitro. Teicoplanin has been recommended in surgical or dental prophylaxis, although advantage over alternate recommendations has not been demonstrated and use for this purpose may be limited by the narrow spectrum of the drug. Clearly, like vancomycin, teicoplanin has potential for parenteral treatment of serious infections caused by otherwise resistant Gram-positive bacteria in animals, but additional information is required on its pharmacokinetic properties and toxicity in animals.

Bibliography

Campoli-Richards DM, et al. 1990. Teicoplanin: a review of its antibacterial activity, pharmacokinetic properties, and therapeutic potential. Drugs 40:449.

Cercenado E, et al. 1996. Emergence of teicoplanin-resistant coagulase-negative staphylococci. J Clin Microbiol 34:1765.

Dutka-Malen S, et al. 1990. Phenotypic and genotypic heterogeneity of glycopeptide resistance determinants in Gram-positive bacteria. Antimicrob Agents Chemother 34:1875.

Avoparcin

Avoparcin has been used extensively as a growth promoter in chickens and pigs in Europe. The recognition that its use selected for vancomycin resistance in *Enterococcus* spp. in these animals, and in a high proportion of meat products derived from these animals, led to its recent withdrawal from use in Denmark and subsequently in Europe. The importance of vancomycin-resistant enterococci (VREs) is that, because of the inherent resistance of many enterococci to antibiotics, they may cause untreatable or difficult-to-treat infections in high-risk patients (eg, neutropenic cancer patients) treated with broad-spectrum antibiotics. Paradoxically, VREs have emerged as significant problems in human hospitals not in Europe but rather in the United States, where avoparcin has never been used in animals. The basis of this paradox may relate to the high level of vancomycin use in human hospitals in the United States relative to use in Europe.

Bibliography

Aarestrup FM, et al. 1996. Glycopeptide susceptibility among Danish *Enterococcus faecium* and *Enterococcus faecalis* isolates of animal and human origin and PCR identification of genes within the VanA cluster. Antimicrob Agents Chemother 40:1938.

Bager F, et al. 1997. Avoparcin used as a growth promoter is associated with the occurrence of vancomycin-resistant *Enterococcus faecium* on Danish poultry and pig farms. Prev Vet Med 31:95.

Bates J, et al. 1994. Farm animals as a putative reservoir for vancomycin-resistant enterococcal infection in man. J Antimicrob Chemother 34:507.

Devreise L, et al. 1996. Presence of vancomycin-resistant enterococci in farm and pet animals. Antimicrob Agents Chemother 40:2285.

Jensen LB. 1998. Differences in the occurrence of two base pair variants of Tn1546 from vancomycin-resistant enterococci from humans, pigs, and poultry. Antimicrob Agents Chemother 42:2463.

Jensen LB, et al. 1998. Molecular analysis of Tn1546 in *Enterococcus faecium* isolated from animals and humans. J Clin Microbiol 36:437.

Kirst HA, et al. 1998. Historical yearly usage of vancomycin. Antimicrob Agents Chemother 42:1303.

Klare I, et al. 1995. *VanA*-mediated high-level glycopeptide resistance in *Enterococcus faecium* from animal husbandry. FEMS Microbiol Lett 125:165.

Van den Braak N, et al. 1998. Molecular characterization of vancomycin-resistant enterococci from hospitalized patients and poultry products in the Netherlands. J Clin Microbiol 36:1927.

Bacitracin

Bacitracin is a polypeptide product of *Bacillus subtilis* that inhibits the formation of bacterial cell wall peptidoglycan by complexing directly with the pyrophosphate carrier and inhibiting the dephosphorylation reaction required for its regeneration. It is bactericidal to Gram-positive bacteria but has little activity against Gram-negative organisms. Resistance develops slowly and is rare. One unit = 26 μg of the United States Pharmacopeia (USP) standard.

Because bacitracin is highly nephrotoxic after parenteral administration, it is generally used only in the topical treatment of superficial infections of the skin and mucosal surfaces, particularly where activity against *Staphylococcus aureus* is required. It is often combined with an aminoglycoside or with polymyxin B for broad-spectrum activity in treating minor skin wounds. It is administered orally as a growth promoter in poultry, cattle, and swine and in the prevention and treatment of enteritis caused by *Clostridium perfringens* (eg, in type C enteritis in suckling pigs or necrotic enteritis in poultry). The drug is not effective in the treatment of swine dysentery. Incorporation in feed may prevent proliferative adenomatosis in swine, although *Lawsonia intracellularis* is resistant in vitro. It might be useful in preventing *C. spiroforme* enteritis in rabbits and *C. difficile* diarrhea in horses, although one study reported complete resistance by equine *C. difficile* isolates to this drug.

Bibliography

Jang SS, et al. 1997. Antimicrobial susceptibilities of equine isolates of *Clostridium difficile* and molecular characterization of metronidazole-resistant strains. Clin Infect Dis 25:S266.

Kyriakis SC, et al. 1996. Clinical evaluation of in-feed zinc bacitracin for the control of porcine intestinal adenomatosis in growing/fattening pigs. Vet Rec 138:489.

Streptogramins

Streptogramin antibiotics are unique among antibiotics, since each member of the class consists of at least two structurally unrelated molecules: group A streptogramins (macrolactones) and group B streptogramins (cyclic hexadepsipeptides). They inhibit protein synthesis by interfering with peptidyltransferase activity in the ribosome, often acting synergistically to produce a rapidly bactericidal effect against Gram-positive and certain Gram-negative bacteria. Their synergistic activity tends to reduce the emergence of bacteria resistance to each component of the combination. Virginiamycin has been developed largely as a growth promoter, but pristinamycin and quinupristin/dalfopristin have been developed for clinical use in human medicine, the former for oral administration and the latter for parenteral use.

Virginiamycin

Virginiamycin is an antibiotic mixture produced as a fermentation product of *Streptomyces virginiae*. Virginiamycin M interferes with protein synthesis by distorting the ribosomal A site to inhibit binding of aminoacyl tRNA and the peptidyl transferase reaction. The action of virginiamycin and virginiamycin S in inhibiting protein synthesis is not well understood.

The drug is mainly active against Gram-positive aerobic and anaerobic bacteria (such as *Clostridium perfringens*). Most Gram-negative bacteria are resistant: *Haemophilus, Lawsonia intracellularis, Leptospira*, and *Serpulina hyodysenteriae* are exceptions. Mycoplasma are often susceptible. A complex pattern of cross-resistance with macrolides and lincosamides occurs of both the constitutive generalized and the inducible types. Resistance is generally to the group B (virginiamycin S) rather than the group A (virginiamycin M) component (Dutta and Devriese, 1982). There is little information on the development and prevalence of resistance to virginiamycin; studies of *C. perfringens* isolated from turkeys and pigs have not identified resistant isolates. Use of virginiamycin as a feed additive may result in the selection of resistant fecal enterococci with cross-resistance to a related streptogramin antibiotic, quinupristin-dalfopristin (Synercid), which has recently been introduced in human medicine for the treatment of vancomycin-resistant enterococci and other infections.

There are few data available on the pharmacokinetic properties of virginiamycin in animals. The drug is not absorbed after oral administration to animals. It is safe if administered orally. Virginiamycin is used to promote growth in animals at the level of 5–20 ppm but has recently been banned for this purpose in the European Union because of resistance in enterococcal isolates. It is administered to swine at 110 ppm in feed to control swine dysentery, but results have sometimes been poor. The drug does not eradicate infection, and duration of treatment should be several weeks. Virginiamycin has been used to control cecal fermentation and prevent laminitis in horses fed high-concentrate rations.

Bibliography

Dutta GN, Devriese LA. 1982. Resistance to macrolide, lincosamide, and streptogramin antibiotics and degradation of lincosamide antibiotics in streptococci from bovine mastitis. J Antimicrob Chemother 10:403.
Johnson KG, et al. 1998. Behavioural changes in stabled horses given nontherapeutic levels of virginiamycin. Equine Vet J 30:139.
Ronne H, Jensen JEC. 1992. Virginiamycin susceptibility of *Serpulina hyodysenteriae* in vitro and in vivo. Vet Rec 131:239.
Thal LA, Zervos MJ. 1999. Occurrence and epidemiology of resistance to virginiamycin and streptogramins. J Antimicrob Chemother 43:171.
Welton LA, et al. 1998. Antimicrobial resistance in enterococci isolated from turkey flocks fed virginiamycin. Antimicrob Agents Chemother 42:705.

Quinupristin/Dalfopristin

The streptogramin antibiotic quinupristin/dalfopristin consists of a mixture of semisynthetic water-soluble derivatives of two naturally occurring pristinamycins. The combination is bactericidal against many Gram-positive bacteria, as well as some fastidious Gram-negative aerobes and Gram-negative anaerobes, and has the advantage over other streptogramins that its water solubility allows parenteral administration. It is usually administered IV. Gram-positive bacteria with acquired resistance to macrolides and lincosamides commonly develop resistance to the streptogramin B rather than to the A component of the combination. These features, as well as the properties of high susceptibility among Gram-positive bacteria, make this combination of considerable interest in human medicine for the treatment of susceptible multiresistant bacteria. Examples include methicillin-resistant *Staphylococcus aureus* (MRSA) and penicillin- or erythromycin-resistant pyogenic streptococci. An important feature is the activity of the combination against vancomycin-resistant enterococci. Since virginiamycin is used extensively as a growth promoter in animals, the continued use of this drug in animals may interfere with the efficacy of the combination for the treatment of vancomycin-resistant enterococcal infections in people.

Pristinamycin, which contains two different pristinamycin molecules as major components, has a similar spectrum of activity to quinupristin/dalfopristin and may be administered to humans orally for the treatment of susceptible pathogens.

Bibliography

Finch RG. 1996. Antibacterial activity of quinupristin/dalfopristin. Drugs 51 (Suppl 1):31.
Pechere J-C. 1996. Streptogramins: a unique class of antibiotics. Drugs 51 (Suppl 1):13.

Rubinstein E, Keller N. 1996. Future prospects and therapeutic potential of strep-togramins. Drugs 51 (Suppl 1):38.

Van den Bogaard AE, et al. 1997. High prevalence of colonization with vancomycin-and pristinamycin-resistant enterococci in healthy humans and pigs in the Netherlands: is the addition of antibiotics to animal feeds to blame? J Antimicrob Chemother 40:454.

Fosfomycin

Fosfomycin (L-[cis]-1,2-epoxypropyl phosphonic acid) is a phospo-noenol pyruvate analog that irreversibly inhibits pyruvyl transferase, the enzyme catalyzing the first step of peptidoglycan biosynthesis. It is pro-duced by various *Streptomyces* spp. and is available for oral or parenteral administration. It is particularly active against many Enterobacteriaceae, including *E. coli* in the 1–8 µg/ml range; *Pseudomonas aeruginosa* is resis-tant. Activity against Gram-positive bacteria such as *Staphylococcus aureus*, enterococci, and streptococci is in the 2–64 µg/ml range. Activity is reduced by alkaline pH and the presence of glucose, sodium chloride, or phosphates in culture media. Resistance, which can be chromosomal or plasmid-mediated, is said to be uncommon. There is no cross-resistance with other antibacterial drugs. Adverse effects are usually minor gas-trointestinal disturbances. Different forms of the drug are available for oral or parenteral use. The drug has been used in human medicine in cer-tain European and Asian countries for a wide variety of infections but is perhaps most commonly used in the single-dose oral treatment or pro-phylaxis of urinary tract infections. Anecdotally, it has been used in vet-erinary medicine, with mixed results, to treat dogs with urinary tract infections caused by multiresistant enterococci.

Bibliography

Aramayona JJ, et al. 1997. Pharmacokinetics of fosfomycin in chickens after a single intravenous and tissue levels following chronic oral administration. Vet Res 28:581.

Patel SS, et al. 1997. Fosfomycin tromethamine. Drugs 53:637.

Stein GE. 1998. Single-dose treatment of acute cystitis with fosfomycin tromethamine. Ann Pharmacother 32:215.

10 | Aminoglycosides and Aminocyclitols

J. F. PRESCOTT

General Considerations

The aminoglycosides and aminocyclitols are mostly bactericidal antibiotics with activity limited to aerobic bacteria and mycoplasma. The newer aminoglycosides (amikacin, netilmicin) have excellent activity against *Pseudomonas aeruginosa*. The development of newer drugs resistant to R plasmid–mediated enzymatic degradation, but with activity equal to or greater than that of their parents, has been an exciting development in this group of antibiotics, although they have been eclipsed by the development of the beta-lactams and fluoroquinolones. Despite this, they remain important drugs in the treatment of severe Gram-negative sepsis, although their highly cationic polar nature means that distribution across membranes is limited. Other disadvantages include problems of toxicity, particularly to branches of the eighth cranial nerve and to the kidneys, poor penetration into cerebrospinal fluid, inhibition by low pH and by divalent cations, inhibition of activity under anaerobic conditions, and inhibition by pus and by necrotic tissue. Single daily dosing is increasingly widely practiced. This is based on the theoretical grounds, supported by animal studies and by human clinical trials, which have demonstrated that such dosing may be clinically slightly more efficacious than divided daily dosing and may also slightly reduce toxicity. This marginally reduced toxicity is not sufficient to support a resurgence in use of aminoglycosides, though it has reduced costs associated with serum drug monitoring in human hospitals.

The date of discovery and order of clinical introduction of aminoglycosides are as follows: streptomycin (1944), neomycin (1949), kanamycin (1957), gentamicin (1963), tobramycin (1967), sisomicin (1970), amikacin

(1972), and netilmicin (1975). No new, less toxic aminoglycosides have been introduced in recent years.

Aminoglycosides remain useful because of their bactericidal activity against aerobic Gram-negative bacteria (including *P. aeruginosa*) and staphylococci and their synergism with beta-lactam drugs. Resistance to older aminoglycosides is, however, widespread and is becoming a problem with the newer drugs.

Chemistry

The aminoglycoside antibiotics—streptomycin, kanamycin, gentamicin, tobramycin, amikacin, and neomycin—are polar organic bases. Their polarity largely accounts for the pharmacokinetic properties that are shared by all members of the group. Chemically, they consist of a hexose nucleus to which amino sugars are attached by glycosidic linkages. This is why these molecules are also referred to as aminocyclitols or aminoglycosidic aminocyclitols. Spectinomycin contains an aminocyclitol but no aminoglycoside.

Mechanism of Action

Aminoglycosides have a rapid, dose-related bactericidal action on susceptible microorganisms. To exert this effect, the agent must first penetrate the cell envelope. This is in part an active, oxidative transport and in part passive diffusion. The active transport does not occur under anaerobic conditions. Penetration can be greatly enhanced by the presence of a drug that interferes with cell wall synthesis, such as a beta-lactam antibiotic. Once the aminoglycoside has entered the cell, it binds to receptors on the 30S subunit of the ribosome, where it induces misreading of the genetic code on the messenger ribonucleic acid (mRNA) template. This causes incorrect amino acids to be incorporated into the peptide and thereby inhibits ribosomal protein synthesis. The extent and type of misreading vary because different members of the group interact with different proteins. Streptomycin acts at a single site, but the other drugs act at several sites. Other effects of aminoglycosides include interference with the cellular electron transport system, induction of RNA breakdown, inhibition of translation, effects on DNA metabolism, and damage to cell membranes. The bactericidal effect is through the formation of abnormal cell membrane channels by misread proteins.

Antimicrobial Activity

The antibacterial action of the aminoglycosides is directed primarily against aerobic Gram-negative bacteria. Their action against many Gram-positive bacteria is limited. Some mycobacteria and some mycoplasma are susceptible. In potency, spectrum of activity, and stability to enzymes with plasmid-mediated resistance, amikacin > tobramycin gentamicin > neomycin = kanamycin > streptomycin. These antibiotics are inactive against anaerobic bacteria and against facultative anaerobic bacteria under anaerobic conditions. The activity of selected aminoglycosides against selected bacteria and mycoplasma is shown in Tables 10.1 and 10.2.

Streptomycin is the most active of these drugs against mycobacteria and the least active against other organisms. Tobramycin, amikacin, and

TABLE 10.1. **Activity (MIC$_{90}$, µg/ml) of selected aminoglycosides against selected bacteria**

Organism	Streptomycin	Neomycin	Kanamycin	Gentamicin
Gram-positive cocci				
Staphylococcus aureus	32	0.5	4	1
Streptococcus agalactiae	128		128	64
S. uberis	64	32	32	
Gram-positive rods				
Arcanobacterium pyogenes	>128	128	64	8
Bacillus anthracis	<8		0.5–4	≤4
Corynebacterium pseudotuberculosis				4
C. renale	64		2	≤0.25
Erysipelothrix rhusiopathiae			>64	≥64
Listeria monocytogenes	32	4	16	16
Mycobacterium tuberculosis	0.5			
Nocardia asteroides	16	4	128	16
Rhodococcus equi	4	≤0.25	2	≤0.25
Gram-negative rods				
Actinobacillus sp.	≤1		4	1
Bordetella bronchiseptica	256		8–16	2
Brucella canis	0.25		0.5	0.12
Campylobacter jejuni			4	0.5
Escherichia coli	>64	>64	>64	2
Haemophilus somnus	8	16–32	8	8
Helicobacter pylori			2	
Klebsiella pneumoniae	256	256	8	4
Leptospira spp.	0.5		4	
Moraxella bovis	16	0.12	0.12	0.5
Pasteurella haemolytica	>128	32	32	8
P. multocida				
Cattle	>128	32	32	8
Pigs	16–32		8–16	8
Proteus spp.	>16	16	4	2
Pseudomonas aeruginosa	>16	64	128	8
Salmonella spp.	>128	4	>32	8
Taylorella equigenitalis	>128	2	1	0.5
Gram-positive cocci				
Staphylococcus aureus	32	0.5	4	1

Note: Some reports are higher because of resistance. This table is designed partly to illustrate the differences in quantitative susceptibility among different aminoglycosides.

TABLE 10.2. **Percentage of aminoglycoside-sensitive bacteria isolated from different species**

Organism	Canada, Dogs and Cats[a]			United States, Dogs, Cats, and Other Species[b]			
	Neomycin	Kanamycin	Gentamicin	Streptomycin	Neomycin	Kanamycin	Gentamicin
Staphylococcus aureus	92	92	98	70	96	95	99
Beta-hemolytic streptococci	11	42	92	8	12	13	74
Escherichia coli	70	71	99	19	57	60	99
Proteus spp.	70	89	97	68	87	91	99
Klebsiella spp.	64	69	95	33	70	72	94
Pseudomonas aeruginosa	64	60	70	17	40	13	90
Bordetella bronchiseptica	100	100	88	4	94	92	99

[a]*Source:* Prescott et al. (1984).
[b]*Source:* Rhoades (1979).

gentamicin are particularly useful for their activity against *Pseudomonas aeruginosa,* with amikacin being the most active of the three drugs.

The bactericidal action of these agents on aerobic Gram-negative bacteria is markedly influenced by pH; the agents are most active in an alkaline environment. Increased local acidity secondary to tissue damage or bacterial destruction may account for failure of aminoglycosides to kill usually susceptible microorganisms. Another factor affecting activity is the presence of purulent debris, which can bind to aminoglycosides and inactivate them. When using an aminoglycoside to treat infections with purulent debris, surgical debridement and/or drainage will increase the efficacy of the drug.

Resistance to Aminoglycoside Antibiotics

Most clinically important resistance to aminoglycosides is caused by R plasmid–specified enzymes, broadly classified as phosphotransferases, acetyltransferases, and adenyltransferases (Table 10.3). At least 11 enzymes have been identified that can inactivate aminoglycosides. These enzymes modify the aminoglycosides at their exposed hydroxyl or amino groups to prevent ribosomal binding. They are present in the periplasmic space of bacteria, so that extracellular inactivation of drug does not occur. Some

TABLE 10.3. **Aminoglycoside- and aminocyclitol-modifying enzymes in R plasmid–bearing bacteria**

Modification	Enzyme[a]	Substrates
Aminoglycoside acetyltransferase (AAC)	AAC(3)-I	Gm
	AAC(3)-II	Gm, Tm
	AAC(3)-III	Gm, Km, Nm, Pm, Tm
	AAC(3)-IV	Gm, Km, Nm, Tm, Ak, Ap
	AAC(2')	Gm, Nm
	AAC(6')-I	Km
Aminoglycoside adenyltransferase (AAD)	AAD(2")	Gm, Km
	AAD(4')	Km, Tm, Nm, Pm, Ak
	AAD(4', 4")	Km, Nm, Tm
	AAD(3")	Sm, Sp
	AAD(6)	Sm
Aminoglycoside phosphotransferase (APH)	APH(3')-I	Km, Nm, Pm
	APH(3')-III	Km, Nm, Pm
	APH(2")	Gm, Km, Tm
	APH(3")	Sm
	APH(6)	Sm

Source: Mitsuhashi and Kawabe (1982) with permission.

Note: Ak, amikacin; Ap, apramycin; Gm, gentamicin; Km, kanamycin; Nm, neomycin; Pm, paramomycin; Sm, streptomycin; Sp, spectinomycin; Tm, tobramycin.

[a]Where enzymes act at the same position but differ in the substrates they degrade they are shown with different Roman numerals. Position of enzyme activity on aminoglycoside is indicated by Arabic numerals in parentheses.

of these enzymes have broad-spectrum activity against aminoglycosides, whereas others are narrow in activity. Complex patterns of cross-resistance occur in individual resistant strains of bacteria.

Strains with reduced permeability and consequently 2- to 4-fold increases in MIC may be selected during treatment with aminoglycosides. Such strains show cross-resistance to all other drugs within the group. Chromosomal mutation resulting in resistance is relatively unimportant except for streptomycin, where it occurs readily, even during treatment, as a result of a single-step mutation to high-level resistance. For the other drugs, chromosomal resistance develops slowly, because there are many 30S ribosomal binding sites. Resistance to aminoglycosides is increasingly important in limiting their effectiveness. Interestingly, the ultimate source of aminoglycoside resistance genes is probably also the microorganism source of aminoglycosides in nature, particularly *Streptomyces* spp. (Davis and Wright, 1997).

Pharmacokinetic Properties

Aminoglycosides are poorly absorbed from the gastrointestinal tract, bind to a low extent to plasma proteins (less than 25%), and have limited capacity to enter cells and penetrate cellular barriers. These drugs do not readily attain therapeutic concentrations in transcellular fluids, particularly cerebrospinal and ocular fluids, although inflammation may increase local concentrations. Poor diffusibility can be attributed to their low degree of lipid solubility. An example of this is the milk-to-plasma equilibrium concentration ratio of 0.5. The apparent volumes of distribution of aminoglycosides are relatively small (<0.35 l/kg) and their half-lives are short (1–2 hours) in domestic animals. Even though these drugs have a small volume of distribution, selective binding to tissues, including kidney cortex, occurs, so that kidney residues persist in animals for extensive periods. Elimination is entirely by renal excretion (glomerular filtration), and unchanged drug is rapidly excreted in the urine. Impaired renal function decreases their rate of excretion and makes it necessary to adjust maintenance dosage to prevent accumulation with attendant toxicity. Either the size of the dose or preferably the dosing interval can be adjusted (see Chapter 19). The significant individual variation in pharmacokinetic parameters among animals of the same species exacerbates problems of toxicity with this drug class.

Liposomal encapsulation of aminoglycosides has been used both clinically and experimentally to assist penetration into macrophages and thus successfully to treat intracellular *Mycobacterium avium* infections (Leitzke et al., 1998).

Drug Interactions

Aminoglycosides are commonly synergistic with beta-lactam drugs. Synergism does not usually occur in the presence of high-level plasmid-mediated or chromosomal resistance. With Gram-negative rods, the beta-lactam drug should be one to which the organisms are susceptible. Combination of newer beta-lactam drugs with newer aminoglycosides provides optimal therapy in seriously ill, particularly neutropenic, patients with bacterial infections. However, these drugs should never be mixed in the same infusion fluids with aminoglycosides.

Toxicity and Adverse Effects

All aminoglycosides can cause varying degrees of ototoxicity and nephrotoxicity. The tendency to produce vestibular damage (streptomycin, gentamicin) or cochlear damage (amikacin, kanamycin, neomycin) varies with the drug. Tobramycin appears to affect both vestibular (balance) and cochlear (hearing) functions equally. The ototoxic effect of aminoglycosides is potentiated by the loop diuretics furosemide and ethacrynic acid and probably other diuretic agents. Table 10.4 summarizes the relative risks of these drugs.

Nephrotoxicity (acute tubular necrosis) occurs in association with prolonged therapy and excessively high trough serum concentrations of the aminoglycoside, particularly neomycin and gentamicin. The saturable nature of renal proximal tubule cell uptake, at least for gentamicin and netilmicin, has been one factor supporting once-daily dosing (see Dosage Considerations, below). Urine characteristically contains protein and tubular casts that increase with continued administration of the drug, resulting in a reduction in the glomerular filtration rate. This reduction decreases the rate of excretion of the aminoglycoside, elevating serum concentrations of the drug and of creatinine and urea. To minimize this, therapy should be limited to the shortest period that will effect a cure. Concurrent therapy with other nephrotoxic drugs, such as the antibiotics cephaloridine or amphotericin B, or the volatile anesthetic methoxyflurane, can potentiate the nephrotoxicity of aminoglycosides. Other risk factors include frequency of dosage (more frequent is worse), total dose, duration of treatment, age (young animals are at greater risk), impaired

TABLE 10.4. **Relative risks of toxicity of different aminoglycosides at usual dosage**

Drug	Vestibular Toxicity	Cochlear Toxicity	Renal Toxicity
Streptomycin	+++	++	(+)
Dihydrostreptomycin	++	+++	(+)
Neomycin	+	+++	+++
Kanamycin	+	++	++
Amikacin	(+)	+	++
Gentamicin	+(+)	+	++
Tobramycin	(+)	(+)	(+)

Source: Pilloud (1983) with permission.

renal function, and prior aminoglycoside therapy. Feeding prior to administration of drug may reduce nephrotoxicity by saturating drug receptor sites with protein.

Serum concentrations of aminoglycosides can be monitored to reduce toxicity and to confirm serum concentrations (since this relates to clinical efficacy and toxicity). In patients at risk, serum concentrations can be checked regularly, 3 times a week if renal function is unstable or in young animals or twice weekly in other patients. Serum trough concentrations of drug should be 0.5–2 µg/ml before the next dosage (gentamicin, tobramycin) or less than 6 µg/ml for amikacin.

The aminoglycosides can produce neuromuscular blockade of the competitive (nondepolarizing) type, which causes acute muscular paralysis and apnea. This blockage is most likely to occur with anesthesia. Treatment consists of applying positive-pressure ventilation and administering calcium gluconate 10% solution IV. Varying success has been associated with administration of a reversible anticholinesterase agent, such as neostigmine methylsulfate, 0.022 mg/kg SC.

All aminoglycosides given rapidly IV slow the heart, reduce cardiac output, and lower blood pressure through an effect on calcium metabolism. These effects are of minor significance. Because aminoglycosides selectively bind to kidney tissue, they are not approved for use in food animals by the U.S. Food and Drug Administration and some other regulatory agencies. Gentamicin is approved for use in cattle as an intrauterine infusion. In the United States, members of the American Veterinary Medical Association have voted on a voluntary ban on extralabel use of all aminoglycosides in cattle.

Dosage Considerations

Aminoglycosides produce rapid, concentration-dependent killing of Gram-negative aerobes and produce a prolonged post-antibiotic effect (PAE), both in marked contrast to beta-lactams. Activity is greatest against growing bacteria. The total dose (serum C_{max}) appears to be the main determinant of efficacy. A high ratio of serum C_{max} to MIC is important in obtaining a positive clinical response and has the added benefit of preventing the emergence of strains with marginally increased resistance. A peak serum concentration:MIC ratio of 8–12:1 appears to optimize bactericidal activity. Higher serum concentrations may also be associated with a longer PAE. Traditionally, aminoglycosides have been administered every 8–12 hours. However, the considerations described above, and evidence that once-daily dosing contributes to reduced toxicity, make it worthwhile to reevaluate dose frequency (Gilbert, 1991). In addition, aminoglycosides have a biphasic mode of bacterial killing—an initial rapid concentration-dependent killing rate and a second, slower killing rate associated with decreased uptake of the aminoglycoside. This is independent of the initial drug concentration. Bacteria surviving the first phase develop temporary and unstable adaptive resistance, mediated by impermeability to all aminoglycosides (Daikos et al., 1991). These observations suggest that doses administered during the refractory period may serve only to enhance toxicity (Daikos et al., 1991).

Renal cortical uptake is a saturable phenomenon for amikacin, gentamicin, and netilmicin, while tobramycin shows a linear pattern. Animal studies have demonstrated several-fold reduced nephrotoxicity when the total daily dose was administered as a single rather than a divided dose (Marra et al., 1996; Freeman et al., 1997).

Understanding of factors involved in bacterial killing by aminoglycosides and recognition that renal uptake is saturable and that renal toxicity is reduced when there is a drug-free interval have been combined to support once-daily aminoglycoside dosing. Meta-analyses comparing single daily total dose versus divided dose administration in humans have found a slight clinical advantage to once-daily dosing, with similar or marginally reduced nephrotoxicity with single daily dose administration (Marra et al., 1996; Munckhof et al., 1996; Freeman et al., 1997; Hatala et al., 1997). Further study of selected groups, including pediatric, geriatric, and pregnant patients, are required before single daily dosage can be fully recommended in people (Freeman et al., 1997) or animals. Apart from experimental laboratory animal studies, there are limited data on the use of single total daily dose administration in veterinary medicine and no field trial comparisons of single versus divided daily dosage, but such pharmacokinetic as there are support single daily dosage (Godber et al., 1995; Magdesian et al., 1997, 1998; Martin-Jiminez et al., 1998). All dosage regimens should take into account kidney function, the exclusive renal excretion route of aminoglycosides, and their toxic potential (see Chapter 19). There are no established dosing schedules in people for once-daily dosing, but the tendency is to use previously recommended total daily dose.

Clinical Usage

The toxicity of aminoglycosides and their ability to produce long-term tissue residues, important in food animals, have largely restricted the use of these drugs to the treatment of severe infections. The more toxic aminoglycosides (neomycin) are largely restricted to oral use for the treatment of infections caused by Enterobacteriaceae, with gentamicin and amikacin being used in the topical treatment of infections caused by *Pseudomonas aeruginosa*. The less toxic aminoglycosides are usually reserved for the treatment of severe sepsis caused by Gram-negative aerobes. Of these, gentamicin is usually the first choice, followed by either amikacin or tobramycin, which are reserved for sepsis caused by organisms resistant to gentamicin. Spectinomycin has been used for treatment of systemic infections in food animals but, like streptomycin, is limited by resistance.

Bibliography

Bragonier R, Brown NM. 1998. The pharmacokinetics and toxicity of once-daily tobramycin therapy in children with cystic fibrosis. J Antimicrob Chemother 42:103.

Brown SA, Riviere JE. 1991. Comparative pharmacokinetics of aminoglycoside antibiotics. J Vet Pharmacol Ther 14:1.

Daikos GL, et al. 1991. First-exposure adaptive resistance to aminoglycoside antibiotics in vivo with meaning for optimal clinical use. Antimicrob Agents Chemother 35:117.

Davis J, Wright GD. 1997. Bacterial resistance to aminoglycoside antibiotics. Trends Microbiol 5:234.

Freeman CD, et al. 1997. Once-daily dosing of aminoglycosides: review and recommendations for clinical practice. J Antimicrob Chemother 39:677.

Gilbert DN. 1991. Once-daily aminoglycoside therapy. Antimicrob Agents Chemother 35:399.

Godber LM, et al. 1995. Pharmacokinetics, nephrotoxicosis, and in vitro antibacterial activity associated with single versus multiple (three times) daily gentamicin treatments in horses. Am J Vet Res 56:613.

Hatala R, et al. 1997. Single daily dosing of aminoglycosides in immunocompromised adults: a systematic review. Clin Infect Dis 24:810.

Leitzke S, et al. 1998. Rationale for and efficacy of prolonged-interval treatment using liposome-encapsulated amikacin in experimental *Mycobacterium avium* infection. Antimicrob Agents Chemother 42:459.

Magdesian KG, et al. 1997. Pharmacokinetics and nephrotoxicity of high dose, once daily administered amikacin in neonatal foals. Am Assoc Equine Pract 43:396.

Magdesian KG, et al. 1998. Pharmacokinetics of high dose of gentamicin administered intravenously and intramuscularly to horses. J Am Vet Med Assoc 213:1007.

Marra F, et al. 1996. Aminoglycoside administration as a single daily dose: an improvement to current practice or a repeat of previous errors? Drugs 52:344.

Martin-Jiminez T, et al. 1998. Population pharmacokinetics of gentamicin in horses. Am J Vet Res 59:1589.

Mattie H, et al. 1989. Determinants of efficacy and toxicity of aminoglycosides. J Antimicrob Chemother 24:281.

Mitsuhashi S, Kawabe H. 1982. Aminoglycoside antibiotic resistance in bacteria. In: Whelton A, New HC, eds. The Aminoglycosides: Microbiology, Clinical Use, and Toxicology. New York: Marcel Dekker, 97–122.

Munckhof WJ, et al. 1996. A meta-analysis of studies on the safety and efficacy of aminoglycosides given either once daily or as divided doses. J Antimicrob Chemother 37:645.

Pilloud M. 1983. Antibiotiques et chemiotherapiques—de la recherche a la pratique: VI. Schweiz Arch Tierheilkd 125:301.

Prescott JF, et al. 1984. Antimicrobial drug susceptibility of bacteria isolated from disease processes in cattle, horses, and dogs and cats. Can Vet J 25:289.

Prins JM, et al. 1996. Validation and nephrotoxicity of a simplified once-daily aminoglycoside dosing schedule and guidelines for monitoring therapy. Antimicrob Agents Chemother 40:2494.

Rhoades HE. 1979. Sensitivity of bacteria to 16 antibiotic agents. Vet Med Small Anim Clin 74:976.

Salauze D, et al. 1990. Aminoglycoside acetyltransferase 3-IV *(aacC4)* and hygromycin B 4-I phosphotransferase *(hphB)* in bacteria isolated from human and animal sources. Antimicrob Agents Chemother 40:2494.

Shinohara T, Briski T. 1998. A comparison of traditional dosing and once-daily aminoglycoside dosing on non-specific antibiotic side-effects in adults. J Antimicrob Chemother 42:114.

Streptomycin

Streptomycin (Fig. 10.1) is the only important member of the streptidine group; dihydrostreptomycin has very similar properties but is more likely to cause deafness. Streptomycin was the earliest aminoglycoside introduced for clinical use.

Antimicrobial Activity

Streptomycin is active against mycobacteria, some mycoplasma, some Gram-negative rods (including *Brucella*), and some *Staphylococcus aureus*. With the exception of mycobacteria, streptomycin is the least active of the aminoglycosides. Among susceptible bacteria are *Leptospira, Francisella tularensis, Yersinia pestis,* and most *Campylobacter fetus* subsp. *venerealis* (see Tables 10.1 and 10.2). Organisms with MIC $\leq$ 4 μg/ml are regarded as susceptible.

Antimicrobial Resistance

Acquired resistance to streptomycin is widespread in veterinary pathogens and has virtually nullified the use of this drug except for special applications. Most clinically important resistance is caused by plasmid-specified enzymes, certain of which specifically inactivate only streptomycin (see Table 10.3). Plasmid-mediated resistance is commonly linked with sulfonamide, ampicillin, and tetracycline resistance genes.

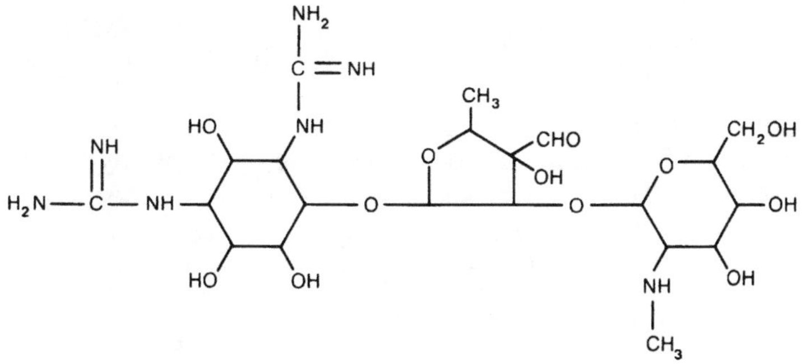

Fig. 10.1. Structural formula of streptomycin.

Chromosomal mutations to resistance arise commonly in vitro and often in vivo within a few days of treatment, although such mutants are sometimes less viable than their parents. Streptomycin is therefore generally combined with other drugs in an attempt to limit chromosomal mutation.

Drug Interactions

Streptomycin is commonly combined with other drugs either to prevent the emergence of chromosomal resistance or for a synergistic effect. Streptomycin is commonly synergistic with cell wall–active antibiotics such as the penicillins. This synergism occurs in Gram-positive bacteria such as streptococci, which are otherwise impermeable to the drug, and in bacteria with chromosomal mutation to low-level resistance. Synergism does not usually occur in the presence of high-level plasmid or chromosomal resistance or in Gram-negative bacteria.

Toxicity and Adverse Effects

Besides resistance, toxicity limits the use of streptomycin. It causes vestibular damage, an effect that increases with the daily and cumulative dose, with the height of peak serum concentrations, and with preexisting renal disease. In general, no toxic effects occur if streptomycin is used at recommended doses for up to 1 week. Streptomycin can cause permanent vestibular damage, producing ataxia that progresses to incoordination, nystagmus, loss of righting reflex, and death. The effects are dose related. Daily IM injection of doses 5–10 times those recommended produce this effect in cats in about 10 days. Cats are particularly sensitive to streptomycin, and usual doses may produce nausea, vomiting, salivation, and ataxia.

Neuromuscular blockade is produced when streptomycin is given at high dosage. Although this effect is insignificant at normal doses, deaths have occurred in dogs and cats given penicillin-streptomycin combinations for prophylaxis of surgical infection after general anesthesia, since general anesthetics and muscle relaxants potentiate the neuromuscular blocking effects. Such fatal effects have generally followed overdosing.

Administration and Dosage

Intramuscular injection is the usual route of streptomycin administration. Rapid and complete absorption takes place from the injection site, with peak serum concentrations occurring within 30 minutes. Dosage of streptomycin is shown in Table 10.5.

Clinical Applications

Streptomycin is used alone in the treatment of leptospirosis, particularly to eradicate the kidney carrier state. Unfortunately, even though it is

TABLE 10.5. Usual dosages of aminoglycosides and aminocyclitols in animals

Drug	Route	Dosage[a] (mg/kg)	Interval (h)	Comments
Amikacin[b]	IM (IV)[b]	21	24	Horses
	IM, SC	15–20	24	Dogs, cats
Apramycin	PO	20	12	Enteric infection
	IM	20	24	Cattle, swine only
Gentamicin	IM, SC (IV)	7–10	24	
Kanamycin	PO	10	6	Enteric infection
	IM, SC	18	24	
Neomycin	PO	10	6	Enteric infection
Spectinomycin	PO	20–40	8	Enteric infection
	IM, SC	20–30	12	Calves, pigs
Streptomycin	IM	20	24	Almost obsolete drug; reserve for specific indications
Tobramycin	IM, SC (IV)	6	24	Need more data

Caution: Because of their narrow margin of safety, aminoglycosides should not be administered to animals with impaired renal function. In human medicine adjustments of gentamicin dosage can be based on serum creatinine concentrations, but such a relationship has not been determined in animals.

[a]Single daily dosing recommendations are based on increasing evidence of the clinical advantage and reduced toxicity associated with such dosage; more clinical experience is needed of such usage in animals.

[b]If administered IV, give slowly diluted in saline.

useful in removing the leptospiral carrier state, streptomycin has been withdrawn from use in food-producing animals in the United States because of its prolonged binding to kidney tissue. In humans it is the drug of choice for *Yersinia pestis, Francisella tularensis,* and (in combination with other drugs) *Mycobacterium tuberculosis* infections. Gentamicin may be an acceptable alternative to streptomycin for the treatment of tularemia (Enderlin et al., 1994). Streptomycin is rarely used alone for infections in animals because of widespread resistance, particularly in Gram-negative bacteria. The newer aminoglycosides are more active against a greater number of organisms and are less toxic. Streptomycin is commonly used in combination with penicillin for the synergistic effect against many Gram-positive bacteria.

It has increasingly fewer applications in veterinary medicine, although for a long time it was used extensively in combination with penicillin for food animals with little clinical data supporting the use of the combination. An area of increasing interest is its value for *Brucella* infections, when combined with tetracyclines.

CATTLE, SHEEP, AND GOATS

A single dose of 25 mg/kg streptomycin IM has been shown to remove *Leptospira pomona* from the kidneys of carrier cattle, probably because of renal persistence of the drug. In one study this dose did not remove *L. hardjo* from the genital tract or kidneys of carrier cattle. The difference may have been related to differences in host adaption of the serovars (Ellis et al., 1985; Prescott, 1991). However, another experimental study and a field study showed that either single or 5-day treatment of cows experimentally infected with *L. hardjo* was effective in stopping shedding for at least 70 days after treatment (Gerritsen et al., 1993; Gerritsen et al., 1994). The drug may also be used in the treatment of acute leptospirosis but should be combined with amoxicillin.

Streptomycin is the drug of choice for the treatment of *Campylobacter fetus* subsp. *venerealis* in the carrier state in bulls. Treatment consists of 3 consecutive daily infusions of 10 ml of drug (500 mg/ml, in a 50% aqueous solution) into the preputial cavity and exterior massage for 5 minutes, with 2 subcutaneous injections of dihydrostreptomycin, 22 mg/kg, at the first and third treatments. Resistance has been described in some *C. fetus* subsp. *venerealis* (Jones et al., 1985).

Streptomycin may be the most effective agent in the treatment of actinobacillosis (wooden tongue). Combination with penicillin may enhance activity against *Arcanobacterium pyogenes* and *Corynebacterium renale*. Penicillin-streptomycin combinations are commonly used in local treatment of staphylococcal or streptococcal mastitis in cows, but the synergism observed in vitro has not been conclusively demonstrated in vivo. Because of this, it has been withdrawn from use in some countries (Whittem and Hanlon, 1997). Although the combination has been recommended as a single IM treatment of dermatophilosis in sheep, not all trials confirm the value of such treatment (Scrivener and Vizard, 1995).

Streptomycin has been combined with tetracycline in the treatment of *Brucella abortus* carriers; the combination has synergistic activity (Nicoletti et al., 1985). In one study 67% of cows were considered cured, but an optimal treatment regimen has not been established. Combination of tetracycline with streptomycin eliminated *B. ovis* from 90% of experimentally infected rams but did not resolve clinical epididymitis in naturally or experimentally infected rams (Marin et al., 1989). Similar synergism has been described in *B. melitensis* infection in sheep (Radwan et al., 1989).

SWINE

Penicillin-streptomycin combinations may be used in the parenteral treatment of Gram-positive infections in swine, such as streptococcal infections or erysipelas. The drug has been used alone to control leptospirosis. Experimentally, a single dose of 25 mg/kg of dihydrostreptomycin administered IM removed *Leptospira pomona* from the kidneys of carrier animals (Stalheim, 1967). Field trials have not always supported the efficacy of single doses to eradicate infection, and better results have been achieved with the same dose given on twice q48 hours (Horsch et al., 1973). Activity against serovar *bratislava* has not been described.

HORSES

Streptomycin has little application in equine medicine because of widespread resistance among bacteria such as *Actinobacillus*, for which it is sometimes recommended. Penicillin-streptomycin combinations should have synergistic effects against streptococcal infections.

DOGS AND CATS

There seems to be little place for streptomycin in infections of dogs. Flores-Castro and Carmichael (1978) described the generally effective treatment of canine brucellosis with combined treatment with streptomycin, 10 mg/kg for 7 days, and minocycline, 15 mg/kg for 14 days. Streptomycin should not be used in cats.

POULTRY

Streptomycin is sometimes used in oral treatment of nonspecific enteritis in chickens and, combined with penicillin, in the parenteral treatment of erysipelas in turkeys.

Bibliography

Dobson KJ. 1971. Eradication of leptospirosis from two commercial piggeries in South Australia. Aust Vet J 47:186.

Ellis WA, et al. 1985. Dihydrostreptomycin treatment of bovine carriers of *Leptospira interrogans* serovar *hardjo*. Res Vet Sci 39:292.

Enderlin G, et al. 1994. Streptomycin and alternative agents for the treatment of tularemia: review of the literature. Clin Infect Dis 19:42.

Flores-Castro R, Carmichael LE. 1978. Canine brucellosis: current status of methods for diagnosis and treatment. Gaines Vet Symp 27:17.

Gerritsen MJ, et al. 1993. Effect of streptomycin treatment on the shedding and the serologic responses to *Leptospira interrogans* serovar *hardjo* subtype *hardjobovis* in experimentally infected cows. Vet Microbiol 38:129.

Gerritsen MJ, et al. 1994. Effective treatment with dihydrostreptomycin of naturally infected cows shedding *Leptospira interrogans* serovar *hardjo* subtype *hardjobovis*. Am J Vet Res 55:339.

Horsch F, et al. 1973. Die Sanierung leptospiroseverseuchter Schweinebestande unter Anwendung von Streptomyzinsulfat. Monatsch Vet Med 28:818.

Jones RL, et al. 1985. Cultural procedures for the isolation of *Campylobacter fetus* ssp. *fetus* from preputial secretions and the occurrence of antimicrobial resistance. Am Assoc Vet Lab Diagn 28:225.

Lein D, et al. 1968. Diagnosis, treatment, and control of vibriosis in an artificial insemination unit. J Am Vet Med Assoc 153:1574.

LeLouedec C. 1978. Efficacite des antibiotiques contre les mammites bovine staphylococciques et streptococciques. Ann Rech Vet 9:63.

Marin CM, et al. 1989. Efficacy of long-acting oxytetracycline alone or in combination with streptomycin for treatment of *Brucella ovis* infections of rams. Am J Vet Res 50:560.

Nicoletti P, et al. 1985. Efficacy of a long-acting oxytetracycline alone or combined with streptomycin in the treatment of bovine brucellosis. J Am Vet Med Assoc 187:493.

Prescott JF. 1991. Treatment of leptospirosis. Cornell Vet 81:7.

Radwan AI, et al. 1989. Experimental treatment of *Brucella melitensis* infection in sheep with oxytetracycline alone or combined with streptomycin. Trop Anim Health Prod 21:211.

Scrivener CJ, Vizard AL. 1995. Efficacy of a single dose of erythromycin or penicillin/streptomycin for the treatment of ovine dermatophilosis. Aust Vet J 72:475.

Stalheim OHV. 1967. Chemotherapy of renal leptospirosis in swine. Am J Vet Res 28:161.

Whittem T, Hanlon D. 1997. Dihydrostreptomycin or streptomycin in combination with penicillin G in dairy cattle therapeutics: a review and re-analysis of published data. Part 1: Clinical pharmacology. N Z Vet J 45:178.

Dihydrostreptamine Aminoglycosides: Neomycin Group

Neomycin is the isomeric mixture of neomycin B and C. Framycetin is identical to neomycin B. Paramomycin (aminosidine) is closely related to neomycin. Its pharmacokinetic and toxic properties and clinical applications are similar to those of neomycin so that, like neomycin, it is best reserved for local applications.

Antimicrobial Activity

Neomycin has similar activity to kanamycin on a weight basis and is several times more active than streptomycin; it is less active than gentamicin, tobramycin, and amikacin (see Table 10.1). Activity against *Staphylococcus aureus* is good, but it is generally low against other Gram-positive bacteria (see Tables 10.1 and 10.2). Many opportunist Gram-negative pathogens are susceptible to neomycin, although the prevalence of susceptible strains is slightly less than for kanamycin and far less than gentamicin. Many *Pseudomonas aeruginosa* are susceptible (see Table 10.2). Bacteria with MIC ≤8 µg/ml are regarded as susceptible.

Resistance

Plasmid-mediated resistance occurs through a variety of enzymes (see Table 10.3). Such resistance, which is often multiple, is relatively common in enteric commensals and pathogens but less common among other opportunist pathogens. Chromosomal mutation to resistance is unimportant.

Drug Interactions

Neomycin shows synergistic activity with beta-lactam antibiotics and bacitracin against Gram-positive bacteria. Neomycin has sometimes been combined with macrolide antibiotics for intramammary treatment of

Gram-positive udder infections, but there is no information on the in vitro effect of the interaction.

Toxicity and Adverse Effects

Neomycin is the most toxic of the aminoglycosides and readily causes nephrotoxicity and deafness. For this reason it should never be used parenterally. Toxic effects are generally not produced when neomycin is administered orally or applied locally, but severe side effects of deafness and tubular necrosis have occurred in humans after oral administration.

Cats given high IM doses (100 mg/kg) daily showed nephrotoxic effects and became deaf in a few days; dogs are about equally susceptible. Total deafness was described in a dog after administration of 500 mg subcutaneously for 5 days (Fowler, 1968). In cattle, parenterally administered neomycin causes nephrotoxicity and deafness, which may be enhanced by dehydration. In pigs, transient posterior paresis and apnea immediately after injection have resulted from neuromuscular blockade. Malabsorption has been described in humans given oral neomycin for prolonged periods.

Administration and Dosage

Neomycin is reserved for local treatment of infections, often combined with bacitracin for broad-spectrum synergistic activity. In some countries neomycin is used as a parenteral injection for food animals and horses. Because of its toxic potential, such usage is strongly discouraged. Neomycin impaired the response of equine neutrophils to chemoattractants in vitro and in vivo, suggesting that the drug should be avoided for horses (Pycock et al., 1988). Paramomycin may be an effective treatment for acute cryptosporidiosis caused by *Cryptosporidium parvum* (Rehg, 1994; Mancassola et al., 1995) but may be less effective than azithromycin for this purpose. Whether neomycin might be equally efficacious remains to be determined. It should be noted that some neomycin appears to be absorbed following oral administration (approximately 3%) and may lead to kidney residues in cattle (Persoli et al., 1994).

Clinical Applications

Neomycin is used for the local treatment of intestinal infections, of wound or skin infections, and of mastitis. Its relatively broad spectrum of activity and the bactericidal effect made the drug popular in some countries for parenteral use in farm animals as an inexpensive "alternative" to gentamicin; safer, considerably less toxic, and more efficacious alternate drugs are now readily available.

CATTLE, SHEEP, AND GOATS

Neomycin has been used successfully in the oral treatment of enteric infections in calves, though resistance increasingly limits its effectiveness. One or 2 g administered orally twice daily has successfully controlled salmonellosis and enterotoxigenic *Escherichia coli* (ETEC) diarrhea in calves. Paramomycin and by implication neomycin might be efficacious in the treatment of cryptosporidiosis, but more work is required to investigate this point. On the other hand, Shull and Frederick (1978) found that routine addition of neomycin to milk powder of neonatal calves increased the frequency of diarrhea, possibly through a suppressive effect on normal intestinal microflora or through an irritant effect on the mucosa. Neomycin is absorbed after oral administration and can lead to violative kidney drug residues. Routine intrauterine administration of neomycin boluses to postparturient cattle was followed by significantly increased number of services per conception compared to controls (Fuquay et al., 1975).

In dry-cow treatment, neomycin alone has given poor cure rates, but combination with penicillin G has produced excellent cure of staphylococcal and streptococcal infections, far superior to penicillin-streptomycin combinations (LeLouedec, 1978). Neomycin has been combined with spiramycin for use in dry-cow treatment with reasonable effect. There is evidence that neomycin dry-cow preparations, particularly those also containing corticosteroids, have predisposed cows to *Nocardia* mastitis. It is unclear if this is a general property of neomycin-corticosteroids or was the result of contamination of batches (Ollis et al., 1991).

Paromomycin is available in some countries for parenteral use in food animals, with one application being the treatment of bovine respiratory disease (Brugere-Picoux et al., 1986).

SWINE

Neomycin is used in the oral treatment of *E. coli* diarrhea, although resistance increasingly limits its use.

HORSES

Neomycin may be used in the local treatment of infections caused by susceptible bacteria. It has been used in Australia in the parenteral treatment of *Rhodococcus equi* pneumonia in foals, often administered for prolonged periods without evidence of toxicity (Barton, 1986), but better alternatives are readily available. Evidence of nephrotoxicity was observed in adult horses within 4 days of parenteral administration (Edwards et al., 1989).

DOGS AND CATS

Neomycin may be used for the local treatment of infections in dogs and cats, such as otitis externa and anal sac infections.

POULTRY

Neomycin is sometimes administered orally to chickens and turkeys in the treatment of *Salmonella* infections.

Bibliography

Barton MD. 1986. Use of neomycin for treatment of *Rhodococcus equi* pneumonia in foals. Aust Vet J 63:163.

Belloli C, et al. 1996. Pharmacokinetics and dosing regimen of aminosidine in the dog. Vet Res Comm 20:533.

Brugere-Picoux J, et al. 1986. Traitement des affections respiratoires du veau par l'aminosidine. Rec Med Vet 162:141.

Crowell WA, et al. 1981. Neomycin toxicosis in calves. Am J Vet Res 42:29.

Edwards DJ, et al. 1989. The nephrotoxic potential of neomycin in the horse. Equine Vet J 21:206.

Fowler NG. 1968. The ototoxicity of neomycin in the dog. Vet Rec 82:267.

Fuquay JW, et al. 1975. Routine postpartum treatment of dairy cattle with intrauterine neomycin sulfate boluses. J Anim Sci 58:1367.

LeLouedec C. 1978. Efficacite des antibiotiques contre les mammites bovine staphylo-cocciques et streptococciques. Ann Rech Vet 9:63.

Mancassola R, et al. 1995. Chemoprophylaxis of *Cryptosporidium parvum* infection with paromomycin in kids and immunological study. Antimicrob Agents Chemother 39:75.

Ollis GW, et al. 1991. An investigation of risk factors for nocardial mastitis in central Alberta dairy herds. Can Vet J 32:227.

Persoli WM, et al. 1994. Disposition and bioavailability of neomycin in Holstein calves. J Vet Pharmacol Ther 17:5.

Pycock JF, et al. 1988. The effect of various antibacterial preparations on the in vitro morphology and chemotactic response of equine neutrophils. J Vet Pharmacol Ther 11:191.

Rehg JE. 1994. A comparison of anticryptosporidial activity of paromomycin with that of other aminoglycosides and azithromycin in immunosuppressed rats. J Infect Dis 170:934.

Shull JJ, Frederick HM. 1978. Adverse effect of oral antibacterial prophylaxis and therapy on incidence of neonatal calf diarrhea. Vet Med Small Anim Clin 73:924.

Kanamycin Group

The kanamycin group contains the kanamycins and semisynthetic derivatives such as amikacin; the nebramycins such as tobramycin and apramycin; and gentamicin, netilmicin, and sisomicin.

Kanamycin

ANTIMICROBIAL ACTIVITY

Kanamycin (Fig. 10.2) has similar activity to neomycin. It is active against many species of mycobacteria and mycoplasma but is inactive against *Pseudomonas aeruginosa* and anaerobes (see Table 10.1). Bacteria with MIC ≤16 μg/ml are regarded as susceptible, of 32 μg/ml as intermediate, and of ≥64 μg/ml as resistant.

RESISTANCE

Plasmid-mediated resistance can occur through a variety of enzymes (see Table 10.3). Chromosomal resistance develops slowly but is far less important. Cross-resistance occurs with neomycin and one-way cross-resistance with streptomycin. Acquired resistance of *Escherichia coli* and other Gram-negative rods occurs frequently (see Table 10.3).

TOXICITY AND ADVERSE EFFECTS

Kanamycin has a larger therapeutic index than neomycin but is less toxic on a weight basis (see Table 10.4). Although excessively high doses are toxic to dogs and cats, cats given 100 mg/kg daily SC over 30 days showed no ill effects, and neither did dogs given the same dose over 9 months (Yeary, 1975).

CLINICAL APPLICATIONS

Kanamycin has largely been replaced for parenteral administration by more active aminoglycosides. For local applications it offers no advantage over neomycin. In animals, kanamycin has potential application in the parenteral treatment of infections caused by Gram-negative bacteria, *Staphylococcus aureus*, and mycoplasma. Gentamicin is generally preferred because of its broader spectrum and increased activity.

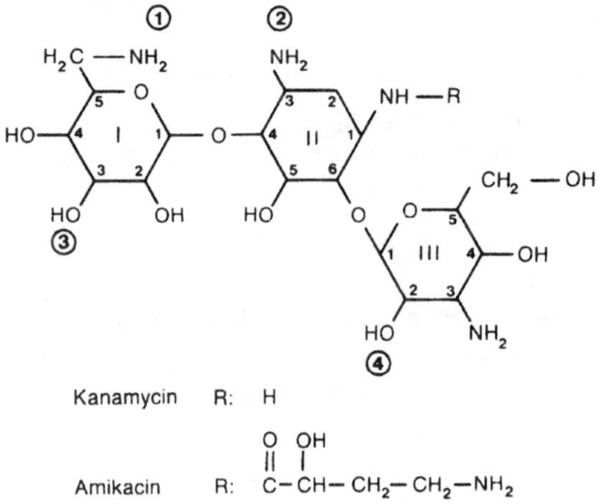

Fig. 10.2. Structural formulas of kanamycin and amikacin.

In cattle, kanamycin (55 mg/kg IM q8 hours) has been suggested for the treatment of *Pasteurella* pneumonia (Hjerpe and Routen, 1976). In combination with penicillin in the intramammary treatment of *Staphylococcus aureus* subclinical mastitis, kanamycin has given excellent cure rates but has the disadvantage of long periods of posttreatment milk withdrawal (Storper, 1984). Kanamycin has been combined with spiramycin for the broad-spectrum intramammary treatment of bovine mastitis, with good results. One other application is in the treatment of ocular *Moraxella bovis* infections by the subconjunctival route (George et al., 1986).

Bibliography

Firth EC, et al. 1988. Effect of induced synovial inflammation on pharmacokinetics and synovial concentration of sodium ampicillin and kanamycin sulfate after systemic administration in ponies. J Vet Pharmacol Ther 11:56.

George LW, et al. 1986. Distribution of kanamycin in ocular tissues of calves. J Vet Pharmacol Ther 9:183.

Hjerpe CA, Routen TA. 1976. Practical and theoretical considerations concerning treatment of bacterial pneumonia in feedlot cattle, with special reference to antibiotic therapy. Proc Am Assoc Bovine Pract, p97.

Storper M. 1984. Experiments with three new intramammary antibiotic combination products for the treatment of subclinical mastitis in lactating cows. Refu Vet 38:154.

Yeary RA. 1975. Systemic toxic effects of chemotherapeutic agents in domestic animals. Vet Clin North Am 5:511.

Amikacin

Amikacin is a chemical modification of kanamycin (Fig. 10.2), with greater activity than kanamycin on a weight basis but with similar activity on a weight basis to that of gentamicin or tobramycin (Table 10.6). The

TABLE 10.6. **Activity (MIC_{90}, µg/ml) of tobramycin, amikacin, and apramycin against selected bacteria**

Organism	Tobramycin	Amikacin	Apramycin
Gram-positive aerobes			
Nocardia spp.	>32	2	
Rhodococcus equi	1	≤0.25	
Staphylococcus aureus	8	4	1.0
Streptococcus pyogenes	64	256	32
Gram-negative aerobes			
Actinobacillus sp.	2	8	16
Bordetella bronchiseptica	2	8	16
Campylobacter jejuni	2	2	
Escherichia coli	0.5	2	8
Klebsiella pneumoniae	8	4	4
Pasteurella multocida	2	8	16
Proteus spp.	1	4	8
Pseudomonas aeruginosa	8	16	16
Salmonella spp.	2	4	8

remarkable property of amikacin is its resistance to most of the enzymes that inactivate the other aminoglycosides, including gentamicin and tobramycin (see Table 10.3). This property is particularly important in the treatment of some *Pseudomonas aeruginosa* infections.

Antimicrobial Activity

Susceptible Bacteria (MIC ≤16 µg/ml) are the Enterobacteriaceae, including gentamicin-resistant *Enterobacter* spp., *E. coli, Klebsiella* spp., *Proteus* spp., and *Serratia* spp. Among Gram-positive bacteria, *Nocardia* spp. and *Staphylococcus aureus* are sensitive (see Table 10.6). *Pseudomonas aeruginosa* has a susceptibility similar to that of gentamicin.

Resistant Bacteria (MIC ≥64 µg/ml) include anaerobes, streptococci, and some *Pseudomonas* spp.

Antimicrobial Resistance

Emergence of resistance to amikacin has been uncommon, relative to that of gentamicin and other newer aminoglycosides (see Table 10.3), but hospital-associated plasmid-mediated resistance in Gram-negative bacteria has been described.

Drug Interactions

Amikacin is synergistic with beta-lactams—for example, with azlocillin or ticarcillin against *Pseudomonas aeruginosa*.

Pharmacokinetic Properties

Amikacin's properties are typical of aminoglycosides. Concerns that decreased glomerular filtration in neonatal foals might lead to a need to reduce dosage to prevent nephrotoxicity were reported to be unfounded by Adland-Davenport et al. (1990), since renal clearance was greater in foals than was observed in adults.

Toxicity and Adverse Effects

Amikacin may be slightly less nephrotoxic and ototoxic than kanamycin, with the frequency of these effects in humans being low. In animals with normal renal function, amikacin administered at recommended doses for 2–3 weeks is unlikely to produce toxic effects. Monitoring of renal function during treatment is recommended. Dosage should be adjusted in cases of preexisting renal impairment, preferably in response to monitored drug levels in serum (see discussion under Gentamicin). Factors predisposing to renal toxicity were discussed under General Considerations, at the beginning of this chapter.

Administration and Dosage

Suggested drug dosages are shown in Table 10.5. The drug has been introduced for use in horses and dogs in the United States.

Clinical Applications

Amikacin is a broad-spectrum bactericidal drug useful for severe illness in animals—for example, in Gram-negative septicemia caused by gentamicin-resistant organisms, as might be encountered in a veterinary hospital. In human medicine, it is often combined with antipseudomonal penicillins in the treatment of *Pseudomonas aeruginosa* infections in neutropenic patients. It is sometimes regarded as an aminoglycoside reserved for use in infections caused by otherwise resistant Gram-negative aerobes.

HORSES

Amikacin has been licensed for use in the United States for the treatment of bacterial endometritis of mares and is used particularly for *Pseudomonas aeruginosa* and *Klebsiella pneumoniae* infections. The drug had no adverse effects on conception in horses when used in a pH-buffered semen extender at 100 μg/ml (Blue and Oriol 1982). An intrauterine infusion of 2 g in 200 ml saline for 3 days gave highest overall cure rates against experimental *Klebsiella* metritis in mares and 94–100% cure rates in *Pseudomonas* or *Klebsiella* metritis under field conditions (Gingerich et al., 1983). Others have successfully used the same treatment for 5 days (Brook, 1982). Pharmacokinetic studies support the use of intrauterine infusions of 2 g once daily rather than IM treatment (Orsini et al., 1996). Routine use of amikacin at breeding in horses is clearly inadvisable.

The drug is used in neonatal foals in the treatment of a variety of conditions, including septicemia, failure of passive immunoglobulin transfer, or pneumonia. Recently, initial dosage of 13 mg/kg q12 hours was suggested for foals, with therapeutic monitoring to ensure peak concentrations of 25–35 μg/ml and trough concentrations of 2–4 μg/ml (Crisman et al., 1997). However, Magdesian et al. (1997) found that a once-daily dose of 21 mg/kg in foals was not associated with nephrotoxicity and suggested that once-daily dosing might be more efficacious than divided daily dosing, for reasons discussed earlier.

DOGS AND CATS

Amikacin has been approved for parenteral use in dogs in the United States. Indications include serious Gram-negative infections (cystitis, skin or soft tissue infections) caused by otherwise resistant Enterobacteriaceae or *Pseudomonas aeruginosa*, for which alternate drugs are not available or appropriate. It should probably not be used in Seeing Eye or similar dogs, because of the danger of cochlear or vestibular damage.

OTHER

A suggested single daily IV dose of amikacin for emus was 7 mg/kg (Helmick et al., 1997).

Bibliography

Adland-Davenport P, et al. 1990. Pharmacokinetics of amikacin in critically ill neonatal foals treated for presumed or confirmed sepsis. Equine Vet J 22:18.

Blue MG, Oriol JG. 1982. Conception in mares following intrauterine therapy with amikacin. J Equine Vet Sci 2:200.

Brook D. 1982. Using amikacin sulfate to treat genital infections in mares. Vet Med Small Anim Clin 77:434.

Crisman MV, et al. 1997. Clinical application of aminoglycoside therapy in neonatal foals. Am Assoc Equine Pract 43:398.

Garlando F, et al. 1992. Successful treatment of disseminated nocardiosis complicated by cerebral abscess with ceftriaxone and amikacin: case report. Clin Infect Dis 15:1039.

Gingerich DA, et al. 1983. Amikacin: a new aminoglycoside for treating equine metritis. Vet Med Small Anim Clin 78:787.

Golenz MR, et al. 1994. Effect of route of administration and age on the pharmacokinetics of amikacin administered by the intravenous and intraosseous routes to 3- and 5-day-old foals. Equine Vet J 26:367.

Green SL, Conlon PD. 1993. Clinical pharmacokinetics of amikacin in hypoxic premature foals. Equine Vet J 25:276.

Helmick KE, et al. 1997. Disposition of single-dose intravenously administered amikacin in emus (Dromaius novaehollandiae). J Zoo Wildl Med 28:49.

Horspool LJI, et al. 1994. Plasma disposition of amikacin and interactions with gastrointestinal microflora in Equidae following intravenous and oral administration. J Vet Pharmacol Ther 17:291.

Jernigan AD, et al. 1988. Pharmacokinetics of amikacin in cats. Am J Vet Res 49:355.

Magdesian KG, et al. 1997. Pharmacokinetics and nephrotoxicity of high dose, once daily administered amikacin in neonatal foals. Am Assoc Equine Pract 43:396.

Orsini JA, et al. 1989. Resistance to gentamicin and amikacin of Gram-negative organisms isolated from horses. Am J Vet Res 50:923.

Orsini JA, et al. 1996. Tissue and serum concentrations of amikacin after intramuscular and intrauterine administration to mares in estrus. Can Vet J 37:157.

Wichtel MG, et al. 1992. Relation between pharmacokinetics of amikacin sulfate and sepsis score in clinically normal and hospitalized neonatal foals. J Am Vet Med Assoc 200:1339.

Apramycin

Apramycin, like tobramycin, is a nebramycin isolated from the fermentation of *Streptomyces tenebrans*. It has not been developed for clinical use in humans but has been used in the oral treatment of Gram-negative bacterial enteritis of farm animals.

Apramycin is active against *Staphylococcus aureus*, many Gram-negative bacteria, and some mycoplasma (see Table 10.6). Additional studies are required to define its spectrum of activity. Bacteria with MIC ≤16 μg/ml are regarded as susceptible.

The unique chemical structure of apramycin resists most of the R plasmid–mediated degradative enzymes. Resistance is thus rare among

Gram-negative bacteria, so that many pathogenic *E. coli* and *Salmonella* isolated from animals are susceptible. Resistance develops only through one enzyme pathway, aminoglycoside 3-*N*-acetyltransferase IV. Such unique resistance has been used as a marker in studies that support the view that resistance in human nonclinical and clinical isolates of bacteria can spread from use of apramycin in animals (Chaslus-Dancla et al., 1991; Hunter et al., 1994; Johnson et al., 1994). Reports from France by Chaslus-Dancla et al. (1986), however, described multiple aminoglycoside resistance in bovine *Salmonella typhimurium* isolates, because of the presence of resistance plasmids encoding AAC(3)IV. Chromosomal cross-resistance does not occur with other aminoglycosides.

Apramycin is used for the treatment of enteritis caused by Gram-negative bacteria *(E. coli, Salmonella)* in calves and *E. coli, Salmonella,* and *Serpulina* infections in piglets. The drug is administered orally or in some countries parenterally.

In calves, administration of 20 or 40 mg/kg orally or 20 mg/kg IM for 5 days significantly reduced losses from experimental salmonellosis (Espinasse et al., 1981). In veal calves with naturally occurring salmonellosis, 40 mg/kg orally was marginally more effective than 20 mg/kg (Bayle et al., 1980). The pharmacokinetic studies of Ziv et al. (1985) led them to suggest a dose of 20 mg/kg IM every 12 or 24 hours for the treatment of *Salmonella* or *E. coli* infections, respectively.

In swine, apramycin is highly effective in prophylaxis and treatment of colibacillosis (Andreotis et al., 1980). The drug is incorporated into water so that pigs consume sufficient amounts to obtain 12.5 mg/kg daily. Efficacy has been reported against naturally acquired *E. coli* infections in broilers (Cracknell et al., 1986).

Tissue residue problems would be expected to be typical of aminoglycosides in general.

Bibliography

Andreotis JS, et al. 1980. An evaluation of apramycin as an in-feed medication for the treatment of postweaning colibacillosis in pigs. Vet Res Comm 4:131.

Bayle R, et al. 1980. L'apramycine: un nouvel antibiotique de la famille aminosides. Bull Mens Soc Vet Prat Fr 64:371.

Chaslus-Dancla E, et al. 1986. Emergence of aminoglycoside 3-*N*-acetyltransferase IV on *Escherichia coli* and *Salmonella typhimurium* isolated from animals in France. Antimicrob Agents Chemother 29:239.

Chaslus-Dancla E, et al. 1991. High genetic homology between plasmids of human and animal origins conferring resistance to the aminoglycosides gentamicin and apramycin. Antimicrob Agents Chemother 35:590.

Cracknell VC, et al. 1986. An evaluation of apramycin soluble powder for the treatment of naturally acquired *Escherichia coli* infections in broilers. J Vet Pharmacol Ther 9:273.

Espinasse J, et al. 1981. Reproduction experimentale de la salmonellose chez le veau: traitement par l'apramycine. Rec Med Vet 157:571.

Hunter JEB, et al. 1992. Apramycin resistance plasmids in *Escherichia coli:* possible transfer to *Salmonella typhimurium* in calves. Epidemiol Infect 108:271.

Hunter JEB, et al. 1994. Apramycin-resistant *Escherichia coli* isolated from pigs and a stockman. Epidemiol Infect 112:473.

Johnson AP, et al. 1994. Gentamicin resistance in clinical isolates of *Escherichia coli* encoded by genes of veterinary origin. J Med Microbiol 40:221.

Ziv G, et al. 1985. Clinical pharmacology of apramycin in calves. J Vet Pharmacol Ther 8:95.

Gentamicin

Gentamicin is one of the fermentation products of *Micromonospora purpurea*. Because it is not a *Streptomyces* product, it is spelled *gentamicin,* not *gentamycin.*

Antimicrobial Activity

Gentamicin is one of the most active aminoglycosides (see Table 10.1). The drug is active against most Gram-negative aerobic rods, including many *Pseudomonas aeruginosa,* against some Gram-positive bacteria, and against mycoplasma. Gentamicin has little activity against mycobacteria or *Nocardia* and none against anaerobic bacteria or against aerobic bacteria under anaerobic conditions. Like all aminoglycosides, it is bactericidal and penetrates phagocytic cells poorly. There is widespread susceptibility among veterinary pathogenic bacteria (see Table 10.2), although resistance is sometimes a problem in veterinary hospital settings. As with other aminoglycosides, its activity is markedly affected by pH, being optimum around 7.4, and is increased by low magnesium and calcium ion concentration.

Susceptible Bacteria (MIC ≤8 µg/ml) are most Enterobacteriaceae, including *Enterobacter* spp., *Escherichia coli, Klebsiella* spp., *Proteus* spp., *Serratia* spp., and *Yersinia* spp.; *Brucella* spp.; *Campylobacter* spp.; *Haemophilus* spp.; and *Pasteurella* spp. Most strains of *Pseudomonas aeruginosa* are susceptible. Among Gram-positive bacteria, *Staphylococcus aureus* are susceptible, but streptococci and many other Gram-positive aerobes are relatively resistant. *Prototheca zopfii* are generally susceptible.

Resistant Bacteria (MIC ≥16 µg/ml) include many Gram-positive aerobes, some *Pseudomonas* spp., and anaerobes. The development of resistance during treatment is rare. Resistant organisms may occur more commonly in veterinary hospitals than in the community (Koterba et al., 1986). Strains of gentamicin-resistant *P. aeruginosa* are commonly susceptible to amikacin or tobramycin (see Table 10.3). In human hospitals, there have been explosive outbreaks of nosocomial infection caused by gentamicin-resistant bacteria of many species.

Pharmacokinetic Properties

Pharmacokinetic properties were discussed earlier in this chapter in the general description of the properties of the aminoglycosides. The larger volume of distribution in young foals and calves suggests that dosage in these animals should be slightly higher than in adults (see Clinical Applications, this chapter).

Drug Interactions

Gentamicin is commonly synergistic with beta-lactam antibiotics against a wide variety of Gram-negative rods, including *Pseudomonas aeruginosa* (azlocillin, piperacillin), as long as the bacteria are susceptible to the beta-lactam and gentamicin. It is commonly synergistic with beta-lactam antibiotics against Gram-positive bacteria such as *Rhodococcus equi* and *Listeria monocytogenes.* Gentamicin is commonly synergistic with trimethoprim-sulfonamide combinations against *E. coli* and *Klebsiella pneumoniae.* Antagonism may occur with chloramphenicol, tetracycline, and erythromycin.

Carbenicillin, a drug with which gentamicin previously was used to treat serious *Pseudomonas* infections in humans, is incompatible with gentamicin in vitro, as are all beta-lactams. Penicillins and gentamicin should not be mixed in vitro.

Toxicity and Adverse Effects

Gentamicin has the usual aminoglycoside toxic effects of neuromuscular blockade, which is exacerbated by anesthetics, and of minor cardiovascular depressive effects; the drug should not be given rapidly IV. Gentamicin is potentially ototoxic, but the major toxic effect is nephrotoxicosis, which limits prolonged use. High trough concentrations are associated with nephrotoxicosis. Because of the nephrotoxic potential of gentamicin, it is best reserved for severe illnesses, but serum creatinine and urine output, or serum drug concentrations, should be monitored in treated animals.

Subclinical renal damage, which occurs with most therapeutic regimens, is generally reversible. This is not of clinical significance if there is no preexisting renal disease. Risk factors enhancing nephrotoxicity include old age, acidosis, concurrent use of diuretics such as furosemide, daily and total dose, fever, dehydration, previous aminoglycoside treatment, concurrent treatment with amphotericin B and possibly phenylbutazone, and, in the dog, pyometra. Fever decreases the volume of clearance and of distribution, thus increasing plasma gentamicin concentrations. Foals and puppies may have enhanced susceptibility. Should it be necessary to administer the drug in the presence of renal impairment, dosage must be modified.

At present, the only recommendation that can be made is to base dose modification on endogenous creatinine clearance and not on serum creatinine concentrations alone (see Chapter 19). Proteinuria and the presence of renal casts are more sensitive indicators of gentamicin nephrotoxicity than creatinine concentration. A better approach is measurement of serum gentamicin and individualization of gentamicin dosage (Frazier et al., 1988). Nomograms based on age and renal function are used in calculating gentamicin dosage in human patients but are not available in veterinary medicine. Recent population pharmacokinetic studies of gentamicin in horses showed that a considerable proportion of the individual variability recognized in gentamicin disposition could be explained by differences in body weight and serum creatinine (Martin-Jiminez et al., 1998) and that such data can be used to estimate dosage for single daily dosing. Renal damage in dogs administered the recommended dosage is usually mild or moderate and reversible.

Factors described earlier enhance risk. Other risk factors identified for nephrotoxicosis include the nature of the diet in horses (Schumacher et al., 1991) and administration in relation to the time of feeding in rats (Beauchamp et al., 1997). The sparing effect of feeding may be related to the competitive inhibition by protein at the proximal tubule or the nephrotoxic-sparing effect of calcium (Brashier et al., 1998).

Foals may be particularly at risk to gentamicin-induced nephrotoxicosis, although precise evidence is lacking (Riviere et al., 1982). Sepsis may enhance the severity of the nephrotoxicosis, possibly because it is associated with anorexia or an inadequate diet (Schumacher et al., 1991). Horses treated with gentamicin for more than 1 week should be monitored as described for dogs. Foals should not be treated for more than 5–7 days without such monitoring.

Cats are susceptible to gentamicin toxicosis, manifested as loss in vestibular function, which precedes nephrotoxicity, although therapeutic dosage is usually safe in cats treated for reasonable periods (5 days). Monitoring of renal function or serum drug levels is advised in seriously ill cats, for which the drug should be reserved.

Gentamicin should be used with caution in unusual species, since dosage cannot necessarily be determined by extrapolation from apparently analogous species (Johnson et al., 1993; Reimschuessel et al., 1996).

Monitoring of serum concentrations should ensure that maximum concentrations lie in the range 20–30 µg/ml ($3–4 \times$ MIC) and that trough concentrations before redosing are <2 µg/ml.

Administration and Dosage

Administration and dosages are shown in Table 10.5. In some species, SC administration may be used in place of IM administration.

TABLE 10.7. Applications of gentamicin to clinical infections in animals

Species	Primary Applications	Comment
Horses	Gram-negative sepsis of foals; keratoconjunctivitis; genital infections caused by *Pseudomonas aeruginosa* or *Klebsiella pneumoniae*	Toxicity limits its use
Dogs and cats	Wide variety of serious infections caused by Enterobacteriaceae and *P. aeruginosa* resistant to other antibiotics	Toxicity limits its use
Cattle, sheep, and goats	Coliform septicemia, uterine infections by local administration	Not useful in meningitis by parenteral administration
Pigs	Neonatal colibacillosis	
Poultry	Treatment of poults to prevent or treat *Salmonella* or *E. coli* infections	

Clinical Applications

Clinical applications of gentamicin are shown in Table 10.7. Gentamicin is a bactericidal drug active against aerobic bacteria, especially Gram-negative bacteria, and is particularly useful for its activity against Enterobacteriaceae and *Pseudomonas aeruginosa*. It is a drug of choice in the treatment of severe sepsis caused by Gram-negative aerobic rods but is rivaled by fluoroquinolones and newer cephalosporins. It has been extensively used in the treatment of sepsis in neonatal foals. It can be combined with a beta-lactam drug for synergistic activity. Combination treatment of severe, undiagnosed sepsis of gentamicin, ampicillin, and metronidazole would be expected to give a broad-spectrum antibacterial effect.

Gentamicin's greatest drawback is its nephrotoxic potential, which is enhanced by a variety of predisposing factors. Its use should probably be reserved for serious infections in animals caused by Enterobacteriaceae or *P. aeruginosa* in which monitoring of renal function or serum drug concentrations is possible, in the case of companion animals, or for short-term use in the case of food animals. Because of the nephrotoxic potential of gentamicin, it is best reserved for severe illnesses, but serum creatinine and urine output, or serum drug concentrations, should be monitored in these animals. Nevertheless, the nephrotoxic potential of gentamicin should be kept in perspective. In the absence of factors predisposing to gentamicin nephrotoxicosis, treatment with recommended dosage for 5–7 days can be regarded as unlikely to produce significant renal damage. There are few circumstances in which gentamicin need be administered for longer than 5 days. Because of its persistence in the kidney following treatment, it is not recommended for systemic use in cattle in the United States. Gentamicin may substitute for streptomycin in the treatment of brucellosis in humans, combined with doxycycline. Gentamicin may also substitute for streptomycin in the treatment of tularemia in people.

Local application in the case of local infections (eye, ear, uterine) usually overcomes the problem of toxicity. Nephrotoxicosis in a cat associated with excessive local topical administration of gentamicin has been described (Mealey and Boothe, 1994).

Gentamicin-impregnated polymethyl methacrylate beads can be used in the treatment of bone and joint infections, since they result in a slow release of gentamicin at the site of infection and thus avoid problems of nephrotoxicity. Beads, 7 mm in diameter, are threaded onto surgical wire inserted into bone or soft-tissue defects and are removed within 2 weeks. Limited experience is reported with their veterinary use (Brown and Bennett, 1988).

Gentamicin, like other aminoglycosides, penetrates poorly into cells, limiting its activity against intracellular pathogens. Penetration and activity can be increased by liposomal incorporation of the drug (Lutwyche et al., 1998).

CATTLE, SHEEP, AND GOATS

Gentamicin has had limited use in cattle, sheep, and goats because of cost and prolonged tissue residues. The only approved use for gentamicin in cattle in the United States is as an intrauterine infusion. Parenteral administration is associated with persistent kidney residues. Gentamicin has been recommended as a parenteral drug of choice in the treatment of coliform mastitis. Distribution into udder tissue from serum is relatively poor, but the great susceptibility of Enterobacteriaceae makes gentamicin a good potential drug. An IM dose of 3 mg/kg was estimated to result in milk drug concentrations exceeding the MIC of many coliforms for 12 hours and of *Staphylococcus aureus* for 6 hours (Ziv, 1980). Nevertheless, one well-conducted field study of cows suffering from coliform mastitis showed no beneficial effects of systemic administration of the drug (Jones and Ward, 1990). The benefit of intramammary application has been questioned (Erskine et al., 1991), and, experimentally, intramammary gentamicin had no beneficial effect on the course of *E. coli* mastitis in cows (Erskine et al., 1992) (see Chapter 31).

The drug has potential use in the treatment of many Gram-negative infections in cattle, particularly in *E. coli* septicemia or diarrhea and salmonellosis in calves. The high cost and problem of kidney residues, however, have limited gentamicin's application to low-dosage use, such as post-insemination infusion in cows. However, it appears contraindicated for this purpose, as it has been associated with reduced conceptions (Daniels et al., 1976) even though it cured the infections (Anetzhofer, 1989).

There is a voluntary moratorium on the extralabel use of gentamicin in cattle in the United States. This is to prevent violative kidney and liver residues that may occur even with intramammary use (Sweeney et al., 1996).

SWINE

Gentamicin is used to treat neonatal colibacillosis. A single IM injection of 5 or 8 mg results in preventing or treating experimental and field cases.

HORSES

Gentamicin is widely used in horses because of its relatively broad activity, the wide prevalence of susceptible bacteria, and the value of some horses relative to many farm animals. Concern for its nephrotoxic potential may limit its use.

In foals, gentamicin is a drug of choice in the treatment of Gram-negative septicemias, although it has no place in the treatment of meningitis. It may be useful in the treatment of *Rhodococcus equi* pneumonia; however, it must be used concurrently with ampicillin or penicillin G for the synergistic activity of the combination and because gentamicin penetrates macrophages and purulent exudate poorly. The drug should not be used for more than 5–7 days without monitoring renal toxicity and trough serum concentrations.

Gentamicin is a drug of choice in the treatment of infectious metritis in mares caused by susceptible *Klebsiella pneumoniae* or *Pseudomonas aeruginosa*. It has given excellent results when infused into the uterus during estrus on a daily basis for 3–5 days (250 ml physiologic saline, 10 mg/ml) (Houdeshell and Hennessey, 1972). Gentamicin should not be used routinely at or before service or insemination, to avoid promoting resistance and destroying normal vaginal microflora. Stallions with *Klebsiella* or *Pseudomonas* infections of the genital tract have been successfully treated with 4.4 mg/kg twice daily IM or IV. The drug produced myositis in these animals after IM injection and was eventually administered IV in 250 ml of dextrose saline (Hamm, 1978).

Gentamicin is the drug of choice in bacterial ulcerative keratitis and other superficial keratitis of the eye. It is sometimes administered intra-articularly in bacterial arthritis in horses. If this is done, the drug must also be given parenterally. Stover and Pool (1985) reported that a mild, reversible synovitis developed after the intra-articular injection of gentamicin sulfate (3 ml, 50 mg/ml), using a commercial product produced for IM injection. Gentamicin has been administered intra-articularly in the treatment of septic arthritis in horses, since concentrations in synovial fluid achieved by this route exceed those achieved by parenteral administration by up to 100 times, thus exceeding the MIC of susceptible pathogens for 24 hours (Lloyd et al., 1990). Administration (3 ml, 50 mg/ml) intra-articularly is a useful adjunct to systemic antibiotic treatment, joint drainage and lavage, and the use of anti-inflammatory drugs. Buffering gentamicin to reduce acid-induced synovitis reduced antibacterial efficacy (Lloyd et al., 1990) and increased local inflammation (Lloyd et al., 1988).

DOGS AND CATS

The widespread susceptibility of common bacterial pathogens of dogs and cats has made gentamicin a popular drug in small animal practice, where it has been used with excellent results in infections of the urinary tract, respiratory tract, skin and soft tissue, eyes (superficial infections), and gastrointestinal tract. Its activity against *Pseudomonas aeruginosa* has made it especially useful in otitis externa caused by that organism and by otherwise resistant Gram-negative bacteria. Over 90% of canine urinary tract isolates are susceptible to gentamicin; urinary alkalinization may prevent the inhibitory effect of acid on gentamicin's activity. Apart from local application, it should be reserved for serious infections for which other drugs are not suitable. Nevertheless, as discussed earlier, the nephrotoxic potential of gentamicin should be kept in perspective. Administration for 5–7 days in animals not predisposed to gentamicin nephrotoxicosis is unlikely to produce significant renal damage. Parenteral administration in animals with factors predisposing to gentamicin nephrotoxicosis should be monitored by renal function or serum drug monitoring.

POULTRY

Gentamicin is administered to 1-to-3-day-old poults in the prevention and treatment of *E. coli, Pseudomonas aeruginosa,* and *Salmonella* infections.

Bibliography

Anetzhofer, J-V. 1989. Die Behandlung der *Actinomyces pyogenes*—Endometritis durch intrauterine Gentaseptin-Applikation. Schweiz Arch Tierheilkd 131:495.

Beauchamp D, et al. 1997. Time-restricted feeding schedules modify temporal variation of gentamicin experimental nephrotoxicity. Antimicrob Agents Chemother 41:1468.

Brashier MK, et al. 1998. Effect of intravenous calcium administration on gentamicin-induced nephrotoxicosis in ponies. Am J Vet Res 59:1055.

Brown A, Bennett D. 1988. Gentamicin-impregnated polymethylmethacrylate beads for the treatment of septic arthritis. Vet Rec 123:625.

Brown SA, et al. 1985. Gentamicin-associated acute renal failure in the dog. J Am Vet Med Assoc 186:686.

Daniels WH, et al. 1976. Effects of intrauterine infusion of gentamicin sulfate on bovine fertility. Theriogenology 6:61.

Erskine RJ, et al. 1991. Theory, use, and realities of efficacy and food safety of antimicrobial treatment of acute coliform mastitis. J Am Vet Med Assoc 198:980.

Erskine RJ, et al. 1992. Intramammary gentamicin as a therapy for experimental *Escherichia coli* mastitis. Am J Vet Res 53:375.

Frazier DL, et al. 1988. Gentamicin pharmacokinetics and nephrotoxicity in naturally acquired and experimentally induced disease in dogs. J Am Vet Med Assoc 192:57.

Greco DS, et al. 1985. Urinary gamma-glutamyl transpeptidase activity in dogs with gentamicin-induced nephrotoxicity. Am J Vet Res 46:2332.

Hamm DH. 1978. Gentamicin therapy of genital tract infections in stallions. J Equine Med Surg 2:243.

Hardy ML, et al. 1985. The nephrotoxic potential of gentamicin in the cat: enzymuria and alterations in urine concentrating capability. J Vet Pharmacol Ther 8:382.

Houdeshell JW, Hennessey PW. 1972. Gentamicin in the treatment of equine metritis. Vet Med Small Anim Clin 67:1348.

Jernigan AD, et al. 1988. Pharmacokinetics of gentamicin after intravenous, intramuscular, and subcutaneous administration in cats. Am J Vet Res 49:32.

Johnson JH, et al. 1993. Gentamicin toxicosis in a North American cougar. J Am Vet Med Assoc 203:854.

Jones GF, Ward GE. 1990. Evaluation of systemic administration of gentamicin for treatment of coliform mastitis in cows. J Am Vet Med Assoc 197:731.

Koterba A, et al. 1986. Nosocomial infections and bacterial antibiotic resistance in a university equine hospital. J Am Vet Med Assoc 189:185.

Lackey ML, et al. 1996. Single intravenous and multiple dose pharmacokinetics of gentamicin in healthy llamas. Am J Vet Res 57:1193.

Lloyd KCK, et al. 1988. Effect of gentamicin sulfate and sodium bicarbonate on the synovium of clinically normal equine antebrachiocarpal joints. Am J Vet Res 49:650.

Lloyd KCK, et al. 1990. Synovial fluid pH, cytologic characteristics, and gentamicin concentration after intra-articular administration of the drug in an experimental model of infectious arthritis in horses. Am J Vet Res 51:1363.

Lutwyche P, et al. 1998. Intracellular delivery and antibacterial activity of gentamicin encapsulated in pH-sensitive liposomes. Antimicrob Agents Chemother 42:2511.

Magdesian KG, et al. 1998. Pharmacokinetics of a high dose of gentamicin administered intravenously or intramuscularly in horses. J Am Vet Med Assoc 213:1007.

Martin-Jiminez T, et al. 1998. Population pharmacokinetics of gentamicin in horses. Am J Vet Res 59:1589.

Mealey KL, Boothe DM. 1994. Nephrotoxicosis associated with topical administration of gentamicin in a cat. J Am Vet Med Assoc 204:1919.

Moore CP, et al. 1983. Bacterial and fungal isolates from Equidae with ulcerative keratitis. J Am Vet Med Assoc 182:600.

Pedersoli WM, et al. 1995. Depletion of gentamicin in the milk of Holstein cows after single and repeated intramammary and parenteral treatments. J Vet Pharmacol Ther 18:457.

Raisbeck MF, et al. 1983. Fatal nephrotoxicosis is associated with furosemide and gentamicin therapy in a dog. J Am Vet Med Assoc 183:892.

Reimschuessel R, et al. 1996. Evaluation of gentamicin-induced nephrotoxicosis in toadfish. J Am Vet Med Assoc 209:137.

Riviere JE, et al. 1982. Gentamicin toxic nephropathy in horses with disseminated bacterial infection. J Am Vet Med Assoc 180:648.

Rubin SI, Papich MG. 1987. Acute renal failure in dogs: a case of gentamicin toxicity. Compend Contin Educ Pract Vet 9:510.

Schumacher J, et al. 1991. Effect of diet on gentamicin-induced nephrotoxicosis in horses. Am J Vet Res 52:1274.

Short CR, et al. 1986. The nephrotoxic potential of gentamicin in the cat: a pharmacokinetic and histopathologic investigation. J Vet Pharmacol Ther 9:325.

Sojka JE, Brown SA. 1986. Pharmacokinetic adjustment of gentamicin dosing in horses with sepsis. J Am Vet Med Assoc 189:784.

Stover SM, Pool RE. 1985. Effect of intra-articular gentamicin sulfate on normal equine synovial membrane. Am J Vet Res 46:2485.

Sweeney RW, et al. 1992. Disposition of gentamicin administered intravenously to horses with sepsis. J Am Vet Med Assoc 200:503.

Sweeney RW, et al. 1996. Systemic absorption of gentamicin following intramammary administration to cows with mastitis. J Vet Pharmacol Ther 19:155.

Ziv G. 1980. Drug selection and use in mastitis: systemic vs. local therapy. J Am Vet Med Assoc 176:1109.

Ziv G. 1981. Concentration and residues of gentamicin in the milk of dairy cows after intramammary infusion. Bovine Pract 16:30.

Spectinomycin

Spectinomycin (Fig. 10.3) is a product of *Streptomyces spectabilis*. It is an aminocyclitol antibiotic that lacks most of the toxic effects of the aminoglycoside antibiotics but unfortunately is limited in application by the ready development of resistance. There are discrepancies between resistance to the drug in vitro and apparent efficacy in some cases clinically, which have not been explained. For example, Goren et al. (1988) observed high efficacy of orally administered spectinomycin or lincomycin-spectinomycin in treating experimentally induced *E. coli* infections in chickens, despite the absence of any antimicrobial activity in the serum of these chickens. To explain this discrepancy, they suggested that a metabolite or degradation product of the drug might reach the respiratory tract and interfere with bacterial attachment. This explanation is speculative, since it has not been shown that the drug undergoes metabolism in any species. In humans, all of an administered dose is recovered in the urine within 48 hours after injection.

Antimicrobial Activity

Spectinomycin is a usually bacteriostatic, relatively broad-spectrum drug that can be bactericidal at increased concentrations (ie, $4 \times$ MIC). It is not particularly active on a weight basis (Table 10.8). Bacteria are usually regarded as susceptible if their MIC is ≤ 20 µg/ml. Susceptibility among aerobic Gram-negative rods is unpredictable because of the

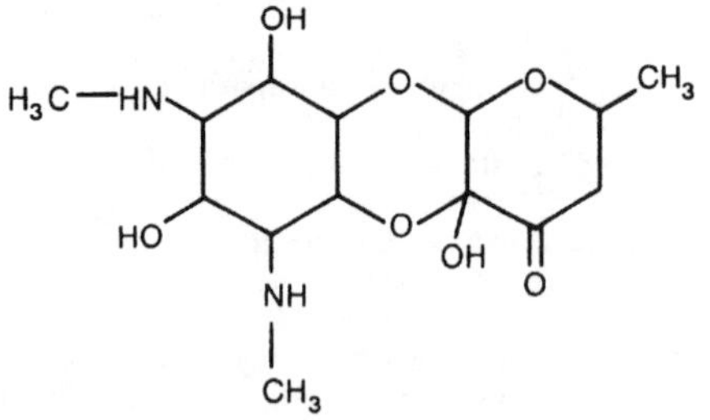

Fig. 10.3. Structural formula of spectinomycin.

presence of naturally resistant strains. Mycoplasma are susceptible, but *Pseudomonas aeruginosa* is resistant. There is little information on the prevalence of susceptibility among animal pathogens.

Resistance

Natural resistance to spectinomycin in many enteric bacteria is widespread. Chromosomal one-step mutation to high-level resistance develops readily in vivo and in vitro, in a manner similar to streptomycin resistance. Chromosomally resistant strains do not show cross-resistance with aminoglycosides. Plasmid-mediated resistance is uncommon. Vaillancourt et al. (1988) reported a marked drop (from 91% to 24%) of in vitro susceptibility of *Actinobacillus pleuropneumoniae* isolated over a 5-year period, associated with the widespread use of the drug to treat pleuropneumonia in swine. They noted, however, discrepancies between in vitro resistance and apparent field efficacy.

Drug Interactions

Combination with lincosamides may marginally enhance spectinomycin's activity against mycoplasmas and *Serpulina hyodysenteriae*.

Toxicity and Adverse Effects

Spectinomycin seems to be relatively nontoxic in animals; it does not induce ototoxicity or nephrotoxicity but may, like the aminoglycosides, cause neuromuscular blockade. The apparent lack of reported toxic effects may reflect lack of long-term usage. Administration of lincomycin-spectinomycin oral preparations, by parenteral injection to cattle, has produced heavy losses associated with severe pulmonary edema. Similar

TABLE 10.8. **Activity (MIC$_{90}$, μg/ml) of spectinomycin against selected bacteria and mycoplasma**

Organism		Organism	
Gram-positive aerobes			
Rhodococcus equi	8	*S. pyogenes*	64
Staphylococcus aureus	64		
Gram-negative aerobes			
Actinobacillus pleuropneumoniae	32	*Ornithobacterium rhinotracheale*	≥64
Bordetella avium	>128	*Pasteurella multocida*	32
B. bronchiseptica	>256	*Proteus* sp.	>128
Brucella canis	1	*Pseudomonas aeruginosa*	>256
Escherichia coli	>400	*Salmonella* sp.	≥64
Haemophilus somnus	25	*Taylorella equigenitalis*	4
Klebsiella pneumoniae	32		
Mycoplasmas			
M. bovis	4	*M. hyorhinis*	1
M. bovigenitalium	4	*M. hyosynoviae*	4
M. hyopneumoniae	1		

problems have been noted with misuse of spectinomycin and attributed to endotoxin contamination (Genetsky et al., 1994).

Pharmacokinetic Properties
Pharmacokinetic properties are similar to those of the aminoglycosides.

Administration and Dosage
Administration and dosages are shown in Table 10.5.

Clinical Applications
Spectinomycin has been largely abandoned in human medicine because of the rapid development of resistance and unpredictable antibiotic susceptibility. The drug is used in animals in the treatment of mycoplasma infections, diseases caused by Enterobacteriaceae (*E. coli*, diarrhea, septicemia), and respiratory disease caused by Gram-negative bacteria. The development of resistance in bacteria limits the drug's long-term use. It is sometimes combined with lincomycin to give a broad-spectrum combination with activity against Gram-positive aerobic as well as anaerobic bacteria.

In cattle, spectinomycin is used to treat pneumonia. A single daily dose of 20 mg/kg was shown to be as effective as the same dose q12 hours in treatment of pneumonia caused by *Pasteurella* sp. and by *Mycoplasma bovis* (Pobel et al., 1997). It has been used successfully to treat *Salmonella dublin* infection in calves at a dosage of 22 mg/kg SC on the first day and 0.5 g PO twice daily for an additional 4 days (Cook, 1973). A dosage of 500 mg IM daily for 5 days successfully treated early cases of *Mycoplasma bovis* pneumonia and arthritis in calves. Combined with lincomycin, the drug was effective in treating *Ureaplasma* infection in rams (Marcus et al., 1994).

For pigs, spectinomycin is available as an oral preparation for the treatment of colibacillosis. It is also administered IM for the treatment of respiratory disease, including *Actinobacillus pleuropneumoniae*. Resistance has limited use for this latter purpose. Although not approved for this use, IM injection of 10 mg/kg BID for 3 days has been used successfully to treat pigs severely affected with proliferative intestinal adenomatosis. The MIC of spectinomycin against *Lawsonia intracellularis* (32 µg/ml) is the lowest among the aminoglycosides but suggests that the organism is barely susceptible, at least in vitro (McOrist et al., 1995). Spectinomycin is available combined with lincomycin for the oral treatment of swine dysentery.

In dogs, spectinomycin has been administered by IM injection for a variety of infections with Gram-negative bacteria, but no reports of efficacy are available. It is available combined with lincomycin for the treatment of streptococcal, staphylococcal, *Mycoplasma*, and *Pasteurella* infections, with dosage based on 20 mg/kg IM of the spectinomycin component administered once or twice daily. Such a combination could give broad-spectrum antibacterial activity that would include activity against Gram-positive as well as anaerobic bacteria.

In poultry, spectinomycin is used parenterally in young poults as a single injection to control salmonellosis, pasteurellosis, *E. coli,* and *Mycoplasma synoviae.* Spectinomycin can be administered in the water to control mortality associated with chronic respiratory disease and infectious synovitis. The activity of spectinomycin against mycoplasma is a particularly useful attribute, but it is surprising that the drug administered orally would have any effect on systemic infections, since it is at best poorly absorbed from the intestine.

Bibliography

Cook B. 1973. Successful treatment of an outbreak of *Salmonella dublin* infection in calves using spectinomycin. Vet Rec 93:80.

Genetsky R, et al. 1994. Intravenous spectinomycin-associated deaths in feedlot cattle. J Vet Diagn Invest 6:266.

Goren E, et al. 1988. Therapeutic efficacy of medicating drinking water with spectinomycin and lincomycin-spectinomycin in experimental *Escherichia coli* infection in poultry. Vet Q 10:191.

Marcus S, et al. 1994. Lincomycin and spectinomycin in the treatment of breeding rams contaminated with ureaplasmas. Res Vet Sci 57:393.

McOrist S, et al. 1995. Antimicrobial susceptibility of ileal symbiont intracellularis isolated from pigs with proliferative enteropathy. J Clin Microbiol 33:1314.

Pobel T, et al. 1997. Comparaison de l'administration quotidienne ou biquotidienne de la spectinomycine (Spectam G. A.) dans le traitement des infections respiratoires des bovins a *Pasteurella haemolytica* ou *Pasteurella multocida* associees ou non a *Mycoplasma bovis.* Rev Med Vet 148:47.

Vaillancourt J-P, et al. 1988. Changes in the susceptibility of *Actinobacillus pleuropneumoniae* to antimicrobial agents in Quebec (1981–1986). J Am Vet Med Assoc 193:470.

Tobramycin

Tobramycin is a naturally occurring deoxykanamycin (Fig. 10.4) with antimicrobial and pharmacokinetic properties similar to those of gentamicin. It is, however, more active against *Pseudomonas aeruginosa,* including perhaps two-thirds of gentamicin-resistant strains. Tobramycin is generally not effective against gentamicin-resistant strains of Enterobacteriaceae. For treatment of serious *P. aeruginosa* infections, tobramycin should be combined with an antipseudomonal penicillin. One other advantage over gentamicin is reduced nephrotoxicity, although ototoxic properties are similar. In a study of tobramycin pharmacokinetics in cats, Jernigan et al. (1988) found persistent elevations of blood urea nitrogen and serum creatinine, suggesting possible renal damage 3 weeks after a single dose

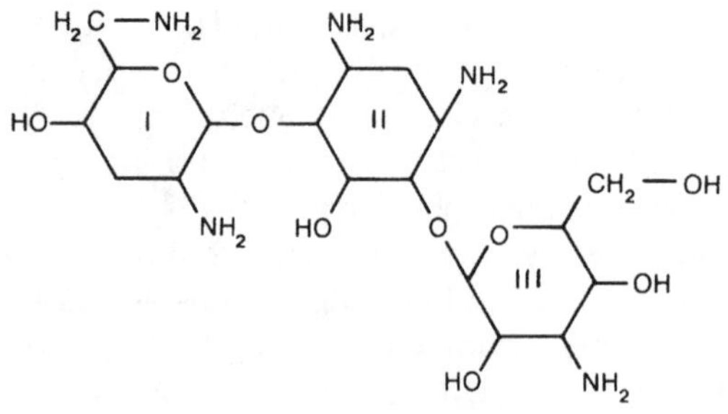

Fig. 10.4. Structural formula of tobramycin.

(5 mg/kg) of tobramycin. The authors suggested that this high dose may have occupied and saturated binding sites in the kidneys from which the drug was only slowly released. Blood urea nitrogen rose in fewer cats after a lower dose (3 mg/kg). Besides evidence of renal toxicity, there was also evidence of dose-dependent differences in pharmacokinetics, suggesting that further studies of toxicity and pharmacokinetics are required in multiple-dosing studies before tobramycin can be recommended in cats.

Bibliography

Hadi, AAA. 1994. Pharmacokinetics of tobramycin in the camel. J Vet Pharmacol Ther 17:48.
Jernigan AD, et al. 1988. Pharmacokinetics of tobramycin in cats. Am J Vet Res 49:608.

New Aminoglycosides

Sisomicin is a derivative of the gentamicin C_{1a} component, with greater activity than gentamicin against certain bacteria, including *Proteus, Pseudomonas aeruginosa,* and some *Citrobacter, Klebsiella,* and *Serratia.* There is incomplete cross-resistance with gentamicin and tobramycin. Pharmacokinetic behavior and toxicity are virtually identical to those of gentamicin.

Netilmicin is a derivative of sisomicin with similar activity to gentamicin but is active against gentamicin-resistant strains, particularly those that produce AAD(2″), including *E. coli, Klebsiella,* and *Serratia.* Most gentamicin-resistant *P. aeruginosa* are netilmicin resistant.

Neither sisomicin nor netilmicin are likely to be introduced into veterinary use, since they have fewer advantages than amikacin and since the introduction of fluoroquinolones in veterinary medicine has largely displaced the need for newer aminoglycosides.

11 | Lincosamides, Macrolides, and Pleuromutilins

J. F. PRESCOTT

Lincosamides, macrolides, and pleuromutilins are structurally distinct antibiotics but share many common properties. They are basic compounds characterized by high lipid solubility, good absorption from the intestine, wide distribution in the body, liver rather than kidney excretion, capacity to penetrate cellular barriers, and other pharmacokinetic features. They have a common site of action on the 50S ribosome. They are bacteriostatic drugs, particularly active against Gram-positive bacteria and mycoplasma and with fair to good activity against anaerobic bacteria. Most aerobic Gram-negative bacteria are resistant, but some important Gram-negative organisms are susceptible. The activity of these drugs against agents of human upper respiratory tract infections and against many intracellular bacteria, together with their sometimes striking concentration in macrophages, have led to the development of newer macrolides that lack the adverse effects of, and may have greater potency than, the classic macrolides.

Lincosamides: Lincomycin, Clindamycin, and Pirlimycin
Chemistry
Lincomycin, the parent compound, is a fermentation product of *Streptomyces* spp. A monoglycoside with an amino acid–like side chain, lincomycin has one derivative, clindamycin (7-chloro-7-deoxylincomycin), which has significantly greater activity than the parent compound (Fig. 11.1).

229

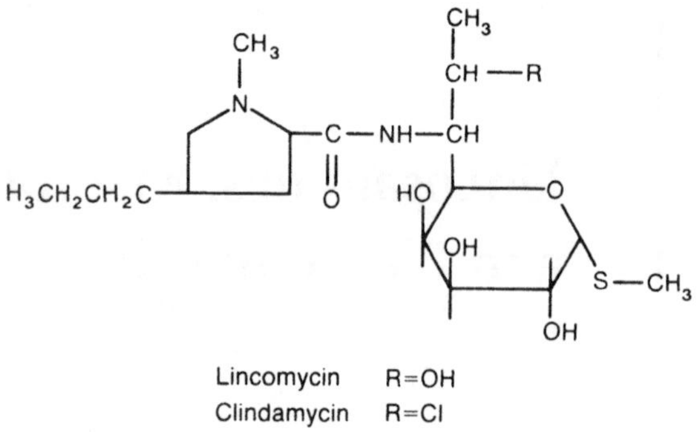

Lincomycin   R=OH
Clindamycin   R=Cl

Fig. 11.1.   Structural formulas of lincomycin and clindamycin.

Mechanism of Action

The lincosamides are bacteriostatic antibiotics. They inhibit protein synthesis by binding to the 50S ribosomal subunit and inhibiting peptidyl transferases. Clindamycin may behave slightly differently. Many Gram-negative bacteria are resistant because of impermeability and methylation of the ribosomal binding site of lincosamides.

Antimicrobial Activity

Lincosamides are moderate-spectrum antimicrobial drugs. Clindamycin is several times more active than lincomycin, especially against anaerobes and *Staphylococcus aureus*. Lincosamides are active against Gram-positive bacteria, anaerobic bacteria, and mycoplasmas but are considerably less active against Gram-negative bacteria than the macrolides.

Good Susceptibility (MIC ≤0.5 µg/ml): Gram-positive aerobes: *Bacillus* spp., *Corynebacterium* spp., *Erysipelothrix rhusiopathiae*, staphylococci, and streptococci (but not enterococci). Gram-negative bacteria: *Campylobacter* spp. Anaerobes: many anaerobes, including *Actinomyces* spp., *Bacteroides* spp. (including *B. fragilis*), and *Clostridium perfringens* (but not all other *Clostridium* spp.). *Fusobacterium* spp., anaerobic cocci, and *Serpulina hyodysenteriae* are particularly susceptible to clindamycin, which may be bactericidal to them. Activity of clindamycin against anaerobes is similar to that of cefoxitin, chloramphenicol, and metronidazole. The antimycoplasma activity of the lincosamides is similar to that of erythromycin but less than that of the other macrolides. Clindamycin has activity against toxoplasmas and certain malarial parasites.

Resistant (MIC ≥4 µg/ml): All aerobic Gram-negative rods, *Nocardia* spp., and *Mycobacterium* spp.

Resistance

Chromosomal resistance develops fairly readily to both the lincosamides and macrolides in a stepwise fashion. Emergence of resistance during treatment is rare in human medicine. Plasmid-mediated resistance is common and more stable. Resistance is the result of methylation of adenine residues in the 23S ribosomal RNA of the 50S ribosomal subunit, which prevents drug binding to the target site. There is usually complete cross-resistance between lincomycin and clindamycin, and cross-resistance with macrolides is also common.

Resistance can develop to the lincosamides alone, but more commonly cross-resistance occurs among macrolides, lincosamides, and streptogramin group B antibiotics (MLS cross-resistance). This cross-resistance is of two types: (1) constitutive resistance, in which bacteria show high-level resistance to all MLS antibiotics; and (2) dissociated inducible cross-resistance, in which bacteria resistant to erythromycin but initially fully susceptible to clindamycin rapidly develop resistance to lincosamides when exposed to erythromycin. Constitutive resistant mutants are rapidly selected from the inducible strains during treatment with either lincosamides or macrolides. Constitutive resistance may be more common among bacteria isolated from food animals fed tylosin or virginiamycin as growth promoters.

Pharmacokinetic Properties

Lincosamides are basic compounds with pK_a values of about 7.6. They have high lipid solubility and consequently large apparent volumes of distribution. They are well absorbed from the intestine of nonherbivores and eliminated mainly by hepatic metabolism, although about 20% is eliminated in active form in the urine. Tissue concentrations consistently exceed serum concentrations by several times because of passage across cell membranes. Because of the lincosamide's basic character, ion trapping also occurs in tissues, such as the udder and prostate, where pH is lower than blood. Extensive binding to plasma proteins and relatively rapid elimination prevent concentrations in cerebrospinal fluid from exceeding 20% of serum concentrations. Clindamycin achieves effective concentrations in bone, although levels are relatively low, perhaps 10–20% of serum concentrations.

Drug Interactions

Combination with spectinomycin appears to give marginally enhanced activity against mycoplasmas in vitro. Clindamycin is commonly combined with an aminoglycoside in human medicine to treat or prevent mixed aerobic-anaerobic bacterial infections, particularly those associated with intestinal spillage into the peritoneum. The combination generally has additive or synergistic effects in vitro against a wide range of bacteria. Clindamycin has synergistic effects with metronidazole against *Bacteroides fragilis* but only additive effects with trimethoprim-sulfamethoxazole combination against common Gram-negative or Gram-positive aerobes. Combination with macrolides or chloramphenicol is antagonistic in vitro.

Toxicity and Adverse Effects

The major toxic effect of the lincosamides is their ability to cause serious and fatal diarrhea in humans, horses, rabbits, and other herbivores.

In humans, mild diarrhea follows the use of lincosamides in up to 10% of patients, but in some (0–2.5% of those treated) this may become severe, resulting in pseudomembranous colitis with profound shock, dehydration, and death. The disease is caused by the rapid colonic growth of lincosamide-resistant *Clostridium difficile* through destruction of competing anaerobic microflora of the colon. Treatment with vancomycin or metronidazole is often successful. Less serious toxic effects in humans include depressed neuromuscular transmission and post-anesthetic paralysis, depression of cardiac muscle after rapid IV injection, mild liver damage, drug rashes, and urticaria.

In cattle, oral administration of lincomycin at concentrations as low as 7.5 parts/million (ppm) in feed has resulted in inappetence, diarrhea, ketosis, and decreased milk production. Inadvertent contamination of feed with 8–10 ppm of lincomycin and 40 ppm of metronidazole caused some affected cows to develop severe diarrhea and to lose consciousness (Lang, 1979). In horses, lincosamides administered by parenteral or oral route can cause hemorrhagic colitis and diarrhea, which may be fatal. In one inadvertent mixing of lincomycin in horse feed, a dose of 0.5 mg/kg caused an outbreak of diarrhea in which one horse died (Raisbeck et al., 1981).

Lincosamides are highly toxic to sheep, rabbits, guinea pigs, and hamsters. Concentrations as low as 8 ppm accidentally added to feed have been followed by severe and fatal cecocolitis in rabbits; ampicillin may have a similar effect (Thilsted et al., 1981). In rabbits the effect is the result of bacterial overgrowth in the large bowel of *Clostridium difficile* or *C. spiroforme* (Borriello and Carman, 1983).

Lincomycin is relatively nontoxic to dogs and cats. Vomiting and diarrhea have sometimes occurred with oral use, and anaphylactic shock has been reported after IM injection. Because of their peripheral neuromuscular blocking and cardiac depressive effects, lincosamides should not be given with anesthetics or by rapid IV injection. Clindamycin given IM is very painful.

TABLE 11.1.   Usual dosages of lincosamides and classic macrolides in animals

Drug	Dosages (mg/kg)	Route	Interval (h)	Comments
Lincomycin	15–25	PO	8–12	Not herbivores
hydrochloride	10–20	IM, IV	12–24	
Clindamycin				
hydrochloride	5–11	PO	12–24[a]	Not herbivores
phosphate	3–5	IM, IV	8–12	
Erythromycin				
estolate	25	PO	8	Not herbivores; *Rhodococcus equi* in foals
gluceptate	5	IV	6	*Rhodococcus equi* in foals
lactobionate	3–5	IM, IV	8–12	IV only horses
Tilmicosin	10	SC	24	Cattle and sheep only; for swine and poultry, see text
Tylosin	20–30	IM	8–12	Not horses; drinking water for swine
Tiamulin	20	IM	24	Cattle
	12	IM	24	Swine
		PO		See text, swine: Chapter 25
Spiramycin	20	IM	24	Cattle

Note: Macrolide antibiotics are highly irritating on injection. They should not be used in adult horses, rabbits, guinea pigs, hamsters, gerbils, and other herbivores with expanded large intestines, because of toxicity.
[a]Use higher dosage of clindamycin for serious infections.

Administration and Dosage

Usual dosages are shown in Table 11.1.

After oral administration to monogastric animals, lincomycin is generally absorbed well, and clindamycin is extremely well absorbed. Food significantly reduces absorption of both drugs, especially lincomycin. Complete absorption occurs from IM injection sites. Clindamycin palmitate, available as a syrup for oral administration, is rapidly hydrolyzed in the intestine before absorption. The drug is also available in capsules as the hydrochloride for oral administration and as the phosphate for IM (painful) or IV injection. Lincomycin is available as the hydrochloride for PO, IM, and IV administration. The dosage should be reduced in patients with hepatic insufficiency.

Clinical Applications

Lincosamides are used in the treatment of staphylococcal infections (dermatitis, osteomyelitis) caused by penicillin G–resistant organisms, for other Gram-positive aerobic infections in penicillin-sensitive individuals, and in the treatment of anaerobic infections. In general, clindamycin is preferred to lincomycin. Clindamycin has excellent activity against anaerobes, equivalent to that of alternatives such as cefoxitin, chloramphenicol, and metronidazole. Clindamycin may be combined with an aminoglycoside in the treatment of mixed anaerobic infections such as those associated with intestinal perforation. Clindamycin may be preferable to penicillin G or ampicillin in the treatment of streptococcal toxic shock syndrome, since it better inhibits superantigen synthesis (Sriskandan et al., 1997). Lincosamides penetrate well into the prostate and eyes. There are some doubts about the efficacy in vivo of clindamycin in the treatment of toxoplasmosis, although combination with pyrimethamine may enhance efficacy. Clindamycin may be useful in treating *Pneumocystis carinii* infection, in combination with primaquine. In swine, lincomycin is used extensively in the prevention and treatment of dysentery and sometimes for mycoplasma infections.

CATTLE, SHEEP, AND GOATS

Lincomycin-spectinomycin combinations are sometimes used in the parenteral treatment of respiratory disease in cattle because lincomycin inhibits mycoplasma, *Arcanobacterium pyogenes*, and anaerobic bacteria, and spectinomycin is often active against *Pasteurella* and *Haemophilus somnus*. A field trial has confirmed the value of the combination (Pobel et al., 1997). Lincomycin (8 g/l) administered as a spray once daily for 5 days was effective in the control of papillomatous digital dermatitis in cattle (Shearer and Elliott, 1998). A single IM injection of the combination (5 mg/kg lincomycin, 10 mg/kg spectinomycin) cured more than 90% of sheep with acute or chronic foot rot and was almost as effective as the same dose given on each of 3 days (Venning et al., 1990). The combination has also been used in the treatment of rams to prevent ureaplasma contamination of semen (Marcus et al., 1994).

Lincomycin and clindamycin can be used in the parenteral treatment of acute staphylococcal or streptococcal mastitis at a dosage of 10 mg/kg q24 hours. The drugs can be given by the intramammary route for the same purpose. Lincomycin has been used parenterally in sheep and cattle. The successful treatment of arthritis and pedal osteomyelitis usually associated with *A. pyogenes* with parenteral lincomycin was reported by Plenderleith (1988). The catastrophic effects of oral administration of lincomycin to sheep were described by Bulgin (1988).

SWINE

Lincomycin is largely used in pigs to control dysentery and mycoplasma infections; control of erysipelas and streptococcal infections may be incidental benefits to incorporating the drug in feed for the principal purposes. Lincomycin is used in feed or water (33 mg/l) to treat (100 ppm feed) or prevent (40 ppm feed) swine dysentery; lincomycin can be administered 11 mg/kg IM for 3–7 days. A drawback has been failure to sterilize *Serpulina hyodysenteriae,* so that withdrawal of drug is followed by recrudescence of infection. Nevertheless, whole herd medication has apparently eradicated swine dysentery from closed herds even in some cases with infection caused by apparently resistant organisms. Lincomycin is effective in reducing losses from *Mycoplasma hyosynoviae* and *M. hyorhinis.* The drug may be given in feed or by injection. Tiamulin is considerably more effective than lincomycin in control of swine dysentery and mycoplasma infections in swine.

HORSES

Lincosamides should not be used in horses because of toxicity, although there are reports of apparently successful use in the treatment of osteomyelitis by IM injection without toxic effects (Plenderleith, 1988).

DOGS AND CATS

Lincosamides are used in the treatment of abscesses, osteomyelitis, periodontal disease, and soft tissue or wound infections that involve Gram-positive coccal or anaerobic bacteria. In experimentally induced *Staphylococcus aureus* osteomyelitis in dogs, a dosage of 11 mg/kg of clindamycin administered q12 hours for 28 days effectively resolved the infection (Braden et al., 1988). Dosage of 5.5 mg/kg q12 hours was less effective. Clindamycin has been administered at low daily oral dosage in the successful prophylaxis of recurrent staphylococcal skin infections (Klempner and Styrt, 1988). Field trials have demonstrated the 94–100% efficacy of single daily dosing with 11 mg/kg orally (average duration 45 days) in the treatment of deep pyoderma in dogs (Harvey et al., 1993; Scott et al., 1998). Lincomycin (22 mg/kg, q12 hours) orally is equally effective in the treatment of staphylococcal skin disease in dogs (Harvey et al., 1993).

In a study of experimental anaerobic infections in dogs, Berg et al. (1984) found that clindamycin, 5.5 or 11 mg/kg administered twice daily IM, was highly efficacious and gave better results than lincomycin, 22 mg/kg twice daily. Clindamycin is used effectively in the treatment of dental infections in dogs, when combined with dental surgery or cleaning (Johnson et al., 1992). Anecdotally, its routine use in periodontal surgery has been associated with problems of salmonellosis in veterinary hospitals. Clindamycin is useful for prostatic infections caused by Gram-positive bacteria. Dosing of 11 mg/kg once daily orally appears to be appropriate, but the same dose could be administered twice daily in serious infections (eg, osteomyelitis).

Clindamycin has been used successfully in the treatment of toxoplasmosis in a dog and in cats, although it was unsuccessful in treating feline chorioretinitis or anterior uveitis in all cases (Greene et al., 1985;

Lappin et al., 1989). Clindamycin administered to cats experimentally infected with toxoplasmosis exacerbated disease, increasing morbidity and mortality from generalized disease (Davidson et al., 1996). This adverse effect was attributed to an effect of the drug in decreasing phagocyte activity. Combination with pyrimethamine was less effective in long-term treatment of toxoplasmic encephalitis in human patients than the combination of pyrimethamine-sulfadiazine (Katlama et al., 1996). Clindamycin was successful in resolving dermatitis caused by *Neospora caninum* in a dog (Dubey et al., 1995).

POULTRY

Lincomycin-spectinomycin combination is administered orally to young chickens for the control of mycoplasmal airsacculitis and complicated chronic respiratory disease caused by *Mycoplasma gallisepticum* and *E. coli*.

Bibliography

Berg JN, et al. 1984. Clinical models for anaerobic bacteria: infections in dogs and their use in the testing of the efficacy of clindamycin and lincomycin. Am J Vet Res 45:1299.

Boothe DM, et al. 1996. Plasma disposition of clindamycin microbiological activity in cats after single oral doses of clindamycin hydrochloride as either capsules or aqueous solution. J Vet Pharmacol Ther 19:491.

Borriello SP, Carman RJ. 1983. Association of iota-toxin and *Clostridium spiroforme* with both spontaneous and antibiotic-associated diarrhea and colitis in rabbits. J Clin Microbiol 17:414.

Braden TD, et al. 1988. Posologic evaluation of clindamycin, using a canine model of post-traumatic osteomyelitis. Am J Vet Res 48:1101.

Brown SA, et al. 1990. Tissue concentrations of clindamycin after multiple oral doses in normal cats. J Vet Pharmacol Ther 13:270.

Bulgin MS. 1988. Losses related to the ingestion of lincomycin-medicated feed in a range sheep flock. J Am Vet Med Assoc 192:1083.

Davidson MG, et al. 1996. Paradoxical effect of clindamycin in experimental acute toxoplasmosis in cats. Antimicrob Agents Chemother 40:1352.

Dubey JP, et al. 1995. Canine cutaneous neosporosis: clinical improvement with clindamycin. Vet Dermatol 6:37.

Greene CG, et al. 1985. Clindamycin for treatment of toxoplasma polymyositis in a dog. J Am Vet Med Assoc 187:631.

Harvey RG, et al. 1993. A comparison of lincomycin hydrochloride and clindamycin hydrochloride in the treatment of superficial pyoderma in dogs. Vet Rec 132:351.

Johnson LA, et al. 1992. Klinische wirksamkeit von clindamycin (Cleorobe) bei infektionen des zahn-, mund- under kieferbereiches des hundes. Prakt Tieraerztl 73:94.

Katlama C, et al. 1996. Pyrimethamine-clindamycin vs. pyrimethamine-sulfadiazine as acute and long-term therapy for toxoplasmic encephalitis in patients with AIDS. Clin Infect Dis 22:268.

Klempner MS, Styrt B. 1988. Prevention of recurrent staphylococcal skin infections with low-dose oral clindamycin therapy. J Am Med Assoc 260:2682.

Lang DC. 1979. Inadvertent inclusion of antibiotics in cattle cake. Vet Rec 104:173.

Lappin MR, et al. 1989. Clinical feline toxoplasmosis: serologic diagnosis and therapeutic management of 15 cases. J Vet Intern Med 3:139.

Marcus S, et al. 1994. Lincomycin and spectinomycin in the treatment of breeding rams with semen contaminated with ureaplasmas. Res Vet Sci 57:393.

Plenderleith RJW. 1988. Treatment of cattle, sheep, and horses with lincomycin: case studies. Vet Rec 122:112.

Pobel T, et al. 1997. Comparaison de l'administration quotidienne ou biquotienne de la spectinomycine (Spectam G. A.) dans le traitement des infections respiratoires des boivins a *Pasteurella haemolytica* ou *Pasteurella multocida* associes ou non a *Mycoplasma bovis*. Rev Med Vet 148:47.

Raisbeck MF, et al. 1981. Lincomycin—associated colitis in horses. J Am Vet Med Assoc 179:362.

Scott DW, et al. 1998. Efficacy of clindamycin hydrochloride capsules for the treatment of deep pyoderma due to *Staphylococcus intermedius* infection in dogs. Can Vet J 39:753.

Shearer JK, Elliott JB. 1998. Papillomatous digital dermatitis: treatment and control strategies 20:S158.

Sriskandan S, et al. 1997. Comparative effects of clindamycin and ampicillin on super-antigenic activity of *Streptococcus pyogenes*. J Antimicrob Chemother 40:275.

Thilsted JP, et al. 1981. Fatal diarrhea in rabbits resulting from the feeding of antibiotic-contaminated feed. J Am Vet Med Assoc 179:360.

Venning CM, et al. 1990. Treatment of virulent foot rot with lincomycin and spectino-mycin. Aust Vet J 67:258.

Pirlimycin

Pirlimycin is an amide of methyl(7,5)-7-chloro-7-deoxythiolin-cosaminide hydrochloride. Activity against aerobes and anaerobes is similar to that of clindamycin but activity in experimental infections has been 2–20 times greater, probably because the drug is markedly concentrated and retained in tissues. The drug is used in local treatment of bovine mastitis caused by Gram-positive bacteria, particularly chronic infections.

Bibliography

Owens WE, et al. 1994. Milk, serum, and mammary tissue concentration of pirlimycin following intramuscular, intramammary, or combination therapy of chronic *Staphylococcus aureus* mastitis. Agri-Practice 15(3):19.

Thornsberry C, et al. 1993. Activity of pirlimycin against pathogens from cows with mastitis and recommendations for disk diffusion tests. Antimicrob Agents Chemother 37:1122.

Macrolides: Erythromycin, Tylosin, Spiramycin, Tilmicosin, Roxithromycin

Macrolides are a large group of similar antibiotics, the metabolic products of *Streptomyces* spp. that are characterized by a macrocyclic lactone ring attached to two or more sugar moieties. The efficacy of this group of drugs against increasingly important human infections including *Campylobacter, Chlamydia, Legionella,* and *Mycobacterium* species has resulted in development of members with increased antibacterial activity, with pharmacokinetic advantages, and with reduced adverse effects. Macrolides with the greatest potential are those with a 14-, 15-, or 16-membered ring, most of which are derivatives of erythromycin.

Azithromycin, a drug with a 15-membered ring and with the greatest therapeutic value, is an azalide rather than a macrolide but has most of the characteristics of a macrolide.

The use of macrolides in animals has been to some extent limited by the toxicity for herbivores of orally administered drugs and pain associated with IM injection. The high intracellular concentrations of these drugs, their broad distribution in tissue, in the case of new drugs their often prolonged half-lives, and their activity against important pathogens are advantages of this important and perhaps underutilized group of antibiotics. Intracellular accumulation within phagocytes may produce the immunomodulatory effect noted with most of the macrolides (and lincosamides), but the precise pharmacodynamic relationships between intracellular concentrations and bacterial killing remain to be defined.

Erythromycin
CHEMISTRY
Erythromycin has a macrocyclic lactone nucleus to which are attached ketones and amino sugars (Fig. 11.2). Its base has a pK_a of 8.8, is poorly soluble in water, and is unstable in gastric acid.

MECHANISM OF ACTION
Erythromycin inhibits protein synthesis by binding to subunits of the 50S ribosome, possibly at the same site as the lincosamides; it inhibits the translocation step. The drug may be bactericidal at high concentrations.

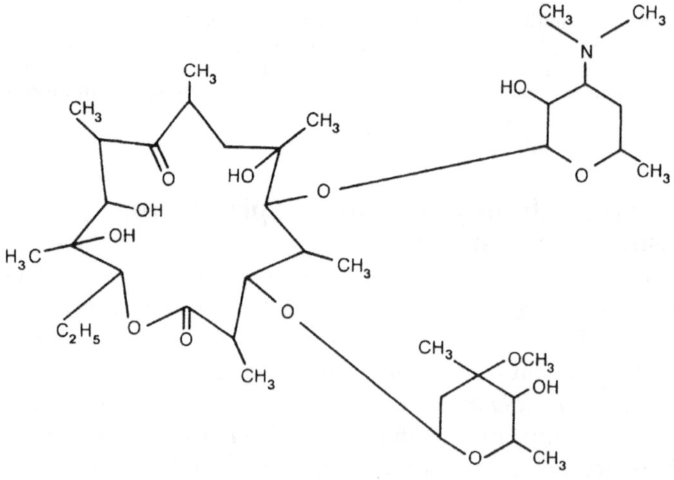

Fig. 11.2.　Structural formula of erythromycin.

ANTIMICROBIAL ACTIVITY

Good Susceptibility (MIC ≤ 0.5 μg/ml) is shown in the following Gram-positive aerobes: *Bacillus* spp., *Corynebacterium* spp., *Erysipelothrix rhusiopathiae*, *Listeria* spp., staphylococci, and streptococci. Among Gram-negative aerobes: *Actinobacillus* spp., *Brucella* spp.; *Campylobacter* spp., and *Leptospira* spp. Anaerobic bacteria: *Actinomyces* spp., *Bacteroides* spp. (except *B. fragilis*), *Clostridium* spp., some *Fusobacterium* sp., and anaerobic cocci (Table 11.2).

Moderate Susceptibility (MIC 1–4 μg/ml) occurs in enterococci, some *Bordetella* spp., *Haemophilus* spp., *Legionella* spp., *Ehrlichia* spp., and *Pasteurella* spp.

Resistant (MIC ≥ 8 μg/ml) bacteria include Enterobacteriaceae, *Pseudomonas* spp., *Nocardia* spp., *Mycoplasma* spp., *Chlamydia psittaci*, and *Mycobacterium* spp. (other than *M. kansasii*).

RESISTANCE

One-step chromosomal mutation to high-level resistance develops fairly readily in macrolides, although such resistance is often unstable. It may occur during treatment. Plasmid resistance is common, the result of methylation of the target site of the drug. Cross-resistance with lincosamides and other macrolides is common, but resistance of *Staphylococcus aureus* and streptococci in animals is less than that with lincomycin.

PHARMACOKINETIC PROPERTIES

Erythromycin is available for oral administration as the free base, the stearate, and esters (estolate). The susceptibility of the base to rapid degradation by stomach acid means that it requires protection by enteric coating, which leads to considerable individual variation in absorption. Various salts and esters have been developed to try to overcome this problem. The stearate is hydrolyzed in the intestine to the base, and the succinate and estolate esters are absorbed as such and hydrolyzed in the body to the active base. The estolate form is preferred for oral administration. Feeding interferes quite markedly with oral absorption. Like all macrolides, erythromycin is well distributed in the body, being concentrated in tissues, although penetration in cerebrospinal fluid is low; prostatic fluid concentration is about half that of serum concentration. The drug is metabolized and excreted largely in the bile and is lost in feces, although some intestinal reabsorption occurs. Urinary excretion is only 3–5% of total administered dose.

Erythromycin is available for parenteral injection as the base, glucoheptonate, or lactobionate. Parenteral administration causes tissue irritation at the site of injection.

TABLE 11.2. **Activity (MIC$_{90}$, µg/ml) of macrolide and pleuromutilin antibiotics against selected bacteria and mycoplasmas**

Organism	Erythromycin	Tylosin	Spiramycin	Tilmicosin	Tiamulin
Gram-positive aerobes					
Arcanobacterium pyogenes	2	2	4	0.03	0.03
Erysipelothrix rhusiopathiae	0.13	<0.13	0.25	0.25	4
Rhodococcus equi	≤0.25	64	128	—	64
Staphylococcus aureus	0.25	1	8	1	0.03
Streptococcus agalactiae	≤1	1		4	
S. uberis	≤0.5	1	0.5	—	
Gram-negative aerobes					
Actinobacillus pleuropneumoniae	8	32	32	2	8
Brucella canis	2	32	64	—	0.5
Haemophilus somnus	2	8	128	8	2
Moraxella bovis		>32		4	
Pasteurella haemolytica	16	128		4	
P. multocida	16	128		16	
Taylorella equigenitalis	≤0.13	0.5	2	—	
Gram-negative anaerobes					
Bacteroides nodosus	0.25	1	—	—	0.016
Fusobacterium necrophorum	8	4	—	4	0.2
Serpulina hyodysenteriae	>128	>128	>128	>64	0.5
S. pilosicoli	—	—	—	—	
Mycoplasmas					
Mycoplasma bovis	0.5	0.5	4	—	—
M. canis	128	0.5	4	—	0.25
M. hyorhinis	128	1.0	0.5	16	0.25
M. hyopneumoniae	4	1.0	1	1	0.25
M. hyosynoviae	—	16	—	—	0.06
M. mycoides mycoides	0.06	0.06	0.5	—	0.5
Ureaplasma spp.		0.13	0.5	—	0.06
Leptospira spp.	0.06	0.06		—	4

Erythromycin has significant anti-inflammatory activity and is used in some countries to treat chronic airway disease in humans through this action, which may involve enhancing neutrophil apoptosis. This immunomodulating effect has also been described in foals (Lakritz et al., 1997).

DRUG INTERACTIONS

There have been few studies of the interactions of macrolide antibiotics with other antimicrobial drugs. Combinations of erythromycin with other macrolides, lincosamides, and chloramphenicol are antagonistic in vitro. Erythromycin has been used alone or with an aminoglycoside to prevent or treat peritonitis after intestinal spillage, but it is not as effective as clindamycin or metronidazole in combination with an aminoglycoside. Combination with penicillin G or rifampin gave synergistic inhibition of *Rhodococcus equi* (Prescott and Nicholson, 1984).

TOXICITY AND ADVERSE EFFECTS

Erythromycin is one of the safest antimicrobial drugs. One problem shared with all macrolides is its irritating nature, which leads to severe pain on IM injection, thrombophlebitis and periphlebitis after IV injection, and an inflammatory reaction after intramammary administration. Dose-related gastrointestinal disturbances (nausea, vomiting, diarrhea, intestinal pain) occur in most animals treated with erythromycin, probably as a result of stimulatory effects on smooth muscle. These are not serious except in the horse, where macrolides, because they are largely excreted in the bile, can lead to serious diarrheic illness. Deaths have occurred because of *Clostridium difficile* in adult horses administered erythromycin (Gustafsson et al., 1997). Interestingly, severe *C. difficile* diarrheal illness has developed in the mares of foals treated orally with erythromycin and rifampin for *Rhodococcus equi* infection. This may be a direct effect of mares ingesting small quantities of antibiotic from the feces of their foals or an indirect effect of mares acquiring erythromycin-resistant *C. difficile* infection from their foals, or a combination of these circumstances (Baverud et al., 1998). Deaths through typhlocolitis have also been reported in rabbits. The drug appears safe in dogs and cats. The estolate form has been associated with self-limiting cholestatic hepatitis and jaundice with abdominal pain, especially with repeated and prolonged use or in patients with preexisting hepatic disease.

Other adverse effects of erythromycin include, in foals, hyperthermia and respiratory distress, which may be more marked in foals under high environmental temperatures (Traub-Dargatz et al., 1996). These adverse effects were speculated to result from absorbed microbiologically inactive anhydroerythromycin formed by degradation of erythromycin base in the stomach (Lakritz and Wilson, 1997).

ADMINISTRATION AND DOSAGE

Dosages of erythromycin are shown in Table 11.1.

CLINICAL APPLICATIONS

Erythromycin is a drug of choice to prevent or treat *Campylobacter jejuni* diarrhea or abortion and to treat *Rhodococcus equi* pneumonia in foals. One drawback to its long-term use is the possible development of chromosomal resistance.

Erythromycin is an alternative to penicillin in penicillin-allergic animals in the treatment of infections caused by susceptible Gram-positive aerobes, a less useful alternative to clindamycin in anaerobic infections, an alternative to ampicillin or amoxicillin in the treatment of leptospirosis, and an alternative to tetracyclines in rickettsial infections. The generally bacteriostatic nature of the drug is a disadvantage of this and other macrolides. Combination with rifampin has been used successfully in the treatment of *Coxiella burnetii* placentitis in a human (Bental et al., 1995).

Cattle, Sheep, and Goats. Erythromycin has moderate use in respiratory disease, given that *Haemophilus somnus*, *Arcanobacterium pyogenes*, and anaerobic bacteria are often moderately susceptible; mycoplasmas are usually resistant and *Pasteurella* only moderately sensitive. Experimental and field trials are required to establish the value and dosage of erythromycin in bovine respiratory disease and the relationship between MIC values for *Pasteurella* and serum concentrations in predicting optimal drug dosage. Pharmacokinetic considerations suggest that erythromycin is not a drug of choice for bovine pasteurellosis. Because of extreme pain associated with parenteral injection, it should be avoided when other antimicrobial drugs are available. This antibiotic is perhaps most useful in its intramammary infusion form for lactating and dry-cow therapy of mastitis where it has a short withdrawal time (36 hours). A single IM injection of 10 mg/kg was effective in the treatment of virulent foot rot in sheep (Ware et al., 1994).

Swine. Erythromycin has little place in the treatment of swine infections. Exceptions may include leptospirosis (Alt and Bolin, 1996) and *Lawsonia intracellularis* infection (McOrist et al., 1995).

Horses. Erythromycin is an alternative to penicillin G or trimethoprim-sulfonamide in the treatment of staphylococcal and streptococcal infections. The potential for inducing diarrhea limits its use in adults, but when it is used, the lactobionate should be given by slow IV infusion at a rate of 3–5 mg/kg at 8-to-12-hour intervals. Duration of treatment should not be more than 3 days. Erythromycin is a drug of choice in the treatment of *Rhodococcus equi* pneumonia in foals and should be used in combination with ampicillin or rifampin, both for the synergistic effect and to prevent the emergence of resistant mutants. A suitable dosage is 25 mg/kg of estolate PO 3 or 4 times daily. The phosphate and stearate could substitute for the estolate and be administered q12 hours (Ewing et al., 1994). Intramuscular injection causes severe local irritation in horses.

The combination of orally administered erythromycin and rifampin successfully treated experimentally induced *Ehrlichia risticii* infection and was advocated as a treatment less likely to cause diarrhea than tetracyclines (Palmer and Benson, 1992).

Dogs and Cats. Erythromycin is a second choice for Gram-positive coccal infections and anaerobic infections. It is the drug of choice in treating *Campylobacter jejuni* enteritis (Monfort et al., 1990).

Poultry. Erythromycin is administered in water for the prevention and treatment of staphylococcal or streptococcal infection, necrotic dermatitis, infectious coryza, and *M. gallisepticum* infection.

Bibliography

Alt DP, Bolin CA. 1996. Preliminary evaluation of antimicrobial agents for treatment of *Leptospira interrogans* serovar *pomona* infection in hamsters and swine. Am J Vet Res 57:59.

Baverud V, et al. 1998. *Clostridium difficile* associated with acute colitis in mares when their foals are treated with erythromycin and rifampicin for *Rhodococcus equi* pneumonia. Equine Vet J 30:482.

Bental T, et al. 1995. Chronic Q fever of pregnancy presenting as *Coxiella burnetii* placentitis: successful outcome following therapy with erythromycin and rifampin. Clin Infect Dis 21:1318.

Edmondson PW. 1989. An economic justification of "blitz" therapy to eradicate *Streptococcus agalactiae* from a dairy herd. Vet Rec 125:591.

Ewing PJ, et al. 1994. Comparison of oral erythromycin formulations in the horse using pharmacokinetic profiles. J Vet Pharmacol Ther 17:17.

Gustafsson A, et al. 1997. The association of erythromycin ethylsuccinate with acute colitis in horses in Sweden. Equine Vet J 29:314.

Lakritz J, Wilson WD. 1997. Erythromycin: pharmacokinetics, bioavailability, nonantimicrobial activity, and possible mechanisms associated with adverse reactions. Am Assoc Equine Pract 43:83.

Lakritz J, et al. 1997. Effect of treatment with erythromycin on bronchoalveolar lavage fluid cell populations in foals. Am J Vet Res 58:56.

McOrist S, et al. 1995. Antimicrobial susceptibility of ileal symbiont intracellularis isolated from pigs with proliferative enteropathy. J Clin Microbiol 33:1314.

Monfort JD, et al. 1990. Efficacies of erythromycin and chloramphenicol in extinguishing fecal shedding of *Campylobacter jejuni* in dogs. J Am Vet Med Assoc 196:1069.

Palmer JE, Benson CE. 1992. Effect of treatment with erythromycin and rifampin during the acute stages of experimentally induced equine ehrlichial colitis in ponies. Am J Vet Res 53:2071.

Prescott JF, Nicholson VM. 1984. The effects of combinations of selected antibiotics on the growth of *Corynebacterium equi*. J Vet Pharmacol Ther 7:61.

Swarbrick O. 1966. The use of parenteral erythromycin in the treatment of bovine mastitis. Vet Rec 79:508.

Traub-Dargatz J, et al. 1996. Hyperthermia in foals treated with erythromycin alone or in combination with rifampin for respiratory disease during hot environmental conditions. Am Assoc Equine Pract 42:243.

Ware JKW, et al. 1994. Efficacy of erythromycin compared with penicillin/streptomycin for the treatment of virulent footrot in sheep. Aust Vet J 71:89.

Tylosin

Tylosin is a macrolide antibiotic isolated from *Streptomyces fradiae*. Its chemical structure and its mechanism of action are similar to those of other macrolide antibiotics.

ANTIMICROBIAL ACTIVITY

Tylosin has a similar spectrum of activity to erythromycin. It is less active against bacteria, except for *Serpulina hyodysenteriae*, but more active against a broad range of mycoplasma (see Table 11.2).

RESISTANCE

Resistance mechanisms are similar to those of erythromycin. Because there is little published information on the prevalence of resistance of common veterinary pathogens, erythromycin resistance is probably the best guide. Resistance to macrolides is widespread in bacteria isolated from swine fed tylosin (Aarestrup et al., 1998). As with most macrolides, chromosomal mutation to resistance develops readily in vitro but is relatively unstable.

PHARMACOKINETIC PROPERTIES

The pharmacokinetic properties of tylosin are characteristic of the macrolides in general. Tylosin is a weak base (pK_a 7.1) and is highly lipid soluble. Half-life in dogs and cattle is about 1 hour, and apparent volumes of distribution are 1.7 and 1.1 l/kg, respectively.

DRUG INTERACTIONS

Interactions may be assumed to be similar to those of erythromycin. Tylosin-sulfonamide combinations have been used in small animal practice to treat upper respiratory tract infections in dogs, but there is no evidence that this combination is synergistic.

TOXICITY AND ADVERSE EFFECTS

Tylosin is a relatively safe drug. Its toxic effects are generally similar to those reported for erythromycin. It was reported to cause fatal diarrhea in a horse. The drug is irritating to tissue when administered IM or SC. Pigs have been reported to react to injection by developing edema, pruritus, edema of rectal mucosa, and mild anal protrusion, effects attributed to the drug vehicle. Inadvertent feeding of dairy cows with a concentrate contaminated with 7–20 ppm of tylosin resulted in ruminal stasis, inappetence, foul-smelling feces, and decreased milk production. Many of the cows became hyperesthetic and some became recumbent (Crossman and Poyser, 1981). Intravenous administration in cattle has produced shock, dyspnea, and depression. Tylosin and spiramycin have induced contact dermatitis in veterinarians.

ADMINISTRATION AND DOSAGE

Tylosin is administered by IM injection (see Table 11.1), by the intramammary route, or for feed incorporation in swine. Tylosin tartrate is readily absorbed from the intestine, but tylosin phosphate is relatively poorly absorbed.

CLINICAL APPLICATIONS

Tylosin is not as active as erythromycin against most bacteria but has greater activity against mycoplasma. In pigs, where it is also used as a growth promoter, its use in the prevention and treatment of swine dysentery and mycoplasma infections is being replaced by the more active tiamulin. The use of tylosin as a swine growth promoter in Europe has recently been recommended to be abandoned. Apart from its use against mycoplasma it is, like erythromycin, a second-choice antibiotic for most clinical uses.

Cattle, Sheep, and Goats. Tylosin is used in cattle to treat pneumonia, foot rot, metritis, pinkeye, and Gram-positive coccal mastitis because of its activity against mycoplasma, anaerobic bacteria, and Gram-positive bacteria. Tylosin may be administered at low concentrations to feedlot cattle on high-concentrate diets to improve weight gain and feed efficiency and to prevent liver abscess. Because of the availability of newer macrolide antibiotics, this is now the major use of tylosin.

In cattle, tylosin (7.5–15 mg/kg IM twice a day) has been successful in controlling and eliminating experimental *Mycoplasma mycoides* pneumonia. In calves the drug has been used effectively to treat *Mycoplasma bovis* pneumonia and arthritis; experimental IM dosage with 10 mg/kg twice a day delayed but did not prevent *M. bovis* arthritis (Stahlheim, 1976). Tylosin has been used by the intramammary route in the treatment of experimentally induced *Mycoplasma californicum* mastitis (Ball and Campbell, 1989). Treatment was most successful when oxytetracycline and tylosin were combined or alternated—426 g of tylosin or 500 g of oxytetracycline given every 12 hours for 3 days.

Tylosin can be administered IM or by the intramammary route in the treatment of mastitis caused by Gram-positive bacteria. Results have been marginally less successful than with erythromycin. A dose of 20 mg/kg IM was used to eliminate ureaplasma from the genital tract of ewes (Ball and McCaughey, 1987). In goats, tylosin is a drug of choice in treating mycoplasma pneumonia, such as that caused by *Mycoplasma mycoides* subsp. *capri*. A high dosage of 25–35 mg/kg IV at 8-to-12-hour intervals is recommended.

Swine. Tylosin is used to promote growth and improve weight gain. For the treatment of atrophic rhinitis, injection of piglets for variable periods has reduced frequency of the disease, suggesting that tylosin inhibits *Pasteurella multocida* (or its production of Pmt toxin), despite the bacteria's relatively high MIC. Injection of neonatal pigs has reduced the frequency of *Mycoplasma hyopneumoniae* lesions (Kunesh, 1981). Tylosin was not as effective as tiamulin in controlling an experimental mixed mycoplasma and bacterial pneumonia (Hannan et al., 1982). Tylosin, 8.8 mg/kg twice a day IM, or tylosin-sulfonamide, 100 ppm of each drug in feed, was effective in treating pigs with experimentally induced *P. multocida* and *Arcanobacterium pyogenes* pneumonia (Matsuoka et al., 1983).

Control of swine dysentery by the drug is hampered by the development of resistance; the in vivo effect of the drug varies with the MIC, which ranges from 2.5 to >40 µg per ml. Derivatives of tylosin may have greater activity against resistant organisms (Jacks et al., 1986). Tylosin (100 ppm) is effective in preventing or treating proliferative hemorrhagic enteropathy (McOrist et al., 1997). Other uses include parenteral treatment of erysipelas and infections involving *A. pyogenes* and anaerobes. Tylosin (44 mg/kg IM once daily for 5 days) effectively treated experimentally induced leptospirosis in swine (Alt and Bolin, 1996).

Horses. Tylosin should not be used parenterally in horses because of its irritating nature. There is no experience with its oral administration but no indication for such use, which might be likely to result in *Clostridium difficile* colitis.

Dogs and Cats. Tylosin has been used successfully in dogs to treat abscesses, wound infections, tonsillitis, tracheobronchitis, and pneumonia caused by pathogens such as staphylococci, streptococci, anaerobes, and mycoplasmas. Occasional pain and swelling at the injection site and vomiting after oral administration have been reported. A tylosin-sulfonamide combination is licensed for the treatment of upper respiratory tract infections in dogs. Tylosin is often effective in the treatment of the upper respiratory tract infection complex of cats, possibly because of its effect against *Chlamydia* and mycoplasmas. Tylosin administered orally has been shown to be 70–90% effective in the treatment of *Staphylococcus intermedius* pyoderma in dogs (Scott et al., 1994; Harvey, 1996); a dose of 10 mg/kg q12 hours was shown to be almost as effective as 20 mg/kg q12 hours (Scott et al. 1996).

Poultry. Tylosin has been used by IM injection in the control of mycoplasma infections and added to the water in the control of avian spirochetosis. Resistance in some *Mycoplasma gallisepticum* isolates may reduce the efficacy of tylosin (Migaki et al., 1993). In one study, tylosin was found to be almost as effective as danofloxacin in control of infection (Jordan et al., 1993).

Bibliography

Aarestrup FM, et al. 1998. Surveillance of antimicrobial resistance in bacteria isolated from food animals to antimicrobial growth promoters and related therapeutic agents in Denmark. APMIS 106:606.

Alt DP, Bolin CA. 1996. Preliminary evaluation of antimicrobial agents for treatment of *Leptospira interrogans* serovar *pomona* infection in hamsters and swine. Am J Vet Res 57:59.

Ball HJ, Campbell JN. 1989. Antibiotic treatment of experimental *Mycoplasma californicum* mastitis. Vet Rec 125:377.

Ball HJ, McCaughey WJ. 1987. Experimental intramuscular inoculation of tylosin in the elimination of ureaplasmas from ewes. Vet Rec 120:557.

Crossman PJ, Poyser MR. 1981. Effect of inadvertently feeding tylosin and tylosin and dimetridazole to dairy cows. Vet Rec 108:285.

Hannan PCT, et al. 1982. Tylosin tartrate and tiamulin effects on experimental piglet pneumonia induced with pneumonic pig lung homogenate containing mycoplasma, bacteria, and viruses. Res Vet Sci 33:76.

Harvey RG. 1996. Tylosin in the treatment of canine superficial pyoderma. Vet Rec 139:185.

Jacks TM, et al. 1986. 3-Acetyl-4'-isovaleryl tylosin for prevention of swine dysentery. Am J Vet Res 47:2325.

Johnston WS. 1975. Eradication of *Str. agalactiae* from infected herds using erythromycin. Vet Rec 96:430.

Jordan FTW, et al. 1993. A comparison of the efficacy of danofloxacin and tylosin in the control of *Mycoplasma gallisepticum* infection in broiler chickens. J Vet Pharmacol Ther 16:79.

Kunesh JP. 1981. A comparison of two antibiotics in treating *Mycoplasma* pneumonia in swine. Vet Med Small Anim Clin 76:871.

Lacey RW. 1988. Rarity of tylosin resistance in human pathogenic bacteria. Vet Rec 122:438.

Matsuoka T, et al. 1980. Orally administered tylosin for the control of pneumonia in neonatal calves. Vet Rec 107:149.

Matsuoka T, et al. 1983. Therapeutic effect of injectable tylosin against induced pneumonia in pigs. Vet Med Small Anim Clin 78:951.

McOrist S, et al. 1997. Oral administration of tylosin phosphate for treatment and prevention of proliferative enteropathy in pigs. Am J Vet Res 58:136.

Migaki TT, et al. 1993. Efficacy of danofloxacin and tylosin in the control of mycoplasmosis in chicks infected with tylosin-susceptible or tylosin-resistant field isolates of *Mycoplasma gallisepticum*. Avian Dis 37:508.

Scott DW, et al. 1994. Efficacy of tylosin tablets for the treatment of pyoderma due to *Staphylococcus intermedius* infection in dogs. Can Vet J 35:617.

Scott DW, et al. 1996. Further studies on the efficacy of tylosin tablets for the treatment of pyoderma due to *Staphylococcus intermedius* infection in dogs. Can Vet J 37:617.

Stahlheim OHV. 1976. Failure of antibiotic therapy in calves with mycoplasmal arthritis and pneumonia. J Am Vet Med Assoc 169:1096.

Spiramycin

Spiramycin is several times less active against bacteria than erythromycin. Its spectrum of activity is similar to that of the other macrolides, but it is not as effective against mycoplasma as tylosin or tiamulin. Resistance, antimicrobial drug interactions, and toxic properties are similar to those of the other macrolides.

Despite relatively poor activity in vitro, spiramycin has quite exceptional ability to concentrate in tissue, in part by tissue binding, resulting in concentrations in organs reaching 25–60 times those of serum. The drug persists even when serum concentrations are negligible. Thus, spiramycin has the paradoxical effect of being less active than erythromycin in vitro but as or more active in vivo. Like other macrolides, it also has a direct effect on phagocytic cells. Spiramycin thus has particular potential against intracellular organisms. In humans, it is used in the treatment of acute toxoplasmosis and may be useful in cryptosporidiosis. In one study (Schilferli et al., 1981), parenteral administration of 50 mg/kg twice a day for 5 days to calves resulted in lung concentrations of approximately 100 µg/g. Not all this drug is active; in mammary tissue about 75% is inactive. One result of its tissue concentration is the persistence of drug residues for prolonged periods, a particular problem in the treatment of mastitis in lactating cows but also more generally in food animals. Spiramycin is used extensively in France for the treatment of infections in farm animals. It has the same applications as tylosin.

Spiramycin has been used extensively in Europe as a broiler chicken growth promoter but has recently been withdrawn for this purpose throughout the European Union. Resistance in bacteria isolated from chickens fed spiramycin is extensive in Europe (Aarestrup et al., 1998).

CATTLE, SHEEP, AND GOATS

Spiramycin (pK$_a$ 8.2) has similar applications to tylosin. The drug has been used successfully to treat contagious bovine pleuropneumonia; 25 mg/kg IM eliminated infection when given on up to three occasions at 2-day intervals (Provost, 1974). In one field trial of the treatment of bovine respiratory disease, spiramycin was considerably less effective than florfenicol (Madelenat et al., 1997). A dose of 20 mg/kg gave mastitic milk concentrations greater than 2.5 µg/ml for 48 hours after IM injection. Intramuscular injection of this dose after the last milking gave effective milk drug concentrations for 6–8 days (Ziv, 1974). In lactating cows, a single intramammary dose of 600 mg gave effective concentrations for 36–48 hours, but persistent residues limit the use of the drug. Spiramycin is administered orally, 100 mg/kg, in the last one-third of gestation to ewes to effectively prevent experimental *Toxoplasma* abortion. Bioavailability after oral administration is limited in ruminants. Spiramycin, 20–30 mg/kg IM, successfully treated ovine infectious rickettsial keratoconjunctivitis; in serious cases the drug should be repeated 5 and 10 days after the first injection (Konig, 1983). One interesting possible application is the use of a single injection of the parenteral dosage form of the drug to treat endometritis in sheep and cattle, because of the extraordinarily long half-life of the drug (Cester et al., 1990).

SWINE AND POULTRY
Spiramycin has the same applications as tylosin in pigs and poultry.

Bibliography

Aarestrup FM, et al. 1998. Surveillance of antimicrobial resistance in bacteria isolated from food animals to antimicrobial growth promoters and related therapeutic agents in Denmark. APMIS 106:606.

Cester CC, et al. 1990. Spiramycin concentrations in plasma and genital-tract secretions after intravenous injection in the ewe. J Vet Pharmacol Ther 13:7.

Chang HR, Pechère J-CF. 1988. Activity of spiramycin against *Toxoplasma gondii* in vitro, in experimental infections, and in human infection. J Antimicrob Chemother 22B:87.

Daffos F, et al. 1988. Prenatal management of 746 pregnancies at risk for congenital toxoplasmosis. N Engl J Med 318:271.

Friis C, et al. 1991. Respiratory tract distribution and bioavailability of spiramycin in calves. Am J Vet Res 52:1269.

Konig CDW. 1983. "Pink eye" or "zere oogjes" or keratoconjunctivitis infectiosa ovis (KIO): clinical efficacy of a number of antimicrobial therapies. Vet Q 5:122.

Madelenat A, et al. 1997. Efficacite comparee du florfenicol et de la spiramycine longue action, associe a la flunixine meglumine, dans le traitement des maladies respiratoires du veau de boucherie. Rec Med Vet 173:113.

Provost A. 1974. Essai de traitement de la spiramycin chez les brebis et les vaches laitieres. Can Med Vet 43:140.

Renard L, et al. 1996. Pharmacokinteic-pharmacodynamic model for spiramycin in staphylococcal mastitis. J Vet Pharmacol Ther 19:95.

Saez-Llorens X. 1989. Spiramycin for treatment of *Cryptosporidium* enteritis. J Infect Dis 160:342.

Schilferli D, et al. 1981. Distribution tissulaire de la penicillin, de l'oxytetracycline et del a spiramycine chez le veau au cours d'une antibiotique courante. Schweiz Arch Tierheilkd 123:507.

Ziv G. 1974. Profil pharmacocinetique de la spiramycine chez les brebis et les vaches laitieres. Can Med Vet 43:371.

Tilmicosin
Tilmicosin, 20-deoxo-20-(3,5-dimethylpiperidin-1-yl) desmycosin, is a chemically modified macrolide derivative of tylosin.

ANTIMICROBIAL ACTIVITY
Tilmicosin has antibacterial and antimycoplasma activity between that of erythromycin and tylosin (see Table 11.2). Typically of macrolides, it

inhibits Gram-positive bacteria, including *Clostridium* spp., *Staphylococcus* spp., and *Streptococcus* spp., and Gram-negative bacteria, including *Actinobacillus* spp., *Campylobacter* spp., *Haemophilus* spp., and *Pasteurella* spp. Enterobacteriaceae are resistant. Mycoplasma susceptibility can be quite variable because of resistance. *Pasteurella* spp. isolated from cattle are regarded as susceptible if their MIC is ≤ 8 μg/ml, intermediate if MIC is 16 μg/ml, and resistant if their MIC is ≥ 32 μg/ml (Shryock et al., 1996). There are repeated observations that macrolides, including tilmicosin, have important subinhibitory activities, which, together with their effects on host immune defenses, may contribute to their clinical efficacy (Shryock et al., 1998). Further study is required to confirm and to define the importance of these effects in determining the clinical efficacy of tilmicosin.

RESISTANCE

Resistance mechanisms are similar to those of erythromycin and tylosin. Cross-resistance between macrolides is extensive.

PHARMACOKINETIC PROPERTIES

The pharmacokinetic properties of tilmicosin are similar to those of macrolides in general and are characterized by low serum concentrations but large volumes of distribution (>2 l/kg), with accumulation and persistence in tissues, including the lung, which may concentrate drug 20-fold relative to serum. The half-life in cows is about 1 hour. Cows administered 10 mg/kg SC as a single dose maintained milk concentrations >0.8 μg/ml for 8–9 days (Ziv et al., 1995).

DRUG INTERACTIONS

Drug interactions may be assumed to be similar to those for erythromycin.

TOXICITY AND ADVERSE EFFECTS

Tilmicosin is potentially toxic to the cardiovascular system, which varies to some extent with species. The drug may be fatal to swine and horses by IM injection, and care should be taken to avoid accidental injection of people. The toxic dose for goats is only about 30 mg/kg SC, or 2.5 mg/kg IV. The toxic effects of tilmicosin are mediated through its effects on the heart, possibly through causing rapid depletion of calcium (Main et al., 1996).

ADMINISTRATION AND DOSAGE

Administration is summarized in Table 11.1.

CLINICAL APPLICATIONS

Tilmicosin has been developed as a long-acting formulation for use in bovine respiratory disease, a single SC dose of 10 mg/kg being claimed to result in lung concentrations exceeding the MIC of *Pasteurella haemolytica* for 72 hours.

Cattle, Sheep, and Goats. Experimental and field data support the value of single-dose SC prophylaxis on arrival of cattle in feedlots and in the treatment in pneumonia of cattle (Ose and Tonkinson, 1988; Schumann et al., 1990, 1991; Young, 1995; Musser et al., 1996). Doses of 20 mg/kg appeared slightly more effective than 10 mg/kg (Gorham et al., 1990). Repeat injections after 3 days are necessary in some animals (Laven and Andrews, 1991; Scott, 1994). In a comparison of florfenicol versus tilmicosin treatment of undifferentiated fever in feedlot cattle in western Canada, florfenicol (administered twice) was superior to tilmicosin (administered once) in reducing mortality overall, including that due to respiratory disease (Jim et al., 1999). These results may not be strictly comparable, since cattle had been previously treated with tilmicosin on arrival at the feedlot. However, they may also reflect differences in length of treatment between the two regimes. Tilmicosin is not approved for use in lactating cattle because of the prolonged period (2–3 weeks) during which violative milk residues can be detected.

Tilmicosin is approved for single-dose SC treatment of pneumonic pasteurellosis in sheep. It can be fatal in goats.

Swine. Tilmicosin has been shown by experimental and clinical studies to be useful as an oral medication in swine (200–400 ppm) in the control of *Actinobacillus* spp. or *Pasteurella multocida* pneumonia. It may also be useful in the control of atrophic rhinitis. There is no information on its effect against mycoplasma pneumonia. It is effective in vitro against *Lawsonia intracellularis* and would likely usefully control proliferative enteropathy. Tilmicosin should be administered only orally to swine.

Rabbits. Tilmicosin at 25 mg/kg SC was effective in treating pasteurellosis in rabbits; this dose may need to be repeated after 3 days to further enhance a clinical cure (McKay et al., 1996).

Poultry. Tilmicosin is effective in the treatment of experimentally induced *Mycoplasma gallisepticum* infection at 50 mg/l administered for 3 or 5 days (Charleston et al., 1998). At 300–500 g/ton, it prevented infection; interestingly, use of the pellet binder bentonite inhibited the effect of tilmicosin in a concentration-dependent manner (Shryock et al., 1994).

Other Species. Tilmicosin is not approved or recommended for use in goats or in species other than those described above, by any route, because of toxicity. It can be immediately fatal on injection in species such as pigs and horses.

Bibliography

Charleston B, et al. 1998. Assessment of the efficacy of tilmicosin as a treatment for *Mycoplasma gallisepticum* infections in chickens. Avian Pathol 27:190.

Gorham PE, et al. 1990. Tilmicosin as a single injection treatment for respiratory disease of feedlot cattle. Can Vet J 31:826.

Jim GK, et al. 1999. A comparison of florfenicol and tilmicosin for the treatment of undifferentiated fever in feedlot calves in western Canada. Can Vet J 40:179.

Laven R, Andrews AH. 1991. Long-acting antibiotic formulations in the treatment of calf pneumonia: a comparative study of tilmicosin and oxytetracycline. Vet Rec 129:109.

Main BW, et al. 1996. Cardiovascular effects of the macrolide antibiotic, tilmicosin, administered alone or in combination with propanolol or dobutamine, in conscious unrestrained dogs. J Vet Pharmacol Ther 19:225.

McKay SG, et al. 1996. Use of tilmicosin for treatment of pasteurellosis in rabbits. Am J Vet Res 57:1180.

Modric S, et al. 1998. Pharmacokinetics and pharmacodynamics of tilmicosin in sheep and cattle. J Vet Pharmacol Ther 21:444.

Moore GM, et al. 1996a. Clinical field trials with tilmicosin phosphate in feed for the control of naturally acquired pneumonia caused by *Actinobacillus pleuropneumoniae* and *Pasteurella multocida* in swine. Am J Vet Res 57:224.

Moore GM, et al. 1996b. Efficacy dose determination study of tilmicosin phosphate in feed for control of pneumonia caused by *Actinobacillus pleuropneumoniae* in swine. Am J Vet Res 57:220.

Musser J, et al. 1996. Comparison of tilmicosin with long-acting oxytetracycline for treatment of respiratory disease in calves. J Am Vet Med Assoc 208:102.

Ose EE, Tonkinson LV. 1988. Single-dose treatment of neonatal calf pneumonia with the new macrolide antibiotic tilmicosin. Vet Rec 123:367.

Schumann FJ, et al. 1990. Prophylactic tilmicosin medication of feedlot cattle at arrival. Can Vet J 31:285.

Schumann FJ, et al. 1991. Prophylactic medication of feedlot calves with tilmicosin. Vet Rec 128:278.

Scorneaux B, Shryock TR. 1998. Intracellular accumulation, subcellular distribution, and efflux of tilmicosin in swine phagocytes. J Vet Pharmacol Ther 21:257.

Scott PR. 1994. Field study of undifferentiated respiratory disease in housed beef calves. Vet Rec 134:325.

Shryock TR, et al. 1994. Effect of bentonite incorporated in a feed ration with tilmicosin in the prevention of induced *Mycoplasma gallisepticum* airsacculitis in broiler chickens. Avian Dis 38:501.

Shryock TR, et al. 1996. Minimum inhibitory concentration breakpoints and disk diffusion inhibitory interpretive criteria for tilmicosin susceptibility testing against *Pasteurella* spp. associated with bovine respiratory disease. J Vet Diagn Invest 8:337.

Shryock TR, et al. 1998. The effects of macrolides on the expression of bacterial virulence mechanisms. J Antimicrob Chemother 41:505.

Thomson TD, et al. 1997. Pharmacology and safety of Pulmotil [tilmicosin phosphate] in swine. 28th Am Assoc Swine Pract p51.

Vogel GJ, et al. 1998. Effects of tilmicosin on acute undifferentiated respiratory tract disease in newly arrived feedlot cattle. J Am Vet Med Assoc 212:1919.

Young C. 1995. Antimicrobial metaphylaxis for undifferentiated bovine respiratory disease. Compend Cont Educ Pract Vet 17:133.

Ziv G, et al. 1995. Tilmicosin antibacterial activity and pharmacokinetics in cows. J Vet Pharmacol Ther 18:340.

Other Classic Macrolides

Uncommon macrolide antibiotics (oleandomycin, josamycin, kitasamycin, rosaramicin) have activity similar to that of erythromycin, spiramycin, and tylosin. There is little reported experience with their use in veterinary medicine, although kitasamycin is used in Japan. The agents appear to have nothing to offer over the commonly used classic macrolide antibiotics, and they lack the excellent activity of tiamulin.

Advanced-generation Macrolide Antibiotics: Azithromycin, Clarithromycin, and Roxithromycin

Interest in the macrolides has been stimulated by their activity against relatively newly recognized or emerging human pathogens, including *Campylobacter* spp., *Helicobacter* spp., and *Legionella* spp., as well as against intracellular organisms that have emerged through the AIDS epidemic, such as *Bartonella* spp. and *Mycobacterium* spp. Newer erythromycin derivatives with enhanced pharmacokinetic and in some cases broader antibacterial activities include azithromycin, clarithromycin, and roxithromycin. For example, roxithromycin is an acid-stable derivative of erythromycin with similar activity to erythromycin that is better absorbed after oral administration and has a considerably longer half-life (13 hours). It is a well-tolerated alternative to erythromycin for daily oral administration. Clarithromycin, a 6-O-methyl derivative of erythromycin, is about twice as active as erythromycin against bacteria on a weight basis, has a half-life about twice that of erythromycin, and includes good activity against *Mycobacterium avium*. Azithromycin, an acid-stable 15-membered ring macrolide (which is technically an azalide and not a macrolide), is more active than erythromycin against Gram-negative bacteria and also has a considerably lengthened half-life relative to erythromycin. The application of these and other newer macrolides for veterinary use will likely take advantage of their long half-lives in the single treatment of mycoplasma infections, of *Campylobacter* infections, and of infections caused by intracellular bacteria.

ANTIMICROBIAL ACTIVITY

All macrolides, including the newer macrolides, share similar antibacterial spectrum of activity (Tables 11.1 and 11.3). Azithromycin has the broadest activity against Gram-negative bacteria, including moderate activity against Enterobacteriaceae, but the others also have activity against important human upper respiratory tract Gram-negative pathogens *(Bordetella pertussis, Haemophilus influenzae, Moraxella catarrhalis)*. Other important antibacterial effects include excellent activity against the genera *Bartonella, Borrelia, Brucella, Campylobacter, Chlamydia (trachomatis), Legionella, Leptospira, Mycoplasma,* members of the

TABLE 11.3. MIC$_{90}$, µg/ml, of erythromycin and newer macrolides against selected pathogens

Bacterium	Erythro-mycin	Roxithro-mycin	Clarithro-mycin	Azithro-mycin
Gram-positives aerobes				
Arcanobacterium pyogenes	≤0.016	≤0.03	≤0.016	≤0.016
Erysipelothrix rhusiopathiae	0.03	0.13	0.06	0.03
Listeria sp.	0.25	0.5	0.13	1
Rhodococcus equi	0.5	0.25	0.06	1
Staphylococcus aureus	0.25	0.25	0.25	0.25
Streptococcus agalactiae	0.13	0.13	0.06	0.13
Viridans streptococci	0.13	—	0.13	0.25
Gram-negative aerobes				
Brucella sp.	16	16	8	2
Pasteurella multocida	4	4	2	1
Gram-negative: other				
Bartonella henselae	0.13	0.13	0.03	0.016
Campylobacter sp.	2	2	2	0.5
Helicobacter pylori	0.5	0.125	1	0.25
Anaerobes				
Bacteroides fragilis	>8	—	16	4
Clostridium perfringens	4	—	4	4
Fusobacterium sp.	16	16	8	1
Peptostreptococcus sp.	>32	>32	>32	>32
Porphyromonas sp.	0.25	0.25	0.13	0.5

Spirochetaceae, and *Ureaplasma*. Mycobacteria such as *Mycobacterium avium* are often moderately susceptible. Activity against anaerobic bacteria is variable (see Table 11.3). Newer macrolides are not more active than erythromycin against staphylococci and streptococci and are ineffective against enterococci. Azithromycin has the most marked and rapid bactericidal activity of the newer macrolides. There are few studies of the spectrum of the newer macrolides against Gram-negative pathogens from animals. Organisms with MIC 2 ≤ µg/ml for newer macrolides are generally regarded as susceptible and those with MIC 8 ≥ µg/ml as resistant.

RESISTANCE

Extensive cross-resistance occurs between macrolides. Its basis has been discussed earlier.

PHARMACOKINETIC PROPERTIES

In comparison with erythromycin, from which they have been developed, newer macrolides are acid stable, produce fewer gastrointestinal side effects, have high bioavailability (40–60%) following oral administration, have considerably lengthened serum half-lives, and produce higher tissue concentrations, so that single daily dosing is appropriate. The long half-lives of these newer drugs, which is particularly marked for azithromycin, apparently results from extensive uptake by, and slow release from, tissues rather than delayed metabolism. The major route of excretion is the bile and intestinal tract, although clarithromycin is more markedly excreted through the kidney. About half the administered azithromycin is excreted unchanged in the bile in dogs and cats; tissue half-lives in cats vary from 13 hours in fat to 72 hours in heart muscle (Hunter et al., 1995). Tissue concentrations of azithromycin in the lung and spleen of cats exceeded 1 μg/ml 72 hours after a single oral dose of 5.4 mg/kg (Hunter et al., 1995). Tissue concentrations of azithromycin are generally 10–100 times those achieved in serum and are concentrated 200–500 times in macrophages. The extensive tissue distribution of azithromycin appears to result from its concentration within macrophages and neutrophils, giving it an intracellular half-life of about 8 days. Clarithromycin macrophage concentrations are 10–20 times greater than serum concentrations. Macrophage concentrations of roxithromycin are less than those of clarithromycin. Such macrophage concentration is not always advantageous, since it may suppress phagocytic activity after a therapeutic dose. Because of this concentration effect, estimated V_d (l/kg) in humans is 23–31 for azithromycin and 3.2–3.8 for clarithromycin; for erythromycin, it is 0.64.

DRUG INTERACTIONS

Azithromycin does not interact with the hepatic cytochrome P450 system and is not associated with the pharmacokinetic drug interactions observed with erythromycin and classical macrolides. Clarithromycin and roxithromycin have lower affinity for the P450 system than erythromycin and other classic macrolides (except spiramycin). Oral absorption is unaffected by food.

TOXICITY AND ADVERSE EFFECTS

Newer macrolides have few of the adverse gastrointestinal effects of erythromycin and are well tolerated in humans. The limited experience in monogastrate animals supports this observation. As with lincosamides and earlier macrolides, in the absence of experience to the contrary, these drugs should not be administered orally and should probably not be administered parenterally to herbivores. Clarithromycin may be fetotoxic and should not be administered to pregnant animals.

ADMINISTRATION AND DOSAGE

Dosage recommendations in animals are currently empiric. For dogs and cats, suggested oral doses are as follows: azithromycin, 10 mg/kg q24 hours (not longer than 5–7 days); clarithromycin, 7.5 mg/kg q12 hours; and roxithromycin, 15 mg/kg q24 hours (not longer than 5–7 days).

CLINICAL APPLICATIONS

There is little experience with the use of newer macrolides in veterinary medicine, but for monogastrates these drugs offer the advantage of oral administration, few adverse effects, and once-daily dosing for a shorter time than classical macrolides. Their particular efficacy against intracellular organisms is a significant advantage. Their current high cost is likely to preclude their use except for special circumstances.

Applications include those described for erythromycin. For example, erythromycin is an alternative to penicillin in penicillin-allergic animals in the treatment of infections caused by susceptible Gram-positive aerobes, a less useful alternative to clindamycin in anaerobic infections, an alternative to ampicillin or amoxicillin in the treatment of leptospirosis, and an alternative to tetracyclines in treatment of *Rickettsia* and *Coxiella* infections. Newer macrolides may have advantage in the treatment of intracellular infections in monogastrates, including *Bartonella, Chlamydia psittaci*, and atypical mycobacterial infections. Their use in the treatment of *Rhodococcus equi* infections of foals deserves to be investigated. Experimentally, treatment with azithromycin of *Brucella* infections in mice has been significantly less effective than treatment with doxycycline. Combination with pyrimethamine has been an effective treatment in people unable to tolerate alternative therapies. Clarithromycin and azithromycin, but not roxithromycin, are effective in the treatment of atypical *Mycobacterium* infections, when combined with other antibiotics (see Chapter 19). Other areas that need to be investigated are use against *Mycoplasma* infections in animals, since medically important *Mycoplasma* are highly susceptible in vitro.

Bibliography

Amsden GW, et al. 1997. The role of advanced generation macrolides in the prophylaxis and treatment of *Mycobacterium avium* complex (MAC) infections. Drugs 54:69.

Charles L, Segreti J. 1997. Choosing the right macrolide antibiotic. Drugs 53:349.

Dunn CJ, Barradell LB. 1996. Azithromycin: a review of its pharmacological properties and use as 3-day therapy in respiratory tract infections. Drugs 51:483.

Hunter RP, et al. 1995. Pharmacokinetics, oral bioavailability, and tissue distribution of azithromycin in cats. J Vet Pharmacol Ther 18:38.

Langtry HD, Brogden RN. 1997. Clarithromycin: a review of its efficacy in the treatment of respiratory tract infections in immunocompetent patients. Drugs 53:973.

Lavy E, et al. 1995. Minimal inhibitory concentrations for canine isolates and oral absorption of roxithromycin in fed and fasted dogs. J Vet Pharmacol Ther 18:382.

Luke DR, et al. 1996. Safety, toleration, and pharmacokinetics of intravenous azithromycin. Antimicrob Agents Chemother 40:2577.

Markham A, Faulds D. 1994. Roxithromycin: an update of its antimicrobial activity, pharmacokinetic properties, and therapeutic use. Drugs 48:297.

Vilmanyi E, et al. 1996. Clarithromycin pharmacokinetics after oral administration with or without fasting in cross-bred beagles. J Small Anim Pract 37:535.

Wenisch C, et al. 1996. Effect of single oral dose of azithromycin, clarithromycin, and roxithromycin on polymorphonuclear leukocyte function assessed ex vivo by flow cytometry. Antimicrob Agents Chemother 40:2039.

Ketolides

Ketolides are members of a new semisynthetic 14-membered ring macrolide, with a 3-keto group instead of an α-L-cladinose on the erythronolide A ring. Their spectrum of activity includes that of classic macrolides, but they appear to have the striking additional advantages of activity against enterococci, methicillin-resistant *Staphylococcus aureus*, and some bacteria with inducible MLS-type resistance. Some members of the class also possess the pharmacokinetic advantages of azithromycin.

Pleuromutilins: Tiamulin and Valnemulin

Tiamulin and valnemulin are semisynthetic derivatives of the naturally occurring diterpene antibiotic pleuromutilin. Pleuromutilins have outstanding activity against anaerobic bacteria and mycoplasma and are used exclusively in animals, largely in swine. Most comments will be confined to tiamulin, which has been used longer clinically. Valnemulin is about twice as active as tiamulin against bacteria and over 30 times more active against swine mycoplasma in vitro (Aitken et al., 1999).

Tiamulin

Tiamulin is used as the hydrogen fumarate in the oral preparation but as the tiamulin base in the parenteral product.

ANTIMICROBIAL ACTIVITY

The antimicrobial spectrum of tiamulin is similar to that of tylosin but has greater activity (Tables 11.2 and 11.4). Tiamulin is active against only a few Gram-negative aerobic species and is inactive against Enterobacteriaceae (Tables 11.2 and 11.4), although subinhibitory concentrations may reduce adhesive properties of enterotoxigenic *E. coli* (Larsen, 1988). Activity against anaerobic bacteria and mycoplasma is better than that of macrolide antibiotics. Organisms with MIC ≤ 4 μg/ml are considered susceptible, of 8–16 μg/ml as moderately susceptible, and of ≥32 μg/ml as resistant (Szancer, 1990).

RESISTANCE

As with the macrolides, chromosomal mutation to resistance of tiamulin emerges readily on in vitro passage of bacteria in the presence of the drug. The rate of emergence is significantly lower than with tylosin.

TABLE 11.4. Activity (MIC$_{90}$, µg/ml) of tiamulin against selected bacteria

Organism	MIC$_{90}$	Organism	MIC$_{90}$
Gram-positive aerobes			
Streptococcus equi	0.5	*S. zooepidemicus*	0.5
S. suis	2		
Gram-negative aerobes			
Actinobacillus pleuropneumoniae	8	*Leptospira* sp.	4
Bordetella bronchiseptica	≥32	*P. haemolytica*	4
Escherichia coli	32	*P. multocida*	32
Klebsiella sp.	>128	*Proteus* sp.	>128
Anaerobic bacteria			
Bacteroides sp.	0.5	*Fusobacterium nucleatum*	0.5
Clostridium perfringens	1	*Serpulina hyodysenteriae*	0.25
C. septicum	>64		
Mycoplasma			
Mycoplasma agalactiae	0.5	*M. gallisepticum*	0.13
M. arginini	0.06	*M. mycoides* subsp. *capri*	0.06
M. flocculare	0.06	*M. ovipneumoniae*	0.5

Note: See also Table 11.2.

There is one-way cross-resistance with tylosin: mycoplasmas resistant to tylosin have slightly increased resistance to tiamulin, but mycoplasmas resistant to tiamulin are completely resistant to tylosin. There is strain variation in bacterial cross-resistance with the other macrolide and lincosamide antibiotics, which may include modest increases in resistance to spectinomycin and chloramphenicol.

PHARMACOKINETIC PROPERTIES

Little information has been published on the pharmacokinetic characteristics of tiamulin, although these generally are similar to the macrolide antibiotics. In ruminants, Ziv et al. (1983) found the drug to be rapidly absorbed after oral administration and to have a half-life, after IV administration, of 25 minutes. Tiamulin is a lipophilic, weak organic base, with a pK$_a$ of 7.6. The drug penetrates cells well and is concentrated several-fold in milk. Concentration in other tissues is several times that in serum. The half-life in dogs after IM administration was 4.7 hours, and serum concentrations were higher and maintained longer when the drug was given by SC injection (Laber, 1988). Tiamulin is almost completely absorbed after oral administration in monogastrates but would be expected to be inactivated by rumen flora if administered orally to ruminants.

DRUG INTERACTIONS

Drug interactions are likely to be similar to those described for lincosamides and other macrolides. Combination at therapeutic concentrations with ionophore drugs (salinomycin, monensin) in recommended doses produces primary ionophore myotoxicity in chickens, calves, and pigs (Miller et al., 1986) (see Chapter 16). On the other hand, use at prophylactic levels in feed has not been shown to produce such interaction problems.

TOXICITY AND ADVERSE EFFECTS

Tiamulin should not be fed at therapeutic concentrations with ionophores such as monensin, narasin, and salinomycin to animals (pigs, poultry) because of the dose-dependent fatal effects of such combinations, which result from tiamulin's potent inducer-inhibiting activity against cytochrome P-450 in the liver.

Intramuscular injection of certain preparations may be irritating, but formulations of tiamulin base in sesame oil are not. Intravenous injection of calves resulted in severe neurotoxicity and death (Ziv et al., 1983). Orally administered tiamulin is transiently unpalatable and irritating in calves.

Acute dermatitis with cutaneous erythema and intense pruritus has been described in pigs following oral administration of tiamulin (Laperle, 1990), where it was associated with poor hygiene and overcrowding. It was suggested that metabolites of tiamulin in urine had a directly irritant effect on the skin.

Tiamulin should not be administered to horses and other herbivores with expanded large intestines because of the danger of destruction of the large bowel flora and predisposition to colitis.

CLINICAL APPLICATIONS

Tiamulin is used extensively in swine against mycoplasma pneumonia and swine dysentery, against leptospirosis, and to a lesser extent against bacterial pneumonias, including *Actinobacillus pleuropneumoniae*. Its potential use in bovine respiratory disease appears good. Because of its excellent activity against bacteria and mycoplasma, tiamulin is preferred over macrolides for many infections.

Cattle, Sheep, and Goats. Tiamulin has similar potential applications as those described for tylosin, with the advantage of better activity. There are few reports of its use in cattle. Tiamulin has been used successfully to prevent *Mycoplasma bovis* fibrinous polyarthritis and synovitis in veal calves after administration in milk at 400 ppm for the fattening period (Keller et al., 1980). In sheep, tiamulin had a beneficial effect on the course of field cases of infectious rickettsial keratoconjunctivitis. A suggested suitable dosage was 20–30 mg/kg IV, repeated on day 3 and, if necessary, days 6 and 9 (Konig, 1983). Ball and McCaughey (1986) found that a single SC injection of aqueous tiamulin eliminated ureaplasma from the genital tract of 18 of 22 sheep.

Swine. Tiamulin is used both as a growth promoter in swine and for its outstanding effectiveness against swine dysentery and chronic pneumonia in swine. It has good activity against *Erysipelothrix rhusiopathiae*, *Leptospira*, and streptococci and moderate activity against *Actinobacillus pleuropneumoniae* and possibly *Pasteurella multocida*. Tiamulin is used in strategic medication in pig production to prevent and treat common infections. Its activity in vitro against *Mycoplasma hyopneumoniae* requires confirmation in vivo.

The drug is highly effective in preventing and treating swine dysentery. Concentrations of 60 ppm in water for 3–5 days apparently eradicated experimental infections; relapses occurred when lower concentrations were used (Taylor, 1980). Tiamulin at 30 ppm in feed has prevented dysentery. Incorporation into water (45 ppm for 5 days, 60 ppm for 3 days) effectively treated swine dysentery and was better than tylosin (Pickles, 1982). A single IM dose of 10–15 mg/kg has successfully treated clinical cases of dysentery (Burch et al., 1983). It is approved for use in the United States for the prophylaxis of swine dysentery. Tiamulin may be used to eradicate swine dysentery from herds, using a variety of approaches. These have included daily injection of carriers with 10 mg/kg IM for 5 consecutive days, combined with management changes and rodent control (Blaha et al., 1987), or oral administration to grower pigs for 10 days followed by carbadox for 42 days (Moore, 1990).

Tiamulin has had good results in treatment of field cases of enzootic pneumonia and other mycoplasma infections. In one study, treatment with 200 ppm in the feed for 10 days at weaning significantly reduced lung lesions (Martineau et al., 1980). Administration in the drinking water at 3 mg/kg to pigs with enzootic pneumonia markedly improved average daily weight gain and feed efficiency (Pickles, 1980). Tiamulin has proved superior to tylosin in treating experimental mycoplasma and bacterial pneumonia in swine (Hannan et al., 1982). It has been used successfully in the early medicated weaning procedure of Alexander et al. (1980) to obtain piglets free of endemic pathogens (Meszaros et al., 1985). Nevertheless, in experimental studies, tiamulin had no effect after oral administration in treating swine in the early stages of induced pure *M. hyopneumoniae* pneumonia (Ross and Cox, 1988). This unexpected discrepancy may be explained by the activity of tiamulin against some of the other bacteria and mycoplasma involved in chronic pneumonia of swine but does not explain the poor activity against *M. hyopneumoniae*. Further studies are required on the use of tiamulin in controlling enzootic pneumonia in pigs. Tiamulin has been used with apparent success in eradicating *A. pleuropneumoniae* infection from herds (Larsen et al., 1990) and also in reducing lesions in pigs treated for chronic *A. pleuropneumoniae* infection (Anderson and Williams, 1990).

Tiamulin fed at 200 ppm in feed for 10 days cured chronic kidney carriage of experimental *Leptospira pomona* infection (Laber and Walzl, 1979). Tiamulin administered in drinking water significantly reduced the effects of experimentally induced *Streptococcus suis* type 2 infection (Chengappa et al., 1990). Tiamulin is effective in the prevention and treatment of proliferative enteropathy (McOrist et al., 1996).

Bibliography

Aitken AA, et al. 1999. Comparative in vitro activity of valnemulin against porcine bacterial pathogens. Vet Rec 144:128.

Alexander TJL, et al. 1980. Medicated early weaning to obtain pigs free of pathogens endemic in the herd of origin. Vet Rec 106:114.

Anderson MD, Williams JA. 1990. Effects of tiamulin base administered intramuscularly to pigs for treatment of pneumonia associated with *Actinobacillus* (*Haemophilus*) *pleuropneumoniae*. Proc 11th Int Pig Vet Soc, p15.

Ball HJ, McCaughey WJ. 1986. Use of tiamulin in the elimination of ureaplasmas from sheep. Br Vet J 142:257.

Blaha T, et al. 1987. Swine dysentery control in the German Democratic Republic and the suitability of injections of tiamulin for the programme. Vet Rec 121:416.

Burch DGS, Goodwin RFW. 1984. Use of tiamulin in a herd of pigs seriously affected with *Mycoplasma hyosynoviae* arthritis. Vet Rec 115:594.

Burch DGS, et al. 1983. Tiamulin injection for the treatment of swine dysentery. Vet Rec 113:236.

Chengappa MM, et al. 1990. Efficacy of tiamulin against experimentally induced *Streptococcus suis* type-2 infection in swine. J Am Vet Med Assoc 197:1467.

Hannan PCT, et al. 1982. Tylosin tartrate and tiamulin effects on experimental piglet pneumonia induced with pneumonic pig lung homogenates containing mycoplasma, bacteria, and viruses. Res Vet Sci 33:76.

Keller H, et al. 1980. Uber Spontan- and Experimentelle von Polyarthritis undsynovitis bei Kalbern, verursacht durch Mycoplasmen: (1) Klinische Aspekte. Schweiz Arch Tierheilkd 122:15.

Konig CDW. 1983. "Pink eye" or "zere oogjes" or keratoconjunctivitis infectiosa ovis (k10): clinical efficacy of a number of antimicrobial therapies. Vet Q 5:122.

Laber G. 1988. Investigation of pharmacokinetic parameters of tiamulin after intramuscular and subcutaneous administration in dogs. J Vet Pharmacol Ther 11:45.

Laber G, Walzl H. 1979. Orientierende Prufung der chemotherapeutischen Wirksamkeit von Tiamulin gegenuber einer experimentellen *Leptospira pomona* Infektion am Schwein. Wien Tieraerztl Monatsh 66:85.

Laperle A. 1990. Dermatite aigue chez des porcs traités à la tiamuline. Med Vet Quebec 20:20.

Larsen H, et al. 1990. Eradication of *Actinobacillus pleuropneumoniae* from a breeding herd. Proc 11th Int Pig Vet Soc, p18.

Larsen JL. 1988. Effect of subinhibitory concentrations of tiamulin on the haemagglutinating properties of fimbriated *Escherichia coli*. Res Vet Sci 45:134.

Martineau GP, et al. 1980. Bronchopneumonie enzootique du porc: Amelioration de l'index pulmonaire apres traitement par la tiamuline. Ann Med Vet 124:281.

McOrist S, et al. 1996. Treatment and prevention of porcine proliferative enteropathy with oral tiamulin. Vet Rec 139:615.

Meszaros J, et al. 1985. Eradication of some infectious pig diseases by perinatal tiamulin treatment and early weaning. Vet Rec 116:8.

Miller DJS, et al. 1986. Tiamulin/salinomycin interactions in pigs. Vet Rec 118:73.

Moore C. 1990. Eradicating disease in the grower-finisher section. Compend Contin Educ Pract Vet 13:329.

Murdoch RS. 1975. Treatment of atrophic rhinitis. Vet Rec 97:251.

Pickles RW. 1980. Field trials in the UK to evaluate tiamulin as a treatment for enzootic pneumonia. Proc Int Pig Vet Soc, p306.

Pickles RW. 1982. Tiamulin water medication in the treatment of swine dysentery under field conditions. Vet Rec 110:403.

Riond JL, et al. 1993. Influence of tiamulin concentration in feed on its bioavailability in piglets. Vet Res 24:494.

Ross RF, Cox DF. 1988. Evaluation of tiamulin for treatment of mycoplasmal pneumonia in swine. J Am Vet Med Assoc 193:441.

Szancer J. 1990. Minimal inhibitory concentrations of antimicrobial agents against *Actinobacillus pleuropneumoniae*. Can J Vet Res 54:198.

Tasker JB, et al. 1981. Eradication of swine dysentery from closed pig herds. Vet Rec 108:382.

Taylor DJ. 1980. Tiamulin in the treatment and prophylaxis of experimental swine dysentery. Vet Rec 106:114.

Ziv G, et al. 1983. Clinical pharmacology of tiamulin in ruminants. J Vet Pharmacol Ther 6:23.

12 | Chloramphenicol, Thiamphenicol, and Florfenicol

J. F. PRESCOTT

Chloramphenicol is a stable, lipid-soluble, neutral compound. It is a derivative of dichloroacetic acid and contains a nitrobenzene moiety (Fig. 12.1). Thiamphenicol has a similar antibacterial spectrum with slightly lower activity to chloramphenicol but differs from the parent compound in that the nitro group attached to the benzene ring is replaced by a sulfomethyl group. Unlike chloramphenicol, this compound has not been clearly implicated in causing aplastic anemia. Florfenicol is a structural analog of thiamphenicol and has the advantage of lacking the *p*-nitro group associated with aplastic anemia as well as being more active than thiamphenicol. Bacteria with acquired resistance to chloramphenicol and thiamphenicol may also be susceptible to florfenicol. Pharmacokinetic properties of thiamphenicol and florfenicol are generally similar to those of chloramphenicol, but metabolism may have important differences in some species.

Chloramphenicol
Mechanism of Action
Chloramphenicol is a potent inhibitor of microbial protein synthesis. It binds irreversibly to a receptor site on the 50S subunit of the bacterial ribosome and interferes with the formation of peptides by blocking the action of peptidyl transferase. Chloramphenicol inhibits mitochondrial protein synthesis in mammalian bone marrow cells.

263

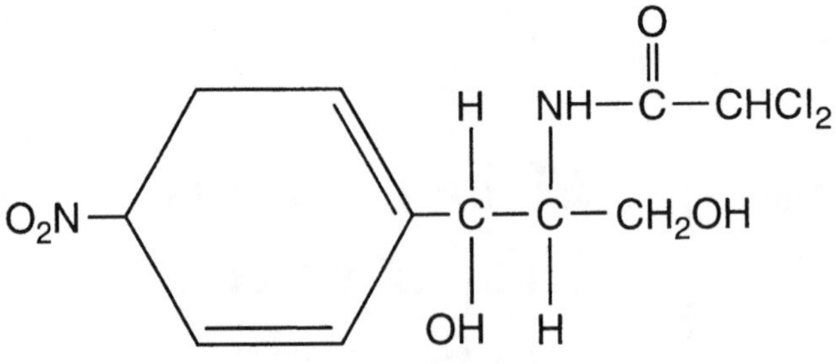

Chloramphenicol

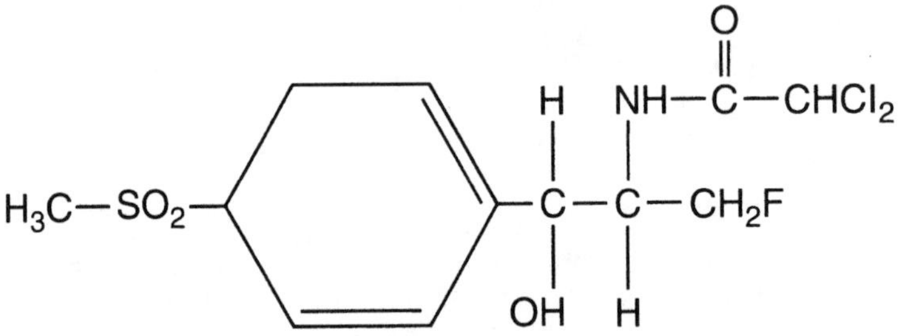

Florfenicol

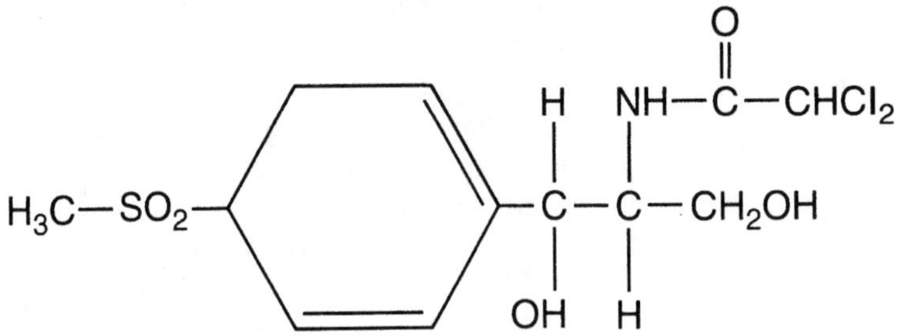

Thiamphenicol

Fig. 12.1. Structural formulas of chloramphenicol, florfenicol, and thiamphenicol.

Antimicrobial Activity

Chloramphenicol is active against a wide range of Gram-positive and many Gram-negative bacteria (Table 12.1), against which it is usually bacteriostatic. All anaerobic bacteria are inhibited at usual therapeutic concentrations (5–15 μg/ml). Chloramphenicol suppresses rickettsial and chlamydial growth. While mycoplasmas often show susceptibility in vitro,

TABLE 12.1. Activity (MIC$_{90}$, µg/ml) of chloramphenicol against selected bacteria and mycoplasmas

Organism	MIC$_{90}$	Organism	MIC$_{90}$
Gram-positive aerobes			
Arcanobacterium pyogenes	1	*Listeria monocytogenes*	8
Bacillus anthracis	2	*Staphylococcus aureus*	8
Corynebacterium renale	4	*Streptococcus dysgalactiae*	4
Enterococcus spp.	>32	*S. uberis*	2
Erysipelothrix rhusiopathiae	2		
Gram-negative aerobes			
Actinobacillus spp.	4	*Klebsiella* spp.	>32
Bordetella bronchiseptica	8	*Pasteurella* spp.	>32
Brucella canis	4	*P. haemolytica*	2
Enterobacter spp.	>32	*P. multocida*	2
Escherichia coli	>32	*Proteus* spp.	>32
Haemophilus somnus	1	*Pseudomonas aeruginosa*	>32
Anaerobes			
Bacteroides spp.	8	*Dichelobacter nodosus*	0.25
B. fragilis	8	*Fusobacterium* spp.	1
Clostridium difficile	4	*F. necrophorum*	2
C. perfringens	4	*Serpulina hyodysenteriae*	4
Mycoplasmas			
Mycoplasma bovis	8	*M. hyopneumoniae*	4
M. bovirhinis	64	*M. ovipneumoniae*	16
M. canis	8		

the outcome of chloramphenicol therapy of pulmonary infections caused by this organism is often disappointing.

Susceptible Organisms (MIC ≤ 8 µg/ml) include among Gram-positive aerobic bacteria: *Actinomyces* sp., *Arcanobacterium pyogenes, Bacillus anthracis, Corynebacterium* spp., *Erysipelothrix rhusiopathiae, Listeria monocytogenes,* many *Staphylococcus* spp., and *Streptococcus* spp. Among Gram-negative aerobic bacteria: *Actinobacillus* spp.; *Bordetella bronchiseptica; Brucella canis;* Enterobacteriaceae, including many *E. coli, Klebsiella* spp., *Proteus* spp., and *Salmonella* spp.; *Haemophilus* spp.; *Leptospira* spp; *Moraxella* spp.; and *Pasteurella* spp. All anaerobes (*Bacteroides* spp., *Clostridium* spp., *Prevotella* spp., *Porphyromonas* spp.) are commonly susceptible.

Intermediately Susceptible Organisms (MIC 16 µg/ml) include *Rhodococcus equi.*

Resistant Organisms (MIC ≥ 32 µg/ml) are *Mycobacterium* spp. and *Nocardia* spp.

Acquired resistance occurs in many Gram-positive and Gram-negative aerobic bacteria, particularly in countries where chloramphenicol is in common use. Resistance is the result of enzymatic inactivation by the enzyme chloramphenicol transacetylase, of which there are several types, and is commonly plasmid mediated. Substitution of the 3-hydroxyl group by fluorine produces an active molecule not affected by the transacetylase enzyme.

Pharmacokinetic Properties

In monogastric animals and preruminant calves, chloramphenicol is well absorbed from the gastrointestinal tract. In ruminant animals, the antibiotic is inactivated in the rumen. The drug's capacity to pass readily through cellular barriers and its moderately low protein binding (30–46%) enable it to attain effective concentrations in most tissues and body fluids, including cerebrospinal fluid, the central nervous system, and aqueous humor, the latter after local ophthalmic application. The drug readily crosses the placenta. This may be of clinical significance, as the liver of the fetus is deficient in glucuronyl transferase activity. Penetration of the blood-prostate barrier is relatively poor and constitutes an exception, as concentration in the uninflamed gland is relatively low.

Consistent with its lipophilic nature, the apparent volume of distribution of chloramphenicol is large (>1 l/kg) in all species. This can be attributed to widespread distribution, given that partitioning of the drug is independent of pH and there is no evidence of selective tissue binding.

The agent's half-life varies widely among species of domestic animal. It is short in horses (1 hour) and longest in cats (5–6 hours). Hepatic metabolism is the principal process of elimination; it takes place mainly by conjugation with glucuronic acid. A fraction of the dose is excreted unchanged by glomerular filtration in the urine of dogs (10%) and cats (20%), while a negligible amount is eliminated by renal excretion in herbivores. The metabolites, which are inactive, are excreted in the urine and to a much lesser extent in the bile. The glucuronide conjugate excreted in bile can be hydrolyzed by intestinal flora to liberate the parent drug.

In newborn animals the half-life of chloramphenicol is considerably longer than in adult animals of the same species. This is due mainly to defective glucuronide conjugation. The rate of conjugation increases with age during the neonatal period, and in calves 10–12 weeks of age the half-life is similar to that in cows (Table 12.2).

Glucuronide conjugation develops most rapidly in foals in that the half-life in the 1-week-old foal approaches that in the adult horse (Table 12.3).

Drug Interactions

Chloramphenicol should not be used concurrently with a bactericidal drug in treating infections where host defenses are poor. For example,

TABLE 12.2. **Relationship between age of cattle and half-life (mean ± SD) of chloramphenicol (50 mg/kg) administered IV as the monosuccinate ester**

Age	Number	Half-life (h)
1 day	6	14 ± 1.4
3 days	6	8.2 ± 0.9
7 days	6	6.5 ± 0.8
14 days	6	6.1 ± 0.6
21 days	6	5.5 ± 0.7
10–12 weeks	6	4.8 ± 0.7
Adult	8	4.2 ± 0.6

TABLE 12.3. **Pharmacokinetic parameter describing disposition of chloramphenicol (25 mg/kg IV) in foals**

Pharmacokinetic Parameter	Age of Foals (days)			
	1	3	7	14
Half-life[a] (h)	5.29	1.35	0.61	0.51
$V_{d(area)}$ (ml/kg)	1,101 ± 284	759 ± 224	491 ± 158	426 ± 65
Cl_B (ml/min × kg)	2.25 ± 0.67	6.23 ± 2.22	8.86 ± 1.90	9.63 ± 1.63

Source: Adamson (1991).
[a]Denotes harmonic mean. Data are expressed as mean ± SD.

well-recognized antagonistic interactions occur between chloramphenicol and penicillin G in treating bacterial meningitis and endocarditis in humans.

Because chloramphenicol inhibits microsomal enzyme activity, hepatic metabolism (oxidative reactions and glucuronide conjugation) of drugs given concurrently takes place more slowly than usual, with prolonged pharmacologic effects as the observed outcome. This interaction assumes clinical importance when chloramphenicol and another drug that is extensively metabolized by microsomal enzymes are used concurrently. Thus chloramphenicol markedly potentiates the effect of barbiturates, and fatal effects have been observed in dogs treated concurrently with low-dose phenobarbital in the control of epilepsy. The drug may prolong the activity of phenylbutazone, as well as xylazine and ketamine in some species. The drug should not be used with ionophores, such as monensin and lasalocid. Combination of the ionophore lasalocid with chloramphenicol has caused severe muscle degeneration in broiler chickens.

Toxicity and Adverse Effects

The main toxic effects of chloramphenicol in humans are bone marrow depression, which can be fatal in a small number of patients, and the gray syndrome in newborn infants because of their deficiency in glucuronic acid conjugation. The development of aplastic anemia is a serious risk associated with chloramphenicol administration in humans by any route, as induction of the condition is not dose related. Aplastic anemia probably represents a genetically determined idiosyncrasy of the individual. The incidence of fatal aplastic anemia has been estimated as 1 in every 25,000 to 60,000 humans who use the drug. A few cases of aplastic anemia in humans have occurred following contact exposure (ophthalmic use, medicated sprays, handling), so that veterinarians and owners should wear protective gloves when handling chloramphenicol and avoid other contact.

In dogs, oral administration of chloramphenicol is safe. In cats, clinical signs of toxicity may be seen when the usual maintenance dosage of 25 mg/kg of base or palmitate ester PO twice daily is administered for 21 days (Watson, 1991). Administration of larger doses for this period caused changes in the peripheral blood and bone marrow of reversible, dose-related disturbances in red cell maturation. It can be concluded that chloramphenicol toxicity is related both to size of dose and duration of treatment and that cats are more likely than dogs to develop toxicity. Administration for less than 10 days using the maintenance dose is not likely to cause toxicity in either dogs or cats, unless the animals have depressed, hepatic microsomal enzyme activity or severely impaired renal function. Anaphylaxis, vomiting, and diarrhea have occasionally been reported in dogs and cats treated with therapeutic doses.

Moderate diarrhea may develop in calves after oral dosing with therapeutic concentrations of chloramphenicol. Rapid IV dosing may be associated with severe hypotension.

Since chloramphenicol can inhibit mammalian protein synthesis, it is inadvisable to immunize animals while they are being treated with chloramphenicol.

Administration and Dosage

Recommended drug dosages of chloramphenicol are given in Table 12.4. Chloramphenicol is a broad-spectrum bacteriostatic drug that

TABLE 12.4. **Usual systemic dosing rate (mg/kg) of chloramphenicol in animals**

Species	Dosage Form	Route	Dose (mg/kg)	Interval (h)	Comments
Dogs and cats	Base, palmitate	Oral, dog	50	12	50–100 mg/kg
		Oral, cat	50 mg/cat	12	priming dose
	Sodium succinate	IV, IM, SC	25–50	8–12	
Horses	Sodium succinate	IM	30–50	6	50 mg/kg priming dose

Note: Owners should be warned of dangers of exposure to chloramphenicol.

can attain effective concentrations at sites of infection that are relatively inaccessible to many antimicrobials. The objective in multiple dosing is to maintain an average steady-state plasma concentration of 5–10 μg/ml.

Chloramphenicol is available for either oral (free base or palmitate ester) or parenteral (sodium succinate) administration. A chloramphenicol base formulation is also available for parenteral use; this may be less irritating and better absorbed than the succinate. For local treatment of eye or ear infections caused by susceptible organisms, ophthalmic preparations can be applied (not the succinate form).

Because the drug is well absorbed from the gastrointestinal tract in small animals, it can be given orally as either the base or the palmitate ester. The ester is hydrolyzed prior to absorption of the free base. The intake of food does not influence systemic drug availability. Subcutaneous injection of chloramphenicol sodium succinate is an alternative to oral administration. While both routes may provide equivalent concentrations, the oral route is preferable because injection of the parenteral preparation causes pain. The regimens for small animals are to initiate therapy with a priming dose of 50 mg/kg and to administer maintenance doses of 25 mg/kg at 8-hour intervals in dogs and 12-hour intervals in cats. The total length of treatment should not exceed 10 days. A precaution is never to administer chloramphenicol to patients with evidence of or suspected bone marrow suppression.

The short half-life of chloramphenicol in horses (1 hour), together with its generally bacteriostatic action, precludes IV dosage. An aqueous suspension of the free drug can be administered PO or the sodium succinate given by IM injection. After absorption from injection sites, the inactive succinate ester is rapidly hydrolyzed to the active drug. The usual regimen for the horse is an initial priming dose of 50 mg/kg followed by maintenance doses of 30–50 mg/kg at 8-hour intervals. This regimen can also be used in foals over 1 week of age.

For most infections in ruminants, a priming dose of 50 mg/kg of the sodium succinate should be followed by maintenance doses of 25 mg/kg at 8-to-12-hour intervals. In sheep, Dagorn et al. (1990) recommended a dosage of 45 mg/kg SC twice daily. Long-acting forms of chloramphenicol have been described for use in cattle, in which dosage is 90 mg/kg IM every 24 hours.

The drug should not be used in the early neonatal period unless plasma concentration is monitored, and it should be used with caution in pregnant animals because of the potential for adverse effects on the fetus.

Clinical Applications

Apart from its bacteriostatic properties and low activity on a weight basis, chloramphenicol has some hallmarks of an ideal antibiotic for animals. It diffuses rapidly into tissues, including brain, cerebrospinal fluid, and aqueous humor of the eyes. Besides being relatively nontoxic and inexpensive, chloramphenicol has broad antimicrobial activity against bacteria, rickettsias, chlamydiae, and possibly mycoplasmas. Two problems, both concerned with human health, have markedly limited its use.

The potential for non-dose-related fatal aplastic anemia in humans has led to prohibition of use of chloramphenicol in food animals in many parts of the world. In Britain the fear at one time that drug resistance might be passed on to human pathogens has also led to restricting use in both farm and companion animals only to local treatment of serious eye infections and to systemic conditions for which clinical and laboratory assessment show no safer antibiotic (Joint RCVS/BVA Statement, 1976). Examples include systemic salmonellosis in cattle and serious respiratory infections in calves, although many suitable alternate drugs are now available.

It appears that use of chloramphenicol should generally be reserved in veterinary medicine for treatment of systemic salmonellosis caused by otherwise resistant organisms, deep infections of the eyes caused by Gram-positive bacteria, and anaerobic infections, although other drugs are equally useful or better for anaerobic infections. Because of the availability of effective bactericidal drugs, chloramphenicol is not indicated for the treatment of meningitis in animals. In spite of its relatively poor penetration into prostatic fluid, it may be useful in dogs to treat prostatic infections caused by Gram-negative bacteria.

There appear to be relatively few primary indications for the use of chloramphenicol in companion animals, but these may include anaerobic infections, serious infections of the eye, prostatitis, and salmonellosis. The issue of human toxicity from handling chloramphenicol should be addressed when prescribing the drug for use in dogs and cats.

Bibliography

Adams HR, Dixit BN. 1970. Prolongation of pentobarbital anesthesia by chloramphenicol in dogs and cats. J Am Vet Med Assoc 156:902.

Adamson PJW, et al. 1991. Influence of age on the disposition kinetics of chloramphenicol in equine neonates. Am J Vet Res 52:426.

Burrows GE, et al. 1989. Interactions between chloramphenicol, acepromazine, phenylbutazone, rifampin, and thiamylal in the horse. Equine Vet J 21:34.

Dagorn M, et al. 1990. Pharmacokinetics of chloramphenicol in sheep after intravenous, intramuscular, and subcutaneous administration. Vet Q 12:166.

Del Giacco GS, et al. 1981. Fatal bone marrow hypoplasia in a shepherd using chloramphenicol spray. Lancet i:945.

Harper RC. 1987. The responsible use of chloramphenicol in small animal practice: clinical considerations. J Small Anim Pract 28:543.

Joint Royal College of Veterinary Surgeons/British Veterinary Association Statement. 1976. Veterinary use of chloramphenicol. Vet Rec 99:152.

Nouws JFM, et al. 1986. Pharmacokinetic, residue, and irritation aspects of chloramphenicol sodium succinate and a chloramphenicol base formulation following intramuscular administration to ruminants. Vet Q 8:224.

Oniviran O. 1974. The comparative efficacy of some antibiotics used to treat experimentally induced mycoplasma infection in goats. Vet Rec 94:418.

Rubhun WC. 1982. Corneal stromal abscess in horses. J Am Vet Med Assoc 181:677.

Spika JS, et al. 1987. Chloramphenicol-resistant *Salmonella newport* traced through hamburger to dairy farms. N Engl J Med 316:565.

Watson ADJ. 1991. Chloramphenicol: (2) Clinical pharmacology in dogs and cats. Aust Vet J 68:2.

Thiamphenicol

Thiamphenicol is a derivative of chloramphenicol, in which the *p*-nitro group has been replaced by a sulfomethyl group. Thiamphenicol is generally 1–2 times less active than chloramphenicol, although it has equal activity against *Haemophilus, Bacteroides fragilis,* and streptococci. Cross-resistance with chloramphenicol is complete in bacteria which possess chloramphenicol transacetylases. Absorption and distribution are similar to those of chloramphenicol, and it is also equally well distributed into tissues. Thiamphenicol is not, however, eliminated by hepatic glucuronide conjugation but is rather excreted unchanged in the urine. Unlike elimination of chloramphenicol, its elimination is therefore unaffected by liver disease and by the use of other drugs metabolized in the liver. Its half-life of elimination appears to be more rapid than that of chloramphenicol in adult cattle and sheep.

One reason for major interest in thiamphenicol is that, because it lacks the *p*-nitro group, it does not induce irreversible bone marrow aplasia in humans, although it may more commonly cause reversible hematopoietic depression than chloramphenicol.

Thiamphenicol is used extensively in Europe and Japan but is not available in North America. Apart from its bacteriostatic character and lower activity than chloramphenicol, thiamphenicol would appear to have underexploited potential for use in the treatment of many infections caused by susceptible organisms, because of its advantages of excellent tissue distribution, broad spectrum of antimicrobial activity, low toxicity, and potential for oral administration in monogastrates. Although detailed dosage is not available because of a relative lack of pharmacokinetic and clinical studies, suitable dosage in animals would appear to be similar to that of chloramphenicol. Dosages for cattle and pigs are 10–30 mg/kg IM every 24 hours, or 50–200 ppm in feed for pigs and 100–500 ppm in feed for chickens.

Bibliography

Abdennebi EH, et al. 1994. Thiamphenicol pharmacokinetics in beef and dairy cattle. J Vet Pharmacol Ther 17:365.

Castells G, et al. 1998. Pharmacokinetics of thiamphenicol in dogs. Am J Vet Res 59:1473.

Ferrari V. 1984. Introductory address. Salient features of thiamphenicol: review of clinical pharmacokinetics and toxicology. Sex Transm Dis 11:336.
Mestorino N, et al. 1993. The pharmacokinetics of thiamphenicol in lactating cows. Vet Res Comm 17:295.

Florfenicol

Florfenicol is a fluorinated derivative of thiamphenicol, in which the hydroxyl group has been replaced with fluorine. Like thiamphenicol, the drug does not cause irreversible aplastic anemia, but, in contrast, it is not susceptible to inactivation by chloramphenicol transacetylases. Its mechanism of action is similar to that of chloramphenicol.

Antimicrobial Activity

Florfenicol has a broad range to activity similar to, but slightly more active than, that of chloramphenicol (see Table 12.1). It may have bactericidal activity against *Haemophilus* and *Pasteurella* spp. at concentrations only 1 dilution above those which are bacteriostatic. Among highly susceptible bacteria, the MIC_{90} for *Actinobacillus pleuropneumoniae*, *Haemophilus somnus*, *Pasteurella haemolytica*, and *P. multocida* is 1 µg/ml, and for *Streptococcus dysgalactiae* and *S. uberis* is 2 µg/ml. The MIC_{90} for Enterobacteriaceae, which are less susceptible, is higher; for example, for *E. coli* it is 8 µg/ml.

Acquired resistance may develop and show cross-resistance with chloramphenicol. Organisms resistant to chloramphenicol through the common transacetylation resistance mechanisms are susceptible to florfenicol.

Pharmacokinetic Properties

Pharmacokinetic properties are generally similar to those of chloramphenicol in the wide tissue distribution and high bioavailability, although pharmacokinetic properties do not appear to be significantly age dependent and the volume of distribution is slightly less than observed for chloramphenicol. There is, however, little data on florfenicol metabolism and renal excretion in animals of veterinary significance. In cattle, florfenicol does not appear to be excreted as the glucuronide conjugate but rather is largely excreted unchanged in the urine. The metabolic fate in other species, including the horse, remains to be determined.

Drug Interactions

There is inadequate data on adverse drug interactions produced by florfenicol. In some species, including the horse, florfenicol may be anticipated to inhibit hepatic microsomal enzymes and therefore like chloramphenicol to interact adversely with drugs metabolized in the liver, but details are lacking.

Toxicity and Adverse Effects

Reversible bone marrow suppression through effects on erythroid cells may result from prolonged florfenicol administration. Transient diarrhea or inappetence has been noted in cattle, which usually returns to normal within a few days after the end of treatment.

Administration and Dosage

Florfenicol is administered to cattle for the treatment of respiratory disease or other infections caused by highly susceptible bacteria (MIC ≤ 1 μg/ml) at 20 mg/kg IM twice at a 48-hour interval. Each injection site should not exceed 10 ml. This dosage would not be expected significantly to inhibit bacteria such as *E. coli*. The drug has recently been approved in some jurisdictions for use as a single SC injection of 40 mg/kg for treatment of bovine respiratory disease.

Clinical Applications

Currently, florfenicol is used as an effective treatment for bovine respiratory disease caused by highly susceptible bacteria such as *Pasteurella* and *Haemophilus*. The same dosage regime has also been used successfully to treat infectious bovine keratoconjunctivitis. Use at this dosage to treat enteric disease in calves, although reported as moderately successful, would be expected to be less successful because of the lower susceptibility of enteric bacteria to this drug. Intramammary administration of 750 mg florfenicol in the treatment of bovine mastitis caused by a variety of pathogens revealed no advantage over cloxacillin in one study (Wilson et al., 1996).

Florfenicol at 50 ppm in feed significantly reduced illness due to experimental *Actinobacillus pleuropneumoniae* pneumonia in pigs, including that caused by a strain resistant to thiamphenicol. Injection at 15 mg/kg 48 hours apart significantly reduced morbidity and illness caused by the same organism (Jackson et al., 1998).

Florfenicol is a drug with potential for use in other species and for infections other than those for which it is currently used. Further studies are required to examine the potential of florfenicol in the treatment of specific infections caused by highly susceptible bacteria in species other than cattle, but the use of this drug for these purposes will depend on toxicity, pharmacokinetic data, and clinical studies in these species. Infections in cattle caused by less susceptible bacteria such as *E. coli* would almost certainly require more frequent dosage than currently used.

Florfenicol is used in the treatment of furunculosis in fish (10 mg/kg body weight administered in the ration) (Samuelsen et al., 1998).

Bibliography

Adams PE, et al. 1987. Tissue concentrations and pharmacokinetics of florfenicol in male calves given repeated doses. Am J Vet Res 48:1725.

Hoar BR, et al. 1998. A comparison of the clinical field efficacy and safety of florfenicol and tilmicosin for the treatment of undifferentiated bovine respiratory disease of cattle in western Canada. Can Vet J 39:161.

Jackson JA, et al. 1998. Comparative efficacy of florfenicol (FFC) and ceftiofur (CEF) in the treatment of naturally occurring swine respiratory disease. Proc 15th Int Pig Vet Congr, p187.

McKellar QA, Varma KJ. 1996. Pharmacokinetics and tolerance of florfenicol in Equidae. Equine Vet J 28:209.

Samuelsen OB, et al. 1998. Efficacy of orally administered florfenicol in the treatment of furunculosis in Atlantic salmon. J Aquat Anim Health 10:56.

Ueda Y, et al. 1995. Efficacy of florfenicol on experimental *Actinobacillus* pleuropneumonia in pigs. J Vet Med Sci 57:261.

Varma KJ, et al. 1986. Pharmacokinetics of florfenicol in veal calves. J Vet Pharmacol Ther 9:412.

Wilson DJ, et al. 1996. Efficacy of florfenicol for treatment of clinical and subclinical bovine mastitis. Am J Vet Res 57:527.

13 | Tetracyclines

J. F. PRESCOTT

Tetracyclines are products of *Streptomyces* spp. (chlortetracycline, oxytetracycline, tetracycline) and their semisynthetic derivatives (doxycycline, minocycline). They are classic broad-spectrum antibiotics because of their activity against Gram-positive and Gram-negative aerobic and anaerobic bacteria, including *Brucella, Coxiella, Ehrlichia,* some *Mycobacterium, Mycoplasma,* and *Rickettsia.* The extraordinarily widespread nature of acquired resistance that has developed in the many common pathogens and particularly Gram-negatives limits the use of tetracyclines in many clinical circumstances. They have generally favorable pharmacokinetic properties, particularly the more lipophilic semisynthetic derivatives, but IM administration is painful, and they produce gastrointestinal disturbances if given orally. They have a number of other uncommon but important adverse effects. They tend to be used as first-line, workhorse antibiotics in ruminants and swine but have some very specific uses in companion animal settings in the treatment of chlamydiosis, coxiellosis, and rickettsiosis, and for some mycobacterial and mycoplasmal infections. Newer derivatives resistant to common resistance mechanisms are on the horizon.

Chemistry

The tetracyclines (chlortetracycline, oxytetracycline, tetracycline, doxycycline, minocycline) are crystalline amphoteric substances that are only slightly soluble in water at pH 7.0. They are available for use, mainly as the hydrochlorides, in a wide variety of dosage forms, both oral and parenteral. Solutions of the hydrochlorides are acidic and, with the exception of

	R	R₁	R₂
Tetracycline	—H	—CH₃	—H
Chlortetracycline	—Cl	—CH₃	—H
Oxytetracycline	—H	—CH₃	—OH
Demeclocycline	—Cl	—H	—H
Methacycline	—H	=CH₂*	—OH
Doxycycline	—H	—CH₃	—OH
Minocycline	—N(CH₃)₂	—H	—H

*No hydroxyl at C6.

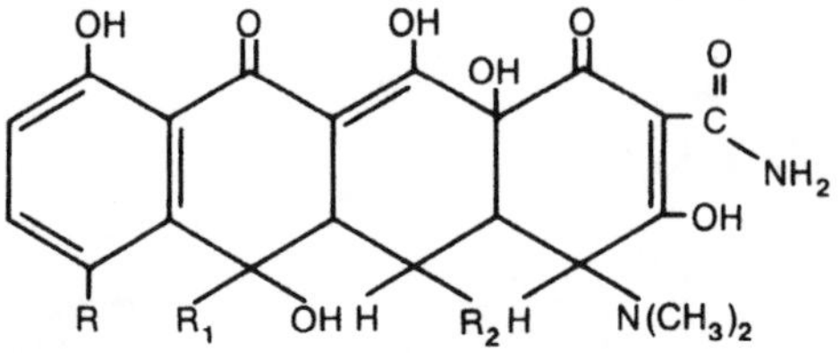

Fig. 13.1. Structural formulas of tetracyclines.

chlortetracycline, fairly stable. All tetracyclines have the same basic structure (Fig. 13.1).

Mechanism of Action

The tetracyclines are bacteriostatic antibiotics that inhibit protein synthesis in susceptible microorganisms. After diffusion through the outer cell membrane, an active carrier-mediated process transports the drugs through the inner cytoplasmic membrane. Once inside the cell, the tetracyclines bind irreversibly to receptors on the 30S subunit of the bacterial ribosome, where they interfere with the binding of the aminoacyl-transfer RNA to the acceptor site on the messenger RNA ribosome complex. This binding effectively prevents the addition of amino acids to the elongating peptide chain, inhibiting protein synthesis.

Antimicrobial Activity

Tetracyclines are classic broad-spectrum antibiotics. They inhibit bacteria, mycoplasmas, chlamydiae, rickettsias, and some protozoa.

Equal amounts of tetracyclines in body fluids or tissues have approximately equal antimicrobial activity. Tetracycline is used as the class drug in determining susceptibility. Minocycline, which is the most lipid soluble, has greater activity than other tetracyclines against *Nocardia,* some mycobacteria, and anaerobes. It has activity against some strains of *Staphylococcus aureus* resistant to other tetracyclines.

TABLE 13.1. Activity (MIC$_{90}$, µg/ml) of tetracycline against bacteria and mycoplasma

Organism	MIC$_{90}$	Organism	MIC$_{90}$
Gram-positive aerobes			
Arcanobacterium pyogenes	64	*Rhodococcus equi*	4
Bacillus anthracis	4	*Staphylococcus aureus*	>64
Corynebacterium pseudotuberculosis	≤0.25	*Streptococcus agalactiae*	0.25[a]
C. renale	4	*S. dysgalactiae*	>32
Erysipelothrix rhusiopathiae	0.25	*S. suis*	64
Listeria monocytogenes	1	*S. uberis*	0.5
Nocardia asteroides		Group C streptococci	2
Gram-negative anaerobes			
Actinobacillus spp.	≤0.25[a]	*Klebsiella pneumoniae*	≥64
A. pleuropneumoniae	≥16	*Leptospira* spp.	4
Bordetella avium	≥16	*Moraxella bovis*	1
B. bronchiseptica (pig)	≥16	*Pasteurella haemolytica*	≥16
Borrelia burgdorferi	1	*P. multocida* (pigs)	1
Brucella canis	0.25	*Proteus* spp.	≥16
Campylobacter fetus	2	*Pseudomonas aeruginosa*	≥16
C. jejuni	≥64	*Pseudomonas* spp.	≥16
Escherichia coli	≥64	*Salmonella* spp.	≥16
Haemophilus parasuis	0.5	*Taylorella equigenitalis*	0.5
H. somnus	2		
Anaerobes			
Actinomyces spp.	1	*Clostridium* spp.	8
Bacteroides asaccharolyticus	2	*C. perfringens*	32
B. fragilis	25	*Dichelobacter nodosus*	0.12
Fusobacterium necrophorum	4		
Mycoplasmas			
Mycoplasma bovirhinis	0.5[a]	*M. hyorhinis*	1
M. bovis	16[a]	*M. hyosynoviae*	32
M. canis	16	*M. ovipneumoniae*	0.5
M. hyopneumoniae	0.03	*Ureaplasma* spp.	0.06

[a]Some reports show resistance.

Good or Moderate Activity (MIC ≤ 4 µg/ml) occurs among the following Gram-positive aerobes: *Bacillus* spp., *Corynebacterium* spp., *Erysipelothrix rhusiopathiae, Listeria monocytogenes,* and streptococci. Among Gram-negative bacteria: *Actinobacillus* spp., *Bordetella* spp., *Brucella* spp., *Francisella tularensis, Haemophilus* spp., *Lawsonia intracellularis, Pasteurella multocida, Yersinia* spp., *Campylobacter fetus, Borrelia* spp., and *Leptospira* spp. Among the anaerobes are *Actinomyces* spp.; *Fusobacterium* spp. (see Table 13.1); *Mycoplasma* spp.; *Chlamydia* spp., including *C. psittaci;* and rickettsias, including *Coxiella burnetii* and *Ehrlichia* spp.; also susceptible are the protozoa *Theileria, Eperythrozoon,* and *Anaplasma.*

Variable Susceptibility, because of acquired resistance, is shown in staphylococci; enterococci; Enterobacteriaceae, including *Enterobacter* spp., *E. coli, Klebsiella* spp., *Proteus* spp., and *Salmonella* spp. Anaerobes such as *Bacteroides* spp. and *Clostridium* spp. show variable susceptibility.

Resistant organisms (MIC ≥ 16 μg/ml) include *Mycobacterium* spp., *Proteus vulgaris, Pseudomonas aeruginosa,* and *Serratia* spp.; some *Mycoplasma* spp., such as *M. bovis* and *M. hyopneumoniae,* are resistant.

Differences in clinical efficacy among tetracyclines are attributable largely to characteristics of absorption, distribution, and excretion of individual tetracyclines, not to differences in susceptibility. These drugs exert their greatest activity in vitro at an acidic pH close to their isoelectric point (5.5 for all tetracyclines, except 6.0 for minocycline).

Resistance

Acquired resistance to tetracyclines, widespread among bacteria and mycoplasma, has considerably reduced the usefulness of these agents (Table 13.1). The basis of this resistance, which is usually plasmid mediated, is often interference with active transport of tetracyclines into, and increased efflux from, the cell. Ribosomal protection, in which protein synthesis machinery is resistant to inhibition through a cytoplasmic protein, is another major mechanism. The transposon Tn*10* is one of several major plasmid-specified resistance determinants and has been reported to incorporate into the bacterial chromosome. At least 12 different genetic determinants (classes) for tetracycline resistance have been described; these code for several mechanisms of drug resistance (efflux, ribosomal protection, or chemical modification).

In recent years, minocycline and tetracycline analogs called glycylcyclines have been identified with activity against strains resistant to conventional tetracyclines due to ribosomal protection or efflux pump mechanisms. These chemicals have potent activity against a wide spectrum of Gram-negative bacteria and may result in rescue of an antibiotic class that appears to be in danger of becoming obsolete because of resistance.

Pharmacokinetic Properties

In dogs and cats most tetracyclines are adequately absorbed from the gastrointestinal tract, but systemic availability can vary widely among different oral preparations. With the exceptions of minocycline and doxycycline, the absorption of tetracyclines is decreased by the presence of food (particularly milk and its products) in the stomach. Divalent cations (calcium, magnesium, iron) decrease absorption by chelating tetracycline. In adult ruminants it is likely that oral dosing with tetracyclines would interfere with normal fermentation processes.

The drugs vary in lipid solubility, and this property largely determines their distribution and rate of excretion. They enter most tissues and body fluids with the exception of cerebrospinal fluid (CSF). The rate at which they penetrate the blood-brain and blood-CSF barriers is related to their degree of lipid solubility and, to a much lesser extent, plasma protein binding. Minocycline and doxycycline are more lipid soluble than other members of the group and are also more highly bound to plasma proteins. The limited evidence available suggests that minocycline has greater capacity than other tetracyclines to penetrate cellular barriers, given that it attains higher concentrations in poorly accessible fluids such as tears and prostatic fluid. Because tetracyclines have approximately equal antimicrobial activity, the higher concentrations attained in tissues by minocycline give this congener greater clinical efficacy. As a result of chelation with calcium, tetracyclines become bound at active sites of ossification and in developing teeth. The drugs cross the placenta to reach the fetus and are secreted in milk, where they reach concentrations approximately those of serum.

The tetracyclines, except minocycline and doxycycline, are excreted unchanged in urine and, to a lesser extent, bile. Because glomerular filtration is their mechanism of urinary excretion, impaired renal function can increase their half-life. Tetracyclines undergo enterohepatic circulation, with much of the compound excreted in bile being reabsorbed from the intestine. This process contributes to the half-life of 6–10 hours, which is long for drugs that are eliminated mainly by renal excretion.

The cumulative recovery of minocycline from urine and feces is much lower than for other tetracyclines, which suggests that this compound is eliminated partly by metabolism. The elimination mechanism for doxycycline differs from that of other tetracyclines in that this agent enters the intestine both by excretion in the bile and directly by diffusion and is excreted in feces. Because doxycycline elimination does not involve renal excretion, it can be recommended for treatment of systemic infection in dogs and cats with renal impairment. The more lipophilic tetracyclines (minocycline and doxycycline) have such high potential for causing digestive disturbances in the colon of the horse that their administration, by any route, to horses and to other animals with expanded large bowels should be avoided.

The long-acting formulations of oxytetracycline available for IM administration to food animals have their long-acting effect because of both the high dosage used and the prolonged drug persistence at the site of IM injection (Nouws et al., 1990).

In swine, there is increasing evidence of poor bioavailability of orally administered tetracycline, so that serum concentrations achieved with therapeutic concentrations in feed or water are equivalent only to those of the most sensitive organisms.

Drug Interactions

Synergism between tetracyclines and tylosin against *Pasteurella* has been described and may occur with other macrolides and other bacteria. Combination with polymyxins may also give synergistic effects by enhancing bacterial uptake of the drugs. Doxycycline is synergistic with rifampin or streptomycin in the treatment of brucellosis. Doxycycline was synergistic with pyrimethamine in the effective treatment of toxoplasmosis in experimentally infected mice.

Toxicity and Adverse Effects

From a pharmacologic viewpoint, the tetracyclines are relatively safe drugs. Adverse effects may be attributed to their severely irritant nature (vomiting after oral administration, tissue damage at injection site), their disturbance of intestinal flora, their ability to bind calcium (cardiovascular effects, deposition in teeth and bone), and their toxic effects on liver and kidney cells. Fatal anaphylaxis has occasionally been recorded. Unless administered slowly, IV injection of a tetracycline is likely to cause an animal to collapse, supposedly because of the cardiovascular effect of the high initial concentration in the systemic circulation. Severe renal tubular damage has been attributed to the administration of outdated or improperly stored preparations and is due to degradation products.

Although the phenomenon is not well documented in veterinary medicine, tetracyclines induce dose-related functional changes in renal tubules in several species (Vaala et al., 1987; Riond and Riviere, 1989). Tetracycline-induced renal toxicosis may be exacerbated by dehydration and debility, hemoglobinuria, myoglobinuria, toxemia, or the presence of other nephrotoxic drugs (Riond and Riviere, 1989).

Severe liver damage can follow overdosage of tetracyclines in animals with preexisting renal failure and may be associated with late pregnancy. In cattle, high doses (33 mg/kg IV) have led to fatty infiltration of the liver and severe proximal renal tubule necrosis (Griffin et al., 1979). Tetracyclines should be administered to cattle only in recommended doses, to avoid problems of nephrotoxicosis (Lairmore et al., 1984). Transient hemoglobinuria with trembling and subnormal temperatures lasting 4 hours has been reported with long-acting formulations (Anderson, 1983). Malabsorption because of moderate diarrhea may occur in calves after oral administration of therapeutic drug doses. Injection IV in cattle has been followed by acute collapse, probably the result of calcium binding and consequent cardiovascular depression (Gyrd-Hansen et al., 1981), although the propylene glycol vehicle may be responsible. Intravenous injections of all forms of tetracyclines should be given slowly to cattle over a period of not less than 5 minutes (Gyrd-Hansen et al., 1981).

In horses, the major toxic effect of tetracyclines is their ability to produce broad-spectrum suppression of the intestinal microflora and to allow superinfection with resistant *Salmonella* or unidentified pathogens, which may include *Clostridium difficile* (Cook, 1973). The result can be a severe and often lethal diarrheic illness. The effect is most common after large doses are given IV but may occur even after low doses administered IM. Many veterinarians have successfully used tetracyclines in horses without observing these effects (other than mild pastiness of feces), but this is best avoided because of the severe potential diarrheic effect.

In dogs, fatal nephrotoxicosis has been reported after the IV administration of tetracyclines at the accidentally high dose of 130 mg/kg on two occasions 24 hours apart (Stevenson, 1980). Administration to growing puppies or pregnant bitches results in yellow discoloration of primary and, to a lesser extent, permanent teeth.

Oxytetracycline irritates tissues. Marked differences have been found in the different formulations of oxytetracyclines in this respect (Nouws et al., 1990). The more irritating the product, the lower the bioavailability and the greater the associated drug persistence at the injection site (Nouws, 1984). The long-acting 20% formulations are particularly irritating. The prolonged action is related to delayed release and hence is associated with increased irritation.

Tetracyclines have anti-anabolic effects that may produce azotemia. Such effects can be exacerbated by corticosteroids. The drugs may also cause metabolic acidosis and electrolyte imbalance.

Administration and Dosage

Recommended dosages are shown in Table 13.2. Tetracyclines are available both in capsular and tablet forms and are usually administered

TABLE **13.2.** **Usual systemic dosages of tetracyclines in animals**

Species	Dosage Form	Route	Dose (mg/kg)	Interval (h)	Comments
Dogs and cats	Tetracycline, oxytetracycline	IV, IM	10	12	
	Doxycycline	IV (not IM)	5–10	12	
Horses	Tetracycline	IV	10	12	Slow IV
	Oxytetracycline	IV	3–5	12	Slow IV
Ruminants	Tetracycline, oxytetracycline	IV, IM	10	12–24	Slow IV
	Long-acting tetracycline	IM	20	48	
Pigs	Tetracycline, oxytetracycline	IM	10–20	12–24	
	Long-acting tetracycline	IM	20	48	

Note: Oral dosages are given in Table 13.3.

TABLE 13.3. **Usual oral dosages of tetracyclines for monogastric animals**

Tetracycline Preparation	Maintenance Dose[a]	Dosage Interval (h)
Tetracycline hydrochloride	15 mg/kg	6–8
Swine	200–800 ppm	
Oxytetracycline hydrochloride	20 mg/kg	8–12
Minocycline hydrochloride	5 mg/kg	12
Doxycycline hyclate	5 mg/kg	12
Swine	200–250 ppm	

[a]One or preferably 2 priming doses should be double this amount.

PO to dogs and cats. Milk, antacids, and ferrous sulfate interfere with absorption. A generally satisfactory approach to PO administration is to initiate therapy with 1 or preferably 2 priming doses and to continue with maintenance doses (each one-half the priming dose) at 12-hour intervals. In the case of tetracycline hydrochloride, a 6-hour interval is recommended (Table 13.3).

Because of poor water solubility, oxytetracycline dihydrate must be given in much higher doses (50 mg/kg) than the hydrochloride to produce equivalent tissue concentrations. In horses, the only route by which the parenteral preparation of oxytetracycline hydrochloride should be administered is by slow (5-minute) IV injection. The regimen that could be expected to maintain therapeutic plasma concentrations (1–5 µg/ml) consists of a priming dose of 5 mg/kg followed by maintenance doses of 3 mg/kg at 12-hour intervals. Because of biliary excretion and passive diffusion into the large bowel, tetracyclines may cause disturbance of the microbial flora of the colon and predispose to salmonellosis or "colitis X." The more lipophilic members of the group (minocycline, doxycycline) are even more likely to have this effect.

Intramuscular injection of tetracyclines cannot be recommended for horses or companion animals because of local tissue damage, local pain, and erratic absorption. The recommended dose in cattle is 10 mg/kg given IM or preferably IV, because of variability in absorption. The long-acting oxytetracycline parenteral preparation, which is oxytetracycline base in 2-pyrrolidone, is approved for IM use in cattle and swine only. A single IM dose of 20 mg/kg provides serum concentrations of oxytetracycline above 0.5 µg/ml for 48 hours but appears to offer no advantage over the same dose of the conventional drug IM (Nouws, 1986). Subcutaneous injection in cattle maintains serum concentrations similar to those following IM administration and appears to be better tolerated. To prevent adverse effects, it is important to differentiate between the conventional and the long-acting formulations in dosage decisions.

Clinical Applications

The primary indications for tetracyclines are in the treatment of borreliosis, brucellosis, chlamydiosis, ehrlichiosis, leptospirosis, listeriosis, rickettsiosis, and tularemia. The older tetracyclines have been used for many years in managing infectious diseases in food animals because of their low cost, broad antimicrobial activity, ease of administration, and general effectiveness. Their widespread use has undoubtedly contributed to resistance in important pathogenic bacteria, which now limits the value of these drugs. The capacity of tetracyclines to attain effective concentrations in most tissues, except those separated by specialized cellular barriers, together with their broad spectrum of activity, makes them particularly useful in the treatment of mixed bacterial infections. The activity of the agents against rickettsias, chlamydiae, *Ehrlichia*, and some mycoplasmas makes them the drugs of choice in treatment of infections caused by these microorganisms. Although recommended for the treatment of plague, results in the treatment of experimental infections in animals have sometimes been disappointing. The tissue irritant effect of these drugs and their potential to cause colonic disturbance largely limit their use in horses. The lipophilic character of the newer tetracyclines (minocycline, doxycycline) allows them to attain concentrations in sites such as the prostate, which is poorly accessible to older members of the group. One disadvantage of tetracyclines over a number of other antimicrobial drugs is their bacteriostatic action, so that treatment may need to be for longer than with bactericidal drugs.

Tetracyclines, particularly doxycycline and minocycline, have antiinflammatory properties independent of their antibacterial action. Experimentally, tetracyclines have protected mice from endotoxin-induced shock by reducing inflammatory cytokine and nitric oxide production.

Tetracyclines are commonly used in the treatment of brucellosis, usually in combination with rifampin or streptomycin. Doxycycline and minocycline are more effective than older tetracyclines because of better penetration into cells. Treatment with doxycycline or minocycline should last 6 weeks and with streptomycin 7–14 days. Tetracyclines (particularly minocycline and doxycycline) are also used in the treatment of infections caused by other intracellular bacteria, including *Ehrlichia* and *Coxiella*.

CATTLE, SHEEP, AND GOATS

Many of the microorganisms that cause bovine pneumonia are susceptible to tetracyclines at concentrations that can be achieved in lung tissue. The drugs are generally useful in the treatment of bovine pneumonias and also in their prophylaxis, especially in feedlots. Nevertheless, increasing resistance in *Pasteurella* and variable susceptibility of *Mycoplasma bovis* limit their effectiveness. The long-acting parenteral formulation, which must be administered by IM injection (or in some formulations SC), 20 mg/kg at 48-hour intervals on 2–4 occasions, may be adequate in treating lower respiratory disease in cattle, sheep, and goats.

If tetracyclines are administered orally to feedlot cattle in the prophylaxis of pneumonia, they should be given in feed and not water. Administration in water may adversely affect mortality (Martin et al., 1982), possibly because of the difficulty of ensuring that even amounts are ingested. Although prophylactic administration of drug in the ration often appears to reduce pneumonia and to improve growth and feed conversion efficiency, the cost-to-benefit ratio may not justify this approach. In addition, such a practice tends to promote resistance among *Pasteurella* organisms. In prophylaxis of feedlot pneumonia, parenteral administration gives better effects than oral administration because of higher bioavailability. An approach shown to be useful is to inject tetracyclines when animals enter feedlots or to inject a single dose of long-acting tetracycline to all animals as soon as some in the lots appear to be developing pneumonia.

Clostridial infections and listeriosis can be treated by tetracyclines. A recommended dosage in neural listeriosis is 10 mg/kg per day IV, but clinical trials are needed to determine whether the same dose given twice daily or the use of ampicillin or penicillin G might not be more effective. In listeriosis, IV administration of the conventional preparation (parenteral aqueous solution) is preferred. In human medicine, minocycline is a recognized alternative to ampicillin.

Oxytetracycline is the drug of choice in anaplasmosis, 20 mg/kg of the long-acting formulation administered IM at 48-hour intervals 3 or 4 times. Taylor et al. (1986) showed the effectiveness of long-acting tetracyclines in preventing *Babesia divergens* infection (redwater) in cattle. Tetracyclines are used in the treatment of, and vaccination against, heartwater disease caused by the rickettsia *Cowdria ruminantium* (Simpson et al., 1987; Mebus and Logan, 1988). The drugs are also used in the prophylaxis of East Coast fever caused by *Theileria parva* (Chumo et al., 1989) and in the prevention of tick-borne fever caused by *Cytoecetes phagocytophilia* (Cranwell, 1990).

For infectious keratoconjunctivitis in cattle, 2 doses of the long-acting preparation, given 3 days apart, can be recommended (George et al., 1988). Long-acting tetracyclines produced moderate cure rates in cattle with dermatophilosis. Long-acting tetracyclines (at 3–4 day intervals for 5 treatments) combined with streptomycin (IM daily for 7 days) successfully treated 14 of 18 cows with *Brucella abortus* infection (Nicoletti et al., 1985). Administration once daily as a topical spray (25 mg/ml) was effective in controlling bovine papillomatous digital dermatitis, with the efficacy increasing with the total number of days of applications (Shearer and Elliott, 1998).

Tetracyclines achieve concentrations in milk approximately those in blood, but because of poor bioavailability after IM injection, they are best given IV. They are second-choice parenteral antibiotics for serious infections of the udder caused by Gram-positive bacteria and possibly by coliforms, although susceptibility among the latter organisms is uncommon. Repeated intramammary administration of tetracycline in combination with tylosin cured experimentally induced *Mycoplasma californicum* mastitis in cows (Ball and Campbell, 1989).

In enzootic abortion in sheep caused by *Chlamydia psittaci*, experimental and field evidence suggests that two treatments of 20 mg/kg of the long-acting preparation at 2-week intervals, starting 6–8 weeks before lambing, will reduce the prevalence of abortions. The drug may be most useful at the start of outbreaks (Greig and Linklater, 1985). Tetracycline is the drug of choice in the prevention and treatment of Q fever. Lambs can be protected from the rickettsial agent of tick-borne fever and associated infections by a single injection of long-acting tetracycline formulation (Brodie et al., 1986). Duration of the effect is between 2 and 3 weeks (Brodie et al., 1988). A single injection of long-acting tetracycline with topical tetracycline is an effective treatment of ovine keratoconjunctivitis caused by *Mycloplasma conjunctivae* (Hosie, 1988; Hosie and Greig, 1995). Long-acting oxytetracycline was highly successful in preventing *Pasteurella haemolytica* pneumonia in sheep (Appleyard and Gilmour, 1990) and has been used successfully in the treatment of ovine foot rot (Grogono-Thomas et al., 1994) and dermatophilosis (Jordan and Venning, 1995).

Long-acting tetracyclines combined with streptomycin were shown to treat successfully about 80% or more of rams with *Brucella ovis* infection (Marin et al., 1989; Dargatz et al., 1990). Daily intraperitoneal injections of 1000 mg oxytetracycline hydrochloride eliminated *B. melitensis* infection from sheep (Radwan et al., 1989).

SWINE

Tetracyclines are commonly used in swine to prevent and treat atrophic rhinitis and lower respiratory disease (*Actinobacillus pleuropneumoniae, Mycoplasma hyopneumoniae, Pasteurella multocida*) and to prevent proliferative adenomatosis. Field outbreaks of *Pasteurella* pneumonia have been controlled by feed medication (200–400 g/ton). Feed medication with chlortetracycline (100 g/ton) has been used to control adenomatosis and at a much higher level (800 g/ton) to eradicate *Leptospira* from the kidneys of swine (Stahlheim, 1967; Love and Love, 1977). Tetracyclines may be effective against erysipelas and *Haemophilus* infections, but because of their bacteriostatic action, they are not drugs of choice for these infections. Enterotoxigenic *Escherichia coli* are usually resistant. Tetracyclines in feed or water have been used successfully to control streptococcal lymphadenitis and *Eperythrozoon suis* infection. Orally administered oxytetracycline in pigs had a bioavailability of only 3% in one study, with tetracycline and chlortetracycline bioavailability being higher (6–18%), particularly in fasted pigs (Nielsen and Gyrd-Hansen, 1996). Orally administered doxycycline may have the advantage in pigs of greater bioavailability. The use of long-acting formulations in experimentally induced *A. pleuropneumoniae* infections showed that these formulations were more effective than conventional ones in preventing infections (when administered 48 hours before challenge) but were no more effective in treatment.

HORSES

Because of the potential for toxic effects, including local necrosis following IM injection in horses, there is little reason to consider administering tetracyclines to horses for bacterial infections, although they have been used extensively in horses with few adverse effects. They are, however, drugs of choice for the rickettsial agent of Potomac horse fever, *Ehrlichia risticii* (Madigan and Gribble, 1987) and for *Ehrlichia equi* infection. Another exception is *Mycoplasma felis* pleuritis. The conventional parenteral preparation of oxytetracycline hydrochloride is the only product that is suitable for administration to horses and must be given by slow IV injection.

DOGS AND CATS

Tetracyclines are drugs of choice for *Ehrlichia canis* and *Rickettsia rickettsii* infections, 66 mg/kg once daily or 33 mg/kg twice daily for 2 weeks. Doxycycline administered orally (5 mg/kg, twice daily, for 2 weeks) is effective in treating acute illness, but even prolonged treatment may not remove the carrier state. In experimental *Brucella canis* infection, the most effective of several treatments was minocycline (22 mg/kg every 12 hours for 14 days) with streptomycin (11 mg/kg every 12 hours for 7 days), but effectiveness must be monitored in the laboratory (Flores-Castro and Carmichael, 1978). Field efficacy of tetracycline and streptomycin was 74% in one study (Nicoletti and Chase, 1987). Tetracycline hydrochloride, 10 mg/kg PO every 8 hours, can be recommended for the treatment of *Pseudomonas aeruginosa* urinary tract infections in dogs because of the high urine concentrations of the drug attained (Ling et al., 1980). Other indications in dogs include treatment of Lyme borreliosis and leptospirosis. Minocycline delivered in a subgingival local delivery system improved the clinical and microbiologic response in dogs with periodontitis following root scaling and planing (Hayashi et al., 1998). Doxycycline administered orally for 3 weeks achieved complete remission of about half of canine patients with superficial pyoderma and partial remission in another 40%, but complete remission in only 14% of patients with deep pyoderma and partial remission in another 51% (Bettenay et al., 1998).

Cats suffering from chlamydial infection of the upper respiratory tract and conjunctiva should be treated with tetracyclines for 14 days to eliminate the organism and to remove the latent carrier state. Tetracyclines are drugs of choice for the treatment of *Haemobartonella felis*. Prolonged oral treatment with doxycycline does not eliminate the carrier state in *Bartonella henselae* or *B. clarridgeiae* infection (Kordick et al., 1997). Treatment by tetracyclines of a cat with *Yersinia pestis* infection was only temporarily effective (Culver, 1987).

POULTRY

Tetracyclines are effective in the treatment of chlamydiosis if administered for prolonged periods. Tetracycline or chlortetracycline can be administered in 1% medicated feed (45 days), and doxycycline has been administered at 100 mg/kg IM at 5-day intervals on 6 or 7 occasions (Gylsdorff, 1987) or orally twice daily for 20 days. Tetracyclines are also used in the treatment of chronic respiratory disease (*Mycoplasma gallisepticum*) and infectious synovitis (*M. synoviae*), as well as of fowl cholera (*Pasteurella multocida*). Prolonged administration of oxytetracycline (250 ppm) in feed is required to control *M. gallisepticum* infection in birds. One report noted the surprising efficacy of tetracycline sorbate in the oral treatment of naturally occurring *Aspergillus fumigatus* infection (Roy et al, 1991).

Bibliography

Anderson WI. 1983. Hemoglobinuria in cattle given long-acting oxytetracycline. Mod Vet Pract 64:997.

Appleyard WT, Gilmour NJL. 1990. Use of long-acting oxytetracycline against pasteurellosis in lambs. Vet Rec 126:231.

Ball HJ, Campbell JN. 1989. Antibiotic treatment of experimental *Mycoplasma californicum* mastitis. Vet Rec 125:377.

Bettenay SV, et al. 1998. Doxycycline hydrochloride in treatment of canine pyoderma. Aust Vet Pract 28:14.

Bousquet E, et al. 1998. Efficacy of doxycycline in feed for the control of pneumonia caused by *Pasteurella multocida* and *Mycoplasma hyopneumoniae* in fattening pigs. Vet Rec 143:269.

Breitschwerdt EB, et al. 1998. Doxycycline hyclate treatment of experimental canine ehrlichiosis followed by challenge inoculation with two *Ehrlichia canis* strains. Antimicrob Agents Chemother 42:362.

Brodie TA, et al. 1986. Some aspects of tick-borne diseases of British sheep. Vet Rec 118:415.

Brodie TA, et al. 1988. Prophylactic use of long-acting tetracycline against tick-borne fever (*Cytoecetes phagocytophilia*) in sheep. Vet Rec 122:43.

Chaslus-Dancla E, et al. 1995. Tetracycline resistance determinants, Tet B and Tet M, detected in *Pasteurella haemolytica* and *Pasteurella multocida* from bovine herds. J Antimicrob Chemother 36:815.

Chumo RS, et al. 1989. Long-acting oxytetracycline prophylaxis to protect susceptible cattle introduced into an area of Kenya with endemic East Coast fever. Vet Rec 124:219.

Cook WR. 1973. Diarrhea in the horse associated with stress and tetracycline therapy. Vet Rec 93:15.

Cranwell MP. 1990. Efficacy of long-acting oxytetracycline for the prevention of tickborne fever in calves. Vet Rec 126:334.

Culver M. 1987. Treatment of bubonic plague in a cat. J Am Vet Med Assoc 191:1528.

Dargatz DA, et al. 1990. Antimicrobial therapy for rams with *Brucella ovis* infection of the urogenital tract. J Am Vet Med Assoc 196:605.

Flores-Castro R, Carmichael LE. 1978. Canine brucellosis: current status of methods for diagnosis and treatment. Gaines Vet Symp 27:17.

Gallo GF, Berg JL. 1995. Efficacy of a feed-additive antibacterial combination for improving feedlot cattle performance and health. Can Vet J 36:223.

George L, et al. 1988. Topically applied furazolidone or parenterally administered oxytetracycline for the treatment of infectious bovine keratoconjunctivitis. J Am Vet Med Assoc 192:1415.

Greig A, Linklater KA. 1985. Field studies on the efficacy of a long-acting preparation of oxytetracycline in controlling outbreaks of enzootic abortion of sheep. Vet Rec 117:627.

Griffin DD, et al. 1979. Experimental oxytetracycline toxicity in feedlot heifers. Bovine Pract 14:37.

Grogono-Thomas R, et al. 1994. The use of long-acting oxytetracycline for the treatment of ovine footrot. Br Vet J 150:561.

Guichon PT, et al. 1993. Comparison of two formulations of oxytetracycline given prophylactically to reduce the incidence of bovine respiratory disease in feedlot calves. Can Vet J 34:736.

Gylsdorff I. 1987. The treatment of chlamydiosis in psittacine birds. Isr J Vet Med 43:11.

Gyrd-Hansen N, et al. 1981. Cardiovascular effects of intravenous administration of tetracycline in cattle. J Vet Pharmacol Ther 6:15.

Hayashi K, et al. 1998. Clinical and microbiological effects of controlled-release local delivery of minocycline on periodontitis in dogs. Am J Vet Res 59:464.

Hosie BD. 1988. Keratoconjunctivitis in a hill sheep flock. Vet Rec 122:40.

Hosie BD, Greig A. 1995. Role of oxytetracycline dihydrate in the treatment of *Mycoplasma*-associated ovine keratoconjunctivitis in lambs. Br Vet J 151:83.

Jordan D, Venning CM. 1995. Treatment of ovine dermatophilosis with long-acting oxytetracycline or a lincomycin-spectinomycin combination. Aust Vet J 72:234.

Kordick DL, et al. 1997. Efficacy of enrofloxacin or doxycycline for treatment of *Bartonella henselae* or *Bartonella clarridgeiae* infection in cats. Antimicrob Agents Chemother 41:2448.

Lairmore MD, et al. 1984. Oxytetracycline-associated nephrotoxicosis in feedlot cattle. J Am Vet Med Assoc 185:793.

Ling GV, et al. 1980. Urine concentrations of chloramphenicol, tetracycline, and sulfisoxazole after oral administration to healthy adult dogs. Am J Vet Res 41:950.

Love RJ, Love DN. 1977. Control of proliferative haemorrhagic enteropathy in pigs. Vet Rec 100:473.

Madigan JE, Gribble D. 1987. Equine ehrlichiosis in northern California: 49 cases (1968–1981). J Am Vet Med Assoc 190:445.

Marin CM, et al. 1989. Efficacy of long-acting oxytetracycline alone or in combination with streptomycin for treatment of *Brucella ovis* infection of rams. Am J Vet Res 50:560.

Martin SW, et al. 1982. Factors associated with mortality and treatment costs in feedlot calves: the Bruce County beef project, years 1978, 1979, 1980. Can J Comp Med 46:341.

Mebus CA, Logan LL. 1988. Heartwater disease of domestic and wild ruminants. J Am Vet Med Assoc 192:950.

Nicoletti P, Chase A. 1987. The use of antibiotics to control canine brucellosis. Compend Contin Educ Pract Vet 9:1063.

Nicoletti P, et al. 1985. Efficacy of long-acting oxytetracycline alone or in combination with streptomycin in the treatment of bovine brucellosis. J Am Vet Med Assoc 187:493.

Nielsen P, Gyrd-Hansen N. 1996. Bioavailability of oxytetracycline, tetracycline, and chlortetracycline after oral administration to fed and fasted pigs. J Vet Pharmacol Ther 19:305.

Nouws JFM. 1984. Irritation, bioavailability, and residue aspects of ten oxytetracycline formulations administered intramuscularly to pigs. Vet Q 6:80.

Nouws JFM. 1986. Factors affecting the oxytetracycline disposition kinetics in ruminants—a review. Ir Vet News (May):9.

Nouws JFM, et al. 1990. A comparative study on irritation and residue aspects of five oxytetracycline formulations administered intramuscularly to calves, pigs and sheep. Vet Q 12:129.

Palmer JE. 1989. Prevention of Potomac horse fever. Cornell Vet 79:20 1.

Potter WL. 1973. Collapse following intravenous injection of oxytetracycline in two horses. Aust Vet J 49:547.

Radwan AI, et al. 1989. Experimental treatment of *Brucella melitensis* infection in sheep with oxytetracycline alone or combined with streptomycin. Trop Anim Health Prod 21:211.

Riond J-L, Riviere JE. 1989. Effects of tetracyclines on the kidney in cattle and dogs. J Am Vet Med Assoc 195:995.

Riond J-L, Riviere JE. 1990. Pharmacokinetics and metabolic inertness of doxycycline in young pigs. Am J Vet Res 51:1271.

Riond J-L, et al. 1990. Comparative pharmacokinetics of doxycycline in cats and dogs. J Vet Pharmacol Ther 13:415.

Roy S, et al. 1991. Use of tetracycline sorbate for the treatment of *Aspergillus fumigatus* infection in broiler chickens. Br Vet J 147:549.

Shaw DH, Rubin SI. 1986. Pharmacologic activity of doxycycline. J Am Vet Med Assoc 189:808.

Shearer JK, Elliott JB. 1998. Papillomatous digital dermatitis: treatment and control strategies—Part I. Compend Cont Educ Pract Vet 20:S158.

Simpson BC, et al. 1987. Protection of cattle against heartwater in Botswana: comparative efficacy of different methods against natural and blood-derived challenges. Vet Rec 120:135.

Stahlheim OHV. 1967. Chemotherapy of renal leptospirosis in swine. Am J Vet Res 28:161.

Stevenson S. 1980. Oxytetracycline nephrotoxicosis in two dogs. J Am Vet Med Assoc 176:530.

Swift BL, Thomas GM. 1983. Bovine anaplasmosis: elimination of the carrier state with injectable long-acting oxytetracycline. J Am Vet Med Assoc 183:63.

Taylor SM, et al. 1986. Inhibition of *Babesia divergens* in cattle by oxytetracycline. Vet Rec 118:98.

Vaala WE, et al. 1987. Acute renal failure associated with administration of excessive amounts of tetracycline in a cow. J Am Vet Med Assoc 191:1601.

Van Donkersgoed J. 1992. Meta-analysis of field trials of antimicrobial mass medication for prophylaxis of bovine respiratory disease in feedlot cattle. Can Vet J 33:786.

Wilson AW, et al. 1979. Chemotherapy of acute bovine anaplasmosis. Aust Vet J 55:71.

Wilson RC, et al. 1985. Compartmental and noncompartmental pharmacokinetic analyses of minocycline hydrochloride in the dog. Am J Vet Res 46:1316.

14 | Sulfonamides, Diaminopyrimidines, and Their Combinations

J. F. PRESCOTT

The value of the sulfonamides as single antimicrobial agents has been greatly diminished by widespread acquired resistance. However, when they are combined with trimethoprim or ormetoprim, resistance occurs less frequently and thus their usefulness has been enhanced.

Sulfonamides

Chemistry

The sulfonamides are derivatives of sulfanilamide, which contains the structural prerequisites for antibacterial activity. The sulfonamides differ in the radical (R) attached to the amido ($—SO_2NHR$) group or occasionally in the substituent on the amino ($—NH_2$) group (Fig. 14.1).

The various derivatives differ in physicochemical and pharmacokinetic properties and in degree of antimicrobial activity. As a group, sulfonamides are quite insoluble; they are more soluble at an alkaline pH than at an acid pH. In a mixture of sulfonamides, each component drug exhibits its own solubility. An example is the trisulfapyrimidine preparation, in which the antibacterial activity of the combined sulfonamides is additive but the agents behave independently with respect to solubility. This mixture was developed to offset the precipitation of sulfonamide crystals in acidic fluid in the distal renal tubules and ureters.

The sodium salts of sulfonamides are readily soluble in water, and parenteral preparations are available for IV injection. These solutions are highly alkaline in reaction, with the notable exception of sodium sulfacetamide, which is nearly neutral and is available as an ophthalmic preparation.

290

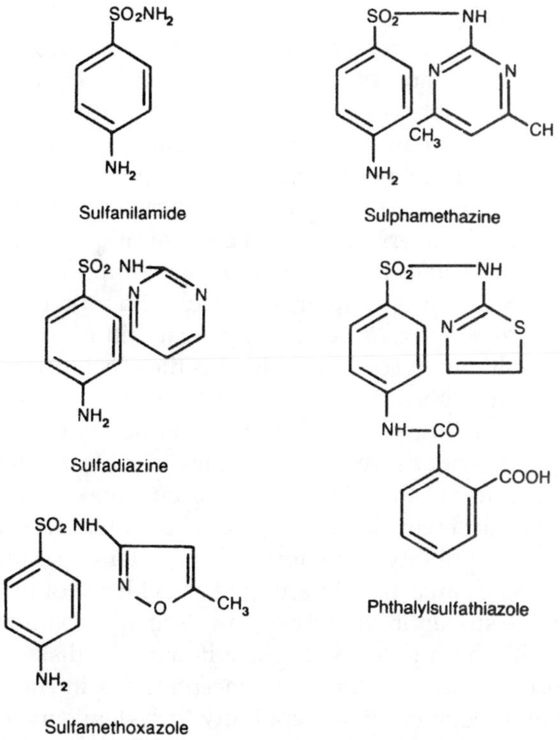

Fig. 14.1. Structural formulas of some sulfonamides.

Certain sulfonamide molecules are designed for low solubility (eg, phthalylsulfathiazole), so they are slowly absorbed and are intended for use in treatment of enteric infections.

Mechanism of Action

Sulfonamides interfere with the biosynthesis of folic acid in bacterial cells by competitively preventing para-aminobenzoic acid (PABA) from incorporation into the folic (pteroylglutamic) acid molecule. Specifically, sulfonamides compete with PABA for the enzyme dihydropteroate synthetase. Their selective bacteriostatic action depends on the difference between bacterial and mammalian cells in the source of folic acid. Susceptible microorganisms must synthesize folic acid, whereas mammalian cells use preformed folic acid. The bacteriostatic action can be reversed by providing an excess of PABA, so that tissue exudates and necrotic tissue should be removed if animals are to be treated with sulfonamides.

Antimicrobial Activity

Sulfonamides are broad-spectrum antimicrobial agents, inhibiting bacteria, toxoplasmas, and other protozoal agents such as coccidia, but their antibacterial activity is significantly limited by the resistance that has developed after more than 50 years of use. Different sulfonamides may show quantitative but not necessarily qualitative differences in activity.

The MIC of sulfonamides is markedly affected by the composition of the medium and the bacterial inoculum concentration. Because of this, in vitro tests may sometimes falsely report a bacterium to be resistant. This will not be the case if proper quality control with a thymidine-sensitive strain of *Enterococcus faecalis* is used. In agar diffusion tests, Mueller-Hinton agar containing lysed horse blood is the ideal medium because it contains thymidine phosphorylase, which decreases the quantity of thymidine in the medium. The criteria of susceptibility for bacteria in systemic infections are not agreed upon because of difficulties in determining MIC and because of the variability in serum concentrations with different drugs and different doses. An MIC of 8–32 µg/ml is a reasonable definition of susceptibility for short-acting systemic sulfonamides; an MIC of ≥ 64–128 µg/ml can be interpreted as evidence of resistance.

Sulfonamide susceptibility testing in veterinary laboratories is sometimes done with high-potency triple-sulfonamide disks, designed to determine susceptibility to the high concentrations in the urinary tract (100 µg/ml); extrapolation of susceptibility to systemic infections is thus not appropriate. The National Committee for Clinical Laboratory Standards (NCCLS) criteria describes susceptibility in bacteria for urinary tract infections as those having an MIC of ≤256 µg/ml.

Good Susceptibility: Bacillus spp., *Brucella* spp., *Erysipelothrix rhusiopathiae, Listeria monocytogenes, Nocardia* spp., pyogenic *Streptococcus* spp., *Chlamydia* spp., coccidia, *Pneumocystis carinii,* and *Cryptosporidium* spp.

Moderate Susceptibility, often variable because of acquired resistance (Table 14.1). Includes among Gram-positive aerobes: staphylococci and some enterococci. Gram-negative aerobes: Enterobacteriaceae, including *Enterobacter* spp., *Escherichia coli, Klebsiella* spp., and *Proteus* spp.; *Actinobacillus* spp.; *Haemophilus* spp.; *Pasteurella* spp.; and *Pseudomonas* spp. Anaerobes such as *Bacteroides* spp. and *Fusobacterium* spp. are often susceptible in vitro if the medium is depleted of thymidine; this is not the case in vivo. *Clostridium* spp. (other than *C. perfringens*) and anaerobic cocci are often resistant.

Resistant: Mycobacterium spp., *Mycoplasma* spp., *Rickettsia* spp., *Pseudomonas aeruginosa,* and spirochetes are resistant.

TABLE 14.1.   Activity (MIC$_{90}$, µg/ml) of sulfonamides, trimethoprim, and trimethoprim-sulfamethoxazole against selected bacteria

Organism	Sulfonamide MIC$_{90}$[a]	Trimethoprim MIC$_{90}$	Trimethoprim-sulfamethoxazole MIC$_{90}$[b]
Gram-positive aerobes			
Arcanobacterium pyogenes	32	8	0.13
Corynebacterium pseudotuberculosis			≤0.5
C. renale	>64		
Erysipelothrix rhusiopathiae	8	0.13	0.06
Listeria monocytogenes	8	0.06	0.03
Nocardia asteroides	128	128	8
Rhodococcus equi	>128	64	32
Staphylococcus aureus	32	2	0.25
Streptococcus agalactiae	32	0.5	0.06
S. dysgalactiae	>256	4	0.06
S. uberis	>128	4	0.5
Beta-hemolytic streptococci	>128	2	2
Gram-positive anaerobes			
Clostridium perfringens	16	64	
Gram-negative aerobes			
Actinobacillus spp.	64		≤0.06
A. pleuropneumoniae[c]	≥128	2	8
Bordetella bronchiseptica[c]	>256		≤0.06
Brucella abortus	16	4	0.06
B. canis	2		
Campylobacter jejuni	≥256	≥512	≥512
Escherichia coli[c]	≥128	1	≤0.5
Haemophilus somnus	≥128		
Klebsiella pneumoniae[c]	≥128	4	≤0.5
Moraxella bovis	>64	>64	>0.15
Pasteurella multocida	>128	4	
Proteus spp.	>256	8	≤0.5
Pseudomonas aeruginosa	>515	512	128
Salmonella spp.	128	4	0.5
Taylorella equigenitalis	>128		
Yersinia enterocolitica	>128	1	8

[a]Mainly sulfadimethoxine.

[b]Single figures refer to trimethoprim concentration; trimethoprim-sulfamethoxazole ratio is 1:19.

[c]Many of these isolates are now reported as resistant to the combination. This table is partly designed to illustrate the synergism that can occur between sulfonamides and trimethoprim.

Resistance

Chromosomal mutation to resistance develops slowly and gradually and results from impairment of drug penetration, production of an insensitive dihydropteroate enzyme, or hyperproduction of PABA. Plasmid-mediated resistance is far more common and is the result of impaired drug penetration or the production of additional sulfonamide-resistant dihydropteroate synthetase enzymes. Resistance to sulfonamides is widespread in bacteria isolated from animals, reflecting extensive use of the drug over many years. There is complete cross-resistance between the sulfonamides.

Pharmacokinetic Properties

The sulfonamides constitute a series of weak organic acids with pK_a values ranging from 10.4 for sulfanilamides to 5.0 for sulfisoxazole. They exist predominantly in the nonionized form in biologic fluids of pH lower than their pK_a. It is the nonionized moiety that diffuses through cell membranes and penetrates cellular barriers.

Most sulfonamides are rapidly absorbed from the gastrointestinal tract and distributed widely to all tissues and body fluids, including synovial and cerebrospinal fluids. The sulfonamides are bound to plasma proteins to an extent varying from 15% to 90%. In addition, there is variation among species in binding of individual sulfonamides. Extensive (>80%) protein binding increases half-life. In any one species, the extent of protein binding, apparent volume of distribution, and half-life vary widely among individual sulfonamides. This information, together with designating 100 µg/ml as the desired steady-state plasma sulfonamide concentration, facilitates calculation of dosages.

Sulfonamides are eliminated by a combination of renal excretion and biotransformation. This combination contributes to species variations in the half-lives of individual drugs. Sulfadimethoxine, for example, has a half-life of 12.5 hours in cattle, 8.6 hours in goats, 11.3 hours in horses, 15.5 hours in swine, 13.2 hours in dogs, and 10.2 hours in cats. These relatively long half-lives have been attributed to extensive binding to plasma albumin and to pH-dependent passive reabsorption of the drug from acidic distal renal tubule fluid.

Sulfonamides undergo metabolic alterations to a variable extent in the tissues, especially the liver. Acetylation (which is the principal metabolic pathway for most sulfonamides), glucuronide conjugation, and aromatic hydroxylation take place in humans and in all domestic animals except dogs. It appears that dogs cannot acetylate aromatic amines. Acetylation takes place in the reticuloendothelial rather than the parenchymal cells of the liver and other tissues such as the lungs. This metabolic reaction has clinical significance, since the acetyl derivative of most sulfonamides (except sulfapyrimidines) has lower aqueous solubility than the parent compound. Acetylation therefore increases the risk of damage to the renal tubules due to precipitation. Aromatic hydroxylation, which may be the principal metabolic pathway for sulfonamides in ruminants, and glucuronide conjugation are microsomal-mediated metabolic reactions. The glucuronide conjugates are highly water soluble and are rapidly excreted.

Renal excretion mechanisms include glomerular filtration of free (unbound) drug in the plasma, active carrier-mediated proximal tubular excretion of ionized unchanged drug and metabolites, and passive reabsorption of nonionized drug from distal tubular fluid. The extent of reabsorption is determined by the pK_a of the sulfonamide and the pH of the fluid in the distal tubules. Urinary alkalinization increases both the fraction of the dose that is eliminated by renal excretion (unchanged in urine) and the solubility of sulfonamides in the urine.

Drug Interactions

The important synergistic interaction of sulfonamides with diaminopyrimidines such as trimethoprim and baquiloprim is discussed under Antibacterial Diaminopyrimidines, below.

The agents appear not to antagonize the bactericidal effect of penicillins, but the procaine of procaine penicillin is an analog of PABA that will antagonize sulfonamides. Combination with pyrimethamine is the treatment of choice for toxoplasmosis and some other protozoal infections.

Toxicity and Adverse Effects

The sulfonamides can produce a wide variety of usually reversible side effects, some of which may have an allergic basis and others due to direct toxicity. The more common adverse effects are urinary tract disturbances (crystalluria, hematuria, or even obstruction), hematopoietic disorders (thrombocytopenia, anemia, leukopenia), and dermatologic reactions. Significant reactions, however, are generally uncommon in animals treated with conventional doses of common sulfonamides (other than sulfaquinoxaline) for less than 2 weeks.

In a small proportion of humans or animals, sulfonamide therapy can produce idiosyncratic drug reactions, which are unpredictable, rare events dependent on the individual response to the drug (Cribb, 1989). These reactions are sometimes described as hypersensitivity reactions (drug fever, urticaria), since they seem to involve immune reactions but may involve a limited capacity to detoxify metabolites of sulfonamides (Cribb and Spielberg, 1990). Idiosyncratic reactions recur if individuals are retreated with sulfonamides. In dogs, serious but reversible sulfadiazine-induced reactions have been described in a number of reports on Doberman pinschers. Nonseptic polyarthritis (with or without glomerulonephropathy), focal retinitis, polymyositis, skin rash, and other manifestations occurred 10 days to 3 weeks after first exposure to trimethoprim-sulfadiazine (Giger et al., 1985; Cribb, 1989).

Idiosyncratic reactions are not restricted to Doberman pinschers, in which sulfonamides should probably be avoided. Adverse reactions occurred in 0.25% of a large number of dogs and cats treated with trimethoprim-sulfonamide combinations. These included stiff gait, polyarthritis, lameness, epistaxis, ulcerative exudative dermatitis, epidermal sloughing, and the development of skin pustules, crusts, scaling, and erosions (Noli et al., 1995).

Some adverse effects are associated with particular sulfonamides. Sulfadiazine and sulfasalazine given for long periods to dogs as a "geriatric stimulant" have caused keratoconjunctivitis sicca (KCS), which was not always fully reversible when the drug was discontinued (Morgan and Bachrach, 1982; Sansom et al., 1985). However, in one study KC—determined by decreased tear production—occurred in 15% of 33 dogs treated with trimethoprim-sulfadiazine combination, within the first week of treatment (Berger et al., 1995). This effect occurred in dogs weighing less than 12 kg, suggesting that dosage must be particularly carefully calculated for small dogs.

Renal tubular damage can be minimized by ensuring that the patient is well hydrated throughout the course of treatment, by administering the most soluble sulfonamides, and by alkalinizing the urine. Prolonged dosage with sulfaethoxypiridine in dogs has produced cataracts. Sulfaquinoxaline has caused hypothrombinemia, hemorrhage, and death in puppies given the drug orally for control of coccidiosis; hemorrhagic diathesis was reported in other species because of the antagonistic effect of this drug on vitamin K.

Rare additional adverse effects reported include hepatic necrosis leading to death or euthanasia, developing in some cases within days of treatment (Twedt et al., 1997), and hypothyroidism associated with prolonged treatment (Hall et al., 1993; Torres et al., 1996). An unusual goitrogenic effect in swine, which increased the number of stillborn or weak piglets born to sows fed sulfadimethoxine and ormetoprim in late gestation, was described by Blackwell et al. (1989).

Administration and Dosage

In treating systemic diseases with sulfonamides, it is desirable to initiate therapy with a priming dose and to administer maintenance doses, each one-half the priming dose, at intervals approximately equal to the half-life of the drug (Table 14.2). When the drug is administered orally, the dose level must compensate for incomplete systemic availability from the oral preparation, that is percent bioavailability of oral preparations.

Although a large number of sulfonamide preparations are available for use in veterinary medicine, many of them are different-dosage forms of sulfamethazine. This sulfonamide is most widely used in food-producing animals and can attain effective plasma concentrations when administered either orally or parenterally. Because of their alkalinity, most parenteral preparations should be administered only by IV injection;

TABLE 14.2. **Examples of usual dosages of sulfonamides in animals**

Drug	Route	Dose (mg/kg)	Dosing Interval (h)	Comments
Short-acting sulfadiazine, sulfamethazine, trisulfapyrimidine (triple sulfas)	IV, PO	50–60	12	Double first dose
Sulfamethoxazole	PO	50	12	Double first dose
Intermediate-acting sulfadimethoxine	PO, IV, IM, SC	27.5	24	Double first dose
(sustained release, cattle)	PO	137.5	96	dose
sulfadiazine	PO, IV	50	12	Double first dose
Sulfisoxazole	PO	50	8	Urinary tract infections
Gut-active phthalylsulfathiazole	PO	100	12	
Special-use salicylazosulfapyridine	PO	25	12	See text
silver sulfadiazine	Topical			

rapid IV injection of high doses of sulfonamide preparations should be avoided. Sulfamethazine therapy should be initiated with an IV priming dose of 100 mg/kg, and effective concentrations can then be maintained by administering maintenance doses of 50 mg/kg PO at 12-hour intervals. At least one prolonged-release oral preparation of sulfamethazine is available for use in calves and could be administered to sheep and goats. This is a convenient form of maintenance therapy in that a single dose provides an effective level for 36–48 hours. Different oral forms have different systemic availability (see Table 4.3).

Sulfadimethoxine preparations are more widely used in companion animals. The parenteral preparation (40%), containing sulfadimethoxine sodium in solution, is suitable for IV administration to horses. Having initiated therapy with a priming dose of 50 mg/kg, effective concentrations can be maintained with maintenance dosage of 25 mg/kg administered IV at 12-hour intervals. In dogs and cats, sulfadimethoxine can be administered either as the parenteral solution IV or as the oral suspension. Therapy should be initiated with a priming dose (55 mg/kg, IV), and therapeutic concentrations can be maintained either by administering maintenance doses IV (27.5 mg/kg) or PO (55 mg/kg) at preferably 12-hour or 24-hour intervals. Selection of the dosing interval should be based on quantitative susceptibility of the pathogenic microorganisms and the site of infection.

Sulfisoxazole has higher aqueous solubility than most other members of the class. Its solubility in urine increases markedly with increase in urinary pH. It has a half-life in dogs of 4.5 hours, and because it is eliminated largely by renal excretion, sulfisoxazole is present in high concentrations unchanged in the urine. This makes sulfisoxazole an effective agent in the treatment of urinary tract infections caused by susceptible organisms. The usual oral dosage is 50 mg/kg administered at 8-hour intervals.

Unlike the sodium salts of other sulfonamides, sodium sulfacetamide is nearly neutral. It is the only sulfonamide available for topical ophthalmic use. When a 30% solution is applied to the conjunctivae, it penetrates well and attains high concentrations in ocular fluids and tissues.

Clinical Applications

Widespread resistance greatly limits the effectiveness of sulfonamides in treating bacterial diseases of animals. Trimethoprim-sulfonamide or other antibacterial diaminopyrimidine-sulfonamide combinations have largely replaced sulfonamides as therapeutic agents used in companion animals. Purulent material must always be removed, since the presence of free purines neutralizes the effect of sulfonamides. Primary uses include treatment of toxoplasmosis (when combined with pyrimethamine), chlamydiosis, *Pneumocystis carinii*, and possibly nocardiosis (combined with minocycline) and the use of sulfasalazine in the treatment of chronic colitis.

CATTLE, SHEEP, AND GOATS

Widespread resistance limits the use of sulfonamides in cattle, sheep, and goats, and it is best to give these agents in combination with trimethoprim. Orally administered, long-acting, sustained-release dosage forms result in effective plasma concentrations for 3–5 days. Such a preparation was useful experimentally in preventing *Pasteurella haemolytica* pneumonia in calves (Janzen et al., 1984) and was effective in clinical trials assessing prevention and treatment of feedlot pneumonia (Hjerpe and Routen, 1976), an unexpected result in view of the resistance reported in bovine *Pasteurella*. Sulfonamides are used successfully to treat bovine interdigital necrobacillosis and coccidiosis. Sulfadimethoxine is the only sulfonamide approved for use in dairy cows over 20 months of age in the United States; extralabel use in dairy cows is prohibited.

Sustained-release oral sulfamethazine and orally administered pyrimethamine, 0.5 mg/kg once daily, might be drugs of choice in preventing outbreaks of *Toxoplasma* abortion in sheep. Sulfonamides have been used with chlortetracyclines in feedlot lambs to improve performance and prevent clostridial enterotoxemias.

SWINE

Sulfonamides have been used to promote growth and to control group E streptococcal infections and atrophic rhinitis in swine. The sulfonamides are often combined with chlortetracycline. In the United States, there have been moves to ban the use of sulfonamides for use in swine because of persistent problems of residues in carcasses in excess of legally permitted concentrations and evidence from chronic toxicity studies in mice that sulfamethazine was linked to the production of thyroid adenomas in rodents. The story of control of sulfonamide residues in swine in the United States is reviewed in Chapter 33.

HORSES

Sulfonamides are only used in horses in combination with trimethoprim.

DOGS AND CATS

Use of sulfisoxazole to treat urinary tract infections in dogs has been largely replaced by antibiotics that are more effective because of their broader spectrum of activity or bactericidal action. Sulfonamides are one of the drugs of choice in the treatment of *Nocardia* infections; effectiveness may be increased by concurrent administration with minocycline (see Chapter 19). Silver sulfadiazine cream has been used as a treatment in chronic otitis externa caused by multiresistant *Pseudomonas aeruginosa*, because the drug acts as a broad-spectrum antimicrobial antiseptic. This preparation has been effective in controlling bacteria that infect burn wounds in human patients.

Sulfasalazine (salicylazosulfapyridine) has been recommended as a drug of choice in the treatment of chronic colitis in dogs (Burrows, 1983). It is hydrolyzed by colonic bacteria to yield sulfapyridine and 5-aminosalicylate; it is likely that the anti-inflammatory effect of the latter is responsible for the therapeutic effect. Comparably high concentrations of salicylate cannot be achieved in the colon by oral administration. The dosage of sulfasalazine for the dog is 25 mg/kg PO 3 times daily. The same dose in cats may induce salicylate poisoning (Burrows, 1983). Some have suggested that a low dose of corticosteroid be administered simultaneously to reduce the overall duration of therapy, which is 3–4 weeks when the drug is administered alone. This dual dosage may decrease the frequency of keratoconjunctivitis sicca. In most cases of sulfasalazine treatment, cure is achieved within 4 weeks, and treatment should not be continued beyond this time without histologic confirmation of colonic inflammation.

Dapsone (diaminodiphenylsulfone) has been used in the treatment of dermatitis herpetiformis in dogs and in the treatment of leprosy in humans.

POULTRY

Sulfonamides have been used in poultry in the prevention and treatment of coccidiosis, infectious coryza, pullorum disease, and fowl typhoid.

Bibliography

Berger SL, et al. 1995. A quantitative study of the effects of Tribrissen on canine tear production. J Am Anim Hosp Assoc 31:236.

Bevill RF. 1989. Sulfonamide residues in domestic animals. J Vet Pharmacol Ther 12:241.

Blackwell TE, et al. 1989. Goitrogenic effects in offspring of swine fed sulfadimethoxine and ormetoprim in late gestation. J Am Vet Med Assoc 194:519.

Burrows CE. 1983. The treatment of diarrhea. In: Kirk RW, ed. Current Veterinary Therapy VIII: Small Animal Practice. Philadelphia: WB Saunders.

Cribb AE. 1989. Idiosyncratic reactions to sulfonamides in dogs. J Am Vet Med Assoc 195:1612.

Cribb AE, Spielberg SP. 1990. An in vitro investigation of predisposition to sulphonamide idiosyncratic toxicity in dogs. Vet Res Comm 14:241.

Giger U, et al. 1985. Sulfadiazine-induced allergy in six Doberman pinschers. J Am Vet Med Assoc 186:479.

Hall IA, et al. 1993. Effect of trimethoprim/sulfamethoxazole on thyroid function in dogs with pyoderma. J Am Vet Med Assoc 202:1959.

Hjerpe CA, Routen TA. 1976. Practical and theoretical considerations concerning treatment of bacterial pneumonia in feedlot cattle, with special reference to antimicrobial therapy. Proc Am Assoc Bovine Pract, p97.

Janzen ED, et al. 1984. Therapeutic and prophylactic effects of some antibiotics on experimental pneumonic pasteurellosis. Can Vet J 25:78.

Miller GE, et al. 1969. Blood concentration studies of a sustained release form of sulfamethazine in cattle. J Am Vet Med Assoc 154:773.

Morgan RV, Bachrach A. 1982. Keratoconjunctivitis sicca associated with sulfonamide therapy in dogs. J Am Vet Med Assoc 180:432.

Noli C, et al. 1995. A retrospective evaluation of adverse reactions to trimethoprim-sulphonamide combinations in dogs and cats. Vet Q 17:123.

Sansom J, et al. 1985. Keratoconjunctivitis sicca in the dog associated with the administration of salicylazosulphapyridine (sulphasalazine). Vet Rec 116:391.

Torres SMF, et al. 1996. Hypothyroidism in a dog associated with trimethoprim-sulphadiazine therapy. Vet Dermatol 7:105.

Twedt DC, et al. 1997. Association of hepatic necrosis with trimethoprim-sulfonamide administration in 4 dogs. J Vet Intern Med 11:20.

Weiss DJ, Klansner JS. 1990. Drug-associated aplastic anemia in dogs: eight cases (1984–1988). J Am Vet Med Assoc 196:472.

Wilson RC, et al. 1989. Bioavailability and pharmacokinetics of sulfamethazine in the pony. J Vet Pharmacol Ther 12:99.

Antibacterial Diaminopyrimidines: Aditoprim, Baquiloprim, Ormetoprim, and Trimethoprim

Diaminopyrimidines interfere with folic acid production by inhibition of dihydrofolate reductase. Some diaminopyrimidines have marked specificity for bacterial dihydrofolate reductases (aditoprim, baquiloprim, ormetoprim, trimethoprim), others for protozoal enzymes (pyrimethamine), and others for mammalian enzymes (methyltrexate). The earliest

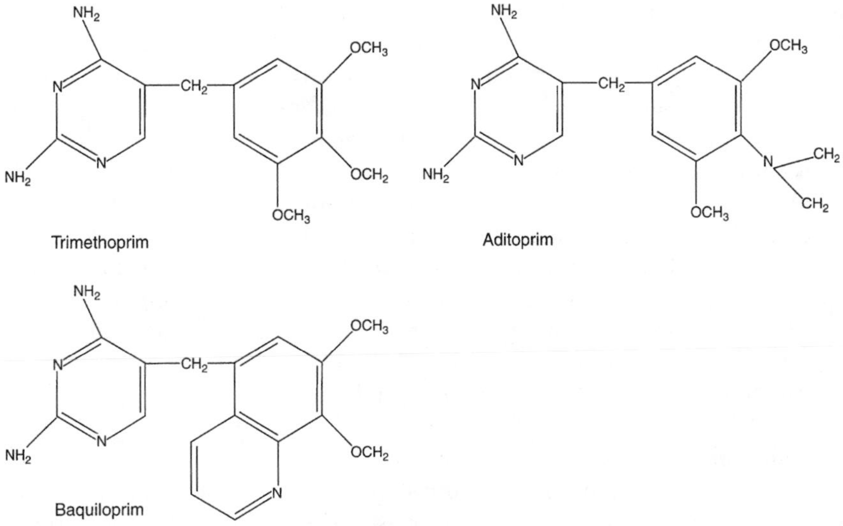

Fig. 14.2. Structural formulas of some diaminopyrimidines.

antibacterial diaminopyrimidine introduced for clinical use was trimethoprim (Fig. 14.2), a synthetic drug that is widely used in combination with sulfonamides. It is a weak base with a pK_a of about 7.6 and is poorly soluble in water. Other antibacterial diaminopyrimidines have antibacterial activities similar to those of trimethoprim but offer significant pharmacokinetic advantages, particularly those of greater half-lives and tissue distribution.

Mechanism of Action

Diaminopyrimidines interfere with the synthesis of tetrahydrofolic acid from dihydrofolate by combining with the enzyme dihydrofolate reductase. Selective antibacterial activity occurs because of greater affinity for the bacterial rather than the mammalian enzyme. Diaminopyrimidines thus inhibit the same metabolic sequence as the sulfonamides, preventing bacterial synthesis of purines and thus of DNA. A synergistic and bactericidal effect occurs when the diaminopyrimidines are combined with sulfonamides (see Antibacterial Diaminopyrimidine-Sulfonamide Combinations, below), and for this reason these drugs are invariably used with a sulfonamide in veterinary medicine.

Interestingly, in the United Kingdom trimethoprim alone rather than the combination is now generally used in human medicine (Hughes, 1997). The reasons for the abandoned use of trimethoprim-sulfonamide combination in favor of trimethoprim alone are (1) bacteriostatic synergy is only demonstrable when the concentration of each drug is less than bacteriostatic, but the bacteriostatic effect of trimethoprim in urinary tract infections, for which the drug is most commonly used, is often detectable in urine for several days; (2) diaminopyrimidines are more widely distributed into tissues than sulfonamides, reaching sites, such as cells, that sulfonamides do not penetrate well; (3) most of the adverse effects of the combination are the result of the sulfonamide component; and (4) the original claim that the combination prevented the emergence of resistance is regarded as dubious, because sulfonamide resistance is widespread and because plasmids conferring resistance to sulfonamides often also confer resistance to trimethoprim (Hughes, 1997). The licensed medical use in the United Kingdom of the combination is therefore restricted largely to the treatment of *Pneumocystis carinii* infection.

Antimicrobial Activity

Antibacterial diaminopyrimidines are generally bacteriostatic, broad-spectrum drugs active against Gram-positive and Gram-negative aerobic bacteria, but not usually against anaerobes (see Table 14.1). Bacteria with MIC ≤1 μg/ml are usually regarded as susceptible. Activity against *Mycoplasma* spp., *Chlamydia* spp., *Mycobacterium* spp., and *Pseudomonas aeruginosa* is negligible. Activity of aditoprim, baquiloprim, and ormetoprim is similar to or very slightly less than that of trimethoprim.

Resistance

Resistance to trimethoprim and other diaminopyrimidines is usually the result of transposon-encoded plasmid or chromosomal synthesis of a resistant dihydrofolate reductase enzyme (Huovinen et al., 1995). Resistance is increasingly reported, particularly among Enterobacteriaceae. Isolates with plasmid-mediated resistance commonly show multiple resistance, which includes sulfonamide resistance. The apparent spread of a trimethoprim resistance gene from porcine to human *E. coli* has been described (Jansson et al., 1992).

Pharmacokinetic Properties

Diaminopyrimidines, including trimethoprim, are lipid-soluble organic bases that are approximately 60% bound to plasma proteins. The drugs distribute widely, penetrating cellular barriers by nonionic diffusion and attaining effective concentrations in most body tissues and fluids. The drug may concentrate in fluids, such as the prostate, that are acidic relative to plasma. The average milk-to-plasma equilibrium concentration ratio is 3:1. The dose, systemic availability from the dosage form, and route of administration determine the plasma concentration profile and tissue levels of the drug. Hepatic metabolism (oxidation followed by conjugation reactions) is the principal process for elimination. Because of this, the half-life and fraction of the dose that is excreted unchanged in the urine vary widely among species (see Table 4.2). In ruminants, the short half-life of trimethoprim is due to rapid demethylation to produce inactive compounds. Replacing the phenyl ring of trimethoprim with the bicyclic ring of baquiloprim resulted in an increase in half-life from 1 hour (trimethoprim) to 10 hours (baquiloprim) in cattle (White el., 1993) and from about 2 to 5 hours in pigs, while replacement of a methyl group in trimethoprim by the dimethylamino group of aditoprim increased its half-life in cattle to 4–7 hours, in horses to 9–14 hours, and in pigs to 8–9 hours, or greater. Greater tissue distribution may be one factor responsible for prolonged half-life relative to that of trimethoprim.

Toxicity and Adverse Effects

The antibacterial diaminopyrimidines are relatively nontoxic drugs. Their main, though clinically unimportant, potential toxic effect, is to induce folic acid deficiency at high doses. Rarely, aseptic meningitis related to trimethoprim therapy has been reported in humans (Carlson and Wiholm, 1987). Hyperkalemia may occur under unusual circumstances (Rubin et al., 1998).

Clinical Applications

Antibacterial diaminopyrimidines are currently used only in combination with sulfonamides in animals, although there may be a need to reassess the benefits of the combination. Alone or in combination they may be a drug of choice for treating prostatic infections caused by Gram-negative bacteria, since prostatic concentrations may reach 10 times those of plasma, at which concentration the drug may be bactericidal. Nevertheless, clinical results in treating chronic prostatitis with trimethoprim may be disappointing, probably because of the nature of the disease process. Trimethoprim administered orally has been used to prevent relapse after treatment of *Listeria monocytogenes* meningitis in humans (Gunther and Philipson, 1988). Antibacterial diaminopyrimidines, including trimethoprim, combined with sulfonamides or dapsone may be the prophylactic drugs of choice for *Pneumocystis carinii* pneumonia (Hughes, 1988).

Bibliography

Brown MP, et al. 1989. Pharmacokinetics and body fluid and endometrial concentrations of ormetoprim-sulfadimethoxine in mares. Can J Vet Res 53:12.
Carlson J, Wiholm B-E. 1987. Trimethoprim associated septic meningitis. Scand J Infect Dis 19:687.
Davies AM, MacKenzie NM. 1994. Pharmacokinetics of baquiloprim and sulphadimidine in pigs after intramuscular injection. Res Vet Sci 57:69.

Gunther G, Philipson A. 1988. Oral trimethoprim as follow-up treatment of meningitis caused by *Listeria monocytogenes*. Rev Infect Dis 10:53.

Hughes DTD. 1997. Diaminopyrimidines. In: O'Grady F, et al., eds. Antibiotic and Chemotherapy. New York: Churchill Livingstone.

Hughes WT. 1988. Comparison of dosages, intervals, and drugs in the prevention of *Pneumocystis carinii* pneumonia. Antimicrob Agents Chemother 32:623.

Huovinen P, et al. 1995. Trimethoprim and sulfonamide resistance. Antimicrob Agents Chemother 39:279.

Jansson C, et al. 1992. Spread of a newly found trimethoprim resistance gene, *dhfrIX*, among porcine isolates and human pathogens. Antimicrob Agents Chemother 36:2704.

Knoppert NW, et al. 1988. Some pharmacokinetic data of aditoprim and trimethoprim in healthy and tick-borne fever infected dwarf goats. J Vet Pharmacol Ther 11:135.

Lohuis ACM, et al. 1992. Effects of endotoxin-induced mastitis on the pharmacokinetic properties of aditoprim in dairy cows. Am J Vet Res 53:2311.

Mengelers MJB, et al. 1990. In vitro susceptibility of some porcine respiratory tract pathogens to aditoprim, trimethoprim, sulfadimethoxine, sulfamethoxazole, and combinations of these agents. Am J Vet Res 51:1860.

Riond J-L, et al. 1992. The influence of age on the pharmacokinetics of aditoprim in pigs after intravenous and oral administration. Vet Res Comm 16:355.

Rubin SI, et al. 1998. Trimethoprim-induced exacerbation of hyperkalaemia in a dog with hypoadrenocorticism. J Vet Intern Med 12:186.

Van Miert ASJPAM. 1994. The sulfonamide-diaminopyrimidine story. J Vet Pharmacol Ther 17:309.

Von Fellenberg R-L, et al. 1990. Plasma disposition and tolerance of aditoprim in horses after single intravenous injection. J Vet Med 37A:253.

West B, White G. 1979. A survey of trimethoprim resistance in the enteric bacterial flora of farm animals. J Hyg 82:481.

White G, et al. 1993. Baquiloprim: a new antifolate antibacterial: in vitro activity and pharmacokinetic properties in cattle. Res Vet Sci 54:372.

Wilson WD, et al. 1987. Ormetoprim-sulfadimethoxine in cattle: pharmacokinetics, bioavailability, distribution to the tears, and in vitro activity against *Moraxella bovis*. Am J Vet Res 48:407.

Antibacterial Diaminopyrimidine-Sulfonamide Combinations

Antibacterial diaminopyrimidines are combined with a variety of sulfonamides (sulfadiazine, sulfamethoxazole, and sulfadoxine) in a fixed (1:5) ratio, which in people produces a 1:20 ratio of drug concentrations in the plasma after oral or parenteral administration. This ratio is desirable since maximum synergy occurs when the drugs are present in the ratio of their MICs; diaminopyridines are 20–100 times more active than the sulfonamides, so that combinations are formulated to give a 1:20 ratio in human serum. This ratio occurs because diaminopyrimidines (lipid-soluble organic bases) are concentrated in tissues, whereas sulfonamides (weak organic acids) remain largely in extracellular fluids. At these MICs and in this ratio, the combination produces a bactericidal effect against a wide range of bacteria, with some important exceptions, and also inhibits certain other microorganisms. Since the combinations of different diaminopyridines, with sulfonamides, give essentially similar antibacterial effects, comments will relate largely to trimethoprim-sulfonamide combinations but can be extrapolated to other combinations.

Veterinary preparations follow medical usage in that they contain diaminopyridines combined with a sulfonamide in the 1:5 ratio. For trimethoprim, the half-lives of the components (sulfadiazine, sulfadoxine, or sulfamethoxazole) do not coincide in any species (except humans), whereas they are more similar for baquiloprim (sulfadimidine, sulfadimethoxine) and ormetoprim (sulfadimethoxine). The dosage aims at maintaining bacteriostatic concentrations of the sulfonamide, which, for a time after each dose, is enhanced by the synergistic bactericidal action of the combination.

Mechanism of Action

The combination of a diaminopyrimidine with a sulfonamide inhibits sequential steps in the synthesis of folic acid and thus of the purines required for DNA synthesis. The interference by the diaminopyrimidine methoprim with recycling of tetrahydrofolic or dihydrofolic acid is probably responsible for the synergistic interaction of the combination.

Antimicrobial Activity

Diaminopyrimidine-sulfonamide combinations have a generally broad and usually bactericidal action against many Gram-positive and Gram-negative aerobic bacteria, including Enterobacteriaceae, *Actinomyces*, *Nocardia*, chlamydia, and protozoa such as *Toxoplasma*. They are not active against anaerobic bacteria in vivo, since thymidine and PABA in the necrotic tissue antagonize their antibacterial effect (Indiveri and Hirsh, 1992). *Pneumocystis carinii* and some malarial parasites are susceptible; mycoplasma and *Pseudomonas aeruginosa* are resistant.

Synergism occurs when the microorganisms are susceptible to both drugs in the combination. Synergism may still be obtained, in up to 40% of cases, when bacteria are resistant to sulfonamides. Synergy often occurs if the organism is resistant to trimethoprim but sensitive to sulfonamides and in nearly 40% of cases in which the organism is resistant to each drug alone. Nevertheless, many organisms described as susceptible to the combination are susceptible to the diaminopyrimidine component only. Clinical response may sometimes be lower than expected from in vitro data, and better understanding of the use of MIC data in prediction of clinical outcome is required. One element of such disappointing responses may also be the presence of thymidine and PABA in infected tissue. Nevertheless, a more important element may be widespread resistance to sulfonamides and consequently the lack of synergism in many cases, so that only the diaminopyrimidine component is active. For trimethoprim, the short half-life in some species may exacerbate a lack of synergism.

Where synergistic interactions occur, a 10-fold increase in activity of the trimethoprim component and a 100-fold increase in activity of the sulfonamide component are common. Synergism occurs at different drug concentration ratios with different bacterial species. Because of differences between the diaminopyrimidine and sulfonamide in distribution and in the case of trimethoprim of elimination, the concentration ratios may differ considerably in tissues and urine from that in plasma. Such variation is said not to be important, because the synergistic interaction may occur over a wide range of concentration ratios of the drugs, but clearly it would not occur in some tissues, since diaminopyrimidines are distributed more widely than sulfonamides. Because of these variations in the pharmacokinetics of diaminopyrimidines and sulfonamides, the length of effective action is difficult to assess based on serum concentrations alone. This gives rise to the suspicion that the manufacturer's recommended dosages may be less than optimal, especially for trimethoprim combinations. Appropriately designed clinical trials could resolve this issue.

Errors in laboratory testing are common because of the presence of PABA or thymidine in media; in one study, half the strains reported as resistant in other laboratories were susceptible when tested in a reference laboratory (West and White, 1979). The use of lysed horse blood, which contains thymidine phosphorylase, will eliminate excess thymidine in the medium.

Good Susceptibility (MIC ≤0.5/9.5 μg/ml) is shown among the following Gram-positive aerobes: *Staphylococcus aureus*, streptococci, *Actinomyces* spp., *Corynebacterium* spp., *Erysipelothrix rhusiopathiae, Listeria monocytogenes*. Gram-negative aerobes: *Actinobacillus* spp.; *Bordetella* spp.; *Brucella* spp.; Enterobacteriaceae such as *Escherichia coli, Klebsiella* spp., *Proteus* spp., *Salmonella* spp., and *Yersinia* spp.; *Haemophilus* spp., and *Pasteurella* spp. Anaerobes: *Actinomyces* spp., *Bacteroides* spp., *Fusobacterium* spp., some *Clostridium* spp., and *Chlamydia* spp.

Moderate Activity (MIC 2/38 μg/ml) includes some *Mycobacterium* spp. and some *Nocardia* spp.

Resistance (MIC ≥4/72 μg/ml) is shown by rickettsias, *Leptospira* spp., *Pseudomonas aeruginosa*, and *Mycoplasma* spp. (see Table 14.1).

Resistance

Mechanisms of resistance were discussed under the individual components of the combination. Resistance to the combination has developed progressively with use. Multiply resistant R factors, which include both sulfonamide and trimethoprim resistance, have been described in *Salmonella typhimurium* and enterotoxigenic *E. coli* isolated from animals.

Pharmacokinetic Properties

In humans the half-lives of trimethoprim and sulfamethoxazole are similar, and maintenance dosage provides continuous, therapeutic concentrations of both drugs in plasma. In animals the half-lives of the drugs are not similar, but the combination is often clinically effective because of the relatively broad range of drug ratio over which synergism occurs. For reasons discussed earlier, the diaminopyrimidine component is concentrated in tissues, whereas the sulfonamide component moves only slowly from plasma into tissues. The longer half-lives of newer diaminopyrimidines (baquiloprim, ormetoprim) give the advantages of better maintenance of the 1:20 ratio said to be desirable, and of less frequent dosing.

Following SC injection in cattle, trimethoprim seems to deposit in a slow-release form, so that serum concentrations remain below MIC (Shoaf et al., 1987). Because of this, the SC route cannot be recommended in cattle and perhaps in other species.

Drug Interactions

Trimethoprim-sulfonamide is sometimes used in conjunction with ampicillin to provide "broad-spectrum bactericidal antimicrobial coverage" before microbiology data are available. However, one study showed that addition of ampicillin to trimethoprim-sulfonamide dosing regimens only marginally increased the spectrum of activity (Hirsh et al., 1990). There is no known mechanism to suggest that such a combination might be synergistic. Rather, such a combination may be effective in treating polymicrobial infections involving aerobic bacteria susceptible to the trimethoprim-sulfonamide combination and anaerobic bacteria susceptible to ampicillin.

Toxicity and Adverse Effects

The combination has a wide margin of safety, and adverse effects can mainly be attributed to the sulfonamide. These effects are discussed in the general description of the adverse effects of each drug class.

In horses, minor tissue damage and pain may occur after IM injection; transient pruritus has been reported to follow the first but not subsequent doses. In isolated incidents a fatal adverse reaction (possibly respiratory failure) followed IV injection of the combination preparation in horses, in some cases in anesthetized horses. A 7% incidence of diarrhea was observed in a study of the effect of twice-daily administration of oral 30 mg/kg trimethoprim-sulfadiazine in horses (Ensink et al., 1996). The prevalence of diarrhea noted following trimethoprim-sulfonamide use in

TABLE 14.3.   Usual dosages of potentiated sulfonamide combinations in animals

Drug (species)	Route	Dose (mg/kg)	Dosing Interval (h)	Comments
Trimethoprim-sulfonamide	PO, IV, IM	(15–)30	12(–24)	Not IM in horses
Ormetoprim-sulfadimethoxine	PO	27.5	24	Double first dose
Baquiloprim-sulfadimethoxine				
Dogs	PO	30	48	
Cats	PO	30	24	
Cattle, swine	IM	10	24	

horses in another study was not significantly different from that observed in horses receiving other antibiotics, including penicillin (Wilson et al., 1996).

Administration and Dosage

Usual dosages are shown in Table 14.3. Dogs and cats can be given the oral form (tablets) at the same dosage. Twice-daily oral dosing of horses with 30 mg/kg trimethoprim-sulfadiazine combination paste rather than once daily was recommended (Bertone et al., 1988). Other studies support the use of twice-daily dosage with trimethoprim-sulfonamide preparations rather than the once-daily administration recommended by the manufacturers, possibly also at higher doses than recommended by the manufacturer (Brown et al., 1988). Oral dosage with ormetoprim-sulfadimethoxine paste in mares recommended for susceptible organisms was a loading dose of 9.2 mg ormetoprim and 45.8 mg sulfadimethoxine/kg followed by half this dose every 24 hours (Brown et al., 1989).

Clinical Applications

Diaminopyrimidine-sulfonamide combinations have the advantages of good distribution into tissues, safety, a relatively broad-spectrum bactericidal activity, and oral administration.

The combination can be recommended in the treatment of urinary tract infections caused by common opportunist pathogens. The combination has a particular place in the treatment of bacterial prostatitis because of good tissue penetration. Other indications include the treatment of enteric infections (*E. coli, Salmonella, Yersinia enterocolitica*). The drug is of value in the treatment of brucellosis, often in combination with rifampin or doxycycline. The combination is a drug of choice in the treatment of *Nocardia* infections, but high oral dosage (3 mg trimethoprim equivalent/kg every 6 hours) must be used for prolonged periods.

Other indications include the treatment of *Pneumocystis carinii* infections, *Chlamydia* infections, certain mycobacterial infections (*Mycobac-*

terium kansasii, M. marinum), and of *Coxiella* infections. The drug is also used in the treatment of acute upper and lower respiratory tract infections caused by susceptible organisms, as well as of infections in other sites.

More clinical trials are needed to establish the optimal dosage of the orally administered combination of trimethoprim-sulfadiazine for different infections in animals, since manufacturers' recommendations may be low.

CATTLE, SHEEP, AND GOATS

Diaminopyrimidine-sulfonamide combinations are widely used in dairy and beef cattle and have been used successfully in the treatment of salmonellosis in calves, as well as in undifferentiated diarrhea, in bacterial pneumonia, in foot rot, and in septicemic colibacillosis. Baquiloprim-sulfadimidine was not as efficacious as danofloxacin in the treatment of experimentally induced *E. coli* diarrhea in calves (White et al., 1998), presumably because the organism is less susceptible to the combination drug. The potential for use in coliform septicemia and meningitis seems excellent but may be limited by resistance. In meningitis the drug should be administered IV 3 or 4 times daily at the usual dosage. The potential for use in the treatment of *Listeria* meningoencephalitis appears excellent. The susceptibility of *Haemophilus somnus*, *Pasteurella multocida*, some *P. haemolytica*, and of *Arcanobacterium pyogenes* suggests a useful application in bovine respiratory disease that has been borne out by field studies (Harland et al., 1991). The drug combination should be administered parenterally (not orally). Clinical trials with undifferentiated bovine respiratory disease have failed to demonstrate improvement when dosage of trimethoprim-sulfadoxine was increased beyond that recommended or when the product was administered IV rather than IM, although pharmacokinetic studies suggested that manufacturer's once-daily recommended dosage of 16 mg/kg is too low (Conlon et al., 1993; but see Dunkley, 1994).

When used to treat acute mastitis, the drug should be given IV at high dose because of poor bioavailability after IM injection and relatively poor udder penetration; a dosage of 48–50 mg/kg every 12 hours is appropriate for acute mastitis. A beneficial effect of trimethoprim-sulfonamide in the treatment of coliform mastitis has been noted (Shpigel et al., 1998).

Other uses in cattle include the treatment of urinary tract infections and mixed aerobe-anaerobe infections such as those occurring in postparturient metritis. The drug has potential but unproven use for the treatment of *L. monocytogenes* encephalitis in ruminants.

A special application in sheep is in preventing *Toxoplasma* abortion; the drug is also potentially useful in preventing chlamydial abortion. In experimental *Toxoplasma* infections in mice, protection by trimethoprim-sulfonamide was inferior to pyrimethamine-sulfadiazine, but clinical results in naturally occurring infections in humans have been excellent (Salter, 1982).

SWINE

Trimethoprim-sulfonamide combinations have been used successfully in controlling a wide variety of conditions in pigs, including neonatal and postweaning colibacillosis, salmonellosis, atrophic rhinitis, greasy pig disease, streptococcal meningitis, and pneumonia. Atrophic rhinitis may be controlled by incorporating the drug in feed or water or by injecting piglets at various times such as the third day of life and again in the third and sixth weeks. The mastitis-metritis-agalactia syndrome has been controlled by the prophylactic administration of 15 mg/kg PO for 3 days before and 2 days after parturition. Guise et al. (1986) showed that feed medication with 500 ppm did not reduce the frequency of *Streptococcus suis* meningitis. The combination has been used in the eradication of *Actinobacillus pleuropneumoniae* infection from herds by treating adults through the water for 3 weeks in combination with removal of serologically positive animals. Other diaminopyrimidine-sulfonamide combinations are available for swine for purposes similar to those for which trimethoprim-sulfonamide combinations are used (see Table 14.3).

HORSES

The combination of trimethoprim-sulfadiazine is popular in horses because it can be administered as an oral antibiotic with few adverse effects; it is painful when administered IM. It is, therefore, used orally to treat acute respiratory infections (including strangles), acute urinary tract infections, and wounds and abscesses and is a drug of choice in salmonellosis. In foals the combination is used in the treatment of *Actinobacillus* and coliform infections, although the latter use may be compromised by resistance. The drug may be used for coliform meningitis, in which high doses should be administered slowly IV 3 or 4 times daily. The drug may otherwise be administered orally, but oral dosage recommended by the manufacturers may be low and there is apparent advantage to twice-daily dosage (30 mg/kg) of oral preparations (Van Duijkeren et al., 1994a). The combination is a drug of choice in the treatment of protozoal encephalomyelitis (Boy et al., 1990), in which it may be combined with pyrimethamine (see Antiprotozoal Diaminopyrimidines, below). It is a drug of choice for *Pneumocystis carinii* infections in foals (Ewing et al., 1994). Direct infusion of the combination into the uterus may cause endometrial inflammation.

DOGS AND CATS

Trimethoprim-sulfonamide or ormetoprim-sulfadimethoxine combinations have wide application in dogs and cats against specific and nonspecific infections. The combination is highly effective against many opportunist bacteria present in canine urinary tract, skin, and ear infections (*Staphylococcus intermedius*, streptococci, and Enterobacteriaceae, including *E. coli* and *Proteus*) (Wilcke, 1988). The drug has the potential for use in prophylaxis of urinary tract infections.

Consideration should be given to twice-daily dosing with trimethoprim-sulfadiazine. A blinded comparison of once-daily versus twice-daily dosing with 30 mg/kg trimethoprim-sulfadiazine in the treatment of canine pyoderma showed an advantage of twice-daily dosing; however, this was not statistically significant, possibly because of small numbers of animals in the trial (Messinger and Beale, 1993). In one study, however, mean serum and skin concentrations using once-daily dosing were considered to achieve therapeutically effective concentrations (Pohlenz-Zertuche et al., 1992).

The combination drug is effective against *Bordetella bronchiseptica*, although relapses after treatment with trimethoprim-sulfadiazine for 5 days were common in experimental kennel cough (McCandlish and Thompson, 1979). The drug has been used successfully in the treatment of canine actinomycosis, often in conjunction with procaine penicillin; the combination may be particularly useful where *Nocardia* and *Actinomyces viscosus* have not been distinguished properly. The combination has been effective in treating coccidiosis in dogs and cats.

The excellent penetration into the prostate makes the combination a treatment of choice in Gram-negative prostatic infections in dogs, equal to or better than minocycline, although now challenged by the fluoroquinolones. Similarly, the excellent penetration (50% of serum concentrations) of the aqueous and vitreous humors of the eyes by both drugs makes the combination suitable in the parenteral treatment of panophthalmitis caused by Gram-negative bacteria.

POULTRY

Trimethoprim-sulfaquinoxaline and sulfamethoxazole-ormetoprim are used in the prophylaxis and treatment of *E. coli*, *Haemophilus*, and *Pasteurella* infections, as well as of coccidiosis.

Bibliography

Bertone AL, et al. 1988. Serum and synovial fluid steady-state concentrations of trimethoprim and sulfadiazine in horses with experimentally induced arthritis. Am J Vet Res 49:1681.

Boy MG, et al. 1990. Protozoal encephalomyelitis in horses: 82 cases (1976–1986). J Am Vet Med Assoc 196:632.

Brown MP, et al. 1988. Pharmacokinetics and body fluid and endometrial concentrations of trimethoprim-sulphamethoxazole in mares. Am J Vet Res 49:918.

Brown MP, et al. 1989. Pharmacokinetics and body fluid and endometrial concentrations of ormetoprim-sulfadimethoxine in mares. Can J Vet Res 53:12.

Conlon PD, et al. 1993. Evaluation of route and frequency of administration of three antimicrobial drugs in cattle. Can Vet J 34:606.

Dunkley MJ. 1994. The use of trimethoprim and sulphadoxine in cattle. Can Vet J 35:71.

Ensink JM, et al. 1996. Side effects of oral antimicrobial agents in the horse: a comparison of pivampicillin and trimethoprim/sulphadiazine. Vet Rec 138:253.

Ewing PJ, et al. 1994. *Pneumocystis carinii* pneumonia in foals. J Am Vet Med Assoc 204:929.

Guise HJ, et al. 1986. Streptococcal meningitis in pigs: field trial to study the prophylactic effect of trimethoprim/sulphadiazine medication in feed. Vet Rec 119:395.

Harland RJ, et al. 1991. Efficacy of parenteral antibiotics for disease prophylaxis in feedlot calves. Can Vet J 32:163.

Hirsh DC, et al. 1990. Lack of supportive susceptibility data for use of ampicillin together with trimethoprim-sulfonamide as broad-spectrum antimicrobial treatment of bacterial disease in dogs. J Am Vet Med Assoc 197:594.

Hughes WT. 1988. Comparison of dosages, intervals, and drugs in the prevention of *Pneumocystis carinii* pneumonia. Antimicrob Agents Chemother 32:623.

Indiveri MC, Hirsh DC. 1992. Tissues and exudates contain sufficient thymidine for the growth of anaerobic bacteria in the presence of inhibitory levels of trimethoprim-sulfamethoxazole. Vet Microbiol 32:235.

McCandlish IA, Thompson H. 1979. Canine bordetellosis: chemotherapy using a sulfadiazine-trimethoprim combination. Vet Rec 104:51.

Messinger LM, Beale KM. 1993. A blinded comparison of the efficacy of daily and twice daily trimethoprim-sulfadiazine and daily sulfadimethoxine-ormetoprim therapy in the treatment of canine pyoderma. Vet Dermatol 4:13.

Pohlenz-Zertuche HO, et al. 1992. Serum and skin concentrations after multiple-dose oral administration of trimethoprim-sulfadiazine in dogs. Am J Vet Res 53:1273.

Salter AJ. 1982. Trimethoprim-sulfamethoxazole: an assessment of more than 12 years of use. Rev Infect Dis 4:196.

Scott DW, et al. 1993. The combination of ormetoprim and sulfadimethoxine in the treatment of pyoderma due to *Staphylococcus intermedius* infection in dogs. Canine Pract 18(2):29.

Shoaf SE, et al. 1987. The effect of age and diet on sulfadiazine/trimethoprim disposition following oral and subcutaneous administration to calves. J Vet Pharmacol Ther 10:331.

Shpigel NY, et al. 1998. Relationship between in vitro sensitivity of coliform pathogens in the udder and the outcome of treatment for clinical mastitis. Vet Rec 142:135.

Spitzer PG, et al. 1986. Treatment of *Listeria monocytogenes* infection with trimethoprim-sulfamethoxazole: case report and review of the literature. Rev Infect Dis 8:427.

Van Duijkeren E, et al. 1994a. A comparative study of the pharmacokinetics of intravenous and oral trimethoprim/sulfadiazine formulations in the horse. J Vet Pharmacol Ther 17:440.

Van Duijkeren E, et al. 1994b. Trimethoprim/sulfonamide combinations in the horse: a review. J Vet Pharmacol Ther 17:64.

Van Duijkeren E, et al. 1995. Pharmacokinetics and therapeutic potential for repeated oral doses of trimethoprim/sulphachlorpyridazine in horses. Vet Rec 137:483.

West B, White G. 1979. A survey of trimethoprim resistance in the enteric bacterial flora of farm animals. J Hyg 82:481.

White DG, et al. 1998. Comparison of danofloxacin with baquiloprim/sulphadimidine for the treatment of experimentally induced *Escherichia coli* diarrhoea in calves. Vet Rec 143:273.

White G, et al. 1981. Use of a calf salmonellosis model to evaluate the therapeutic properties of trimethoprim and sulfadiazine and their mutual potentiation in vivo. Res Vet Sci 31:27.

Wilcke JR. 1988. Therapeutic application of sulfadiazine/trimethoprim in dogs and cats: a review. Companion Anim Pract 2(9):3.

Wilson WD, et al. 1996. Case control and historical cohort study of diarrhea associated with administration of trimethoprim-potentiated sulfonamides to horses and ponies. J Vet Intern Med 10:258.

Antiprotozoal Diaminopyrimidines

Some diaminopyrimidines such as pyrimethamine have high activity against protozoa by inhibiting dihydrofolate reductase and thus preventing purine synthesis. These drugs are used in the treatment of systemic protozoal infections such as toxoplasmosis, neosporosis, and equine protozoal myelitis.

Pyrimethamine and sulfadiazine are the most effective drugs in the treatment of toxoplasmosis in humans and are generally preferred over alternatives such as azithromycin and trimethoprim-sulfamethoxazole. The adult human dosage is 75 mg pyrimethamine and 4 g sulfadiazine PO/day in 4 divided doses, administered for up to 4 weeks. Dapsone combined with pyrimethamine has good activity experimentally against *Toxoplasma* (Derouin et al., 1991).

Pyrimethamine combined with trimethoprim-sulfadiazine or with an oral sulfonamide alone (12–24 mg/kg q12 hours) has become the standard treatment for equine protozoal myeloencephalitis (EPM). Current maintenance dosage is 1 mg/kg daily given orally with trimethoprim-sulfadiazine or trimethoprim-sulfamethoxazole (20 mg/kg daily) for a minimum of 4 months (Fenger, 1998). The trimethoprim component is unnecessary. Anti-inflammatory drugs may also be administered. A small proportion of horses may develop anemia during treatment. Such animals can be treated with folic acid (40 mg daily). Alternate drugs for the treatment of EPM are required, since pyrimethamine is teratogenic for animals and may lead to myeloid, erythroid, or lymphoid hypoplasia with epithelial dysplasia and renal hypoplasia or nephrosis in newborn foals. Such effects may be exacerbated by administering folic acid to mares being treated for EPM (Toribio et al., 1998).

Pyrimethamine and diaveridine are commonly combined with sulfaquinoxaline for their synergistic effect against coccidia. Pyrimethamine (1 mg/kg daily) combined with a sulfadoxine (20 mg/kg daily) or trimethoprim-sulfadiazine has been used successfully in the treatment of *Neospora caninum* infection in dogs (Ruehlmann et al., 1995; Thate and Laanen, 1998).

Bibliography

Boy MG, et al. 1990. Protozoal encephalomyelitis in horses: 82 cases (1976–1986). J Am Vet Med Assoc 196:632.

Clarke CR, et al. 1992. Pharmacokinetics, penetration into cerebrospinal fluid, and hematologic effects after multiple oral administrations of pyrimethamine to horses. Am J Vet Res 53:2296.

Derouin F, et al. 1991. Anti-*Toxoplasma* effects of dapsone alone and combined with pyrimethamine. Antimicrob Agents Chemother 35:252.

Fenger CK. 1998. Treatment of equine protozoal myeloencephalitis. Compend Cont Educ Pract Vet 21:1154.

Ruehlmann D, et al. 1995. Canine neosporosis: a case report and literature review. J Am Anim Hosp Assoc 31:174.

Thate FM, Laanen SC. 1998. Successful treatment of neosporosis in an adult dog. Vet Q 20:S113.

Toribio RE, et al. 1998. Congenital defects in newborn foals of mares treated for equine protozoal myeloencephalitis during pregnancy. J Am Vet Med Assoc 212:697.

15 | Fluoroquinolones

R. D. WALKER

The introduction of fluoroquinolones into clinical medicine, approximately 14 years ago, ushered in an important era in the evolution of antimicrobial agents. These compounds were regarded as almost the "ideal" antimicrobial agents because of their broad spectrum of activity, clinically advantageous pharmacokinetic properties, and low toxicity, which represents a considerable advance over other classes of antimicrobial agents (Dalhoff and Bergan, 1998; Segev and Rubinstein, 1998). Chemically, they are totally synthetic, and a large number of analogs and derivatives have been synthesized from the basic 4-quinolone nucleus (Grohe, 1998). Microbiologically, although they were initially primarily active against aerobic Gram-negative bacteria, chemical modifications have increased their spectrum to include Gram-positive bacteria and atypical bacteria, including mycobacteria, and mycoplasmas. Some of the newer compounds now in use in human medicine exhibit good activity against anaerobic bacteria (Goldstein et al., 1998). The fluoroquinolones are well absorbed following oral administration, have a large volume of distribution, penetrate nearly every tissue and cell in the body, and have extended elimination half-lives, allowing for q12- or q24-hour dosing. At appropriate concentration:MIC ratios, the fluoroquinolones are rapidly bactericidal, exhibit concentration-dependent killing, and may exhibit a prolonged in vivo post-antibiotic effect (PAE) on certain bacteria. The potential for fairly rapid selection of resistance in some pathogens is, however, a disadvantage of this class of drugs but can be minimized by appropriate dose selection.

Because the fluoroquinolones are relatively new antimicrobial agents, extensive research is needed to identify factors that will contribute

315

TABLE 15.1. **Fluoroquinolones used in veterinary medicine**

Fluoroquinolone	Species
Enrofloxacin	Dogs, cats, chickens, turkeys, beef cattle, horses, pigs
Orbifloxacin	Dogs, cats
Difloxacin	Dogs, chickens, turkeys
Danofloxacin	Cattle, pigs
Marbofloxacin	Dogs, cats, pigs, cattle
Sarafloxacin	Chickens, turkeys

Note: These drugs are marketed for veterinary medicine use only.

to maximizing their clinical efficacy for use in animals. Considerable information relating to their optimal use is available from human medicine. This knowledge can be applied in veterinary medicine to develop and implement appropriate dosing regimens that can reduce the selection for resistant bacterial pathogens, thus ensuring the continued future of this powerful class of antimicrobial agents.

This chapter reviews chemical, microbiological, pharmacokinetic, pharmacodynamic, and clinical aspects of the fluoroquinolone antibacterial agents, with specific attention to those agents approved for use in animals (Table 15.1).

Chemistry

The fluoroquinolones, like sulfonamide and nitrofurans, are totally synthetic compounds (Grohe, 1998). The first clinically approved 4-quinolone–type compound was nalidixic acid (a naphthyridone molecule with a nitrogen atom at position 8 instead of a carbon atom), marketed in 1965. Since its discovery in 1962, more than 10,000 compounds have been designed from the parent bicyclic 4-quinolone molecule (Fig. 15.1). Clinically, nalidixic acid had several limitations, including a narrow spectrum of activity, poor pharmacokinetic properties, toxic effects, and a tendency to select for resistant organisms. Replacing the hydrogen atom at position 6 of the 4-quinolone molecule with a fluorine atom resulted in increased activity against both Gram-positive and Gram-negative bacteria. The increased activity is attributed, in part, to increased penetration of the bacterial cell membrane (Petersen and Schenke, 1998). Substituting a piperazinyl ring for the methyl group at position 7 increased Gram-negative activity, including antipseudomonal activity. These modifications led to the development of the first broad-spectrum fluoroquinolone, norfloxacin, marketed in 1986. Additional studies demonstrated that substantial changes in potency could be obtained by variations at the N-1 and C-7 positions. For example, ciprofloxacin is similar in structure to norfloxacin but has a cyclopropyl group in place of the ethyl group at N-1. This substitution enhances its Gram-positive and

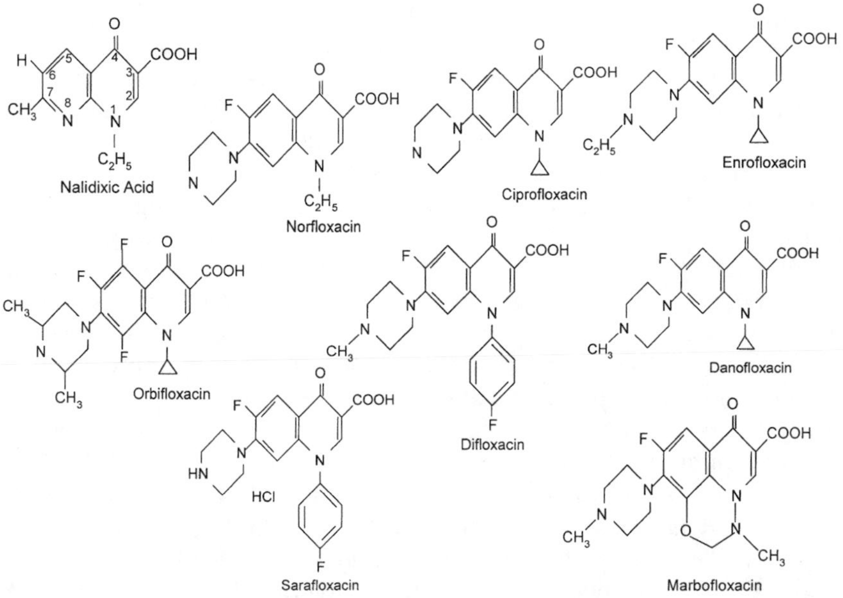

Fig. 15.1. Structural formulas of fluoroquinolones used in veterinary medicine.

Gram-negative activity. Difloxacin has a phenyl ring at position N-1 that reportedly gives it enhanced activity against Gram-positive bacteria, relative to enrofloxacin activity. Difloxacin has a second fluorine atom in its structure, whereas orbifloxacin has a total of three fluorine atoms. These additional fluorine atoms do not appear to influence the antibacterial activity of these compounds. Overall, there have been several chemical modifications at each of the 8 positions in the 4-quinolone molecule. Some have been found to increase absorption, some have increased antibacterial activity, and others have increased toxicity. For example, ciprofloxacin and enrofloxacin are similar molecules except for the ethyl group on the piperazinyl ring of enrofloxacin. This group enhances the absorption of enrofloxacin over ciprofloxacin but decreases its antipseudomonal activity (Walker et al., 1990, 1992). In addition to enrofloxacin, five other fluoroquinolones (sarafloxacin, orbifloxacin, difloxacin, danofloxacin, and marbofloxacin) have been marketed exclusively for use in veterinary medicine. These fluoroquinolones and their clinical uses in veterinary medicine are listed in Table 15.1.

Mechanism of Action

The bacterial chromosome is a continuous, circular, double-stranded DNA molecule approximately 1,000 times longer than the bacteria in which it is contained. In order for such a long molecule to fit into the cell, it is densely packed in a negative supercoil, twisted in the opposite direction to the right-handed double helix of DNA. This supercoiled configuration is so highly strained that, to improve function, the chromosome is divided into approximately 50 topologically independent domains. Topoisomerase enzymes catalyze changes in coiling of the molecule. Topoisomerase I is characterized by reactions involving single-stranded DNA, whereas topoisomerase II is involved in reactions with double-stranded DNA. Topoisomerase II, also known as DNA gyrase, consists of two subunits, GyrA and GyrB. The *gyr*A gene encodes two α-subunits while the *gyr*B gene encodes two β-subunits; the active DNA gyrase is an A_2B_2 complex. DNA gyrase binds to DNA; a segment of approximately 130 nucleotides wraps around the DNA gyrase. This wrapped DNA is cleaved in both strands, forming a DNA-protein covalent bond between the GyrA subunit and the 5′-phosphates of the DNA molecule. Another segment of DNA is passed through this double-stranded break, which may then be resealed. The α-subunit of the DNA gyrase has been shown to be important in the breakage and reunion that allow for this relaxation of the DNA molecule. The 4-quinolone molecule interrupts the DNA breakage-reunion step by binding to the DNA gyrase–DNA complex. Magnesium concentrations affect the binding of fluoroquinolones to the gyrase-DNA complex.

Recent data suggest that fluoroquinolones have a second intracellular target, DNA topoisomerase IV (Topo IV) (Kato et al., 1990, 1992). This is a bacterial type II DNA topoisomerase that is also composed of two subunits. However, unlike the DNA gyrase, Topo IV cannot supercoil DNA. Instead it is involved in the ATP-dependent relaxation of DNA. It is a more potent decantenase than DNA gyrase (Hoshino et al., 1994). Topo IV may be the primary target of fluoroquinolones in *Staphylococcus aureus* and streptococci (Ferrero et al., 1994; Kaatz and Seo, 1998), suggesting that the primary target of fluoroquinolones could vary in different bacteria. However, the role of Topo IV as a target for fluoroquinolones has not been clearly defined and is an important area for continued research, including drug development.

Antimicrobial Activity

The fluoroquinolones have excellent activity in vitro against a wide range of aerobic Gram-negative bacteria, including the Enterobacteriaceae, *Actinobacillus pleuropneumoniae, Haemophilus somnus, Mannheimia (Pasteurella) haemolytica,* and *Pasteurella multocida.* They are also active against *Bordetella bronchiseptica, Brucella* spp., *Chlamydia* spp., *Mycoplasma* spp., and *Ureaplasma.* Activity against *Pseudomonas aeruginosa* is dependent on the fluoroquinolone, with ciprofloxacin being the most potent agent against this bacterium. For the most part, the older fluoroquinolones are less active against Gram-positive bacteria, especially enterococci, and have poor activity against anaerobic bacteria. Newer fluoroquinolones are addressing this deficiency. Trovafloxacin is a new-generation agent that is highly active against Gram-positive bacteria and against anaerobes, while maintaining a Gram-negative aerobe spectrum similar to that of ciprofloxacin (Goldstein et al., 1998).

The in vitro activities of fluoroquinolones used in veterinary medicine are listed in Table 15.2. Because the susceptibility of some bacterial isolates of animal origin to the fluoroquinolones decreases over time (see Table 2.2) (Walker and Thornsberry, 1998), the values listed in Table 15.2 need to be evaluated in relation to the date of isolation of the organisms.

The antibacterial activity of the fluoroquinolones is dependent on the drug concentration and the MIC of the bacterium, but it appears to be relatively independent of the concentration of organisms, or inoculum effect. Only minor differences in the MIC are observed when the bacterial concentration increases from 10^3 to 10^7 colony-forming units/ml for most organisms (Fernandez-Guerrero et al., 1987). *Pseudomonas* and enterococci may be notable exceptions. Fluoroquinolones exhibit a biphasic dose response curve, since they are less active at concentrations below or much higher than the MIC (Brown, 1996).

Fluoroquinolones exhibit concentration-dependent killing. As the ratio of fluoroquinolone concentration to MIC increases from 1:1 to the optimal bactericidal concentration (usually shown to be approximately 10:1 but may be drug-bacterium dependent), bacterial killing increases and is usually very rapid (Maxwell and Critchlow, 1998; Preston et al., 1998). As illustrated in Figure 15.2, when a strain of *M. (Pasteurella) haemolytica* is exposed to a fluoroquinolone at concentrations that are 25% of its MIC, the drug exhibits a slight stationary effect, but then the bacterium resumes growth at a rate similar to that of the untreated control. As the concentration of the drug is increased above the MIC, there is a decrease in the number of viable organisms. For drug concentrations that are 1–4 times the MIC, this decrease in viable organisms continues for at least the first 6 hours of exposure. However, by 24 hours of continuous exposure, the number of viable organisms has increased to the point that the total number of viable organisms is equal to or exceeds the number present in the suspensions after a 2-hour exposure to the drug. At drug concentrations that are 8 times the MIC, there is a rapid bactericidal effect. After a 24-hour exposure there was no detectable regrowth of the bacterium, suggesting that there was a 100% cidal effect. The concentration-dependent killing effect may plateau off when the ratio of fluoroquinolone concentration to MIC reaches 15:1 to 20:1 and at ratios greater than 20:1 the fluoroquinolones may become bacteriostatic (Schentag and Scully, 1999). Others, however, have not observed this paradoxical (Eagle)

TABLE 15.2. Microbiological activity (MIC$_{90}$, µg/ml) of the fluoroquinolones to common bacterial pathogens isolated from animals

Organism	Enrofloxacin[a]		Orbifloxacin[b]		Difloxacin[c]		Ciprofloxacin[d]		Sarafloxacin[e]		Marbofloxacin[f]		Danofloxacin[g,h]	
	MIC$_{90}$ Range	No. Isolates	MIC$_{90}$ Range	No. Isolates	MIC$_{90}$ Range	No. Isolates	MIC$_{90}$ Range	No. Isolates	MIC$_{90}$ Range	No. Isolates	MIC$_{90}$ Range	No. Isolates	MIC$_{90}$ Range	No. Isolates
Staphylococcus intermedius	0.12–0.5	349	0.5	81	1.0	164	0.25	64			0.25	160	0.12	25
S. aureus	0.12–0.25	202	0.5[i]	15			0.5	50					0.12–0.25	88
Streptococcus canis			1.0–2.0	36										
Enterococcus spp.	1.0–2.0	59	16–32	35			1.0	20					1.0	20
Arcanobacterium pyogenes	0.5	104											4.0	36
Escherichia coli	0.03–0.125	529	0.5	78	0.25	78	≤0.015–0.06	95	0.06	499			≤0.015–0.25	350
Klebsiella pneumoniae	0.06–0.12	104	0.25[i]	12	0.5	20	0.06	37	0.06	52			0.06	20
Proteus spp.	0.12–0.5	147	1.0–2.0	24	1.0	38	0.03–0.06	58	0.25	89			0.12	20
Pasteurella multocida	≤0.016–0.125	434	0.06	52					0.03	133			0.06–0.12	266
Pseudomonas aeruginosa	1.0–8.0	246	8–16[i]	17	4.0	24	0.12	50	0.5–≥0.5	177				

Organism	MIC90 range	n	MIC90	n	MIC90	n	MIC90 range	n
Mannheimia (Pasteurella) haemolytica	0.03–0.06	283	≤0.015	26	0.03	38	≤0.015–0.12	169
Haemophilus somnus	0.03–0.06	223	0.03	26			0.06–0.12	91
Salmonella spp.	0.06–0.125	276	≤0.015	82	0.06	194	0.03–0.5	317
Actinobacillus pleuropneumoniae	0.06	108					0.12	127
Bordetella bronchiseptica	0.5–1.0	127					2.0	41

[a] *Sources:* Richez et al. (1994); Walker and Thornsberry (1998); Stegemann et al. (1996); Ewert (1997); Watts et al. (1997); Walker (1998–99), unpubl. data.
[b] *Source:* Technical monograph, values adjusted to NCCLS dilution schemes.
[c] *Source:* Package insert, values adjusted to NCCLS dilution schemes.
[d] *Sources:* Walker et al. (1990) and Watts et al. (1997), adjusted to NCCLS dilution values.
[e] *Sources:* Package insert, values adjusted to NCCLS dilution schemes; Walker (1998–1999), unpubl. data from numerous animal species.
[f] *Source:* Stegemann et al. (1996).
[g] *Source:* Watts et al. (1997).
[h] *Source:* Technical monograph.
[i] MIC90 is presented for all organisms where more than 20 isolates were tested. MIC90 range is presented if the data were generated from more than one study and each study presented a different MIC90.

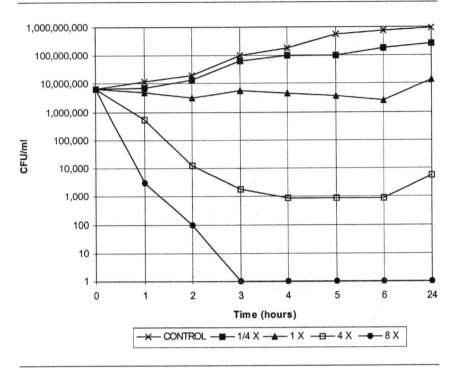

Fig. 15.2. Concentration-dependent killing effect of a fluoroquinolone tested against *Mannheimia (Pasteurella) haemolytica.*

effect, even at concentrations 200 times the MIC (Gould et al., 1990). The decrease in antibacterial activity at high drug concentrations is thought to be caused by inhibition of protein or RNA synthesis, resulting in a bacteriostatic effect (Smith and Zeiler, 1998).

Fluoroquinolones are thought to possess three mechanisms of bacterial killing: mechanism A, common to all fluoroquinolones, requires RNA and protein synthesis and is effective only against bacteria involved in cell division; mechanism B can act on cells that are not actively dividing and does not require RNA or protein synthesis; and mechanism C requires RNA or protein synthesis but not cell division (Howard et al., 1993). The clinical importance of these different killing mechanisms is being explored in new drug development.

Bacterial Resistance

Resistance to the fluoroquinolone can occur by three mechanisms. These mechanisms, in increasing importance are (1) decreased permeability of the bacterial cell wall caused by alterations of the hydrophilic pores (outer membrane proteins); (2) an efflux pump, which actively transports the fluoroquinolone molecule out of the cell as it approaches or passes through the bacterial membrane; and (3) mutation of the DNA gyrase, or topoisomerase IV, thus altering the 4-quinolone molecule's binding site. Selection of resistant mutants by the first two mechanisms generally means a 2-to-8-fold increase in MIC, whereas alteration of the DNA gyrase binding site may result in high-level resistance. Resistance to one fluoroquinolone frequently results in resistance to all. This is especially true for the older compounds and for high-level resistance. Some mutations that confer resistance to the fluoroquinolones, via alterations in permeability or activation of the efflux pump, can also confer resistance to other antimicrobial agents such as the cephalosporins and tetracyclines.

Selection of resistant organisms is related to the concentration of bacteria at the site of infection. Kaatz et al. (1987) demonstrated in an experimental model of *Staphylococcus aureus* endocarditis that at ciprofloxacin concentrations 2 times the MIC, resistance occurred in 4 in 10^7 bacteria. At drug concentrations that were 4 times the MIC, resistance occurred in 6 in 10^{10} bacteria. However, at drug concentrations that were 10 times the MIC, resistance could not be detected. In any given bacterial population, even within a single species, the MIC for a specific antimicrobial agent varies (see Table 15.2 and Figure 2.2). Initially, bacteria with the higher MICs may form a tiny percentage of the total population. When exposed to high concentrations of a fluoroquinolone, susceptible organisms are killed rapidly (Figure 15.2). The higher the drug concentration, the higher the percentage of organisms that are susceptible and are therefore killed. On the other hand, when bacteria are exposed to a lower concentration of the fluoroquinolone, fewer are susceptible and thus killed. Those that survive do so because they have a higher MIC. These bacteria then have the potential to become the dominant population within 24 hours after exposure (Preston et al., 1998; Schentag and Scully, 1999). Since fluoroquinolone resistance is chromosomally mediated, and thus stable and not energy dependent, these resistant bacteria have the potential to persist even after the removal of the drug from their environment. High-level, stable resistance can thus be selected by repeated exposure to sublethal concentrations of drug.

In vitro models have shown that, to minimize the selection of resistant organisms, a 10:1 ratio of peak serum (C_{max}) to MIC and a 125:1 ratio of the 24-hour area under the serum concentration curve (AUC_{0-24}) to MIC are necessary for rapid bacterial eradication and prevention of regrowth of resistant subpopulations of the pathogen (Forrest et al., 1993; Hyatt et al., 1995; Schentag and Scully, 1999). The AUC_{0-24}:MIC has also been described as area under the inhibitory curve, or AUIC, but this may not be an accurate term. Animal and patient studies have confirmed the importance of these C_{max}:MIC and AUC_{0-24}:MIC ratios (Forrest et al.,

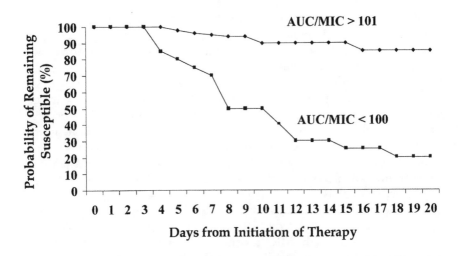

Fig. 15.3.   Relationship between AUC_{0-24}:MIC and the probability of selecting for resistant bacteria (in humans). After Thomas et al. (1998); reproduced with permission.

1993; Stein, 1996; Preston et al., 1998). In other words, the bacteria must survive the exposure to the antimicrobial agent in order to emerge resistant. It should be noted that there is a high correlation between C_{max}:MIC ratios and AUC_{0-24}:MIC ratios (R > 0.9) and that clinical studies have shown that AUC_{0-24}:MIC ratios of less than 100 increase the chance of selecting for resistant organisms (Figure 15.3) (Thomas et al., 1998).

The conclusion from these studies is that effective use of the fluoroquinolones against clinically important animal pathogens is dependent on designing dosing regimens that attain serum C_{max}:MIC ratios of 10:1 or AUC_{0-24}:MIC ratios of 125:1. Figure 15.4 illustrates how this may be accomplished by using knowledge of the serum C_{max} or AUC_{0-24} and the MIC of the pathogen. It is the responsibility of the drug manufacturer to provide sufficient pharmacokinetic data—that is, appropriate serum C_{max}, AUC_{0-24}, and perhaps bioavailability curves—on the product package insert, as well as current MIC data (which may also come from the diagnostic laboratory). Such data can assist the clinician in treating animals optimally with fluoroquinolones, thus prolonging their use for numerous animal species.

Resistance to the fluoroquinolones has stimulated considerable political debate concerning the use of these compounds in animals, especially animals that will enter the human food chain (see Chapter 3). This followed the appearance of ciprofloxacin-resistant *Campylobacter jejuni* shortly after the approval of enrofloxacin for use in chickens in the

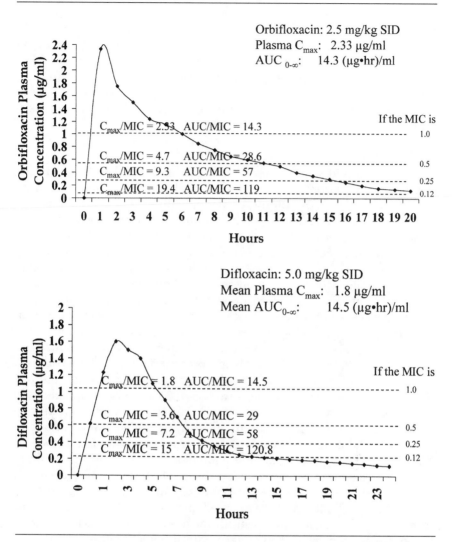

Fig. 15.4. Determining peak MIC ratios and AUC_{0-24}:MIC ratios for orbifloxacin and difloxacin. Bioavailability curves and plasma C_{max} and AUC are from the sponsor's package insert (Orbifloxacin, 1997; Difloxacin, 1997).

Netherlands (Endtz et al., 1991) and the decrease in susceptibility of *Salmonella typhimurium* DT104 to ciprofloxacin shortly after enrofloxacin was approved for use in cattle in the United Kingdom. The debate has focused on responsibility for this increase in resistance, with several consequences. The most far-reaching is the call for new regulations in the approval of new antimicrobial agents for use in food animals. Other subjects of debate include programs for the national and international monitoring of antibiotic resistance of pathogenic and sentinel bacteria of animal origin (see Chapter 34). Another consequence may be to improve understanding of how resistance occurs and how optimal use of antimicrobial drugs, such as that described here, can slow the selection of resistant organisms.

Pharmacokinetic Properties

Orally administered fluoroquinolones are rapidly absorbed (depending on the fluoroquinolone and animal species) in monogastrates, with peak serum concentrations occurring within 2 hours after administration. The bioavailability of the fluoroquinolones may vary from 30% to 90%, depending on the fluoroquinolone and animal species. The pharmacokinetic parameters of fluoroquinolones administered to dogs, cattle, horses, and pigs are given in Table 15.3. Ingestion with food may delay the occurrence of the peak serum concentrations without affecting total serum concentrations, unless the food is rich in magnesium or aluminum ions. Increases in oral dose usually produce linear increases in serum concentrations. Following absorption, fluoroquinolones exhibit rapid and extensive tissue distribution because of their hydrophilic nature and low (<50%) protein binding. Their apparent volume of distribution exceeds the total body water. In general, fluoroquinolone concentrations in interstitial fluid, skin, and bones are 35–100% of those obtained in the serum, whereas bronchial secretions and prostatic concentrations may be 2–3 times the corresponding serum concentrations. Penetration into cerebrospinal fluid is approximately 25% of serum concentration. However, this may vary with individual fluoroquinolones. High concentrations are found in bile and organs of excretion (liver, intestine, and urinary tract). Fluoroquinolones are partially metabolized in the liver to produce a number of metabolites and are excreted in an active form in the bile and urine. The major metabolite of enrofloxacin is ciprofloxacin. The amount of ciprofloxacin produced may vary with different species, with some producing ciprofloxacin concentrations that exceed the MIC of some pathogens (Kung et al., 1993). The elimination half-life of the fluoroquinolones is dependent on the drug, the animal species, and possibly the dose. For example, the elimination half-life of enrofloxacin ranges from 3.6 hours in beef calves to 6.1 hours in the horse (Table 15.3), whereas the elimination half-life of marbofloxacin in the dog may be as long as 14 hours. These long elimination half-lives make the fluoroquinolones ideal for q12- or q24-hour dosing regimens. Oral administration of fluoroquinolones to ruminants is associated with inactivation of the drug in the rumen.

TABLE 15.3. **Pharmacokinetic parameters of fluoroquinolones administered orally to dogs, horses, and cattle**

Fluoroquinolone	Animal Species	Route	Dose (mg/kg)	C_{max} (ug/ml)	T_{max} (h)	$T_{1/2\beta}$	$AUC_{0-\infty}$
Enrofloxacin	Dogs	PO	2.75[c]	0.7	1.2	3.7	7.2
			5.5[c]	1.4	1.7	5.8	15.7
			11.0[c]	2.1	1.9	5.6	27.1
			20.0	5.2[d]	3.6[d]		57.0[d]
	Cattle (adult)[e]	SC	5	0.7	3.5	7.8	8.4
	Calves[e]	SC	5	0.9	1.9	3.6	6.1
	Horses[f]	IV	2.5	1.9		5.9	10.1
			5.0	5.4	1.2	6.1	35.6
	Pigs[g]	SQ	2.5	0.8	5–6		8.3
			5.0	1.6	5–6		15.4
			7.5	1.8	5–6		21.7
Orbifloxacin	Dogs[h] (Cats)	PO	2.5	2.3[b] (2.1)	0.8[b] (1.0)	5.6, (5.5)	14.3,[a] (10.8)
			7.5	6.9[b]	0.8[b]	5.6[b]	42.9[a,b]
Difloxacin	Dogs[h]	PO	5.0	1.8	2.8	9.3	14.5[a]
			10.0	3.6[b]	2.8[b]	9.3[b]	29.0[a,b]
Ciprofloxacin	Dogs[c]	PO	11.0	0.9	1.2	4.6	11.9
			23.0	2.3	1.8	4.0	29.6
Marbofloxacin	Dogs[d]		1.0	0.8	1.7	14.7	11.8[a]
			2.0	1.4	2.5	14.0	22.0[a]
			4.0	2.9	2.0	12.5	45.6[a]
Danofloxacin[i]	Calves	IV	1.25	0.7		7.4	2.71[a]

[a] $AUC_{0-\infty}$.
[b] *Source:* Extrapolated from package insert.
[c] *Source:* Walker et al. (1990, 1992).
[d] *Source:* Eberhard Rosen, pers. comm. (1997).
[e] *Source:* Richez et al. (1994).
[f] *Source:* Giguere et al. (1996).
[g] *Source:* Ewert (1997).
[h] *Source:* Package insert.
[i] *Source:* Technical monograph.

Pharmacodynamic Properties

Given the favorable pharmacokinetic properties of the fluoroquinolones, along with their potential to select for resistant bacteria, the pharmacodynamic aspects of fluoroquinolone action assume major importance in designing dosing regimens. Pharmacodynamic parameters describe the interaction of drug concentration, which is dependent on dose and pharmacokinetic parameters, with the bacterial killing ability of the drug. The bacterial killing ability of a fluoroquinolone is related to the MIC, because the MIC and the minimal bactericidal concentration (MBC) are usually within 1 dilution of each other. Although low MICs generally indicate greater in vitro potency, these values must be interpreted in relation to achievable serum and tissue concentrations of the drug. By simultaneously considering the pharmacokinetic properties—that is, serum concentration, or $AUC_{0-\infty}$ of a drug and the MIC of the pathogen, an index of beneficial effect can be determined. In the examples given in Figure 15.4, peak plasma concentrations and AUC_{0-24} values are from the low doses of these two drugs listed in Table 15.3. (Note that in these bioavailability curves, $AUC_{0-\infty}$ values are used instead of AUC_{0-24} values, resulting in slightly higher AUC values and thus AUC:MIC values.) The MIC proposed values are in accordance with NCCLS dilution schemes and may represent an MIC value received from a package insert or from a microbiology report, provided that the lab reports MICs. The index of beneficial effect is an AUC_{0-24} of approximately 125 or greater (or C_{max} of 10 or more). Thus, for those bacterial pathogens with low MICs (0.12 μg/ml or less), the low doses of orbifloxacin or difloxacin should be adequate. On the other hand, to treat pathogens with higher MICs will require higher doses, or more frequent dosing, to achieve the desired clinical outcome. This point is illustrated in Table 15.4. As discussed above, AUC_{0-24} depends on dose or frequency of dosing. For those pathogens with low MICs—that is, 0.06 μg/ml or less—dosing regimens that result in AUC_{0-24}:MIC ratios of 100 or more are adequate to achieve an appropriate index of beneficial effect (Table 15.4). On the other hand, for pathogens with higher MICs, the dose or frequency of dosing needs to be increased in order to achieve an effective AUC_{0-24}:MIC ratio. These data illustrate why pathogens with higher MIC values require higher doses for clinical success, whereas an organism with a lower MIC could be treated successfully with the same drug but at a much lower dose.

The continued efficacy of the fluoroquinolones depends on designing dosing regimens that attain serum AUC_{0-24}:MIC ratios of 125 or C_{max}:MIC ratios of 10:1. By using the MIC data provided on the package insert, in Table 15.2, or in the microbiological report resulting from the submitted sample, along with the pharmacokinetic parameters from the package

TABLE 15.4.   **Relationship between serum AUC_{0-24} and MIC values**

If the AUC_{0-24} is . . .	MIC ($\mu g/ml$)							
	0.03	0.06	0.12	0.25	0.5	1.0	2.0	4.0
5	167	83	42	20	10	5	2.5	1.25
10	333	167	83	40	20	10	5	2.5
15	500	250	125	60	30	15	7.5	3.75
20	667	333	167	80	40	20	10	5
25	833	417	208	100	50	25	12.5	6.25
30	1,000	500	250	120	60	30	15	7.5

Note: Values listed are the AUC_{0-24}:MIC ratios, at various AUC_{0-24} values with commonly reported MICs, that could pertain to any fluoroquinolone at the appropriate dose. These ratios are dependent not on any specific fluoroquinolone but rather on the relationship between the AUC and the MIC.

insert or from Table 15.3, a practitioner should be able to determine the optimal dose to use. Failure to use this approach may result in therapeutic failure, which will inevitably lead to the selection of resistance of bacterial pathogens that are the norm, not the exception.

Drug Interactions

The fluoroquinolones have shown synergism when used with beta-lactams, aminoglycosides, and vancomycin against some bacterial pathogens. Some examples include *Staphylococcus aureus* (ciprofloxacin and azlocillin; levofloxacin and oxacillin); *Pseudomonas aeruginosa* (ciprofloxacin and imipenem or azlocillin or amikacin); and enterococci (ciprofloxacin and ampicillin or vancomycin) (Eliopoulos and Moellering, 1996). Antagonistic interactions have been demonstrated in vitro between ciprofloxacin and chloramphenicol, and ciprofloxacin and rifampin have been described in human medicine (Eliopoulos and Moellering, 1996). Fluoroquinolones have been used with metronidazole to expand the antibacterial spectrum in the treatment of polymicrobial infections. There are few reported drug interactions with the fluoroquinolones, and most are of no veterinary significance. Decreased absorption occurs in the presence of antacids containing magnesium or aluminum. Products of metabolized fluoroquinolones in the liver can depress hepatic microsomal enzyme activity, resulting in reduced elimination of drugs that depend on liver metabolism for excretion. For example, the fluoroquinolones decrease the hepatic clearance, and thus increase the elimination half-life, of theophylline and caffeine. In a veterinary context, adverse interactions with barbiturates, chloramphenicol, rifampin, and ionophore antibiotics may therefore be anticipated. By inhibiting renal tubular secretion, probenecid has been shown to reduce the renal clearance of ciprofloxacin by 50% in humans (Stein, 1988).

Toxicity and Adverse Effects

Fluoroquinolones are relatively safe antimicrobial drugs. Administered at therapeutic doses, toxic effects are mild and generally limited to
gastrointestinal disturbances such as nausea, vomiting, and diarrhea. At
very high doses (50 mg/kg), the fluoroquinolones have been associated
with arthropathies in young experimental animals, especially Beagle dogs.
It is therefore currently recommended that fluoroquinolones not be administered to growing young animals of any species that are expected to perform as an adult, especially dogs, which may be the species most susceptible to this effect. Photosensitivity in humans has occasionally been
associated with the use of fluoroquinolones; minor differences occur in
phototoxicity between the different fluoroquinolones. Occasionally, mild
interstitial inflammation of the kidney tubular walls has been associated
with precipitation of fluoroquinolone complexes. Crystalluria, leading to
obstructive uropathy, has been reported in human studies, but it is uncommon. Other renal toxicities may include acute renal failure, associated with
interstitial nephritis. In human medicine, however, most cases of renal toxicity have been associated with the use of fluoroquinolones at doses well
above the therapeutic range. Rarely, ocular toxicities include retinal degeneration and subcapsular cataracts, which may be related to the specific fluoroquinolone and the dose, have been reported. Neurotoxic effects causing
central nervous system disturbances (seizures, dizziness, ataxia, insomnia,
restlessness, somnolence, tremors) are common side effects in human medicine. These usually depend on dose and specific fluoroquinolone and
occur most frequently with the more-lipophilic drugs used in human medicine, such as fleroxacin and ofloxacin. Higher doses have also been associated with convulsions, defecation, urination, and emesis (Brown, 1996).
Enrofloxacin has been associated with increased frequency and intensity of
seizures in epileptic dogs (Van Cutsem et al., 1990).

The introduction of fluoroquinolones for use in dogs has been associated with the emergence of canine toxic shock syndrome and necrotizing fasciitis caused by *Streptococcus canis* (Miller et al., 1996). Minor infections caused by this organism have developed into very severe illness in
dogs treated with a fluoroquinolone, an illness that can be exacerbated by
the use of corticosteroids or nonsteroidal anti-inflammatory drugs. In
some cases the isolates have been susceptible to fluoroquinolones in vitro.

Administration and Dosage

Fluoroquinolones are usually administered orally in monogastrates
(IV preparations are available and are occasionally used, especially in the
horse) or preruminants and parenterally (IV, IM, and SC) in ruminants, or
subcutaneously in day-old chicks. The usual dosages of currently available fluoroquinolones are shown in Table 15.5.

TABLE 15.5. **Usual dosages of fluoroquinolones in animals**

Drug	Species	Route	Dose Range (mg/kg)	Interval	Comment
Enrofloxacin	Dogs, cats	PO (dogs, cats), IM (dog only)	5.0–20	24	Do not use in growing animals
	Cattle	IV, IM, SC	2.5–5.0 7.5–12.5 5.0	SID 3–5 days Once 24 h	
	Horses[a]	IV			Do not use in growing animals
	Pigs	IV, SC	2.5–7.5	24 h	Do not use in growing animals
Orbifloxacin	Dogs, cats	PO	2.5–7.5	24 h	Do not use in growing animals
Difloxacin	Dogs	PO	5–10	24 h	Do not use in growing animals
	Chickens, turkeys	PO	10	Continuous medication in drinking water	
Ciprofloxacin[b]	Dogs	PO	11–23	12 h	Do not use in growing animals
Marbofloxacin	Dogs				Do not use in growing animals
Danofloxacin	Calves	IV, IM, SC	1.25	SID 3–5 days	Do not use in growing animals
Sarafloxacin	Chickens, turkeys	PO	20–40 ppm	Continuous medication in drinking water	

Sources: Drug sponsors, package insert, or published data as indicated.
[a]Giguere et al. (1996).
[b]Walker et al. (1990).

Perhaps more than with any other class of antimicrobial agent, dosage of fluoroquinolones should be based on the susceptibility of the bacterial target. Clinical efficacy of the fluoroquinolone is dependent on dose and bacterial pathogen. To maximize clinical efficacy and reduce selection of resistant bacteria, C_{max}:MIC ratios ≥10:1 or AUC_{0-24}:MIC ratios ≥125:1 may be required. There is argument as to whether it is the C_{max}:MIC or the AUC_{0-24}:MIC ratio that determines maximum clinical efficacy. Although these two parameters are closely associated, there are subtle differences. As an example, when a fluoroquinolone is administered at q12-hour dosing intervals, the C_{max} and the AUC_{0-12} for each dose may remain essentially the same. (There may be slight increases, depending on the elimination half-life.) However, it is AUC_{0-24} that has been shown to be important. The AUC value should double when a drug is administered q12 hours ($AUC_{0-12} \times 2$), whereas the C_{max} remains essentially the same. Because the fluoroquinolones exhibit concentration-dependent killing, this uncertainty as to whether C_{max} or AUC_{0-24} is more important can be addressed by knowledge of the MIC of the bacterial pathogen. For pathogens with low MICs (ie, ≤0.06 µg/ml), AUC_{0-24}:MIC ratios are important in determining clinical efficacy. For pathogens with high but still susceptible MICs, since there is an increased chance of selecting for resistant organisms, the C_{max}:MIC ratio may be the better predictor of clinical efficacy because of the concentration killing effect (Craig and Dalhoff, 1998).

When the fluoroquinolones are used, designing appropriate and optimal dosing regimens requires three things: (1) knowledge of the selected agents' C_{max} or AUC_{0-24} within the recommended dosing range; (2) knowledge of the MIC of the selected fluoroquinolone for the pathogen; and (3) understanding pharmacodynamic relationships.

Use of the C_{max}:MIC ratio approach involves the following. If the MIC is known, the peak serum concentration should be ≥10 times the MIC—that is, the C_{max}:MIC ratio is ≥10:1. For example, if the MIC is 0.12 µg/ml, 10 times that would require a peak serum concentration of at least 1.2 µg/ml. From Table 15.3 it can be seen that enrofloxacin and difloxacin produce serum C_{max} of >1.2 µg/ml when administered at 5.0 mg/kg, whereas marbofloxacin and orbifloxacin exceed this concentration when administered at doses of 2.0 and 2.5, respectively. If the MIC is 0.25 µg/ml, a higher dose (from Table 15.3) of 15 mg/kg for difloxacin, approximately 11.0 mg/kg for enrofloxacin, and 23 mg/kg for ciprofloxacin would be required to reach the desired C_{max}:MIC ratio of 2.5 µg/ml. If the pharmacokinetic parameters are available for a single dose but not for a dosing range, then, generally speaking, doubling the dose results in a corresponding doubling of the serum C_{max}.

Using the AUC_{0-24}:MIC ratio approach involves the following. Relate the AUC_{0-24} to the MIC. For example, if the MIC for enrofloxacin is

0.06 µg/ml, the required dose is between 2.75 mg/kg and 5.0 mg/kg. (Table 15.3 illustrates that when enrofloxacin is administered at a dose of 2.75 mg/kg, the AUC_{0-24} is 7.2. Therefore, 7.2 divided by the MIC of 0.06 µg/ml results in an AUC_{0-24}:MIC ratio of 120. A dose of 5 mg/kg would result in an AUC_{0-24}:MIC ratio of 262.) These ratios have been shown to be important in maximizing the clinical efficacy and minimizing selection of resistant organisms, since a ratio of 125:1 is required for optimal use (Forrest et al., 1993; Thomas et al., 1998). Figure 15.3 illustrates the AUC_{0-24}:MIC relationship and the probability of selecting for resistant organisms, whereas Figure 15.5 illustrates the AUC_{0-24}:MIC relationship of ciprofloxacin and eradication of the pathogen. As was stated above, if the organism is killed, it cannot be resistant.

In using these approaches, the dosing interval must prevent serum concentrations from dropping below the MIC of the pathogen for more than 20% of the dosing interval. This is not usually a problem when AUC_{0-24}:MIC ratios are used.

Clinical Applications

Fluoroquinolones in veterinary use offer the advantages of oral administration, high potency against many Gram-negative aerobic pathogens, moderate activity against Gram-positive aerobes, widespread distribution throughout the body, and low toxicity. Their disadvantages include their tendency to select for resistant bacteria if they are not used

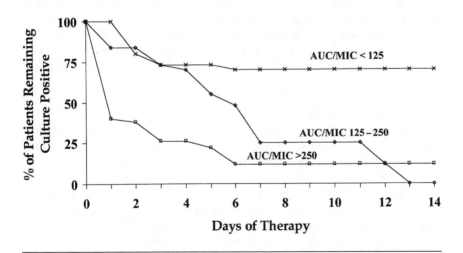

Fig. 15.5. Relationship among time, days of therapy to bacterial eradication (in humans), and AUC_{0-24}:MIC, illustrated by a time-to-event (survival) plot. After Forrest et al. (1993); reproduced with permission.

to produce optimal killing, and their moderate activity against Gram-positive aerobes, such as pyogenic streptococci (eg, *Streptococcus canis*). They are very effective in the treatment of urinary tract infections in animals and can be useful for serious infections such as septicemia and pneumonia caused by susceptible Gram-negative bacteria (*E. coli, Pasteurella* spp.), for the treatment of skin and many soft-tissue infections caused by Gram-negative or some Gram-positive aerobic bacteria, and for intra-abdominal infections caused by Gram-negative aerobes. Fluoroquinolones may be the most effective antimicrobial agent for the treatment of chronic bacterial prostatitis caused by susceptible Gram-negative bacteria. They are effective in the treatment of *Mycoplasma* infections. Because of their potency and ability to enter phagocytes, they have the potential to be valuable for the treatment of infections caused by atypical bacteria, including mycobacteria, *Brucella* spp., *Chlamydia* spp., *Coxiella* spp., *Ehrlichia* spp., and *Rickettsia* spp. However, documentation is required in veterinary medicine of their efficacy for treating infections caused by many of these pathogens. Veterinarians should not prescribe these drugs for use in growing animals, particularly dogs, because of their tendency to cause severe arthropathy.

The introduction of fluoroquinolones for the treatment of bacterial infections in companion animals was associated with their promotion as drugs of choice for numerous infectious disease processes. One justification was that plasmid-mediated resistance was not likely to occur, or if it did, it would not be transferable. Indeed, since the introduction of these drugs into clinical medicine, plasmid-mediated resistance has been described in only one case (Schentag and Scully, 1999). However, resistance and decreased susceptibility to fluoroquinolones have emerged rapidly. Unless they are used with optimal dosing strategies, the fluoroquinolones may soon be ineffective in treating anything but the simplest infections, despite the promise they offered only a decade ago.

CATTLE, SHEEP, AND GOATS

Fluoroquinolones are quite active when tested against bacteria associated with acute respiratory disease in cattle, sheep, and goats (*Mannheimia (Pasteurella) haemolytica, Pasteurella multocida*, and *Haemophilus somnus*). They also have the potential to be effective against several other species of bacteria known to cause disease in these animals, especially Gram-negative bacteria such as *E. coli* and *Salmonella*, although the MICs of these pathogens will most likely be higher than the MICs of the bacteria associated with acute respiratory disease, thus requiring higher doses and longer withdrawal times. Other indications could include mastitis, metritis, conjunctivitis, and infections caused by *Mycoplasma*, such as pneumonia and otitis media. Unfortunately, details on the efficacy of the fluoroquinolones for treating these infections are lacking.

Although fluoroquinolones should be effective in treating most of the indications noted above, in the United States they have been approved only for the treatment of acute pneumonia in beef cattle and are prohibited from any extralabel use. Extralabel use includes any alteration of dose, frequency of dosing, or dosing duration in any animal that may enter the human food chain. Traditionally, in the approval process for the use of an antibiotic in a food animal, the emphasis has been more on drug residues than on consideration of whether the dose would select for resistant bacteria. In actuality, these are two opposed positions associated with drug approval. To minimize drug residues, the lowest possible dose is used for the shortest length of time. Conversely, to prevent selection of resistant bacteria, a high dose is needed to kill the pathogen rapidly. When an antimicrobial agent, such as a fluoroquinolone, is approved for use in food animals, which position weighs heavier in determining the dosage regimen—residues or resistance? It is apparent that a higher dosing regimen would both reduce handling of beef cattle and reduce the potential for selection of resistant bacteria.

SWINE

Fluoroquinolones have established value in the treatment of *Mycoplasma hyopneumoniae* infections and have the potential for the prevention or treatment of *Actinobacillus pleuropneumoniae, E. coli,* and *Pasteurella multocida* infections. Their use should be optimized to the individual pathogen and infection. Fluoroquinolones should never be administered in feed, because this will result in residues that will contaminate the environment from the feed mill to the farm. Low concentrations of the drug have the potential of selecting for resistant bacteria. In addition, sick animals do not eat well. Because of concern about resistance, fluoroquinolones are prohibited from use in pigs in the United States and several other countries.

HORSES

Because of the potential of fluoroquinolones to cause cartilage erosion, their use is not recommended in young, growing horses. In one study of the pharmacokinetics of enrofloxacin in adult horses, Giguere and Belanger (1997) did not observe any adverse joint reactions during IV or oral administration of enrofloxacin. However, Kaartinen et al. (1997) found intramuscular administration to be very irritating, resulting in swelling or tenderness at the injection site, with elevated creatine kinase activity for up to 32 hours after injection. Because fluoroquinolones can be administered orally, they may be useful in horses for the treatment of a variety of Gram-negative infections caused by susceptible bacteria resistant to alternative, first-choice drugs. For example, enrofloxacin was used in the successful treatment of chronic *E. coli* pleuritis caused by an otherwise resistant organism (Heath et al., 1989).

DOGS AND CATS

Fluoroquinolones have provided small-animal clinicians with a truly exciting new class of anti-infectives. Never before have they had an antimicrobial agent with such a broad spectrum of activity as the fluoroquinolones, combined with the pharmacokinetic properties that allow for oral administration on a once-a-day basis. This has allowed clinicians to treat a larger number of patients as outpatients with more assurance that there would be owner compliance because of the once-a-day dosing requirement. Because fluoroquinolones can penetrate nearly every tissue in the body, these drugs can be used to treat urinary tract infections, including prostatitis caused by susceptible bacteria; respiratory infections such as rhinitis and pneumonia, including those caused by *Bordetella bronchiseptica*; deep and superficial pyoderma, otitis media and externa, and wound infections cause by susceptible organisms; peritonitis (used in combination with metronidazole if anaerobic bacteria are suspected); osteomyelitis caused by susceptible Gram-negative aerobes; and infections caused by mycoplasmas, such as conjunctivitis and soft-tissue infections. At therapeutic doses, the fluoroquinolones have proven to be relatively safe, with few reported side effects. If adverse reactions do occur, they are not as frequent as those reported in human medicine, or at least they are not reported as frequently. As with any animal species, this class of antimicrobial agents should not be administered to animals less than 8 months of age or to large-breed dogs less than 12 months of age.

POULTRY

In intensive poultry production, antimicrobial agents that have the ability to rapidly kill any bacterial pathogen that invades a poultry house are needed. The most critical of such infections is *E. coli* septicemia and cellulitis (see Chapter 27), but other important Gram-negative aerobic infections include salmonellosis and *Haemophilus paragallinarum* and *Pasteurella multocida* infections (Bauditz, 1987). Two fluoroquinolones, sarafloxacin and enrofloxacin, have been developed for poultry use and approved as water medication. In the United States, these drugs may be used only under labeled conditions. Sarafloxacin and enrofloxacin are approved for treating *E. coli* infections in chickens and turkeys, and enrofloxacin is also approved for treating *P. multocida* infections in turkeys. Unfortunately, their labeled dosage has not addressed the pharmacokinetic and pharmacodynamic properties determining clinical efficacy. Neither recommends pulse dosing, which would maximize bacterial killing and therefore would also maximize clinical efficacy and decreased selection of resistant bacteria. Instead both drugs are administered in water as a continuous medication over the entire treatment period. Fluoroquinolones are also used in some countries for the control of *Mycoplasma* infections by SC administration to day-old poults.

Bibliography

Bauditz R. 1987. Results of clinical studies with Baytril in poultry. Vet Med Rev 2:130.

Brown SA. 1996. Fluoroquinolones in animal health. J Vet Pharmacol Ther 19:1.

Craig WA, Dalhoff A. 1998. Pharmacodynamics of fluoroquinolones in experimental animals. In: Kuhlman J, et al., eds. Quinolone Antibacterials. New York: Springer-Verlag.

Dalhoff A, Bergan T. 1998. Pharmacokinetics of fluoroquinolones in experimental animals.

Eliopoulos GM, Moellering RC, Jr. 1996. Antimicrobial combinations, Chapter 9. In: Lorian V, ed. Antibiotics in Laboratory Medicine, 4th ed. Baltimore: Williams and Wilkins.

Endtz HP, et al. 1991. Quinolone resistance in *Campylobacter* isolated from man and poultry following the introduction of fluoroquinolones in veterinary medicine. J Antimicrob Chemother 27:199.

Ewert K. 1997. Pharmacokinetics and in vitro antimicrobial activity of enrofloxacin. Am Assoc Swine Pract, p153.

Fernandez-Guerrero M, et al. 1987. In vitro and in vivo activity of ciprofloxacin against enterococci isolated from patients with infective endocarditis. Antimicrob Agents Chemother 31:430.

Ferrero L, et al. 1994. Cloning and primary structure of *Staphylococcus aureus* DNA topoisomerase IV: a primary target of fluoroquinolones. Mol Microbiol 13:641.

Forrest A, et al. 1993. Pharmacodynamics of intravenous ciprofloxacin in seriously ill patients. Antimicrob Agents Chemother 37:1073.

Giguere S, Belanger M. 1997. Concentration of enrofloxacin in equine tissues after long term oral administration. J Vet Pharmacol Ther 20:402.

Giguere S, et al. 1996. Pharmacokinetics of enrofloxacin in adult horses and concentration of the drug in serum, body fluid, and endometrial tissues after repeated intragastrically administered doses. Am J Vet Res 57:1025.

Giles CJ, et al. 1991. Efficacy of danofloxacin in the therapy of acute bacterial pneumonia in housed beef cattle. Vet Rec 128:296.

Goldstein EJC, et al. 1998. Trovafloxacin compared with levofloxacin, ofloxacin, ciprofloxacin, azithromycin, and clarithromycin against unusual aerobic and anaerobic human and animal bite-wound pathogens. J Antimicrob Chemother 41:391.

Gould IL, et al. 1990. Concentration-dependent bacterial killing, adaptive resistance, and post-antibiotic effect of ciprofloxacin alone and in combination with gentamicin. Drugs Exper Clin Res 26:621.

Grohe K. 1998. The chemistry of the quinolones: methods of synthesizing the quinolone ring system. In: Kuhlman J, et al., eds. Quinolone Antibacterials. New York: Springer-Verlag.

Heath SE, et al. 1989. Chronic pleuritis in a horse. Can Vet J 30:69.

Hoshino K, et al. 1994. Comparison of inhibition of *Escherichia coli* topoisomerase IV by quinolones with DNA gyrase inhibition. Antimicrob Agents Chemother 38:2623.

Howard BMA, et al. 1993. Function of the SOS process in repair of DNA damage induced by modern 4-quinolones. J Pharm Pharmacol 45:658.

Hyatt JM, et al. 1995. The importance of pharmacokinetics/pharmacodynamic surrogate markers to outcome: focus on antimicrobial agents. Clin Pharmacokinet 28:143.

Kaartinen L, et al. 1997. Pharmacokinetics of enrofloxacin in horses after single intravenous and intramuscular administration. Equine Vet J 29:378.

Kaatz GW, Seo SM. 1998. Topoisomerase mutations in fluoroquinolone-resistant and methicillin-susceptible and -resistant clinical isolates of Staphylococcus aureus. Antimicrob Agents Chemother 42:197.

Kaatz GW, et al. 1987. The emergence of the resistance to ciprofloxacin during treatment of experimental Staphylococcus aureus endocarditis. J Antimicrob Chemother 20:753.

Kato J, et al. 1990. New topoisomerase essential for chromosome segregation in E. coli. Cell 63:393.

Kato J, et al. 1992. Purification and characterization of DNA topoisomerase IV in Escherichia coli. J Biol Chem 267:25676.

Kung K, et al. 1993. Pharmacokinetics of enrofloxacin and its metabolite ciprofloxacin after intravenous and oral administration of enrofloxacin in dogs. J Vet Pharmacol Ther 16:462.

Maxwell A, Critchlow SE. 1998. Mode of action. In: Kuhlmann J, et al., eds. Quinolone Antibacterials. New York: Springer-Verlag, p119.

Miller CW, et al. 1996. Streptococcal toxic shock in dogs. J Am Vet Med Assoc 209:1421.

Petersen U, Schenke T. 1998. The chemistry of the quinolones: chemistry in the periphery of the quinolones. In: Kuhlman J, et al., eds. Quinolone Antibacterials. New York: Springer-Verlag, p63.

Preston SL, et al. 1998. Levofloxacin population pharmacokinetics and creation of a demographic model for prediction of individual drug clearance in patients with serious community-acquired infection. Antimicrob Agents Chemother 42:1098-1104.

Richez, et al. 1994. Pharmacokinetics of enrofloxacin in calves and adult cattle after single and repeated subcutaneous injections. Proc 6th Eur Assoc Vet Pharm Ther, p232.

Schentag JJ, Scully BE. 1999. Quinolones. In: Yu VL, et al., eds. Antimicrobial Therapy and Vaccines. New York: Williams and Wilkins, p875.

Segev S, Rubinstein E. 1998. Future aspects. In: Kuhlman J, et al., eds. Quinolone Antibacterials. New York: Springer-Verlag, p455.

Smith JT, Zeiler H-J, 1998. History and introduction. In: Kuhlmann J, et al., eds. Quinolone Antibacterials. New York: Springer-Verlag, p1.

Stegemann M, et al. 1996. Kinetics of antibacterial activity after administration of enrofloxacin in dog serum and skin: in vitro susceptibility of field isolates. Compend Contin Educ Pract Vet 18 (Suppl):30.

Stein GE. 1988. The 4-quinolone antibiotics: past, present, and future. Pharmacotherapy 8:301.

Stein GE. 1996. Pharmacokinetics and pharmacodynamics of newer fluoroquinolones. Clin Infect Dis 23 (Suppl 1):S19.

Thomas JK, et al. 1998. Pharmacodynamic evaluation of factors associated with the development of bacterial resistance in acutely ill patients during therapy. Antimicrob Agents Chemother 42:521.

Van Cutsem PM, et al. 1990. The fluoroquinolone antimicrobials: structure, antimicrobial activity, pharmacokinetics, clinical use in domestic animals, and toxicity. Cornell Vet 80:173.

Walker RD, Thornsberry C. 1998. Decrease in antibiotic susceptibility or increase in resistance. J Antimicrob Chemother 41:1.

Walker RD, et al. 1990. Serum and tissue cage fluid concentrations of ciprofloxacin after oral administration of the drug to healthy dogs. Am J Vet Res 51:896.

Walker RD, et al. 1992. Pharmacokinetic evaluation of enrofloxacin administered orally to healthy dogs. Am J Vet Res 53:2315.

Watts JL, et al. 1997. In vitro activity of premafloxacin, a new extended-spectrum fluoroquinolone, against pathogens of veterinary important. Antimicrob Agents Chemother 41:1190.

Miscellaneous Antibiotics: Ionophores, Nitrofurans, Nitroimidazoles, Rifamycins, and Others

J. F. PRESCOTT

This chapter discusses a variety of miscellaneous antimicrobial agents used in veterinary medicine—the ionophores, nitrofurans, nitroimidazoles, and rifampin, in detail—and briefly comments on other agents, including arsenicals, quinoxalines, fusidic acid, isoniazid, methenamine, and novobiocin.

Ionophore Antibiotics

Carboxylic ionophore polyether antibiotics are *Streptomyces* products used in agriculture largely as growth promoters and for their anticoccidial activity. They behave as an alkali metal ionophore in altering bacterial cell permeability, complexing with sodium in the cell membrane to cause passive transport of potassium ions out of the cell and their replacement by hydrogen ions, which kill the cell by lowering intracellular pH. Examples include lasalocid, maduramicin, monensin, and narasin. These drugs are not used in human medicine.

Monensin

Monensin is a fermentation product of *Streptomyces cinnamonensis*. It is active against Gram-positive bacteria, some *Campylobacter* spp., and *Serpulina hyodysenteriae* (MIC 0.1 µg/ml), as well as against coccidia and *Toxoplasma*. When fed to ruminants in small quantities, monensin changes the rumen microflora toward a more Gram-negative flora, which shifts volatile fatty acid production to increase propionic acid production, decrease rumen protein breakdown, inhibit primary hydrogen or formic

339

acid production, and decrease lactate production. The net effect is to improve feed conversion efficiency in ruminants.

Because of the drug's toxicity, considerable care must be taken to avoid accidental overdosage with monensin or its concurrent use with potentiators of toxicity, and to prevent accidental incorporation into rations for horses and other unintended species for which it is toxic.

TOXICITY AND ADVERSE EFFECTS

Monensin intoxication occurs in a wide variety of species. Monensin is highly toxic to horses, ruminants, and other animals at doses 5–10 times those recommended or when mixed with certain incompatible drugs. Care should be taken not to feed rations to livestock for which they are not intended, to carefully compute doses of monensin for ruminants, and to prevent accidental contamination in feed mills. The LD_{50} (mg/kg) of monensin for different species is as follows: horses, 2–3; sheep, 12; pigs, 16; dogs, 20; and chickens, 200 (Langston et al., 1985). Monensin toxicity should be suspected when a recent feed change is associated with anorexia, ataxia, depression, mild diarrhea, dyspnea, stiffness, weakness, recumbency, and death (Langston et al., 1985). Muscle weakness and myoglobinuria are marked features of monensin poisoning in dogs, pigs, and sheep. Monensin causes cell membrane disruption, with damage particularly to skeletal and cardiac muscle. There may be species differences in whether monensin causes cardiomyopathy (Baird et al., 1997). Monensin transports cations and particularly sodium across cell membranes, exchanging sodium preferentially for potassium and indirectly also increasing intracellular calcium, producing severe cell damage. The clinicopathologic changes observed vary with the species affected. Toxicosis by monensin and other ionophores in animals is potentiated by drugs that interfere with hepatic metabolism, including chloramphenicol, erythromycin, sulfonamides, and tiamulin. Furazolidone potentiates the toxicity of monensin in turkeys (Czarnecki, 1990).

Cattle, Sheep, and Goats. Poisoning has been reported in cattle fed 5–10 times the recommended doses of monensin. The LD_{50} is about 22 mg/kg, over 20 times the recommended daily dose for cattle (Schweitzer et al., 1984). Initial signs of toxicity are inappetence and refusal to eat treated feed. Progressive cardiomyopathy develops, and animals die with generalized heart failure, often with individuals of a group dying over a period of several weeks. In sheep, striated muscle, not cardiac muscle, is the target of monensin poisoning, so that affected animals show signs of lethargy, muscle weakness, stiffness, posterior incoordination, and atrophy of the hind limb muscle mass.

Horses. Monensin has an LD_{50} for horses of only 2–3 mg/kg. Horses fed diets containing 125 ppm have died in about 1 week (Matsuoka, 1976).

In acute poisoning, heart irregularities result from specific effect of monensin on the mitochondria of cardiac muscle. Symptoms in acutely poisoned horses include complete or partial anorexia within 12 hours of eating contaminated feed, profuse intermittent sweating, restlessness, and recumbency. Delayed cardiac failure, because of cardiac myodegeneration and fibrosis, was described in horses with a history of poor performance and ill health several months after acute monensin poisoning (Muylle et al., 1981). Extreme care should be taken not to feed cattle or poultry rations or supplements to horses and to avoid accidental contamination in feed mills.

Dogs and Cats. In dogs, monensin causes both cardiac and striated muscle degeneration and is characterized clinically by anorexia, ataxia, paresis, and profound muscle weakness. Monensin should never be administered to dogs or cats.

Swine. Pigs fed 100 ppm of monensin combined with 200 ppm of tiamulin became anorexic within 2 days; drowsiness, ataxia, paraplegia, coma, and death occurred within 5–10 days (Potts and Skov, 1981). Vitamin E administration reduced the skeletal muscle damage of tiamulin-potentiated monensin toxicosis in swine but did not ameliorate the acute clinical signs (Van Vleet et al., 1987).

Poultry. The predominant lesions of monensin toxicosis in chickens and turkeys are necrosis of skeletal and cardiac muscle associated clinically with posterior paresis, inability to rise, incoordination, leg weakness, and reluctance to move. Gross lesions may be absent, but microscopic lesions include muscle fiber necrosis and degeneration and sarcolemmal nuclear proliferation. Outbreaks of monensin intoxication following ingestion of feed containing therapeutic levels of drug were described by Wages and Ficken (1988).

CLINICAL APPLICATIONS

Monensin is used to control coccidiosis in poultry and in other species and to improve the efficiency of feed conversion in ruminants. It improves feed efficiency and weight gain when fed to cattle at 11–33 ppm feed, the dosage depending on the stage of feeding. A slow-release capsule bolus form of monensin is available that gives sustained release in the rumen for about 4 months. Besides improving weight gain and feed conversion efficiency, it is also used to prevent the incidence of and mortality resulting from bloat in cattle on leguminous pasture. More recently, the sustained release form has been licensed for use in the prevention and treatment of ketosis in lactating dairy cows. Monensin also prevents coccidiosis in calves if administered at concentrations that stimulate weight gain. Experimentally, monensin fed at 100 mg twice daily or 200 mg once daily prevented tryptophan-induced acute bovine pulmonary edema and emphysema by reducing 3-methyl-indole production. Effective prevention of fog fever requires continuous administration of monensin for 10 days after exposure to tryptophan or during a change of pasture (Hammond et al., 1982).

Monensin has been shown experimentally to considerably reduce abortion and loss due to toxoplasmosis in ewes fed 15–16 mg/day (Buxton et al., 1988; Mathieson et al., 1990). Monensin is effective in the control of swine dysentery and porcine intestinal adenomatosis and hemorrhagic enteropathy. An effective dose may be 100 ppm daily for 3 weeks followed by 50 ppm for a further 3 weeks.

Bibliography

Baird GJ, et al. 1997. Monensin toxicity in a flock of ostriches. Vet Rec 140:624.
Buxton D, et al. 1988. Further studies in the use of monensin in the control of ovine toxoplasmosis. J Comp Pathol 98:225.
Carlson JR, et al. 1983. Effect of monensin on bovine ruminal 3-methylindole production after abrupt change to lush pasture. Am J Vet Res 44:118.
Czarnecki, CM. 1990. Effect of including lasalocid or monensin singly or in combination with furazolidone on the growth and feed consumption of turkey poults. Res Vet Sci 49:256.
Doonan GR, et al. 1989. Monensin poisoning in horses—an international incident. Can Vet J 30:165.
Duffield TF, et al. 1998. Effect of prepartum administration of monensin in a controlled-release capsule on postpartum energy indicators in lactating dairy cows. J Dairy Sci 81:2354.
Hammond AC, et al. 1982. Effect of monensin pretreatment on tryptophan-induced acute bovine pulmonary edema and emphysema. Am J Vet Res 43:753.
Langston VC, et al. 1985. Toxicity and therapeutics of monensin: a review. Vet Med 80:75.
Mathieson AO, et al. 1990. Monensin and ovine toxoplasmosis. Vet Rec 126:20.
Matsuoka T. 1976. Evaluation of monensin toxicity in the horse. J Am Vet Med Assoc 169:1098.
Miller RE, et al. 1990. Acute monensin toxicosis in stone sheep (*Ovis dalli stonei*), blesbok (*Damaliscus dorcus phillipsi*), and a bactrian camel (*Camelus bactrianus*). J Am Vet Med Assoc 196:131.
Muylle E, et al. 1981. Delayed monensin sodium toxicity in horses. Equine Vet J 13:107.
Potts JM, Skov B. 1981. Monensin-tiamulin interactions in pigs. Vet Rec 109:545.
Schweitzer D, et al. 1984. Accidental monensin sodium intoxication of feedlot cattle. J Am Vet Med Assoc 184:1273.
Smyth JBA, et al. 1990. Effects of concurrent oral administration of monensin on the toxicity of increasing doses of selenium in lambs. J Comp Pathol 102:443.
Van Vleet JF, et al. 1987. Monensin toxicosis in swine: potentiation by tiamulin administration and ameliorative effect of treatment with selenium and/or vitamin E. Am J Vet Res 48:1520.
Wages DP, Ficken MD. 1988. Skeletal muscle lesions in turkeys associated with the feeding of monensin. Avian Dis 32:583.

Other Ionophore Antibiotics: Lasalocid, Maduramicin, Narasin, and Salinomycin

Lasalocid, maduramicin, narasin, and salinomycin, like monensin, possess anticoccidial activity and are also used for their effect in improving the efficiency of ruminal fermentation and in some cases for their effect against *Clostridium perfringens*. Extralabel (as well as inadvertent) use should be avoided in all cases. Salinomycin is used as a growth promoter in swine and is effective in the prevention and treatment of proliferative enteropathy. All have similar usages to those of monensin, a similar mode of action, and equivalent potential for toxicity if incorrectly mixed in feed or (in most species) if used concurrently with toxicity-potentiating drugs, including tiamulin. Extreme care should be taken not to include lasalocid and salinomycin in the rations of laying birds, because of their toxic effects on laying hens and on embryos. Horses appear particularly susceptible to the toxic effects of ionophores.

Bibliography

Bastionello SS, et al. 1995. Cardiomyopathy of ruminats induced by the litter of poultry fed rations containing the ionophore antibiotic, maduramicin. II. Macropathology and histopathology. Onderstepoort J Vet Res 62:5.

Bastionello SS, et al. 1996. A chronic cardiomyopathy in feedlot cattle attrributed to toxic levels of salinomycin in the feed. Tydskr S Afr Vet Ver 67:38.

Benson JE, et al. 1998. Lasalocid toxicosis in neonatal calves. J Vet Diagn Invest 10:210.

Blanchard PC, et al. 1993. Lasalocid toxicosis in dairy calves. J Vet Diagn Invest 5:300.

Hoop RK. 1998. Salinomycin toxicity in layer breeders. Vet rec 142:550.

Kyriakis SC, et al. 1996. Effect of salinmoycin in the control of *Clostridium perfringens* type C infection in suckling pigs. Vet Rec 138:281.

Perelman B, et al. 1993. Effects of the accidental feeding of lasalocid sodium to broiler breeder chickens. Vet rec 132:271.

Plumlee KH, et al. 1995. Acute salinomycin toxicosis in pigs. J Vet Diagn Invest 7:41

Rollinson J, et al. 1987. Salinomycin poisoning in horses. Vet Rec 121:126.

Safran N, et al. 1993. Paralytic syndrome attributed to lasalocid residues in a commercial ration fed to dogs. J Am Vet Med Assoc 202:1273.

Shlosberg A, et al. 1997. Acute maduramicin toxicity in calves. Vet Rec 140:643.

Nitrofurans

Nitrofurans have broad antibacterial activity, but their toxicity largely limits their use to topical application, to the treatment of intestinal infections, and to the treatment of urinary tract infections. Because of suspected carcinogenicity, they are not available in some countries.

Chemistry

Nitrofurans are a group of synthetic nitrofurane derivatives with broad-spectrum antibacterial action; thousands of derivatives have been developed since the 5-nitrofuraldehyde basic structure was described in

1930. They are stable compounds, slightly soluble in water. Nitrofurantoin is a weak acid (pK_a 7.2), but nifuratel has no ionizable group. Five compounds are sometimes used in veterinary medicine: nitrofurazone, nitrofurantoin, nifuratel, nifuroquine, and furazolidone.

Mechanism of Action

Bacterial nitroreductase enzymes degrade nitrofurans to a variety of poorly characterized reduction products that differ depending on the nitrofuran involved. The antibacterial effect of nitrofurans results from these reduction products, which among other effects prevent mRNA translation by disrupting codon-anticodon interactions.

Antimicrobial Activity

Nitrofurazone, nitrofurantoin, nifuratel, and furazolidone have similar antimicrobial activity. They are relatively broad-spectrum drugs, active against bacteria, some protozoa, and some fungi. Nitrofurans are bactericidal at concentrations just over MIC. The antibacterial activity of many is markedly reduced by alkaline conditions. The activity of nitrofurantoin is greatly enhanced at pH 5.5 or below but diminished by very high concentrations of bacteria in urine.

Gram-positive bacteria such as *Staphylococcus aureus*, streptococci, and many corynebacteria are susceptible. Among Gram-negative bacteria, *Escherichia coli* and *Salmonella* are usually susceptible, as are *Klebsiella*; *Proteus* species are often, and *Pseudomonas aeruginosa* are always, resistant (Table 16.1). Nitrofurans have moderate activity against anaerobic bacteria and are most active under anaerobic conditions. Some aerobic bacteria that are resistant under aerobic conditions are susceptible when tested under anaerobic conditions. Nitrofurans are active against mycoplasmas, and some have antiprotozoal activity (coccidia, trypanosomes). Nifuratel, 0.1–1.0 µg/ml, has good activity against *Trichomonas vaginalis* and presumably also *Tritrichomonas foetus* of cattle. Furazolidone has good activity against *Giardia lamblia*.

Furazolidone has the greatest antibacterial activity, followed by nitrofurazone and nitrofurantoin. In one study, the MIC_{50} of *Salmonella dublin* was 1.25 µg/ml for furazolidone, 10 µg/ml for nitrofurazone, and 40 µg/ml for nitrofurantoin.

Most information on susceptibility relates to urinary tract concentrations of the drug in humans. In the disk diffusion procedure, the National Committee for Clinical Laboratory Standards (NCCLS) regards bacteria with an inhibitory zone equivalent to MIC ≤64 µg/ml as susceptible. There are no agreed criteria to define susceptibility when furazolidone or nitrofurazone is administered parenterally, but maximum blood concentrations after nontoxic doses in humans are about 2–4 µg/ml. The MIC of

TABLE 16.1. Antimicrobial activity (MIC_{90}, µg/ml) of nitrofurans against selected bacteria

Organism	Nitrofurazone MIC_{90}	Furazolidone MIC_{90}
Gram-positive bacteria		
Clostridium perfringens		4
Enterococcus spp.	16	2
Staphylococcus aureus	8	2
Streptococcus uberis	16	16
Beta-hemolytic streptococci	8	
Gram-negative bacteria		
Actinobacillus pleuropneumoniae		0.13
Bacteroides nodosus	4	
Campylobacter jejuni		0.25
Escherichia coli	4	1
Helicobacter pylori	0.5	
Klebsiella spp.	64	8
Moraxella bovis	1	
Proteus spp.	64	64
Pseudomonas spp.	>256	>256
Salmonella spp.	8	4
Serpulina hyodysenteriae	16	
Mycoplasmas		
Mycoplasma hyorhinis	8	
Ureaplasma spp.		0.25

susceptible bacteria can thus be regarded as ≤2–4 µg/ml when the drugs are used systemically.

Resistance

Like other antibiotics that affect DNA synthesis, resistance is almost exclusively chromosomal. Resistance involves either absence of intracellular reductase enzymes or the development of a permeability barrier. The latter is sometimes associated with the presence of R factors specifying resistance to unrelated antibiotics. Cross-resistance occurs among the nitrofurans and has been reported with the nitroimidazoles, which may share a common mechanism of action.

Chromosomal mutation to resistance develops in a gradual, stepwise manner. Such resistance often represents a slight shift, perhaps only 4-fold; however, even slight increases may have important in vivo effects. For example, a decrease in susceptibility of Salmonella gallinarum to furazolidone from 0.3 µg/ml to 1.3–2.5 µg/ml was sufficient to neutralize the clinical effect of the drug in chickens (Smith et al., 1981).

There is a general impression that antibacterial resistance to nitrofurans has not changed much over the years, but most testing is done with high-potency disks to determine susceptibility to high concentrations of drugs, such as are present in the urinary tract. Subtle but important shifts in resistance are not detected by these tests. The high frequency of susceptibility in enterotoxigenic *E. coli* and *Salmonella* reported in some countries may thus be more apparent than real, although a recent report from Australia confirmed the high susceptibility of *Salmonella enteritidis* isolates in vitro (Cox et al., 1996).

Pharmacokinetic Properties

Nitrofurantoin is well absorbed after oral administration. The half-life is short because the drug is rapidly excreted through the kidneys in the urine; blood and tissue concentrations are too low for treatment of systemic infections. Mean urine concentrations are between 50 and 250 µg/ml. Maximum excretion occurs within 3–4 hours. Nitrofurazone and furazolidone are poorly soluble and are not absorbed after oral administration. The metabolism of nitrofurans is poorly understood because of the production of many extremely unstable metabolites in tissues (Nouws et al., 1987).

Drug Interactions

Nitrofurans are antagonistic with nalidixic acid, which acts at the same site. It seems likely that the same is true with other nucleic acid inhibitors.

Toxicity and Adverse Effects

Since nitrofurans are mutagenic and procarcinogenic, their use has been prohibited in some countries, including in food animals in the United States. High oral doses of furazolidone or nitrofurantoin result in central nervous effects in animals, and lower doses in calves and dogs have caused hemorrhagic diathesis with thrombocytopenia, anemia, leukocytopenia, and prolonged bleeding times. Anorexia, nausea, and vomiting occur with high doses in all species. Other serious adverse effects, reported in humans, include peripheral neuropathy, which occurs days or even years after continuous or intermittent administration; acute or chronic pulmonary reactions may also occur. Although these drugs may be mutagenic, no long-term adverse carcinogenic effects have been detected in humans.

Administration orally of 7.1 mg/kg daily of nitrofurazone to calves is nontoxic; higher doses result in inappetence, irritability, and convulsions. For furazolidone, fatal dose-related hemorrhagic diathesis develops in calves and dogs administered the drug over long periods; dosage of furazolidone only twice that recommended has, however, caused granulocytopenia in calves (Sheldon, 1994). Accidental administration of more than 3,000 ppm in feed caused nervous symptoms in pigs (Borland, 1979). Dose-related congestive cardiomyopathy has been described clinically or induced experimentally in turkeys, chickens, and ducklings fed excessive amounts of furazolidone. Furazolidone is directly cardiotoxic in these species.

Administration and Dosage

In countries where the use of nitrofurans in food animals is allowed, they are administered to livestock at dosages of about 10–12 mg/kg for 5–7 days. Concentrations used in feed for pigs vary from 100 to 500 ppm and 100 mg/l are used in water. In dogs, 4 mg/kg nitrofurantoin has been administered 3 times daily PO for 5–7 days to treat urinary tract infections.

Clinical Applications

The clinical use of nitrofurans is limited by poor solubility and by toxicity. Their use is prohibited in food animals in some countries. Nitrofurantoin is occasionally used for urinary tract infections and nitrofurazone or furazolidone for enteric infections in farm animals. All, but especially furazolidone, are potentially useful for local treatment of infections in the udder, uterus, and skin, where their broad bactericidal activity is not hampered by toxicity or solubility problems. Care should be taken in mixing nitrofurans in milk replacer for calves, in order to avoid accidental overdosing, and the drug should not be used for prolonged periods.

Repeated treatment with nifuroquine of *Mycoplasma bovis* mastitis resulted in complete disappearance of infection from a herd in which other drugs had failed (Hartman et al., 1981). Nifuroquine has been used successfully in the treatment of bacterial mastitis and in dry-cow therapy (Ziv et al., 1987).

The drugs have also been effective in topical treatment of infections— for example, uterine infections. Although sometimes used in the treatment of infectious bovine keratoconjunctivitis *(Moraxella bovis)* in cattle, a field trial of topically applied furazolidone showed no significant difference from untreated controls. In addition, a progressive increase in MIC of *M. bovis* isolates was observed over the course of treatment (George et al., 1988).

In swine, furazolidone and other nitrofurans have been used extensively in the prevention and treatment of colibacillosis and salmonellosis in swine. The nitrofurans have been used in enteric infections in horses, in which they are also used in the topical treatment of bacterial infections. In dogs and cats, nitrofurantoin is sometimes used to treat bacterial urinary tract infections caused by otherwise resistant organisms.

Nitrofurazone and furazolidone have been used in the prevention of coccidiosis in poultry and furaltadone in the treatment of salmonellosis and *M. gallisepticum* infections. Nitrofurans are sometimes used in the treatment of nonspecific enteritis in poultry.

Bibliography

Borland ED. 1979. An incident of suspected furazolidone toxicity in pigs. Vet Rec 105:169.
Cox JM, et al. 1996. Sensitivity of Australian isolates of *Salmonella enteritidis* to nitrofurantoin and furazolidone. Vet Microbiol 9:305.
George LW, et al. 1988. Topically applied furazolidone or parenterally administered oxytetracycline for the treatment of infectious bovine keratoconjunctivitis. J Am Vet Med Assoc 192:1415.
Hartman EG, et al. 1981. *Mycoplasma bovis* alj oorzaak van een mastitisuitbraak bij runderen in Nederland. Tijdschr Diergeneeskd 106:3.
Hayashi T, et al. 1976. Hematological and pathological observations of chronic furazolidone poisoning in calves. Jap J Vet Sci 38:225.
Nouws JFM, Laurensen J. 1990. Postmortal degradation of furazolidone and furaltadone in edible tissues of calves. Vet Q 12:56.
Nouws JFM, et al. 1987. Some pharmacokinetic data about furaltadone and nitrofurazone administered orally to preruminant calves. Vet Q 9:208.
Sheldon IM. 1994. A field case of granulocytopenic disease of calves. Vet Rec 135:408.
Smith HW, et al. 1981. Furazolidone resistance in *Salmonella gallinarum*: the relationship between in vitro and in vivo determinations of resistance. J Hyg Camb 87:71.
Ziv G, et al. 1987. Efficacy of an intramammary nifuroquine dry cow product in the elimination and prevention of udder infections. Isr J Vet Med 43:3.

Nitroimidazoles

A variety of nitroimidazoles (Fig. 16.1)—metronidazole, dimetridazole, ronidazole, tinidazole, ipronidazole—are used in veterinary medicine, particularly for their activity against anaerobic bacteria. They are similar to the nitrofurans in spectrum of activity and mechanism of action but are not active against aerobic bacteria. Metronidazole has particularly useful activity against protozoa, such as *Tritrichomonas foetus* and *Giardia*. Because of potential carcinogenicity of uncertain significance, nitroimidazoles are no longer used in food-producing animals in certain countries, including the United States, or are selectively used in others.

Chemistry

Nitroimidazoles are heterocyclic compounds based on a five-membered nucleus similar to that of the nitrofurans.

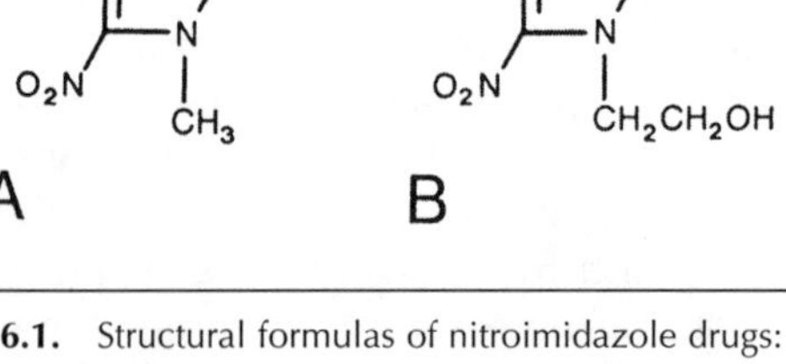

Fig. 16.1. Structural formulas of nitroimidazole drugs: *A*, metronidazole; *B*, dimetridazole.

Mechanism of Action

After entry into the cell, nitroimidazoles undergo reduction of the nitro group to produce a variety of unstable intermediates, among which are the antibacterial products. Reduction occurs under anaerobic conditions but, unlike that of the nitrofurans, is not enzymatically controlled. The reduction system of aerobic bacteria is insufficiently low for reduction to occur, but there is the suggestion that these agents or their metabolites, produced by anaerobic bacteria, may have some activity against aerobic bacteria under anaerobic conditions. Nitroimidazoles cause extensive breakage of DNA strands and inhibition of the DNA repair enzyme DNAase 1.

Antimicrobial Activity

The antimicrobial activity of the clinically useful nitroimidazoles is similar. They are bactericidal to most Gram-negative and many Gram-positive anaerobic bacteria (Table 16.2). They are highly active against *Serpulina hyodysenteriae* and a variety of protozoa *(Tritrichomonas foetus, Giardia lamblia, Histomonas meleagridis)*. In vitro studies show decreasing activity against *T. foetus* in the following order: dimetridazole, metronidazole, and ronidazole. *Campylobacter* spp. are moderately susceptible. *Helicobacter pylori* are commonly susceptible, but the susceptibility of animal-derived *Helicobacter* species has not been sufficiently investigated to be able to make any statement regarding their activity.

Resistance

Resistance is rare among usually susceptible bacteria, a characteristic shared with the nitrofurans. Resistance involves reduced intracellular drug activation. Clinical experience is that swine dysentery shows increased resistance to dimetridazole in some herds, but surveys of the susceptibility of *Serpulina hyodysenteriae* have not seemed to support this

TABLE 16.2. Activity (MIC$_{90}$, µg/ml) of metronidazole against selected anaerobic bacteria

Organism	MIC$_{90}$	Organism	MIC$_{90}$
Gram-positive anaerobes			
Actinomyces spp.	>128	*Clostridium* spp.	4
Clostridium difficile	0.5	*Eubacterium* spp.	4
C. perfringens	2	*Peptococcus* spp.	1
C. septicum	2	*Peptostreptococcus* spp.	≥64
Gram-negative anaerobes			
All anaerobes	2	*Fusobacterium* spp.	0.5
Bacteroides spp.	2	*Porphyromonas asaccharolytica*	2
B. fragilis	2	*Serpulina hyodysenteriae*	0.5

finding (Jenkinson and Wingar, 1983). Cross-resistance between nitroimidazoles is complete; some occurs with nitrofurans. Resistance in *Trichomonas vaginalis* was reported to metronidazole as the result of a several-fold increase in MIC (Lossick et al., 1986). Equine isolates of *Clostridium difficile* resistant to metronidazole have been described, apparently the result of exposure of horses to a common source (Jang et al., 1997).

Pharmacokinetic Properties

Metronidazole is completely absorbed after oral administration in monogastric species and has a half-life in humans of 6–10 hours. The drug is extensively oxidized and conjugated in the liver to less active forms, but about two-thirds of the dose is excreted in the urine, mostly in the active form. Tissue penetration is excellent, including penetration into brain and cerebrospinal fluid (CSF). Other nitroimidazoles have similar properties, although their half-lives in humans and animals are often longer.

The half-life in horses of metronidazole following IV administration was 3.9 hours (Baggot et al., 1988). The drug was well-absorbed after oral administration to horses and was distributed well to tissues. The half-life of tinidazole in horses after IV administration was 5.2 hours (Pyorala et al., 1990b) but in cows was 2.4 hours (Pyorala et al., 1990a). Tinidazole was well absorbed after oral administration to horses but (as expected) poorly absorbed in cattle after oral administration (Pyorala et al., 1990a,b).

Drug Interactions

No interference with the susceptibility of anaerobic bacteria has been reported in vitro when metronidazole is combined with a variety of other anaerobe-active drugs, such as clindamycin, erythromycin, penicillin G, amoxicillin-clavulanic acid, cefoxitin, and rifampin. Combined with gentamicin or tobramycin, metronidazole has been used successfully in humans in the treatment of serious peritonitis caused by intestinal spillage.

Toxicity and Adverse Effects

There are rare reports of adverse reactions to nitroimidazoles in domestic animals. The most serious potential hazard is the marginal and contentious carcinogenic effect observed in some laboratory animal studies. No significant increase in cancer-related morbidity was observed in women treated with metronidazole for vaginal trichomoniasis (Beard et al., 1988). The drug should not be used in early pregnancy. In humans, nausea is a common side effect of treatment with metronidazole; rashes, peripheral neuropathy, epileptiform seizures, and dark urine are reported rarely. Neurotoxicity has been reported in ducklings. Vomiting, nausea, and nervousness are sometimes noted in dogs and cats, as is inappetence in horses. Cats often salivate profusely after oral administration of metronidazole. Acute central nervous toxicosis was reported in 5 dogs administered dosages of 67–129 mg/kg per day after 6–12 days of treatment (Dow et al., 1989). The clinical signs were dose-related response and included severe ataxia, positional and vertical nystagmus, seizures, and head tilt. Similar neurologic symptoms have been described in cats between 5 days and many months of starting high dose (>48–62 mg/kg daily) metronidazole treatment (Saxon and Magne, 1993). Dosage in dogs and cats should probably not exceed 30 mg/kg daily. Oral daily dosing of bulls with 60 mg/kg for 5 days was well tolerated, although a small proportion of animals showed mild digestive disturbances.

Administration and Dosage

Dosage recommendations are shown in Table 16.3. Since antibacterial effect is concentration dependent, twice rather than three times daily administration is recommended. The drugs are not approved by the U.S. Food and Drug Administration for any use in food animals. If bulls are treated for trichomoniasis, they cannot be slaughtered in the United States for food.

In cattle, Skirrow et al. (1985) reported on the apparent 100% efficacy of an inexpensive imidazole, ipronidazole (30 g dissolved in 60 ml sterile water, administered IM on day 1 and 15 g in 30 ml water on days 2 and 3) for the treatment of *Tritrichomonas foetus* infection. Procaine penicillin G was administered for 2 days before treatment to prevent preputial commensal bacteria from metabolizing the drug, as this pretreatment significantly enhances the effectiveness of imidazole treatments. Abscesses developed at injection sites in 12% of bulls (BonDurant, 1985). Topical administration of a 5% ointment with a urethral douche containing 30 ml

TABLE 16.3. Usual systemic dosages of metronidazole and tinidazole in animals

Species	Drug	Route	Dose (mg/kg)	Interval (h)	Comment
Dogs, cats	Metronidazole	PO (IV, SC)	22 loading dose, then 15	12	Anaerobic infections
Dogs	Metronidazole	PO	10	12	Colitis, stomatitis
Cats	Metronidazole	PO	10	12–24	Giardiasis
Dogs	Metronidazole	PO	15	12	Giardiasis
Dogs, cats	Tinidazole	PO	15	12 (dogs), 24 (cats)	Anaerobic infections
Horses	Metronidazole	PO	15	12	Adult
	Tinidazole	PO	12	12	
Bulls	Metronidazole	IV	75	12	3 doses only: *Tritrichomonas foetus* infection

of a 1% solution has been effective against *Tritrichomonas* infection. At a dosage of 100 mg/kg intraruminally for 5 days, natural *Campylobacter fetus* infection in bulls was apparently cured (Stoessel and Haberkorn, 1977).

Dimetridazole incorporated in feed at 0.007–0.02% or in water at 0.006–0.0125% is often successful in preventing or treating swine dysentery. Ronidazole in feed (60–120 ppm) or water (0.006%) has a similar effect. Concentrations in feed of 90–120 ppm are required to eliminate infection (Taylor, 1976).

Dimetridazole is administered in water to prevent (150–200 ppm) or treat (600–800 ppm) blackhead in turkeys. A lower dose is used for ipronidazole or ronidazole.

Clinical Applications

Nitroimidazoles are not approved by the U.S. Food and Drug Administration for any use in food animals. The drugs are important for their efficacy against anaerobic bacteria and protozoa. They are used extensively in some countries to prevent and treat swine dysentery, to treat *Tritrichomonas foetus* infections in bulls, and to treat anaerobic infections and *Giardia lamblia* enteritis in dogs and cats. Concentrations in brain and CSF are excellent, so nitroimidazoles have a special place in the treatment of anaerobic brain abscess.

Metronidazole is used to treat a wide variety of anaerobic infections, such as postoperative or posttraumatic abdominal and genitourinary infections, pleuropulmonary infections, dental infections, and abscesses. The drug has the advantage of oral administration but the drawback of inactivity against aerobic bacteria. For this reason it is often combined with an aminoglycoside, particularly when Gram-negative aerobes are likely to be present. Metronidazole has activity equal to that of clindamycin and penicillin G, and sometimes better than that of erythromycin. In the treatment of peritonitis associated with intestinal spillage in humans, the superiority of metronidazole over clindamycin or erythromycin (all combined with an aminoglycoside) has not been demonstrated convincingly (Bartlett, 1982). Metronidazole is active against penicillinase-producing *Bacteroides fragilis* and is the drug of choice in acute ulcerative gingivitis. Metronidazole, combined with bismuth (or acid-suppressing drugs) and amoxicillin or tetracycline, is used in people in the treatment of *Helicobacter* gastritis.

CATTLE

Nitroimidazoles have been used to treat *Tritrichomonas foetus* infections in bulls. The drugs cause severe necrosis at the IM injection sites and are therefore given IV or PO. They have also been used successfully to treat genital *Campylobacter* infections (Campero et al., 1987). Pyometra in cows caused by mixed aerobic and anaerobic bacteria was treated by a single intrauterine infusion of metronidazole with ampicillin or neomycin with approximately 50% and 70% success in complete bacteriological and clinical cure (Stephens and Slee, 1987). However, the use of this class of drugs in animals destined for the human food chain is forbidden in the United States.

SWINE

Dimetridazole, ronidazole, and ipronidazole are used to prevent and treat swine dysentery. The higher doses are required to eliminate infection. Because of possible human health hazard through meat residues, the use of these agents in food animals is not approved in the United States. Clinical experience suggests that resistance develops in *Serpulina hyodysenteriae* with prolonged use, although in vitro studies may not support this suggestion.

HORSES

Metronidazole is used orally in the treatment of anaerobic or mixed aerobic-anaerobic infections, particularly involving the respiratory and gastrointestinal tract (Sweeney et al., 1991). In the treatment of mixed aerobic-anaerobic infections, it should be combined with other drugs, such as aminoglycosides. Metronidazole was used successfully to treat anaerobic pleuropneumonia when administered at 20 mg/kg IM once daily (Mair and Yeo, 1987). Metronidazole (oral or IM) appears particularly useful in anaerobic pleuropneumonia in horses. Metronidazole administered orally is used in the effective treatment of *Clostridium difficile* or acute idiopathic toxemic colitis in horses (McGorum et al., 1998), although resistant *C. difficile* have been described.

DOGS AND CATS

Metronidazole or tinidazole is effective in the treatment of anaerobic infections such as acute gingivitis and periodontal disease (for which they are a drug of choice, like clindamycin), abscesses, and anal sac infections. Metronidazole is highly effective in the treatment of *Giardia* enteritis in dogs (for 5–7 days) and has been used successfully to treat undiagnosed chronic diarrhea in dogs and cats, possibly associated with *Campylobacter jejuni* or *Clostridium difficile* (Berry and Levett, 1986).

Bibliography

Baggot JD, et al. 1988. Clinical pharmacokinetics of metronidazole in horses. J Vet Pharmacol Ther 11:417.
Bartlett JG. 1982. Anti-anaerobic antibacterial agents. Lancet ii:478.

Beard CM, et al. 1988. Cancer after exposure to metronidazole. Mayo Clin Proc 63:147.

Berry AP, Levett PN. 1986. Chronic diarrhea in dogs associated with *Clostridium difficile* infection. Vet Rec 118:102.

BonDurant RH. 1985. Diagnosis, treatment, and control of bovine trichomoniasis. Compend Contin Educ Pract Vet 7:S179.

Campero CM, et al. 1987. Dual infection with campylobacteriosis and trichomoniasis: bulls with treatment with dimetridazole chlorhydrate. Aust Vet J 64:320.

Dow SW, et al. 1989. Central nervous system toxicosis associated with metronidazole treatment of dogs: five cases (1984–1987). J Am Vet Med Assoc 195:365.

Freeman CD, et al. 1997. Metronidazole: a therapeutic review and update. Drugs 54:679.

Jang SS, et al. 1997. Antimicrobial susceptibilities of equine isolates of *Clostridium difficile* and molecular characterization of metronidazole-resistant strains. Clin Infect Dis 25:S266.

Jenkinson SR, Wingar CR. 1983. Sensitivity to dimetridazole of field isolates of *Treponema hyodysenteriae*. Vet Rec 112:58.

Lossick JG, et al. 1986. In vitro drug susceptibility and doses of metronidazole required for cure of refractory vaginal trichomoniasis. J Infect Dis 153:948.

Mair TS, Yeo SP. 1987. Equine pleuropneumonia: the importance of anaerobic bacteria and the potential value of metronidazole in treatment. Vet Rec 121:109.

McGorum BC, et al. 1998. Use of metronidazole in equine acute idiopathic toxaemic colitis. Vet Rec 142:635.

Pyorala S, et al. 1990a. Pharmacokinetics of tinidazole in cows—preliminary study. J Vet Pharmacol Ther 13:425.

Pyorala S, et al. 1990b. Pharmacokinetics of tinidazole in the horse. J Vet Pharmacol Ther 13:76.

Pyorala S, et al. 1994. Pharmacokinetics of single-dose administration of tinidazole in unweaned calves. Am J Vet Res 55:831.

Roe FJC. 1983. Toxicologic evaluation of metronidazole with particular reference to carcinogenic, mutagenic, and teratogenic potential. Surgery 93:158.

Sarkiala EM. 1993. Treatment of periodontitis in dogs with tinidazole. J Small Anim Pract 34:90.

Sarkiala-Kessel EM, et al. 1996. Concentrations of tinidazole in gingival crevicular fluid and plasma in dogs after multiple dose administration. J Vet Pharmacol Ther 19:171.

Saxon B, Magne ML. 1993. Reversible central nervous system toxicosis associated with metronidazole therapy in three cats. Prog Vet Neurol 4:25.

Skirrow S, et al. 1985. Efficacy of ipronidazole against trichomoniasis in bulls. J Am Vet Med Assoc 187:405.

Stephens LR, Slee KJ. 1987. Metronidazole for the treatment of bovine pyometra. Aust Vet J 64:343.

Stoessel FR, Haberkorn SEM. 1977. Efecto del metanosulfanato de dimetridazole inyectado por via intraruminal como tricomonicida en los toros. Gac Vet 39:5060 (Vet Bull 1978:3608).

Sweeney RW, et al. 1991. Clinical use of metronidazole in horses: 200 cases (1984–1989). J Am Vet Med Assoc 198:1045.

Taylor DJ. 1976. Ronidazole in the treatment and prophylaxis of experimental swine dysentery. Vet Rec 99:453.

Rifamycins

Rifampin (Fig. 16.2) is the most important synthetically modified member of the family of the rifamycins, antibiotic products of *Amycolatopsis mediterranei*. Rifampin is a highly active first-line oral drug for the treatment of tuberculosis in humans and, until recently, had been largely

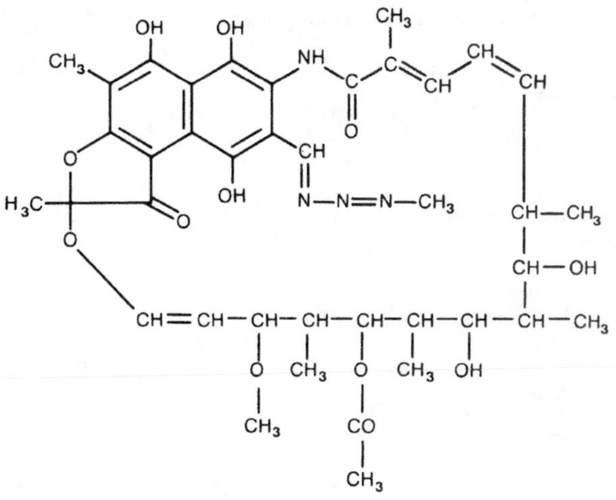

Fig. 16.2. Structural formula of rifampin.

reserved for that purpose in human medicine, so that its value in treatment of other infections may have been underestimated. It is always combined with other antibiotics because of the ready development of resistance to the drug. It has good activity against Gram-positive bacteria and anaerobes and some unimportant antiviral and antifungal activity. Other semisynthetic derivatives of rifamycin (rifabutin, rifapentine) are in clinical use and have the slight advantage over rifampin of less induction of hepatic enzymes. Only rifampin will be discussed.

Chemistry

Rifampin is an ansamycin, possessing an aromatic ring system spanned by an aliphatic bridge. It is soluble in organic solvents and in water at acid pH.

Mechanism of Action

Rifampin has the action unique among antibiotics of inhibiting RNA polymerase. Rifampin binds to the beta subunit of the enzyme and causes abortive initiation of RNA synthesis. Gram-negative bacteria are relatively impermeable to the drug.

Antimicrobial Activity

Rifampin is a bactericidal antibiotic with a wide spectrum of antimicrobial activity; it is inhibitory to bacteria, *Chlamydia*, *Rickettsia*, some protozoa, and poxviruses. Particularly active against Gram-positive bacteria

TABLE 16.4. Activity (MIC$_{90}$, µg/ml) of rifampin against selected bacteria

Organism	MIC$_{90}$	Organism	MIC$_{90}$
Gram-positive aerobes			
Bacillus anthracis	0.03	*Nocardia* spp.	>256
Corynebacterium pseudotuberculosis	≤0.25	*Rhodococcus equi*	0.06
Enterococcus spp.	≥4	*Staphylococcus aureus*	0.03
Listeria monocytogenes	0.25	Beta-hemolytic streptococci	8
Mycobacterium avium complex	4		
M. fortuitum	>64		
M. tuberculosis	<0.03		
Gram-positive anaerobes			
Actinomyces spp.	0.06	*C. septicum*	≤0.13
Clostridium difficile	≤0.25	*Clostridium* spp.	1
C. perfringens	0.13	*Peptostreptococcus*	32
Gram-negative aerobes			
Actinobacillus pleuropneumoniae	0.5	*Escherichia coli*	16
Bordetella bronchiseptica	≥128	*Klebsiella pneumoniae*	32
Brucella abortus	2	*Pasteurella* spp.	1
B. canis	1	*Proteus* spp.	32
Campylobacter jejuni	>128	*Pseudomonas aeruginosa*	64
Gram-negative anaerobes			
Bacteroides fragilis	1	*Porphyromonas asaccharolytica*	0.25
Fusobacterium spp.	2		

and some mycobacteria, rifampin is the most active drug known against *Staphylococcus aureus* and is very active against *Mycobacterium tuberculosis*, but most other mycobacteria are resistant. It is the most active drug known against *Chlamydia trachomatis* (MIC <0.25 µg/ml) and is very active against *Coxiella burnetii*. Gram-negative bacteria are generally resistant, although *Brucella* and other fastidious organisms are susceptible. Both Gram-positive and Gram-negative anaerobic bacteria are inhibited by low concentrations, and the drug is active against *Bacteroides fragilis* (Table 16.4).

Bacteria with MIC ≤2 µg/ml are regarded as susceptible and those with MIC 2–4 µg/ml as moderately susceptible.

Resistance

Chromosomal mutation to high-level resistance to rifampin develops readily in most bacteria. Such mutants show stable changes in RNA polymerase that prevent binding. Because the mutation rate is so high, about 1 in 10^7 or 10^8 bacteria, the drug should never be used alone to treat infections. Resistance to rifampin is not transferable, and there is no cross-resistance with other antibiotics.

Pharmacokinetic Properties

Absorption of rifampin is good after oral administration in monogastrates, with peak blood concentrations occurring within 2–4 hours (see

Fig. 4.6). The half-life in humans is about 4 hours, in horses 6 hours, in calves 3 hours, in sheep 4.5 hours, and in dogs 8 hours. The drug is highly lipophilic and diffuses rapidly into tissues, reaching concentrations exceeding those in serum. Penetration into phagocytic cells is excellent, achieving concentrations several times those of serum. Penetration into CSF is poor but is improved by inflammation (10–90% of serum concentrations). Excretion in humans is partially in bile (40%) and partially in the urine. Enterohepatic recirculation occurs, so that therapeutic concentrations may be maintained in plasma for relatively long periods. After intestinal absorption, rifampin is metabolized in the liver largely to 25-desacetylrifampin, a bioactive form. Desacetylation is a rate-limiting process in the metabolism of rifampin. Peak serum concentrations following oral administration of 10 mg/kg are 10 μg/ml in humans, 40 μg/ml in dogs, and 2.9 μg/ml in horses, reflecting differences in oral bioavailability in these species (Frank, 1990). Metabolism in foals is significantly slower than in adult horses (Castro et al., 1986). Serum concentrations of about 1 μg/ml were achieved in adult sheep for about 8 hours following oral dosage with 10 mg/kg (Sweeney et al., 1988). Rifampin metabolites may color urine, saliva, and feces orange red.

Drug Interactions

Concurrent use with other antibiotics reduces the development of mutants resistant to rifampin, which should never be used alone. Studies of the in vitro interaction of rifampin with other drugs have shown, as expected, effects varying from synergism to antagonism, although even antagonistic combinations may prevent the emergence of rifampin-resistant strains. Combination with trimethoprim produced apparent synergy against many organisms isolated from the human urinary tract (Brumfitt et al., 1983). The interactions with other antibiotics are complex and unpredictable; for example, in one study of the interaction of rifampin with cloxacillin in the treatment of experimental *Staphylococcus aureus* endocarditis, both synergism and antagonism were observed, depending on dosage (Zak et al., 1983).

Despite the uncertainty of the in vitro effect of some drug combinations, clinical response in humans with staphylococcal infections to treatment with vancomycin-rifampin, nafcillin-rifampin, or oxacillin-rifampin has been good. Clinical results suggest that combination with kanamycin, gentamicin, erythromycin, or fusidic acid in the treatment of *S. aureus* infections appears most promising. Against *Rhodococcus equi* in vitro, rifampin exhibits synergism with erythromycin and penicillin G but is antagonistic with gentamicin.

Rifampin is a potent hepatic enzyme inducer and produces clinically important increases in the rate of metabolism of other drugs, including oral anticoagulants, digitoxin, barbiturates, theophylline, ketoconazole, corticosteroids, and other steroid hormones, so that increased dosage of these drugs may be required.

Toxicity and Adverse Effects

Side effects reported in humans are uncommon. A small number of patients have developed self-limiting hepatotoxicity of varying degrees. The drug acts as a hapten, so that antibody formation has occurred after several months, resulting in effects varying from mild skin eruptions to, rarely, thrombocytopenia, hemolytic anemia, shock, and acute renal insufficiency. The immunoallergic effect occurs most commonly in patients treated with large doses given intermittently over long periods. The drug may be teratogenic and should not be administered to pregnant animals. It should not be administered to patients with liver disease.

In dogs, increases in hepatic enzyme activities may be relatively common and can progress to clinical hepatitis, which may be fatal in dogs with a history of liver disease (Frank, 1990). More information is required on adverse effects, which may relate to increased bioavailability in dogs.

Administration and Dosage

Rifampin is available in capsule form for oral administration. A dosage of 10 mg/kg PO q12 hours is recommended in adult horses and 5 mg/kg q24 hours in foals; in dogs and cats a suitable dosage is 10 mg/kg q24 hours; in sheep and calves an oral dosage of 20 mg/kg q24 hours may be suitable. Administration to adult ruminants is, however, preferably by IM or IV injection (10 mg/kg q24 hours).

Clinical Applications

Rifampin has been used extensively in treating human tuberculosis and for many years was reserved for that purpose. It has also been used in humans to treat carriers of *Neisseria meningitidis* and for serious staphylococcal infections. When used to treat staphylococcal infections, it is combined with penicillinase-resistant penicillins, vancomycin, or trimethoprim. It may be used in this manner to treat serious staphylococcal infections (eg, osteomyelitis) in animals.

An attractive feature of rifampin is its ability to kill intracellular bacteria. There is veterinary interest in its use against macrophage-associated bacteria such as *Brucella*, *Rhodococcus equi*, *Corynebacterium pseudotuberculosis*, and intracellular *Staphylococcus aureus*, including those associated with bovine mastitis. The drug has been used with reasonable success in treating human brucellosis *(Brucella melitensis)* when combined with doxycycline and is effective when combined with oral erythromycin in the treatment of *R. equi* pneumonia of foals. *Mycobacterium paratuberculo-*

sis is susceptible to rifampin, which has been shown to reduce experimental infection in mice (Chiodini et al., 1993). A combination of streptomycin-isoniazid-rifampin seemed to be effective in treating Johne's disease in a goat (Slocombe, 1982), but postmortem findings suggested that the therapy had only a palliative effect. Rifampin is often used with clarithromycin in the treatment of atypical mycobacterial infections (see Chapter 19).

Rifampin has been found to be as effective as tetracyclines in the treatment of *Chlamydia trachomatis* in humans and might be useful in *C. psittaci* infections in animals, as well as in *Coxiella burnetii* infections. A combination of rifampin and erythromycin has been used in the successful medical treatment of *Coxiella* placentitis (Bental et al., 1995). Similarly, the combination has been used successfully in the treatment of experimentally induced *Ehrlichia risticii* infection (Palmer and Benson, 1992). The drug may be efficacious alone or in combination in the treatment of *Bartonella henselae* infection in cats (Breitschwerdt and Greene, 1998). However, the potential for selecting resistant strains must be considered when rifampin is used as a single agent.

More information is needed about the clinical efficacy of rifampin in a variety of infections in animals, including brucellosis, caseous lymphadenitis, chlamydiosis, listeriosis, mycobacterial infections, and anaerobic infections.

Bibliography

Bental T, et al. 1995. Chronic Q fever of pregnancy presenting as *Coxiella burnetii* placentitis: successful outcome following therapy with erythromycin and rifampin. Clin Infect Dis 21:1318.

Breitschwerdt EB, Greene CE. 1998. Bartonellosis. In: Greene CE, ed. Infectious Diseases of the Dog and Cat. Philadelphia: WB Saunders, p337.

Brumfitt W, et al. 1983. Use of rifampin for the treatment of urinary tract infections. Rev Infect Dis 5:S573.

Burrows GE, et al. 1992a. Rifampin disposition in the horse: effects of age and method of oral administration. J Vet Pharmacol Ther 15:124.

Burrows GE, et al. 1992b. Rifampin disposition in the horse: effects of repeated dosage of rifampin or phenylbutazone. J Vet Pharmacol Ther 15:305.

Castro LA, et al. 1986. Pharmacokinetics of rifampin given as a single oral dose in foals. Am J Vet Res 47:2584.

Chiodini RJ, et al. 1993. Use of rifabutin in treatment of systemic *Mycobacterium paratuberculosis* infection in mice. Antimicrob Agents Chemother 37:1645.

Frank LA. 1990. Clinical pharmacology of rifampin. J Am Vet Med Assoc 197:114.

Gillis JC, Brogden RN. 1995. Rifamixin. Drugs 49:467.

Jernigan AD, et al. 1991. Pharmacokinetics of rifampin in adult sheep. Am J Vet Res 52:1626.

Kohn CW, et al. 1993. Pharmacokinetics of single intravenous and single and multiple dose oral administration of rifampin in mares. J Vet Pharmacol Ther 16:119.

Palmer JE, Benson CE. 1992. Effect of treatment with erythromycin and rifampin during the acute stages of experimentally induced equine ehrlichial colitis in ponies. Am J Vet Res 53:2071.

Slocombe RF. 1982. Combined streptomycin-isoniazid-rifampin therapy in the treatment of Johne's disease in goats. Can Vet J 23:160.
Sweeney RW, et al. 1988. Pharmacokinetics of rifampin in calves and adult sheep. J Vet Pharmacol Ther 11:413.
Wilson WD, et al. 1988. Pharmacokinetics, bioavailability, and in vitro antibacterial activity of rifampin in the horse. Am J Vet Res 49:2041.
Zak O, et al. 1983. Rifampin in experimental endocarditis due to *Staphylococcus aureus* in rabbits. Rev Infect Dis 5:S481.

Arsenicals

Arsenic-containing compounds (arsanilic acid, sodium arsanilate, 3-nitro-4-hydroxyphenylarsonic acid) are used to promote growth in pigs and poultry and to treat swine dysentery. They are sometimes used to control chronic diarrhea of unknown etiology in swine. Sodium arsanilate is used at 100 ppm in feed as a growth promoter and at 200–400 ppm for 7 days to control swine dysentery. There is little recent information on the efficacy of arsenicals in swine. The drugs must be withdrawn 10 days before slaughter. Toxicity is likely to occur if the drugs are administered at therapeutic doses for more than 7 days. The 3-nitro derivative is particularly toxic. Symptoms of poisoning or overdosage include diarrhea followed by constipation, hyperemia of the skin, ataxia and incoordination (especially of the hindquarters), paresis of the hindquarters, recumbency, and blindness. Pigs poisoned with 3-nitro may show no symptoms until made to move, at which time they become hyperexcitable and a proportion show violent muscle tremors, which stop when they become recumbent within a few minutes; other pigs are ataxic and incoordinate and become paraplegic.

Bibliography

Blakley BR, et al. 1990. Roxarsone (3-nitro-4-hydroxyphenylarsonic acid) poisoning in pigs. Can Vet J 31:385.
Shapiro JL, et al. 1988. An unusual necrotizing cholangiohepatitis in broiler chickens. Can Vet J 29:636.

Carbadox

Carbadox is a quinoxaline *NN* dioxide derivative used to promote growth and prevent dysentery in swine. Other quinoxalines used as growth promoters in animals include olaquindox and cyadox. Carbadox inhibits bacterial DNA synthesis and denatures preexisting DNA. It is more active under anaerobic than aerobic conditions, and its effect on DNA, like that of the nitrofurans, is believed to be caused by an unstable quindoxin-reduction product.

Carbadox is highly active against clostridia (MIC ≤ 0.25 µg/ml) and *Serpulina hyodysenteriae* (MIC <0.005 µg/ml) and against aerobic bacteria under anaerobic conditions. Quindoxins have some activity against chlamydia and protozoa. Resistance in field cases of swine dysentery has been described, but its basis has not been clarified.

Carbadox is used as a growth promoter in pigs at levels in feed of 10–25 ppm. Concentrations of 50–55 ppm in feed are used in the prevention and treatment of swine dysentery and proliferative intestinal adenomatosis. The drug is administered in feed over 6–8 weeks and may eradicate infection. There are, however, some reports of ineffectiveness. It is not licensed for use in breeding pigs.

Carbadox induces hypoaldosteronism by causing dose- and time-related damage to the glomerular zone of the adrenal cortex (Van der Molen, 1988), with effects occurring at levels as low as 50 ppm. At 50 ppm, mild effects of increased fecal dryness may be observed, but at higher doses (100–150 ppm) fecal dryness, urine drinking, growth retardation, and poor condition occur, which may result in posterior paresis and death in acute poisoning (300 ppm). Olaquindox has toxicity for pigs similar to that of carbadox, but cyadox is less toxic (Nabuurs et al., 1990).

Carbadox and olaquindox have recently been withdrawn from use in Europe, because they may cause photosensitization in people exposed to them.

Bibliography

DeGraaf GJ, et al. 1988. Some pharmacokinetic observations of carbadox medication in pigs. Vet Q 10:34.

Nabuurs MJA, et al. 1990. Clinical signs and performance of pigs treated with different doses of carbadox, cyadox, and olaquindox. J Vet Med 37A:68.

Olson LD. 1986. Probable elimination of swine dysentery after feeding ronidazole, carbadox, or lincomycin and verification by feeding sodium arsanilate. Can J Vet Res 50:365.

Power SB, et al. 1989. Accidental carbadox overdosage in pigs in an Irish weaner-producing herd. Vet Rec 124:367.

Van der Molen EJ. 1988. Pathological effects of carbadox in pigs with special emphasis on the adrenal. J Comp Pathol 98:55.

Fusidic Acid

Fusidic acid is a lipophilic steroid antibiotic, a fusidane (like cephalosporin P_1 and helvolic acid). It is a product of *Fusidium coccineum* and available as a readily soluble sodium salt. It prevents protein synthesis by inhibiting the binding of aminoacyl tRNA to the ribosomal A site. Sodium fusidate is active mainly against Gram-positive bacteria; it has conspicuous bactericidal activity (MIC ≤0.03 µg/ml) against *Staphylococcus aureus* and reasonable activity against *Mycobacterium tuberculosis* (MIC 0.5–2 µg/ml). Gram-negative rods are resistant. Resistant strains of

S. aureus emerge readily in vitro and sometimes during treatment. Combination with penicillin prevents the emergence of such mutants. Fusidic acid has been used successfully in the oral treatment of serious staphylococcal infections in humans when other drugs have failed and is used almost exclusively for this purpose. It is apparently not well absorbed in dogs but is available as a topical application in the treatment of local staphylococcal infection (Saijonmaa-Koulumies et al., 1998). It is available in some countries as an ophthalmic preparation for the treatment of conjunctivitis in dogs and cats.

Bibliography

Greenwood D. 1988. Fusidic acid. In: Peterson PK, Verhoef J, eds. The Antimicrobial Agents Annual. Amsterdam: Elsevier.

Reeves DS. 1987. The pharmacokinetics of fusidic acid. J Antimicrob Chemother 20:467.

Saijonmaa-Koulumies L, et al. 1998. Elimination of *Staphylococcus intermedius* in healthy dogs by topical treatment with fusidic acid. J Small Anim Pract 39:341.

Isoniazid

Isoniazid is the hydrazide of isonicotinic acid, a low-molecular-weight, water-soluble drug. It is the most potent antituberculosis drug used in humans, being bactericidal to *Mycobacterium tuberculosis* at concentrations of 0.05–0.2 µg/ml. *M. bovis* is similarly susceptible, but *M. avium-intracellulare* and other atypical mycobacteria are resistant. Many *M. kansasii* are susceptible. Among other genera, *Rhodococcus equi*, *Corynebacterium pseudotuberculosis*, and *Streptococcus zooepidemicus* are resistant. *Actinomyces bovis* appears to be susceptible. The drug is never administered alone, because resistant bacteria develop readily (about 1 in 10^6). The mechanism of action of isoniazid is unknown.

The drug is well absorbed from the intestine and distributes well into tissues, including cerebrospinal fluid. The dosage used in humans is 200–300 mg PO once daily.

Toxic effects occur in that proportion of the human population genetically predisposed to slow inactivation of the drug. These neurotoxic effects, which occur in up to 20% of people, result from a relative deficiency of pyridoxine as a result of competitive inhibition. Symptoms include restlessness, insomnia, peripheral neuritis, and psychosis. Severe hepatocellular damage develops in about 2% of patients treated for long periods. Administration of 11–22 mg/kg to a cow orally for 28 days produced no ill effects; higher doses caused anorexia and depression. Accidental ingestion of 66 mg/kg by a dog resulted in rapid development of convulsions, which were controlled by barbiturates. The dog recovered (Doherty, 1982).

The drug has been used at 11–22 mg/kg PO once daily to treat actinomycosis in cattle; lesion activity was controlled, and in some cases lesions regressed (Watts et al., 1973). No relapses were reported. *Mycobacterium paratuberculosis* is moderately susceptible to isoniazid, 2 µg/ml, but treatment of Johne's disease in cattle has been unsuccessful. Combination with rifampin or use of isoniazid alone in paratuberculosis in goats has also been unsuccessful (Gezon et al., 1988). Isoniazid has been used with moderate success in the prevention and treatment of *M. bovis* infection in cattle in South Africa (Konyha, 1992) and other countries but cannot be recommended as the method of control.

Bibliography

Doherty T. 1982. Isoniazid poisoning in a dog. Vet Rec 111:460.
Gezon HM, et al. 1988. Identification and control of paratuberculosis in a large goat herd. Am J Vet Res 49:1817.
Konyha LD. 1992. Tuberculosis. In: Howard JL, ed. Current Veterinary Therapy: Food Animal Practice, 3rd ed. Philadelphia: WB Saunders.
Specht TE, et al. 1991. Skin pustules and nodules caused by *Actinomyces viscosus* in a horse. J Am Vet Med Assoc 198:457.
Watts TC, et al. 1973. Treatment of bovine actinomycosis with isoniazid. Can Vet J 14:223.

Mupirocin

Mupirocin (pseudomonic acid) is a novel antibiotic, isolated from *Pseudomonas fluorescens*. By preventing incorporation of isoleucine into protein chains, this powerful inhibitor of bacterial isoleucyl transfer RNA synthetase stops protein synthesis. It has excellent activity in vitro against staphylococci and streptococci but less activity against other Gram-positive and Gram-negative bacteria. Its activity is slowly bactericidal. Activity against multiple antibiotic–resistant *Staphylococcus aureus* is slightly less than its excellent activity against most skin isolates (<0.12 µg/ml). Cross-resistance with other antibiotics is unlikely because of its distinct mechanism of action. Its activity increases with decreasing pH, a particularly useful feature in topical application to skin, since it is slightly acid. The drug is rapidly metabolized after systemic administration and so is available only for topical application. Mupirocin is inactivated by body fluids, including pus and mucosal secretions.

A 2% formulation is available for thrice daily application to unbroken skin in the effective treatment of primary skin infections caused by *S. aureus* or streptococci. The drug has been used successfully in human medicine for intranasal application to treat the staphylococcal carrier state. Other applications, for which efficacy is less well demonstrated, have included secondary infection of skin lesions, including burns, ulcers, and wounds.

Low- and high-level resistance to mupirocin, the latter plasmid mediated, have been reported in staphylococci (Cookson, 1990). To attempt to avoid the selection of resistant bacteria, it is recommended to use the drug for a maximum of 10 days. White et al. (1997) used the drug twice daily for 3 weeks in the good to excellent treatment of feline acne.

Bibliography

Cookson BD. 1990. Mupirocin resistance in staphylococci. J Antimicrob Chemother 25:497.
Doebbeling BN, et al. 1993. Elimination of *Staphylococcus aureus* nasal carriage in health care workers: analysis of six clinical trials with calcium mupirocin ointment. Clin Infect Dis 17:466.
Ward A, Campoli-Richards DM. 1986. Mupirocin: a review of its antibacterial activity, pharmacokinetic properties, and therapeutic use. Drugs 32:425.
White SD, et al. 1997. Feline acne and results of treatment with mupirocin in an open clinical trial: 25 cases (1994–96). Vet Dermatol 8:157.

Methenamine

Methenamine (hexamine) is a highly soluble, basic substance of chemical formula $(CH_2)_6N_4$, which decomposes under acid conditions to release formaldehyde. It is available as a salt of mandelic acid or hippuric acid. After administration of enteric-coated tablets, the drug is well absorbed and excreted unchanged in the urine. If the urine is strongly acidic (pH <5.5), methenamine releases formaldehyde, which acts as a nonspecific urinary antiseptic. It is usual to ensure urine acidity by concurrent administration of ascorbic acid or ammonium chloride. The drug is used for the long-term prophylaxis of recurrent urinary tract infections in dogs and cats at a dosage of 0.25 mg/15 kg 4 times daily. Microorganisms such as *Proteus* that make urine strongly alkaline through release of ammonia from urea are usually not susceptible.

Novobiocin

Novobiocin (Fig. 16.3) is an antibiotic product of *Streptomyces*, occasionally used in the local treatment of *Staphylococcus aureus* infections,

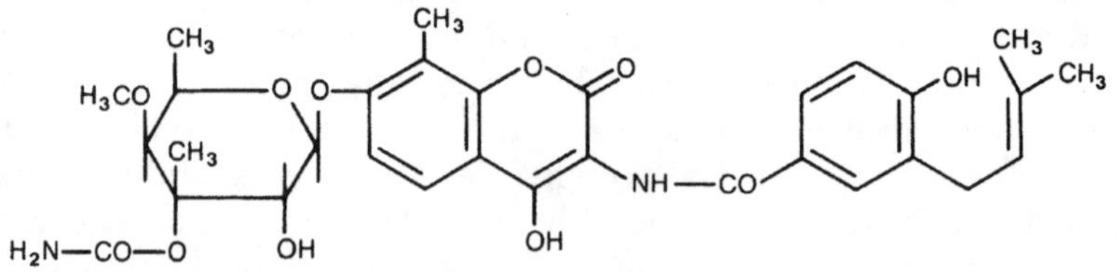

Fig. 16.3. Structural formula of novobiocin.

particularly in mastitis in cows. It is a drug of minimal importance. Novobiocin is a coumarin antibiotic, a dibasic acid available as a poorly water-soluble calcium salt or as the more soluble monosodium salt.

Novobiocin inactivates the beta subunit of DNA gyrase, inhibiting supercoiling, DNA-dependent adenosine triphosphatase, and catenation/uncatenation.

Novobiocin is very active against *S. aureus*, less active against streptococci and the more fastidious Gram-negative bacteria *(Haemophilus, Brucella)*, and least active against Enterobacteriaceae and *Pseudomonas* (Table 16.5). In a study of bovine mastitis isolates, 95% of *S. aureus*, 60% of *Streptococcus dysgalactiae*, and 40% of *S. agalactiae* were susceptible to the drug; many mycoplasmas are moderately susceptible.

Novobiocin is usually bacteriostatic; activity is decreased by alkaline conditions and the presence of magnesium. Bacteria with MIC ≤4 μg/ml are regarded as susceptible, with MIC 8 μg/ml as intermediate, and with MIC ≥16 μg/ml as resistant. Chromosomal resistance develops fairly readily in vitro and has been reported during treatment of *S. aureus* infection.

Moderate synergism with penicillin G against bovine *S. aureus* and streptococci has been described. The claim that novobiocin is synergistic with tetracycline may be a laboratory artifact associated with magnesium chelation by tetracycline.

Novobiocin is well absorbed from the gastrointestinal tract in humans and has a half-life of 2–4 hours. Penetration into tissues is relatively modest. The drug is mainly excreted in the bile, and enterohepatic

TABLE 16.5. **Antimicrobial activity (MIC$_{90}$, μg/ml) of novobiocin against selected bacteria**

Organism	MIC$_{90}$	Organism	MIC$_{90}$
Gram-positive aerobes			
Arcanobacterium pyogenes	64	*Rhodococcus equi*	>64
Corynebacterium bovis	1	*Staphylococcus aureus*	2[a]
Enterococcus faecalis	64	*Streptococcus agalactiae*	16
Erysipelothrix rhusiopathiae	>64	*S. pyogenes*	4
Listeria monocytogenes	2	*S. uberis*	2[a]
Gram-positive anaerobes			
Actinomyces spp.	16	*Clostridium perfringens*	1
Gram-negative aerobes			
Brucella canis	2	*P. multocida*	16
Escherichia coli	>64	*Proteus* spp.	64
Haemophilus somnus	≤0.13	*Pseudomonas aeruginosa*	>64
Pasteurella haemolytica	64	*Taylorella equigenitalis*	2
Mycoplasma			
M. ovipneumoniae	8		

[a]Some reports are far higher because of resistance.

circulation occurs. Skin eruptions in humans are common. The drug has a profound depressing effect on liver metabolism. Eosinophilia, thrombocytopenia, and leukopenia are occasional side effects. Skin rashes may occur in cows treated with intramammary infusions of the drug.

The main application of novobiocin is in the local treatment of *S. aureus* infections. The drug is combined with procaine penicillin G in dry-cow therapy, with reasonable results. It is not used alone. The drug is used in poultry by oral administration to treat staphylococcal infections and to control fowl cholera.

Combination with tetracycline has given apparently better clinical results in the treatment of nonspecific upper respiratory tract infections in dogs than has tetracycline alone (Maxey, 1980).

Bibliography

Hamdy AH, et al. 1975. Activity of penicillin and novobiocin against bovine mastitis pathogens. Am J Vet Res 36:259.

Maxey BW. 1980. Efficacy of tetracycline/novobiocin combination against canine upper respiratory tract infections. Vet Med Small Anim Clin 75:89.

17 | Antifungal Chemotherapy

J. F. PRESCOTT

The destruction of normal host microbial flora by broad-spectrum bactericidal antibacterial drugs, the increased numbers of neutropenic patients, the use of intravascular catheters, and the rise of the numbers of patients with AIDS are all factors responsible for the considerable increase in infections with *Candida* and other fungi in people. It can be anticipated that fungal infections may increase in animals for some of the same reasons.

Until relatively recently, the range of antifungal drugs available for systemic use was limited to a few agents, the most effective of which (amphotericin B) was highly toxic. The progressive development in the 1980s of the azole drugs for systemic use revolutionized antifungal therapy. These and earlier systemic agents targeted fungal cell membrane structures, notably interfering with ergosterol incorporation. Unrelated, nontoxic antifungal drugs are now being evaluated for clinical use. Some have the advantage, unusual among systemic antifungal drugs, of fungicidal rather than fungistatic activity. The major target of the antifungal drugs under development is the fungal cell wall, which has unique features. These new drugs include echinocandin B analogs, which target a unique fungal cell wall structure through inhibition of 1,3-β-D-glucan synthase; nikkomycins, which inhibit chitin synthase; pradimicins, which complex cell wall mannoproteins; and sordarins, which interfere with fungal elongation factor 2.

Antifungal Susceptibility Testing

The susceptibility of fungi to different drugs is not always predictable. Both acquired resistance and constitutive resistance have been described. Susceptibility testing of fungi has been marked by highly discrepant results among laboratories. In addition, development of interpretive criteria of MIC data based on in vivo–in vitro correlation has been slow. This may be in part because the underlying immunocompromised state of many patients with fungal infections treated with the currently available fungistatic drugs is an important determinant of the outcome of treatment. The situation has been largely though not completely resolved in medical microbiology for yeasts by the formation of a subcommittee within the National Council for Clinical Laboratory Standards (NCCLS) to address the issue of in vitro antifungal testing (NCCLS, 1997). In addition, acceptable methods for susceptibility testing of filamentous fungi and criteria for MIC interpretation are under development (Denning et al., 1997; Espinel-Ingroff et al., 1997). In the absence of veterinary-specific criteria, the standards developed in human medicine may be useful.

Antifungal Drug Resistance

Antifungal drug resistance can be intrinsic or acquired. Resistance can follow acquisition of intrinsically resistant fungi, selection of a resistant strain from a population of many strains, or mutation of an initially susceptible fungus that renders it resistant. Resistance following antifungal drug use is well recognized. The precise mechanism associated with resistance depends on the mode of action of the class of antifungal drug and includes reduced drug uptake, drug export through efflux pumps, or reduced affinity of target enzymes. Unlike in bacteria, transferable drug resistance has not been recognized in fungi, so that the spread of resistance has been considerably slower among fungi. Prevention of emergence and spread of resistant fungi depends on taking maximal advantage of the pharmacodynamic properties of the particular drug class; on use of local rather than systemic treatment, thus reducing general exposure of the animal's fungal flora to antifungal agents; and on hygienic precautions. In the case of flucytosine, combination antifungal therapy is a well-recognized strategy to prevent emergence of flucytosine resistance.

Bibliography

Denning DW, et al. 1997. Correlation between in-vitro susceptibility testing to itraconazole and in-vivo outcome of *Aspergillus fumigatus* infection. J Antimicrob Chemother 40:401.

Espinel-Ingroff A, et al. 1997. Multicenter evaluation of proposed standardized procedure for antifungal susceptibility testing of filamentous fungi. J Clin Microbiol 35:139.

Georgopapadakou NH, Walsh TJ. 1996. Antifungal agents: chemotherapeutic targets and immunologic strategies. Antimicrob Agents Chemother 40:279.

Ghannoum MA, et al. 1996. Susceptibility testing of fungi: current status of correlation of in vitro data with clinical outcome. J Clin Microbiol 34:489.

Groll AH, et al. 1998. Emerging targets for the development of novel antifungal therapeutics. Trends Microbiol 6:117.

Johnson EM, Warnock DW. 1995. Azole resistance in yeasts. J Antimicrob Chemother 36:751.

Kauffman CA, Carver PL. 1997. Antifungal agents in the 1990s. Drugs 53:539.

National Committee for Clinical Laboratory Standards. 1997. Reference method for broth dilution antifungal susceptibility testing of yeasts. Tentative standard M27-T. Villanova, PA: National Committee for Clinical Laboratory Standards.

Antifungal Drugs for Topical Application

An extensive range of antifungal drugs, some described in Table 17.1, is available for topical application. Clotrimazole, itraconazole, miconazole, and natamycin are drugs of choice for topical treatment of fungal infections. Many other chemicals have antifungal properties, including phenolic antiseptics such as thymol and hexachlorophene; iodides; 8-hydroxyquinoline; quaternary ammonium and bisquaternary antiseptics; salicylamide; propionic, salicylic, and undecanoic acids; and chlorphenesin. All these compounds and others have been used for the topical treatment of fungal infections of the skin and sometimes of mucosa. The topical antifungal drugs discussed here are of interest for their potency or their broad-spectrum activity.

Natamycin

Natamycin is a fungicidal polyene antibiotic with action against the fungal cell membrane. It is effective against a wide range of filamentous and dimorphic fungi and yeasts (Table 17.2). Natamycin is used for local application against ringworm, in the udder for yeast mastitis, and on the

TABLE 17.1. **Some antifungals for topical use**

Drug	Antifungal Activity	Drug Form
Amorolfine	Dermatophytes	0.25% cream
Amphotericin B	Broad spectrum, some *Aspergillus* resistance	3% cream
Clotrimazole	Broad spectrum, especially *Aspergillus*	1% cream, solution
Cuprimycin	Broad spectrum, antibacterial	1% cream, solution
Enilconazole	Broad spectrum; treatment of choice in canine nasal aspergillosis	5% solution
Fluconazole	Most *Candida*; yeasts; not *Aspergillus*	1% cream
Haloprogin	Dermatophytes, *Candida*	2% cream, solution
Ketoconazole	Broad spectrum	1% solution
Natamycin	Broad spectrum, high potency, fungicidal	2.5–5% solution, 100 ppm spray
Nystatin	Broadish spectrum, especially yeasts	100,000 units/ml cream
Tolnaftate	Dermatophytes	1% cream, solution, powder

TABLE 17.2. Activity (MIC_{90}, µg/ml) of three topical antifungal antibiotics against selected fungi

Organism	Natamycin	Clotrimazole	Nystatin
Filamentous fungi			
Alternaria spp.	2	—	32
Aspergillus fumigatus	8	8	≥64
Fusarium spp.	1	8	≥64
Microsporum canis	8	2	4
Mucor spp.	1	1	8
Trichophyton spp.	8	8	16
Yeasts			
Candida spp.	8	0.5	4
Cryptococcus neoformans	8	4	2
Malassezia pachydermatis	8	2	0.25

eyes for mycotic keratitis. It is recommended in humans as the initial therapy for fungal keratitis while awaiting identification of the organism and results of susceptibility testing. In terms of in vitro activity against fungal isolates from the eye of horses with ulcerative keratomycosis, natamycin is equal to miconazole, which is better than itraconazole, which is better than ketoconazole (Brooks et al., 1998). Natamycin is not effective against deep mycotic infections of the eyes, because of poor absorption.

Natamycin has been used successfully to treat cows with *Candida* mastitis (20 ml of a 2.5% solution, or 10 ml of a 5% solution, into the affected udder quarter once daily for 3 days). Total-body spraying or sponging is effective in treatment of ringworm in cattle and horses. It is important that all grooming utensils be thoroughly cleansed or immersed in the natamycin suspension, which should be prepared in plastic or galvanized containers. The drug is used successfully to treat filamentous fungal keratitis in horses and is the drug of choice for this purpose. A recommended treatment is 1 drop of a 5% suspension every 1 or 2 hours, decreasing to 6 or 8 times daily after a few days (Bistner and Riis, 1979). Some clinicians have found natamycin to be locally irritating. Topical application in the treatment of nasal aspergillosis in horses has been clinically effective. Natamycin has potential application in the local treatment of *Candida* metritis in mares.

Nystatin

Nystatin is a polyene antibiotic that disorganizes the membrane of fungi, occupying ergosterol-binding sites and altering membrane permeability, so that intracellular ions leak from the cell. The drug is effective against *Candida*, *Malassezia*, *Cryptococcus*, dermatophytes, some filamentous fungi, and some dimorphic fungi. Several *Candida* species other than *C. albicans* are resistant. Nystatin is fungicidal at concentrations about 4 times MIC. *Prototheca* are reported to be susceptible. Nystatin is used clinically as a topical, broad-spectrum antifungal drug. Clotrimazole has a broader spectrum and is more active. In one study, about one-fifth of yeasts isolated from bovine mastitis were resistant to the drug. A recommended dose is 300,000 units/quarter on three occasions as a single daily dose; the drug can be diluted in saline to 5,000 units/ml and 50 ml administered. Nystatin has been used in dogs to treat *Malassezia* infections of the outer ear and in horses to treat *Candida* metritis.

Azole Antibiotics: Clotrimazole, Enilconazole, Itraconazole, Ketoconazole, and Miconazole

Clotrimazole is an azole with chemical structure and mechanism of action described under the systemic azoles. It is inhibitory in vitro to a wide range of filamentous fungi, including *Aspergillus* and dermatophytes; yeasts such as *Candida;* and dimorphic fungi. Concentrations above 10 µg/ml are fungicidal. Few naturally occurring strains of fungi are resistant.

Clotrimazole is reserved for topical administration, as a broad-spectrum antifungal. Local application in mycotic keratitis in horses is well tolerated; the 1% solution is used for *Aspergillus* infections of the cornea. A 1-hour application of 100 ml of a 1% solution is used in the effective treatment of nasal aspergillosis in dogs under general anesthetic. In one study, a single topical application by either surgically implanted catheters or catheters placed nonsurgically in the nose resulted in cure in 65% of dogs; a second treatment increased cure rate to 87% (Mathews et al., 1998). Prolonged recovery in a dog after barbiturate anesthesia and intranasal treatment with clotrimazole for nasal aspergillosis was attributed to hepatic microsomal enzyme induction by clotrimazole (Caulkett et al., 1997).

The drug is used in humans to treat *Candida* vaginitis. In the local treatment of mycotic endometritis in cows or horses, infusions of 400–600 mg clotrimazole every other day for 12 days has been recommended, using sufficient volume of saline diluent to gently fill the uterus. It may be the drug of choice for yeast mastitis in cows. Intramammary administration of 100–200 mg/quarter per day of 1% solution or cream, on one to four occasions as a single daily dose, has given good clinical results in mycotic mastitis in cows.

Miconazole has similar activity to clotrimazole and has also proven useful for topical treatment of dermatophyte, candidal, *Aspergillus* spp., and *Malassezia* infections.

Enilconazole is effective in the treatment of canine nasal aspergillosis both following surgical removal of necrotic and foreign material and on its own, and it has become the treatment of choice for nasal aspergillosis in dogs. After bilateral placement of indwelling catheters in the frontal sinuses, a 5% enilconazole solution (dose 10 mg/kg, total volume 5–10 ml) is administered twice daily for 10 days (Lanthier and Chalifoux, 1991; Sharp et al., 1993). Total drug contact time is 45–60 minutes. Administration of enilconazole via nonsurgically placed catheters was ineffective compared with administration via surgically placed catheters (Bray et al., 1998). A technique for endoscopic placement of tubes in the frontal sinuses and nasal cavity, requiring fewer treatments, has been described (McCullough et al., 1998). Itraconazole should be an effective alternative to clotrimazole and enilconazole for local treatment of nasal aspergillosis.

Enilconazole has been used successfully in environmental decontamination of poultry houses to prevent aspergillosis. Local infusion of enilconazole has been used successfully in the treatment of guttural pouch mycosis in the horse.

Ketoconazole is also available for topical antifungal therapy, though it is less active in vitro than clotrimazole, itraconazole, and miconazole. Like other topical azoles, it is used in the treatment of *Malassezia pachydermatis* ear and skin infections. Miconazole combined with chlorhexidine was more effective as a shampoo than selenium sulfide in dogs for treatment of seborrheic dermatitis caused by *M. pachydermatis* (Bond et al., 1995).

Amorolfine

Amorolfine is a morpholine fungicidal drug that inhibits ergosterol biosynthesis. It is active against dermatophytes, some yeasts, and some filamentous fungi. The major use in human medicine is in topical treatment of moderate dermatophytic infections.

Bibliography

Bistner SI, Riis RC. 1979. Clinical aspects of mycotic keratitis in the horse. Cornell Vet 69:634.
Bond R, et al. 1995. Comparisons of two shampoos for treatment of *Malassezia pachydermatis*–associated seborrheic dermatitis in basset hounds. J Small Anim Pract 36:99.
Bray JP, et al. 1998. Treatment of canine nasal aspergillosis with a new non-invasive technique: failure with enilconazole. J Small Anim Pract 39:223.
Brooks DE, et al. 1998. Antimicrobial susceptibility patterns of fungi isolated from horses with ulcerative keratomycosis. J Am Vet Med Assoc 59:138.
Caulkett N, et al. 1997. Upper-airway obstruction and prolonged recovery from anesthesia following intranasal clotrimazole administration. J Am Anim Hosp Assoc 33:264.
Lane JG. 1989. The management of guttural pouch mycosis. Equine Vet J 21:321.
Lanthier T, Chalifoux A. 1991. Enilconazole as an adjunct to the treatment of four cases of canine nasal aspergillosis. Can Vet J 32:110.
Mathews KG, et al. 1998. Comparison of topical administration of clotrimazole through surgically placed versus nonsurgically placed catheters for treatment of nasal aspergillosis in dogs: 60 cases (1990–1996). J Am Vet Med Assoc 213:501.
McCullough SM, et al. 1998. Endoscopically placed tubes for administration of enilconazole for treatment of nasal aspergillosis in dogs. J Am Vet Med Assoc 212:67.

McDonald JS, et al. 1980. In vitro antimycotic sensitivity of yeasts isolated from infected bovine mammary glands. Am J Vet Res 41:1987.

Nappert G, et al. 1996. Successful treatment of a fever associated with consistent pulmonary isolation of *Scopulariopsis* sp. in a mare. Equine Vet J 28:421.

Oldenkamp EP. 1979. Treatment of ringworm in horses with natamycin. Equine Vet J 11:36.

Sharp NJH, Sullivan M. 1986. Treatment of canine nasal aspergillosis with systemic ketoconazole and topical enilconazole. Vet Rec 118:560.

Sharp NJH, et al. 1993. Treatment of canine nasal aspergillosis with enilconazole. J Vet Intern Med 7:40.

Uchida Y, et al. 1990. In vitro activity of five antifungal agents against *Malassezia pachydermatis*. Jap J Vet Sci 52:851.

Van Damme DM. 1983. Use of miconazole in treatment of bovine mastitis. Vet Med Small Anim Clin 78:1425.

Antifungal Drugs for Systemic Administration
Griseofulvin
CHEMISTRY

Griseofulvin (Fig. 17.1) is a benzofuran cyclohexene antibiotic, a product of *Penicillium griseofulvum*. It is poorly soluble in water.

MECHANISM OF ACTION

Griseofulvin is a fungistatic antibiotic that inhibits mitosis, probably by disorganizing the spindle microtubules. It may also interfere with cytoplasmic microtubules.

ANTIMICROBIAL ACTIVITY

Virtually all dermatophytes of animal origin are inhibited by griseofulvin concentrations of 0.2–0.5 µg/ml. Other hyphal fungi, yeasts, dimorphic fungi, and bacteria are unaffected. Resistance (MIC ≥ 3 µg/ml) to griseofulvin has been described in dermatophytes of human origin.

PHARMACOKINETIC PROPERTIES

Absorption, after oral administration, depends greatly on particle size. It is enhanced in humans after a high-fat meal. Half-life in humans is

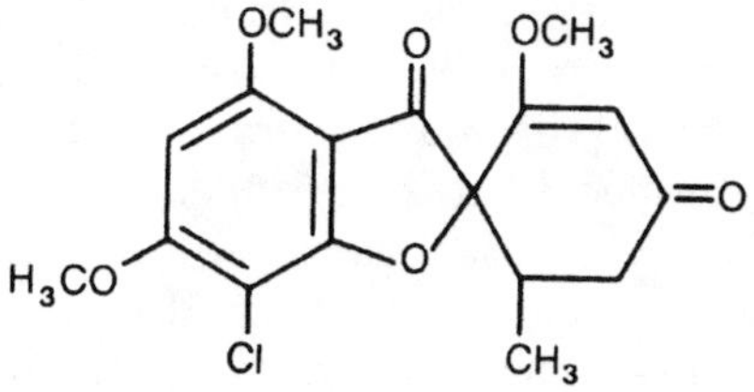

Fig. 17.1.   Structural formula of griseofulvin.

about 20 hours but is considerably shorter (<6 hours) in dogs. Most of the drug is excreted in the stool. The drug appears to be metabolized in the liver, and increased metabolism may be caused by drugs that induce liver enzymes (eg, rifampin). It is selectively deposited in the newly formed keratin of hair, nails, and skin and gradually moves from these deep layers to the site of infection in the superficial keratinized epithelium, where keratinized cells mature and are progressively desquamated. Actively growing fungus may be killed, but dormant cells are only inhibited, so that cure occurs when infected keratinized cells are shed. For this reason, treatment is prolonged.

TOXICITY AND SIDE EFFECTS

Prolonged medication in humans has occasionally been associated with mild and transient side effects, such as mild central nervous effects (headaches, dizziness, fatigue), photosensitivity, and gastrointestinal disturbances (nausea, vomiting, diarrhea).

Griseofulvin is teratogenic in cats, particularly in the first weeks of gestation. The drug's use results in numerous congenital defects, including brain malformations, skeletal abnormalities, spina bifida, anophthalmia, and atresia ani (Scott et al., 1975). High doses in cats have also been associated with anemia, a possibly idiosyncratic reaction (Kunkle and Meyer, 1987). This may relate to feline immunodeficiency virus infection (Shelton et al., 1990). FIV-positive animals should probably be treated with another drug, such as itraconazole. Signs of toxicosis in cats of all types include anorexia, vomiting, ataxia, anemia, leukopenia, anorexia, depression, jaundice, pruritus, and pyrexia (Helton et al., 1986; Wack et al., 1992). These signs are usually, but not always, reversible. Because of the teratogenic effect for all species (Schutte and van den Ingh, 1997), griseofulvin should not be given to any pregnant animal. Dogs and cats may vomit if given griseofulvin on an empty stomach.

ADMINISTRATION AND DOSAGE

The drug should be given for 1 or 2 weeks beyond clinical or mycologic cure and may therefore require 4–12 weeks for ringworm and 6–12 months for nail infections. A single daily dose of 50 mg/kg can be reduced to 25 mg/kg once clinical response occurs. The optimal dose in cats has not been firmly established, but toxicity appears to be idiosyncratic rather than dose related (Levy, 1991). Because of the unpredictable nature of griseofulvin toxicosis in cats, however, this drug should be used in cats only for serious infections unresponsive to topical application or to other systemic drugs. Griseofulvin is administered orally to ringworm-infected cattle as a 10% mycelial mix, 7.5–10 mg/kg for 7 days.

CLINICAL APPLICATIONS

Griseofulvin is effective only against dermatophytic infections and effective against ringworm only if administered orally. The drug reaches the superficial, dead, parasitized epithelium only through progressive maturation of basal cells. Treatment is thus slow, 3–6 weeks in dogs and cats. In cattle, probably because of economic considerations, a short treatment of only 7 days has been found to render animals free of lesions 4 weeks or so after treatment. This dosage in larger animals is lower than that used in dogs and cats but is apparently equally effective. Unresponsive ringworm infections in dogs and cats may sometimes be treated successfully by doubling or tripling the dosage, although high doses should be used with caution in cats (see Toxicity and Side Effects, above). A single large dose may be given to animals for prophylactic purposes.

Bibliography

Helton KA, et al. 1986. Griseofulvin toxicity in cats: literature review and report of seven cases. J Am Anim Hosp Assoc 22:453.

Kunkle GA, Meyer DJ. 1987. Toxicity of high doses of griseofulvin in cats. J Am Vet Med Assoc 191:322.

Levy JK. 1991. Ataxia in a kitten treated with griseofulvin. J Am Vet Med Assoc 198:105.

Rottmann JB, et al. 1991. Bone marrow hypoplasia in a cat treated with griseofulvin. J Am Vet Med Assoc 198:429.

Schutte JG, van de Ingh TSGM. 1997. Microphthalmia, brachygnathia superior, and palatocheiloschisis in a foal associated with griseofulvin administration to the mare during early pregnancy. Vet Q 19:58.

Scott FW, et al. 1975. Teratogenesis in cats associated with griseofulvin therapy. Teratology 11:79.

Shelton GH, et al. 1990. Severe neutropenia associated with griseofulvin therapy in cats with feline immunodeficiency virus. J Vet Intern Med 4:317.

Wack RF, et al. 1992. Griseofulvin toxicity in four cheetahs (Acinonyx jubatus). J Zoo Wild Med 23:442.

Allylamines: Naftifine and Terbinafine

Allylamines are synthetic drugs that inhibit ergosterol biosynthesis by their effect against an important enzyme (squalene epoxidase) involved in its synthesis. Naftifine is used topically to treat dermatophyte infections, whereas terbinafine is available for oral use in human medicine. Terbinafine is used in the treatment of dermatophytic, *Malassezia*, and *Sporothrix schenckii* infections, and there is interest in it for its activity against *Candida* and dimorphic and filamentous fungi. It is used in people in the systemic treatment of persistent or intractable dermatophyte infections, in which it is more effective than ketoconazole, itraconazole, or griseofulvin. It concentrates in the nails and stratum corneum. It is generally nontoxic. There is no experience with its use in animals.

Amphotericin B

Amphotericin is a polyene broad-spectrum and active antifungal antibiotic, which was the mainstay of systemic treatment for many years, although its place in systemic treatment of yeast or dimorphic fungal infections is challenged by the azole antifungal drugs. It is still the mainstay for systemic treatment of filamentous fungal infections. A major advantage of this drug is its fungicidal nature, so that it is often used in treatment of life-threatening yeast or dimorphic fungal infections. Its toxicity has been circumvented in recent years by development of lipid formulations that, though expensive, are just coming into clinical use in animals.

CHEMISTRY

Amphotericin is a heptaene product of *Streptomyces nodosus* belonging, like nystatin, to the polyenes (Fig. 17.2). It is an amphoteric polyene macrolide that is poorly soluble in water and unstable at 37° C. The antifungal effects of the antibiotic are maximal between pH 6.0 and 7.5 and decrease at low pH. The amphotericin B sodium deoxycholate compound with phosphate buffer is more water soluble and is used for IV administration. Lipid-based formulations (liposomal, colloidal, or lipid complex) are less toxic than the micellar suspension, which is the conventional formulation.

MECHANISM OF ACTION

Amphotericin B binds to ergosterol, the principal sterol of the fungal cell membrane, causing leakage of cell contents. The drug binds cholesterol in mammalian cell membranes less avidly, but its ability to bind to mammalian cells makes this the most toxic of the clinically useful systemic antifungal drugs.

ANTIMICROBIAL ACTIVITY

Amphotericin B is a broad-spectrum antifungal antibiotic with the advantage of generally fungicidal activity against most pathogenic fungi.

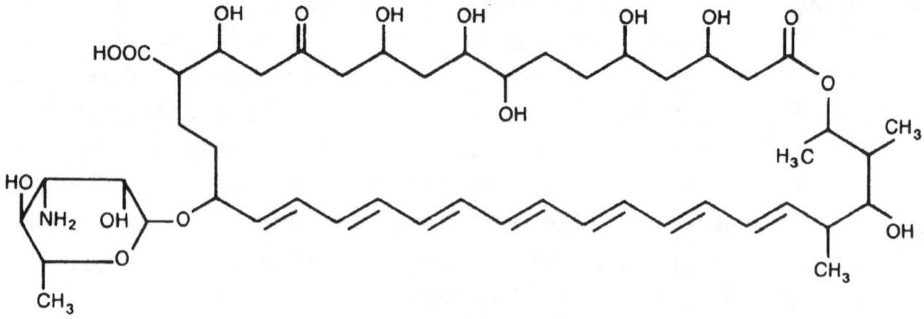

Fig. 17.2. Structural formula of amphotericin B.

Organisms with MIC ≤1 µg/ml are regarded as susceptible. *Blastomyces dermatitidis, Histoplasma capsulatum, Cryptococcus neoformans, Candida* spp., *Sporothrix schenckii,* and *Coccidioides immitis* are susceptible, in decreasing order (Table 17.3). Some resistant *Candida, Coccidioides immitis,* and *Mucor* have been described. Strains of filamentous fungi, although commonly susceptible, can vary from extreme susceptibility to resistance. Of the filamentous fungi, *Aspergillus* are the most frequently resistant, although most are susceptible. McDonald et al. (1980) reported half the yeasts isolated from bovine mastitis to be susceptible. *Prototheca* are susceptible. Lipid-based formulations have similar activity to the conventional preparation.

RESISTANCE

Although rare, development of resistance during treatment of susceptible fungi such as *Candida* spp. with amphotericin B has been described. *Pseudallescheria boydii, Trichosporon beigelii,* and some dematiaceous fungi are intrinsically resistant to amphotericin B.

PHARMACOKINETIC PROPERTIES

Amphotericin B is a macrolide with lipophilic and hydrophilic parts, which confer curious pharmacokinetic properties on the drug that have not been fully elaborated. There is virtually no absorption after oral administration. The half-life in humans after IV injection is about 20 hours. The drug is thought to bind to plasma or cellular lipoproteins and to be released slowly from these sites. Only about 5% of the injected dose is excreted in the kidneys, but the agent continues to be excreted in the urine of humans for several weeks after therapy is stopped. Penetration into cerebrospinal fluid (CSF) is poor (5%) but increases in meningitis. Absorption from the lungs following aerosol administration is poor, so that this route has been used successfully in the treatment of pulmonary aspergillosis. The most marked characteristic pharmacokinetic property of lipid-based formulations is the reduced volume of distribution, which allows greater drug concentration in serum. This is probably the result of decreased interaction of the amphotericin with host proteins or membrane cholesterol. Lipid-based formulations appear to be taken up extensively by the reticuloendothelial system, which may give them significant therapeutic advantage.

DRUG INTERACTIONS

Because of both the serious nature of systemic fungal infections and the toxicity of amphotericin B, considerable effort has been expended to find synergistic combinations of drugs that will reduce dosage and speed cure.

Flucytosine and amphotericin B show additive or synergistic effects in vitro against *Candida, Cryptococcus,* and *Aspergillus.* Flucytosine reduces

TABLE 17.3. Activity (MIC$_{90}$, μg/ml) of selected systemic antifungal agents against selected fungi

Organism	Amphotericin B	Flucytosine	Ketoconazole	Fluconazole	Itraconazole
Filamentous fungi					
Aspergillus fumigatus	1	>64	16	>64	0.25
A. flavus	1	>64	8	>64	0.25
Cladosporium spp.	0.5	>64	16	32	0.12
Mucor spp.	0.25	—	>64	>64	4
Rhizopus spp.	0.25	—	>64	>64	2
Yeasts					
Candida albicans	0.5	0.13	0.13	0.25	0.03
C. glabrata	1	—	>64	>64	>16
C. tropicalis	1	0.25	0.06	0.5	0.25
Cryptococcus neoformans	0.25	—	0.25	2	0.008
Dimorphic fungi					
Blastomyces dermatitidis	1	—	0.5	32	≤0.03
Coccidioides immitis	0.25	—	0.5	—	—
Histoplasma capsulatum	0.25	—	0.25	2	0.06
Sporothrix schenckii	4	—	4	—	4

the concentration of amphotericin B necessary to inhibit growth of *Candida* and *Cryptococcus* in vitro. The combination is synergistic in cryptococcal meningitis in humans, producing faster cure, fewer relapses, more rapid sterilization of CSF, and less nephrotoxicity.

Combination with imidazole antibiotics, such as ketoconazole, against *Candida albicans* and *Cryptococcus neoformans*, produces complex interactions in vitro that are hard to interpret. In experimental cryptococcal infection, combination with ketoconazole significantly increased the rate of killing in cerebrospinal fluid. Combination with ketoconazole has been used successfully to treat systemic mycoses in dogs (Richardson et al., 1983), but such use may be premature until it is shown that such a combination produces optimal effects. Combination with ketoconazole in experimentally disseminated aspergillosis antagonized the effect of amphotericin.

TOXICITY AND ADVERSE EFFECTS

Renal toxicity inevitably accompanies treatment with micellar, conventional amphotericin B. In humans, the damage is reversible below a total dose of 4 g. Monitoring of blood urea nitrogen (BUN) or creatinine shows the extent of renal damage, which can be reversed either by temporarily stopping treatment or by decreasing the dosage. Dosing every other day reduces nephrotoxic effects that result from administering the same dose daily (Butler and Hill, 1964). Other side effects include thrombophlebitis at the injection site and hypokalemia with resulting cardiac arrhythmias, sweating, nausea, malaise, and depression. In dogs and cats, signs of nephrotoxicity develop within 3–4 weeks of starting treatment, associated with BUN levels of 60–70 mg/dl. The effect is reversible, and the drug should be discontinued until BUN falls below 40 mg/dl. Blood urea nitrogen should be monitored twice weekly during treatment. In addition, serum potassium should be monitored and hypokalemia corrected by oral supplementation; it does not seem to be as common in dogs and cats as in humans. Concurrent use of flucytosine decreases the dosage required to treat cryptococcal infection.

Lipid-based formulations reduce the toxicity of amphotericin B, reducing the infusion-related toxicities (nausea, fever, chills) and markedly reducing nephrotoxicity. Because of reduced toxicity, daily doses of the lipid-based formulations range in humans up to 3–5 mg/kg daily, whereas doses of the conventional form are 0.5–1 mg/kg q48 hours. More clinical efficacy comparisons of lipid-based with conventional formulations are needed, although current data suggest that lipid-based formulations are equally or slightly more effective.

Doses >5 mg/kg in dogs resulted in death due to cardiac abnormalities; doses of 2–5 mg/kg occasionally caused cardiac arrhythmias in dogs; but doses of <1 mg/kg were without effect on the heart.

TABLE 17.4. Suggested dosage of systemic antifungal agents

Agent	Dosage (mg/kg)	Comment
Amphotericin B	0.5 IV 3 times weekly	See text; 2-hour infusion ideal
Fluconazole	50 PO q12–24 hours	
Flucytosine	50 PO q6 hours	Always combine with another systemic antifungal drug
Griseofulvin	50 PO q24 hours	Reduce to 25 mg/kg once clinical response
Itraconazole	5 PO q12 hours, or 10 PO q24 hours	Dosage varies with severity and type of infection
Ketoconazole	10–20 PO q12 hours; cats, 10–15 PO q24 hours	Dosage varies with severity and type of infection

Note: Treatment duration varies with drug, but for systemic infections it is at least 2–3 months, and 1 month past resolution of disease.

ADMINISTRATION AND DOSAGE

Dosage is summarized in Table 17.4. There is no general agreement as to the optimum dosage, total dose, or duration of treatment required for amphotericin B. The dosage generally used is 0.3–1.0 mg/kg per day; it is lower in patients with normal defenses and more-susceptible organisms.

For otherwise healthy animals, IV dosage is 0.5 mg/kg 3 times a week; BUN is monitored for evidence of kidney damage. On the first day the total dose is diluted in 20 ml of 5% dextrose and 5 ml given; if no acute anaphylactic response develops in 1 minute, the remainder is given over 45 seconds. Thereafter the total dose is given over 1 minute in 20 ml of 5% dextrose for 6–12 weeks, 3 times a week. If BUN exceeds 60 mg/dl, the dose is discontinued or reduced 25–50% until BUN falls below 40 mg/dl. Administration by slow IV infusion, in 1 liter of 5% dextrose over 5 hours, though inconvenient, is preferable because it causes less severe systemic toxicity (vomiting, diarrhea, weight loss) and less renal damage (Legendre et al., 1984; Rubin et al., 1989). In severely debilitated dogs, an initial dosage is 0.2 mg/kg IV, increasing by 0.1 mg/kg daily until day 4 (0.5 mg/kg), then using this maintenance dosage as described. In cats with cryptococcal infection, combination with flucytosine reduces the time required for successful treatment.

Subcutaneous administration of amphotericin in 0.45% saline with 0.5% dextrose (0.5–0.8 mg/kg in 500 ml in dogs) and cats (same dose, in 400 ml) 2 or 3 times weekly was described as a way of administering large quantities of amphotericin without producing the marked azotemia associated with bolus IV injection (Malik et al., 1996). The drug was administered in combination with a triazole drug for the treatment of cryptococcal infection.

Amphotericin B lipid complex (Albecet) has been used to treat dogs with blastomycosis at 1 mg/kg q48 hours, for a total cumulative dose of

8–12 mg/kg. Most dogs given a cumulative dose of 12 mg/kg became clinically free of blastomycosis; the 2 dogs in the study receiving a total dose of 8 mg/kg had a relapse of blastomycosis. No dogs developed evidence of renal damage. There is no reported experience with other lipid-based formulations in animals (such as cholesteryl, Amphotec; colloidal, Amphocil; liposomal, AmBisome), but recommended human IV dosage might be appropriate in dogs. Dosage of most lipid-based formulations is approximately 3 mg/kg IV daily, but optimum duration is not well defined. The advantages of lipid-based formulations may be offset by their high cost.

Treatment duration with conventional amphotericin varies with clinical response but may be up to 12 weeks. For blastomycosis the total cumulative dose used is about 12 mg/kg.

CLINICAL APPLICATIONS

Amphotericin B is the most toxic antibiotic in clinical use, but its fungicidal action makes it the drug of choice for most systemic fungal infections (*Candida, Blastomyces, Coccidioides, Histoplasma*) in immunocompromised hosts. In noncompromised hosts, the less toxic, though fungistatic, ketoconazole and the newer triazole drugs may be equally valuable for yeast infections. Comparative clinical trials are required to support this statement. Amphotericin B was the only reliable antifungal drug for systemic aspergillosis and zygomycosis (*Mucor, Rhizopus*), but itraconazole is challenging amphotericin's use for this purpose. Aerosol treatment of pulmonary aspergillosis may be one way to assure high lung levels and low toxicity.

For systemic infections caused by dimorphic fungi, amphotericin may be combined with, precede, or be replaced in nonimmunocompromised hosts by itraconazole or ketoconazole treatment. The drug should not be combined with ketoconazole in the treatment of infections caused by filamentous fungi.

In horses, amphotericin B is not suitable for the local treatment of mycotic keratitis because of its poor activity against some filamentous fungi and its locally irritating nature. The drug was used successfully in treating localized cutaneous phycomycoses (Florida horse leech), in regimens that lasted up to 6 weeks (McMullan et al., 1977). It has not always been effective in nasal or disseminated *Aspergillus* infections in animals, possibly because of their lack of susceptibility. Amphotericin B may be a drug of choice in the treatment of *Prototheca* infections.

Bibliography

Brogden RN, et al. 1998. Amphotericin-B colloidal suspension. Drugs 56:365.
Butler WT, Hill GJ. 1964. Intravenous administration of amphotericin B in the dog. J Am Vet Med Assoc 144:399.

Coukell AJ, Brogden RN. 1998. Liposomal amphotericin B. Drugs 55:585.
Craven PC, Graybill JR. 1984. Combination of oral flucytosine and ketoconazole as therapy for experimental cryptococcal meningitis. J Infect Dis 149:584.
Krawiec DR, et al. 1996. Use of an amphotericin B lipid complex for treatment of blastomycosis in dogs. J Am Vet Med Assoc 209:2073.
Legendre AM, et al. 1984. Treatment of canine blastomycosis with amphotericin B and ketoconazole. J Am Vet Med Assoc 184:1249.
Madison JB, et al. 1995. Amphotericin B treatment of *Candida* arthritis in two horses. J Am Vet Med Assoc 206:338.
Malik R, et al. 1996. Combination chemotherapy of canine and feline cryptococcosis using subcutaneously administered amphotericin B. Aust Vet J 73:124.
McDonald JS, et al. 1980. In vitro antimycotic sensitivity of yeasts isolated from infected bovine mammary glands. Am J Vet Res 41:1987.
McMullan WC, et al. 1977. Amphotericin B for the treatment of localized subcutaneous phycomycoses in the horse. J Am Vet Med Assoc 170:1293.
Niki Y, et al. 1990. Pharmacokinetics of aerosol amphotericin B in rats. Antimicrob Agents Chemother 34:29.
Pyle RL. 1981. Clinical pharmacology of amphotericin B. J Am Vet Med Assoc 179:83.
Reilly LK, Palmer JE. 1994. Systemic candidiasis in four foals. J Am Vet Med Assoc 205:464.
Richardson RC, et al. 1983. Treatment of systemic mycoses in dogs. J Am Vet Med Assoc 183:335.
Rubin SI, et al. 1989. Nephrotoxicity of amphotericin B in dogs: a comparison of two methods of administration. Can J Vet Res 53:23.
White MH, et al. 1997. Amphotericin B colloidal dispersion vs amphotericin B therapy for invasive aspergillosis. Clin Infect Dis 24:635.

Flucytosine

Flucytosine (or 5-fluorocytosine) is a fluorinated pyrimidine, a low-molecular-weight compound slightly soluble in water but readily soluble in alcohol. After permease-mediated entry into the fungal cell, flucytosine is deaminated to 5-fluorouracil, which is incorporated into messenger RNA. This perverted mRNA functions poorly, garbling codon sequences and producing faulty proteins.

Flucytosine has a narrow spectrum of antifungal activity, being active against most *Cryptococcus neoformans*, 80–90% of *Candida,* and most *Torulopsis* and *Cladosporium*. The majority of yeast isolates from bovine mastitis are resistant. Although a few *Aspergillus* strains are susceptible, dermatophytes, other filamentous fungi, and dimorphic fungi are resistant. A strain with MIC ≤16 µg/ml is considered susceptible. The drug is fungicidal at concentrations 5 times the MIC.

About 10–20% of *Candida* but only 1–2% of *Cryptococcus neoformans* show primary resistance. Resistance develops readily in vitro and in vivo; up to two-thirds of fungal isolates change from susceptible to resistant during treatment, and therefore flucytosine should be used only in combination with other antifungal agents. Combination with amphotericin B is commonly synergistic, because amphotericin B increases fungal permeability to flucytosine.

Flucytosine is well absorbed from the intestine after oral administration in humans, giving peak plasma concentrations of 70–80 µg/ml 1–2 hours after a dose of 37.5 mg/kg (Bennett et al., 1979). Half-life in humans is about 4 hours; in the presence of renal impairment the half-life is increased. Penetration into tissues, including cerebrospinal fluid, is excellent. The drug is largely excreted in the urine by glomerular filtration in unchanged form.

Flucytosine is well tolerated. Occasional side effects reported are reversible anorexia, nausea, vomiting, diarrhea, mild elevations of liver enzymes, and bone marrow depression resulting in leukopenia. Intestinal perforation is a rare complication.

Dosage is summarized in Table 17.4. The drug is given in capsule form at a dosage of 200–600 mg/kg daily in 4 divided doses. Successful treatment was achieved in one cat by giving 250 mg/kg q12 hours, when the same dose given q24 hours had failed (Moore, 1982). Flucytosine should be used in conjunction with amphotericin B or ketoconazole.

The major application is in the treatment of cryptococcal infection in cats. Its use for this purpose has now largely been replaced by triazole drugs. The drug should be combined with amphotericin B (or ketoconazole) to prevent the emergence of resistant mutants. The usual dose of amphotericin B can be reduced by half or less, or the normal dose be administered for a shorter period. Ketoconazole can substitute for amphotericin B and significantly reduces the length of treatment required with either drug alone (Shaw, 1988), as do other azole drugs experimentally. Moore (1982) and Wilkinson et al. (1983), however, described successful treatment of cryptococcosis in cats treated with flucytosine alone, given over 4–9 weeks, but because of the likelihood of resistance, this cannot be recommended.

Bibliography

Bennett JE, et al. 1979. A comparison of amphotericin B alone and combined with flucytosine in the treatment of cryptococcal meningitis. N Engl J Med 301:126.

Moore R. 1982. Treatment of feline nasal cryptococcosis with 5-flucytosine. J Am Vet Med Assoc 181:816.

Shaw SE. 1988. Successful treatment of 11 cases of feline cryptococcosis. Aust Vet Pract 18:135.

Wilkinson GT, et al. 1983. Successful treatment of four cases of feline cryptococcosis. J Small Anim Pract 24:507.

Azole Antifungal Drugs for Systemic Use: Imidazoles and Triazoles

Imidazole and triazole drugs have the common antifungal action of inhibiting cytochrome P-450-dependent ergosterol synthesis leading to disruption of fungal membranes and membrane-bound enzymes, as well as other antifungal effects. All are fungistatic drugs, so that prolonged

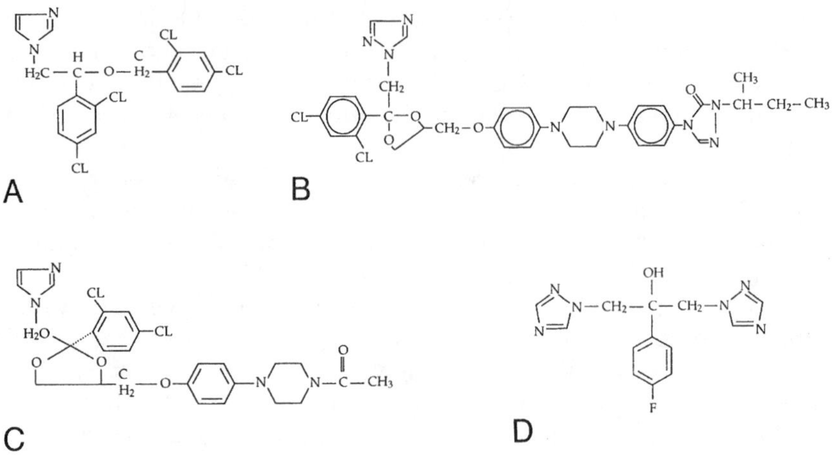

Fig. 17.3. Structural formulas of representative antifungal azole compounds: *A*, miconazole; *B*, itraconazole; *C*, ketoconazole; *D*, fluconazole.

treatment regimens are required, especially in immunocompromised patients.

Azole drugs were first extensively evaluated in the early 1970s for antifungal activity. Clotrimazole could not be administered parenterally, since it rapidly induced hepatic-metabolizing enzymes, and the toxicity of the solubilizing agent required for IV injection of miconazole limited its use. Both drugs are successful topical antifungal agents. Developed in the late 1970s, ketoconazole became a major addition in antifungal therapy, with the advantages of broad antifungal properties, oral administration, and low toxicity. Substitution of the imidazole ring by a triazole ring has produced compounds (fluconazole, itraconazole) (Fig. 17.3) with greatly increased half-lives, oral activity, lower toxicity, and possibly greater antifungal activity than observed with imidazole drugs.

Imidazoles: Ketoconazole

CHEMISTRY

Ketoconazole is a poorly water-soluble, highly lipophilic, weak dibasic compound that requires an acid pH for dissolution, which precedes absorption from the stomach. There are conflicting reports on the effect of feeding on absorption of the drug.

ANTIMICROBIAL ACTIVITY

Ketoconazole is generally fungistatic against a wide range of filamentous fungi, including dermatophytes, yeasts, and dimorphic fungi.

Most strains of *Candida albicans* are sensitive in the range of 0.5–10 μg/ml, but *C. tropicalis* strains are resistant. *Malassezia pachydermatis* is susceptible. Some strains of *Aspergillus* are resistant, and the drug is not usually recommended for *Aspergillus* infections. In one study of fungal isolates from keratomycosis in horses, however, all isolates, which were mainly *Aspergillus*, were susceptible to ketoconazole and miconazole. The drugs are active against some Gram-positive bacteria, and ketoconazole has activity against *Leishmania, Plasmodium,* and other protozoa. The in vitro resistance of *Prototheca* is apparently contradicted by in vivo response to ketoconazole treatment. About three-fourths of yeasts isolated from bovine mastitis were susceptible to ketoconazole and one-third to miconazole, whereas they showed nearly complete susceptibility to clotrimazole (McDonald et al., 1980).

RESISTANCE

Acquired resistance has been reported with ketoconazole but has not been well documented, in part because of the lack of standardization of susceptibility tests.

PHARMACOKINETIC PROPERTIES

Ketoconazole is well absorbed after oral administration; in dogs, plasma concentration after an oral dose of 10 mg/kg peaks at 8.9 μg/ml within 1–2 hours (Moriello, 1986). The drug requires an acid environment for full dissolution and absorption and should be given with food. Ketoconazole is extensively metabolized in the liver to inactive compounds, which are excreted in the bile. The distribution of ketoconazole is limited, and its penetration into cerebrospinal fluid is minimal. The drug does, however, enter milk. Little active drug is excreted in urine. In horses, oral administration of ketoconazole dissolved in 0.2N hydrochloric acid was required for oral absorption of the drug; no absorption of drug suspended in corn syrup occurred (Prades et al., 1989).

DRUG INTERACTIONS

There are conflicting reports about the interactions of imidazoles with amphotericin B. Combination of amphotericin B with ketoconazole gives additive effects in the treatment of cryptococcal infection. It has been suggested, based on consideration of the site of action of the drugs, that the combination does not result in antagonism but rather prevents the fungicidal effect of amphotericin B. Experimentally, however, ketoconazole antagonizes the activity of amphotericin against *Aspergillus.* Combination with flucytosine in the treatment of cryptococcal infections may prevent the emergence of resistance to flucytosine and reduce time required for treatment. Significant drug interactions occur with drugs that inhibit or induce hepatic metabolizing enzymes (eg, barbiturates, rifampin).

TOXICITY AND ADVERSE EFFECTS

Ketoconazole produces no significant adverse effects in humans, although long-term experience with its use is insufficient. Nausea, vomiting, dizziness, itching, and increases in liver enzyme levels are side effects in humans. In dogs the most common side effects are inappetence, pruritus, alopecia, and reversible lightening of the hair (Moriello, 1986). Long-term treatment of dogs (mean 13.6 months, range 3.5–37) has been associated with the development of cataracts (da Costa et al., 1996). Mean time from onset of treatment to development of cataracts was 15 months. Cats appear more sensitive to ketoconazole and may develop anorexia, depression, weight loss, diarrhea, and fever. In a few human patients (1 in 15,000), more severe hepatitis may develop. This reaction does not appear to be dependent on dose. High doses in dogs (greater than 80 mg/kg per day) for prolonged periods have produced severe hepatitis (Moriello, 1986). Cats treated concurrently with flucytosine have shown evidence of liver damage and developed leukopenia, possibly because of additive or synergistic toxicity. Significant inhibition occurs of mammalian P_{450} systems responsible for cholesterol, cortisol and testosterone synthesis. Gynecomastia, decreased libido, and azoospermia have been reported in a small percentage of men but not in dogs or cats. Ketoconazole at therapeutic dosage suppressed plasma cortisol and testosterone but increased progesterone concentrations in dogs (Willard et al., 1986b). Similar effects were not observed in cats (Willard et al., 1986a). Care should therefore be taken when using the drug in male breeding dogs. Ketoconazole may be embryotoxic and teratogenic and should not be given to pregnant animals.

ADMINISTRATION AND DOSAGE

Dosage is summarized in Table 17.4. Absorption from the gastrointestinal tract may be erratic. The oral dosage of ketoconazole in dogs and cats for the treatment of ringworm was extrapolated from human clinical studies and varies from 5–10 mg/kg daily for 4–6 weeks. Recommended dosages of ketoconazole are 10–20 mg/kg for dogs and 10–15 mg/kg for cats, given once daily or in divided doses. Lower doses (11 mg/kg) have been used in the successful treatment of ringworm in dogs (Angarano and Scott, 1987). The relatively slow fungistatic action of ketoconazole requires that rapidly progressing mycotic diseases, such as blastomycosis, be treated initially (or concurrently) with amphotericin B. Coccidioidomycosis, histoplasmosis, and cryptococcosis have, however, been treated successfully in dogs and cats with ketoconazole alone (Dunbar et al., 1983; Marks, 1983; Moriello, 1986). Treatment of coccidioidomycosis requires at least 6 months. In all systemic mycoses, treatment with ketoconazole should last at least 4 weeks after apparent clinical cure, and relapses should be anticipated.

CLINICAL APPLICATIONS

Ketoconazole is the most widely used antifungal drug in veterinary medicine, because of its efficacy, safety, oral dosing, and cost. It is being eclipsed by fluconazole and itraconazole, because of their greater activity and improved pharmacokinetic properties. It is an attractive alternative to amphotericin B in the treatment of systemic mycotic infections (dimorphic fungi, candidiasis, cryptococcosis) in nonimmunocompromised animals. Because of its fungistatic nature, prolonged (3–6 months) treatment is necessary in systemic mycoses to prevent relapse. Although ketoconazole has been used successfully alone in treatment of blastomycosis, coccidioidomycosis, cryptococcosis, and histoplasmosis, current recommendations are to use it in conjunction with amphotericin in the treatment of these systemic mycoses. In the treatment of canine blastomycosis, Legendre et al. (1984) suggested that amphotericin was better than ketoconazole (10 mg/kg daily), but that a course of amphotericin (total 4 mg/kg) followed by ketoconazole (10 mg/kg daily for 2 months) was as effective as more prolonged treatment with amphotericin (total 8–9 mg/kg) and produced less kidney damage.

Ketoconazole is a drug of choice in humans for chronic mucocutaneous candidiasis and in the systemic or topical treatment of vulvovaginal candidiasis. It is not useful in zygomycosis, and its efficacy against *Aspergillus* infections is problematic. Only about 50% of dogs treated for nasal aspergillosis were cured by the use of ketoconazole alone (5 mg/kg, q12 hours) (Sharp and Sullivan, 1989). Combination with 5-flucytosine reduced the dose and duration of treatment required for feline cryptococcosis compared to either drug alone (Shaw, 1988).

Ringworm in dogs and cats has been treated successfully with 10 mg/kg of ketoconazole daily for 10–20 days (DeKeyser and Van den Brande, 1983). Because of ketoconazole's adverse effects (especially in cats) and the lower cost and greater efficacy in vitro of griseofulvin, the latter is preferred for the treatment of ringworm. Animals with lesions may require 6 weeks (range 4–10) for complete resolution (Medleau and Chalmers, 1992). Ketoconazole is effective in the oral treatment of soft tissue sporotrichosis in humans, but high doses are required and relapses may occur. Ketoconazole is the systemic treatment of choice for *Malassezia* infections, although topical treatment with ketoconazole or miconazole is more usual.

Bibliography

Angarano DW, Scott DW. 1987. Use of ketoconazole in treatment of dermatophytosis in a dog. J Am Vet Med Assoc 190:1433.

Coad TC, et al. 1985. Antifungal sensitivity testing for equine keratomycosis. Am J Vet Res 46:676.

da Costa PD, et al. 1996. Cataracts in dogs after long-term ketoconazole therapy. Vet Comp Ophthamol 6:176.

DeBoer DJ, Moriello KA. 1995. Clinical update on feline dermatophytosis—Part II. Compend Cont Educ Pract Vet 17:1471.

DeKeyser H, Van den Brande M. 1983. Ketoconazole in the treatment of dermatomycosis in cats and dogs. Vet Q 5:142.

Dunbar MR, et al. 1983. Treatment of canine blastomycosis with ketoconazole. J Am Vet Med Assoc 182:156.

Legendre AM, et al. 1984. Treatment of canine blastomycosis with amphotericin B and ketoconazole. J Am Vet Med Assoc 184:1249.

Marks DL. 1983. Treatment of coccidioidomycosis with ketoconazole. Canine Pract 10:35.

Mason GD, et al. 1989. Ketoconazole therapy in a dog with systemic cryptococcosis. J Am Vet Med Assoc 195:954.

McDonald JS, et al. 1980. In vitro antimycotic sensitivity of yeasts isolated from infected bovine mammary glands. Am J Vet Res 41:1987.

Medleau L, Chalmers SA. 1992. Ketoconazole for treatment of dermatophytosis in cats. J Am Vet Med Assoc 200:77.

Moriello KA. 1986. Ketoconazole: clinical pharmacology and therapeutic recommendations. J Am Vet Med Assoc 188:303.

Noxon JO, Schmidt DA. 1986. Disseminated histoplasmosis in a cat: successful treatment with ketoconazole. J Am Vet Med Assoc 181:817.

Prades M, et al. 1989. Body fluid and endometrial concentrations of ketoconazole in mares after intravenous injection or repeated gavage. Equine Vet J 21:211.

Sharp NJH, Sullivan M. 1989. Use of ketoconazole in the treatment of canine nasal aspergillosis. J Am Vet Med Assoc 194:782.

Shaw SE. 1988. Successful treatment of 11 cases of feline cryptococcosis. Aust Vet Pract 18:135.

Willard MD, et al. 1986a. Effect of long-term administration of ketoconazole in cats. Am J Vet Res 47:2510.

Willard MD, et al. 1986b. Ketoconazole-induced changes in selected canine hormone concentrations. Am J Vet Res 47:2504.

Triazoles: Itraconazole

CHEMISTRY

Like ketoconazole, itraconazole is a poorly water-soluble, highly lipophilic, weakly dibasic triazole compound that also requires an acid pH for absorption from the stomach.

ANTIMICROBIAL ACTIVITY

Itraconazole is a potent inhibitor of most fungal pathogens of animals, because of its greater selectivity for the fungal cytochrome system than ketoconazole (see Table 17.3). The spectrum includes dimorphic fungi, *Cryptococcus, Sporothrix, Alternaria,* most *Aspergillus,* and *Candida tropicalis,* but activity against other *Candida* spp., the dermatophytes, and the agents of phaeohyphomycoses is variable. It is fungicidal at low concentrations against some fungi. For *Candida* spp. and *Cryptococcus neofor-*

mans, organisms with MIC ≤0.12 µg/ml are regarded as susceptible, those with MIC 0.25–0.5 µg/ml as susceptible depending on dose, and those with MIC ≥1 µg/ml as resistant.

PHARMACOKINETIC PROPERTIES

A lipophilic drug, itraconazole is well absorbed after oral administration and widely distributed to tissues (except the CSF), where it achieves concentrations several times those in plasma. Skin concentrations exceed plasma concentrations and marked keratin binding occurs; this is significant in the treatment of dermatophyte infections. Food significantly enhances absorption. The half-life in humans is 17 hours. It is cleared mainly by intrahepatic metabolism and virtually no drug appears in the urine or cerebrospinal fluid, even though the drug has been successfully used in the treatment of cryptococcal meningitis. A steady state in serum concentration was achieved in cats after 2–3 weeks of administration of 10 mg/kg q24 hours (Boothe et al., 1997). As with other azoles, concurrent administration of rifampin will increase hepatic metabolism of itraconazole and ketoconazole.

TOXICITY AND ADVERSE EFFECTS

Because of greater selective effects of itraconazole than ketoconazole against fungi, toxicity reported in humans is minimal and limited to nausea in a small proportion of patients and rare, transient increases in hepatic enzymes. Blockage of adrenal steroid or testosterone synthesis has not been described. No adverse effects developed in cats treated with 10 mg/kg per day for 3 months, whereas cats treated with the same dosage of ketoconazole developed anorexia and weight loss (Medleau et al., 1990). Adverse effects reported in dogs and cats have, apart from occasional anorexia and vomiting, been minimal. Dosage can be progressively decreased in animals that vomit or become anorectic until these effects are no longer observed. Fatal hepatotoxicity was reported in one cat treated with over 20 mg/kg (Medleau et al., 1995). Drug eruption has been described in a dog (Plotnick et al., 1997). Itraconazole is contraindicated in pregnancy.

ADMINISTRATION AND DOSAGE

Recommended dosage is summarized in Table 17.4. Itraconazole is administered orally to monogastrates, preferably with food. Dosage in animals has not been determined, but a dosage of 10 mg/kg q24 hours or 5 mg/kg q12 hours would seem appropriate. Duration of treatment should be tailored to clinical and mycological response.

Dosage of 5 mg/kg q24 hours for 60 days was as effective as 10 mg/kg q24 hours for the treatment of canine blastomycosis and was associated with fewer adverse effects (Legendre et al., 1996); about 20% of treated dogs relapsed. Dosage in humans is ≤400 mg/day, but higher doses (600 mg) have been used in infections that have not responded to the lower dose, although toxicity was observed in long-term use of high dosage (Sharkey et al., 1991). Dosage of 5 mg/kg q12 hours for 60 days or more was used to treat histoplasmosis in cats; recurrence of disease occurred in 2 of 8 treated cats, which required further treatment (Hodges et al., 1994). The dosage of 5 mg/kg q12 hours in cats can safely be increased to 10 mg/kg q12 hours (Boothe et al., 1997). Dosage of 1.5–3 mg/kg q24 hours, usually for 15 days (but sometimes for longer), was effective in controlling dermatophytosis in cats (Mancianti et al., 1998).

CLINICAL APPLICATIONS

Because of its potency, pharmacokinetic advantages, clinical efficacy, and safety, itraconazole has become the systemic treatment of choice for aspergillosis, blastomycosis, coccidioidomycosis, histoplasmosis, and sporotrichosis. It has similar application to that of ketoconazole, but its broader spectrum includes *Aspergillus* and the agents of phaeohyphomycosis. It has greater activity against *Sporothrix*. It is as effective as but less toxic than ketoconazole in the treatment of cryptococcosis and dermatophyte infections. It is as effective as griseofulvin in the treatment of dermatophyte infection in cats (Moriello and DeBoer, 1995). Treatment of serious infections with this generally fungistatic drug needs to be prolonged (>3 months), and relapses anticipated. The effectiveness of treatment may be monitored by serology, for cryptococcal (Jacobs et al., 1997) and possibly for other systemic mycoses. In the treatment of serious systemic mycoses, combination with amphotericin in the initial stages of treatment is advisable.

Although itraconazole has been used successfully to treat disseminated *Aspergillus* infections in dogs (Kelly et al., 1995), its oral administration has been found to be ineffective in treatment of canine nasal aspergillosis. In high doses, it has successfully treated cerebral aspergillosis in humans (Verweij et al., 1997). The drug has a particularly useful place in the systemic treatment of aspergillosis in pet birds; pharmacokinetic studies in blue-fronted Amazon parrots suggested that a dosage of 10 mg/kg q24 hours was appropriate (Orosz et al., 1996).

In horses, topically applied 1% itraconazole with 30% dimethyl sulfoxide (DMSO) ointment gave considerably higher corneal concentrations than drug without DMSO (Ball et al., 1997a); applied every 4 hours for a median of 35 days, it was effective in resolving keratomycosis in the majority of cases (Ball et al., 1997b). Administered orally at 3 mg/kg q12 hours for 3.5–5 months, itraconazole was effective in the treatment of mycotic rhinitis in horses (Korenek et al., 1994). Oral administration of 5 mg/kg q24 hours was combined with locally applied enilconazole in the successful treatment of guttural pouch mycosis (Davis and Legendre, 1994).

Bibliography

Ball MA, et al. 1997a. Corneal concentrations and preliminary toxicological evaluation of an itraconazole/dimethyl sulphoxide ophthalmic ointment. J Vet Pharmacol Ther 20:100.
Ball MA, et al. 1997b. Evaluation of itraconazole-dimethyl sulfoxide ointment for treatment of keratomycosis in nine horses. J Am Vet Med Assoc 211:199.
Boothe DM, et al. 1997. Itraconazole disposition after single oral and intravenous and multiple oral dosing in healthy cats. Am J Vet Res 58:872.
Davis EW, Legendre AM. 1994. Successful treatment of guttural pouch mycosis with itraconazole and topical enilconazole in a horse. J Vet Intern Med 8:304.
Heit MC, Riviere JE. 1995. Antifungal therapy: ketoconazole and other azole derivatives. Compend Cont Educ Pract Vet 17:21.
Hodges RD, et al. 1994. Itraconazole for the treatment of histoplasmosis in cats. J Vet Intern Med 8:409.
Jacobs GJ, et al. 1997. Cryptococcal infection in cats: factors influencing treatment outcome, and results of sequential serum antigen titers in 35 cats. J Vet Intern Med 11:1.
Kelly SE, et al. 1995. Long-term survival of four dogs with disseminated Aspergillus terreus infection treated with itraconazole. Aust Vet J 72:311.
Korenek NL, et al. 1994. Treatment of mycotic rhinitis with itraconazole in three horses. J Vet Intern Med 8:224.
Legendre AM, et al. 1996. Treatment of blastomycosis with itraconazole in 112 dogs. J Vet Intern Med 10:365.
Mancianti F, et al. 1998. Efficacy of oral administration of itraconazole to cats with dermatophytosis caused by Microsporum canis. J Am Vet Med Assoc 213:993.
Medleau L, et al. 1990. Evaluation of ketoconazole and itraconazole for treatment of disseminated cryptococcosis in cats. Am J Vet Res 51:1454.
Medleau L, et al. 1995. Itraconazole for the treatment of cryptococcosis in cats. J Vet Intern Med 9:39.
Moriello KA, DeBoer DJ. 1995. Efficacy of griseofulvin and itraconazole in the treatment of experimentally induced dermatophytosis in cats. J Am Vet Med Assoc 207:439.
Orosz SE, et al. 1996. Pharmacokinetic properties of itraconazole in Blue-fronted Amazon parrots (Amazona aestiva aestiva). J Avian Med Surg 10:168.
Plotnick AN, et al. 1997. Primary cutaneous coccidioidomycosis and subsequent drug eruption to itraconazole in a dog. J Am Anim Hosp Assoc 33:139.
Sharkey PK, et al. 1991. High-dose itraconazole in the treatment of severe mycoses. Antimicrob Agents Chemother 35:707.
Verweij PE, et al. 1997. High-dose itraconazole for the treatment of cerebral aspergillosis. Clin Infect Dis 23:1196.

Triazoles: Fluconazole

Fluconazole is a specific inhibitor of the fungal enzyme lanosterol 14α-demethylase, preventing conversion of fungal cell lanosterol to the membrane lipid ergosterol. It is highly selective for fungal cytochrome P-450 enzymes.

CHEMISTRY

Fluconazole is a water-soluble bis-triazole compound with marked pharmacokinetic differences from ketoconazole and itraconazole.

ANTIMICROBIAL ACTIVITY

Fluconazole has broad antifungal activity and is effective against *Blastomyces dermatitidis, Candida albicans* and many other *Candida* spp., *Cryptococcus neoformans, Coccidioides immitis,* and *Histoplasma capsulatum* (see Table 17.3). It is usually ineffective against *Aspergillus.* For *Candida* and *Cryptococcus,* organisms with MIC ≤8 μg/ml are regarded as susceptible, with MIC 16–32 μg/ml as susceptible dependent on dose, and with MIC ≥64 μg/ml as resistant.

RESISTANCE

Candida glabrata and *C. krusei* are resistant. Progressive development of acquired resistance in *C. albicans* has been reported in isolates from AIDS patients and occurs during long-term treatment.

PHARMACOKINETIC PROPERTIES

In contrast to other azoles, fluconazole is a water-soluble, weakly protein-bound drug, and oral absorption is unaffected by acid. It is well absorbed after oral administration, and because of its low molecular weight, water solubility, and lack of protein binding, it distributes widely to tissues. Its ability to reach high concentrations (50–90% of serum) in cerebrospinal fluid is a particular advantage in treating yeast (eg, *Cryptococcus*) infections in the brain. Food does not affect absorption. The drug is excreted unchanged in the urine. Half-life in humans is 25–30 hours, so that single oral dosing is used for some types of infections. Half-life in cats has been reported as 14 or 25 hours (Malik et al., 1992; Vaden et al., 1997). In contrast to ketoconazole and itraconazole, fluconazole can be administered IV.

TOXICITY AND ADVERSE EFFECTS

Fluconazole is well tolerated after oral or IV administration, with minimal side effects other than nausea, skin rash, and headaches in some human patients. There is no evidence of interference with steroid biosynthesis, but elevations in hepatic enzymes, which are usually mild, have been reported. It can interfere with the metabolism of drugs whose metabolism is dependent on hepatic P-450 enzymes. Drug eruption has been described in dogs a median of 20 days after start of fluconazole treatment (median dose 50 mg/kg q8 hours, combined with other antifungal drugs) (Malik et al., 1996). Healing took more than 2 weeks after discontinuation of the drug, up to 2 months in some cases.

ADMINISTRATION AND DOSAGE

Dosage recommendations for fluconazole in animals are largely empirical. Cryptococcal infections in cats were successfully treated with

50 mg/cat q12 hours (Malik et al., 1992); in one animal, 100 mg q12 hours was required. Pharmacokinetic considerations led Vaden et al. (1997) to suggest a dose in cats of 50 mg/cat q24 hours. A dose of 11 mg/kg q24 hours was used in the effective treatment of cryptococcosis in a dog and was reduced to 4.2 mg/kg several weeks later, when anorexia developed (Tiches et al., 1998).

CLINICAL APPLICATIONS

Fluconazole has had excellent success in oral treatment of local or systemic candidiasis in humans and is a drug of choice for this purpose. In severe candidiasis, it should be combined with amphotericin. In vaginal candidiasis in women, treatment with a single oral dose has been effective. Fluconazole is also the treatment of choice for cryptococcal meningitis in AIDS patients. It is as effective as amphotericin B in treatment of acute cryptococcal meningitis in all patients and is more effective in maintenance therapy in AIDS patients. Initial concurrent treatment with amphotericin B is recommended. It is a drug of choice for candidal cystitis. In animals, fluconazole is probably the drug of choice for cryptococcal infections and for the systemic treatment of candidal infections (which are rare). It may be useful in the treatment of *Prototheca* infections.

Efficacy against blastomycosis, histoplasmosis, and sporotrichosis in humans has been moderate at the dosages assessed; fluconazole is not as effective as itraconazole for these infections. Its effectiveness against *Aspergillus* pneumonia in humans has been variable. Fluconazole was administered PO at 2.5–5 mg/kg per day to dogs in a divided dose in the successful treatment of nasal aspergillosis or penicilliosis. Treatment was for a minimum of 8 weeks and was successful in 6 of 10 dogs (Sharp et al., 1991).

Bibliography

Bennett JE. 1990. Fluconazole: a novel advance in therapy for systemic fungal infections. Rev Infect Dis 12:S263.

Craig AJ, et al. 1994. Pharmacokinetics of fluconazole in cats after intravenous and oral administration. Res Vet Sci 57:372.

Malik R, et al. 1992. Cryptococcosis in cats: clinical and mycological assessment of 29 cats and evaluation of treatment using orally administered fluconazole. J Med Vet Mycol 30:133.

Malik R, et al. 1996. Suspected drug eruption in seven dogs during administration of flucytosine. Aust Vet J 74:285.

Sharp NJH, et al. 1991. Treatment of canine nasal aspergillosis/penicilliosis with fluconazole (UK-49,858). J Small Anim Pract 32:513.

Tiches D, et al. 1998. A case of canine central nervous system cryptococcosis: management with fluconazole. J Am Anim Hosp Assoc 34:145.

Vaden SL, et al. 1997. Fluconazole in cats: pharmacokinetics following intravenous and oral administration and penetration into cerebrospinal fluid, aqueous humour, and pulmonary epithelial lining fluid. J Vet Pharmacol Ther 20:181.

Triazoles: Voriconazole

Voriconazole is a triazole drug active against opportunist fungi resistant to fluconazole, including *Aspergillus* spp. and *Candida glabrata* and *C. krusei*. It is less active on a weight basis than itraconazole against filamentous fungi, more potent than itraconazole against fluconazole-susceptible *Candida* spp., and as potent as itraconazole against fluconazole-resistant *Candida*. It is fungicidal against *Aspergillus* and has proven more efficacious than itraconazole in the systemic treatment of some experimental infections with *Aspergillus* spp. in animals.

Other Antifungal Agents

Echinocandins and Pneumocandins

Echinocandins and pneumocandins are novel lipopeptide antifungal agents which are 1,3-D-glucan synthase inhibitors, preventing production of an essential polysaccharide in the cell wall of many fungi. The first echinocandin, cilofungin, failed in clinical development, but echinocandin B and pneumocandin B are likely to be introduced into clinical use. Pneumoncandin is named for its activity against *Pneumocystis* and *Candida*. These drugs are active against fluconazole-resistant *Candida* as well as against *Aspergillus* spp. and other important filamentous fungi but are not active against *Blastomyces dermatitidis*, *Cryptococcus neoformans*, or *Fusarium* spp., since these lack 1,3-D-glucan synthase.

Iodides

Iodides have been used for many years to treat mycotic infections. Their action is unknown, but action may result from enhancement of the immune response of the host, by spurring the halide-peroxide killing system of phagocytic cells. Amphotericin B and imidazoles also affect the immune system. Sodium iodide has been the treatment of choice in sporotrichosis, but itraconazole is probably preferable. Ketoconazole and sodium iodide administered together appear to have additive effects. The dose is 20 mg/kg in cats and 40 mg/kg in dogs. The drug is administered orally once or twice daily, and a response occurs in 1–4 weeks; treatment should be continued for several weeks past clinical cure. Treatment should be temporarily stopped if signs of iodism occur. Sodium iodide has been used as an adjunct in the treatment of nasal aspergillosis in dogs (Barrett et al., 1977). Sodium iodide has been administered IV, 1 g/15 kg in a 10% solution, in the treatment of ringworm in cattle. The use of iodine preparations in animals that will enter the human food chain is discouraged because of the residue such preparations leave.

Bibliography

Barrett RE, et al. 1977. Treatment and immunological evaluation of three cases of canine aspergillosis. J Am Anim Hosp Assoc 13:328.
Burke MJ, et al. 1983. Successful treatment of cutaneolymphatic sporotrichosis in a cat with ketoconazole and sodium iodide. J Am Anim Hosp Assoc 19:542.

18 | Antiviral Chemotherapy

D. YOO

Viruses are the simplest of organisms, with a genome size between only 1.5 to 200 kilobases of DNA or RNA. Because of the limited capacity of their genome, viruses do not carry all the genes required for multiplication but rather carry only the most essential genes. For multiplication, viruses therefore pirate the cellular machinery of the infected cell, so that virus multiplication is strictly dependent on the metabolic pathway of the host cell. Despite the simple nature of viruses, development of antiviral agents has been very slow, the major reason being the inability to distinguish viral-specific multiplication pathways from normal cellular metabolic processes. Since the inhibitory effect of an antiviral agent may be general for both viral and cellular processes, the efficacy demonstrated in vitro is far remote from the clinical efficacy, mainly because of toxic effects of the antiviral agents. In the past two decades, however, improved understanding of the replication cycles of viruses has led to the development of selective antiviral drugs to inhibit specific stages of virus replication.

A general overview of virus life cycle reveals some stages that may be useful to target for chemotherapeutic inhibition of virus replication (Fig. 18.1).

Virus replication starts with attachment of the virus to specific receptors on the cell surface, followed by penetration into the cell either by direct fusion of viral membrane with plasma membrane and/or by endocytosis, depending on the particular virus involved. The attachment and penetration steps include specific interactions between viral proteins and cellular proteins, specific interactions that can be targeted for antiviral inhibitors. Once internalized into the cell, the viral genome is released for synthesis of viral proteins and for replication of viral DNA or RNA. Repli-

396

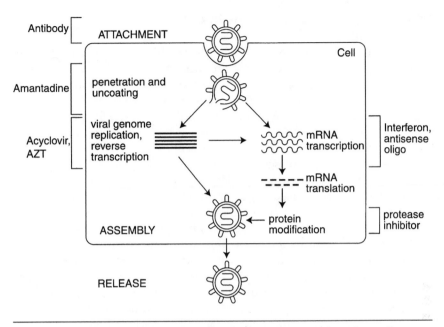

Fig. 18.1.   Schematic of viral replication process within a host cell, indicating targets for antiviral drugs.

cation of viral nucleic acids is generally mediated by virally encoded enzymes, either by DNA or RNA polymerases or by nucleoside kinases, processes that can also be a target for specific inhibition of the virus. Many of the licensed drugs currently used in antiviral chemotherapy are directed against the synthesis of viral DNA or RNA. When viral messenger RNAs (mRNAs) are synthesized, translation of the viral mRNAs can be a target to block virus multiplication. Translation of mRNAs can be blocked either in a general fashion to block both viral and cellular mRNAs, or in a rather selective way to block only the viral-specific mRNA using a specific antisense oligonucleotide. Once mRNAs are translated, the proteins are often processed further to yield smaller subunit proteins by a specific proteolytic cleavage or to add carbohydrates, lipids, or phosphate groups to the protein. Inhibition of proteolytic cleavage or of the addition of carbohydrates has also been a target for antiviral therapy. Specific inhibition of protease activity is an attractive target, and antiprotease drugs have been recently licensed to treat HIV infection for AIDS patients.

    This chapter describes basic strategies for developing antiviral drugs, the modes of action of some of the successful drugs, and their veterinary application.

Inhibitors of Virus Attachment to Cells
Immunoglobulin

Administration of immunoglobulin can block the initial stage of virus life cycle by preventing the attachment of virus to cells. Immunoglobulins are prepared from pooled plasma to contain predominantly IgG selected for high titers of antibody (hyperimmune) for specific viruses. Immunoglobulins are more effective when used for prophylactic purpose than therapeutic purpose, because the passively administered immunoglobulins are present in the extracellular phase where the antibodies can neutralize viruses before they enter into cells. In veterinary medicine, oral administration of colostrum containing high titers of specific antibody has been used to prevent transmissible gastroenteritis virus infection in swine. A similar approach has been practiced in newborn calves to prevent neonatal scours caused by bovine rotavirus and bovine coronavirus. Vaccination of dams with appropriate antigens increases the specific antibody titers in the colostrum, and the suckling offspring is protected from enteric virus infections during the nursing period (Lee et al., 1995). In human medicine, immunoglobulins have been available predominantly for IM administration. Since large volumes of immunoglobulin cannot be administered IM, the amount that can be given by this route is limited. It is not possible to administer immunoglobulin IV, because of the tendency for IgG to form aggregates and to fix complement in the body. Recent advances in cold fractionation procedures have made it possible to prevent the IgG aggregation, and newer preparations are available for IV administration (Pennington, 1990). Immunoglobulins are safe, with very few side effects. In people, immunoglobulins are used for preexposure prevention of hepatitis A and for postexposure prevention of hepatitis B and rabies virus infections. Intravenous administration of immunoglobulin is useful to treat the immunodeficiency state. In AIDS patients, the immunoglobulin itself does not contain antibodies for HIV, but rather it contains antibodies to other infectious agents, which function to prevent opportunistic infections during the immunodeficiency state.

Receptor Homologs

A number of compounds inhibit initial attachment of virus to cell receptors. Among the most extensively studied is the WIN compound for picornavirus (Rueckert, 1996). This drug inserts into a hydrophobic pocket within the canyon floor on the surface of the virus particle. Binding of the drug triggers deformation of the receptor binding site of the virus, leading to inhibition of the virus attachment to the cellular receptor. Since most of the many serotypes of human rhinovirus utilize a single cellular receptor (ICAM-1), the drug is effective against most rhinoviruses.

Rhinoviruses are the major cause of common cold, and the drug is therefore most effective when delivered intranasally.

Inhibitors of Uncoating of Virus
Amantadine and Rimantadine (Ion Channel Blocking Agents)

Amantadine and its structural analog, rimantadine, were first recognized to possess antiviral activity for influenza A virus in cell culture and in mouse and ferret models in the 1960s. The spectrum of these drugs was limited to type A influenza virus only, with no activity for type B influenza virus, parainfluenza virus, or other respiratory viruses. It was two decades later before the molecular basis for the inhibitory mechanisms was precisely elucidated. Influenza virus contains single-stranded RNA as a genome consisting of eight RNA segments. Individual RNA segments are packaged into viral ribonucleoprotein complex (vRNP) in association with M1 protein and the nucleocapsid protein (NP). Following attachment to the cellular receptor to initiate infection, influenza virus is internalized by receptor-mediated endocytosis and is delivered to endosomes. The M2 protein, a small protein associated in the membrane of the virus, appears to function as an ion channel for proton influx from the endosome into the interior of the virion before viral membrane and endosomal membrane fusion occurs. Low pH in the virion causes dissociation of the M1 protein from the RNP complex. In parallel, low pH in the endosome triggers fusion of viral membrane with the endosomal membrane. This fusion allows entry of the viral RNP complex and the M1 protein into the cytoplasm, where the vRNP is further transported to the nucleus to initiate replication and transcription of viral RNA. The M2 protein is the target of amantadine, which binds to the protein and blocks its ion channel activity. In consequence, the pH in the virion is not changed and the M1 protein is therefore not dissociated from the vRNP complex. Association of the M1 protein with the RNP complex prevents transport of the RNP to the nucleus, thereby inhibiting the subsequent replication transcription of the viral genome. Amantadine is highly specific for influenza virus type A. The sequence of the M2 protein is conserved in the transmembrane domain for both human and avian strains of influenza A virus, and thus the drug is effective for both strains of virus.

Clinical Application

Both amantadine and rimantadine are available in oral formulations. The drugs are absorbed well in the body, with peak plasma concentration occurring 2–4 hours after oral administration. Amantadine is metabolically stable, and adequate antiviral levels can be achieved in the lungs, nasal mucus, and saliva. Protection efficacy against influenza A virus infection is up to 90% in humans. Amantadine has been evaluated in horses to treat equine influenza virus infection (Rees et al., 1997). Intravenous injection of amantadine at 15 mg/kg of body weight can yield plasma concentrations of safe and effective levels for antiviral therapy in the treated horse. However, commercial preparation is available only in a tablet form and an oral syrup, and the oral administration of amantadine appears to be generally poor in yielding effective plasma concentrations. Rimantadine has been demonstrated to be more effective than amantadine in that oral administration of rimantadine at 30 mg/kg of body weight twice daily provided safe and effective serum concentration to prevent the infection. Neurotoxicity in the central nervous system has been observed at a higher dose administration in horses. The cost to treat one mature Thoroughbred horse with oral amantadine syrup may, however, be up to $600 per day.

Inhibitors of DNA or RNA Synthesis
Nucleoside Analogs
IDOXURIDINE, VIDARABINE, AND TRIFLURIDINE

Antiviral drugs used in the early years were mostly nucleoside analogs synthesized as anticancer drugs. Since smallpox and herpesvirus infections were among the most important viral diseases during that time, the anticancer drugs were tested for antiviral activities for these viruses. Idoxuridine, vidarabine, and trifluridine are potent inhibitors of herpesvirus DNA synthesis. During the synthesis of the DNA strand, these drugs are incorporated into the growing chain of viral DNA, resulting in the misinterpretation of the genetic codes. However, the blocking effect is not restricted to the virus alone but is also directed toward the normal cells to cause a significant cytotoxicity, such as loss of hair, anemia, and neutropenia. Therefore, these drugs are recommended for use as topical applications.

ACYCLOVIR AND RELATED DRUGS

The discovery of acyclovir was a major breakthrough in antiviral chemotherapy. Acyclovir appears to be selective for viral rather than normal cellular functions, specific selectivity that results in fewer cytotoxic effects. The molecular target for acyclovir is the viral DNA polymerase. Acyclovir has potent activity against herpesviruses but not against other viral families. In herpesvirus-infected cells, acyclovir is phosphorylated by thymidine kinase to become acycloguanosine monophosphate (ACG-P). The thymidine kinase encoded by herpesviruses has broader specificity than cellular kinase, and thus acycloguanosine is selectively phosphorylated by the herpesvirus thymidine kinase (Fig. 18.2).

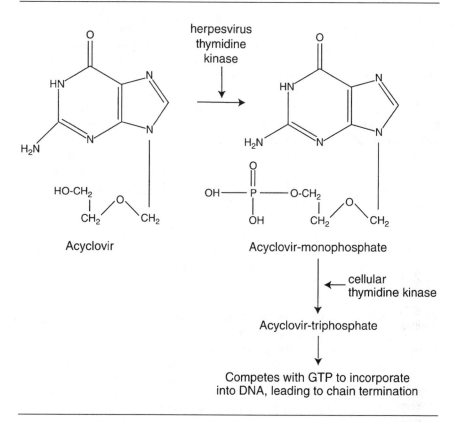

Fig. 18.2. Mechanism of metabolism of acyclovir in the cell to produce the active antiviral drug.

ACG-P is then further phosphorylated to acycloguanosine triphosphate (ACG-PPP) by a normal cellular kinase. ACG-PPP competes with guanosine triphosphate (GTP) to incorporate into a DNA chain. Since acyclovir lacks the 3' hydroxyl group, once ACG-PPP is incorporated into the growing DNA strand, further elongation of the DNA chain is terminated. In normal cells, acyclovir is not phosphorylated, because of the lack of herpesvirus-encoded thymidine kinase, and thus acyclovir is essentially nontoxic to uninfected cells. In humans, acyclovir and its derivatives are drugs of choice for treating the herpes simplex virus types 1 (HSV-1) and 2 (HSV-2) and varicella-zoster virus (VZV, chickenpox) infections.

Ganciclovir is a guanosine analog structurally similar to acyclovir but approximately 100 times more potent against cytomegaloherpesvirus (CMV) than acyclovir. The reason for its greater activity against CMV is not clear. Since more than 90% of the administered acyclovir is recovered intact in urine, several prodrugs have been developed to increase the bioavailability. Valaciclovir is a valyl ester of acyclovir and is an oral prodrug that is rapidly converted to acyclovir and L-valine, the essential amino acid, by intestinal and hepatic metabolism. Therefore, valaciclovir is similar to acyclovir in therapeutic efficacy but has greater bioavailability. Penciclovir is a synthetic acyclic guanine derivative, chemically similar to ganciclovir but functionally closer to acyclovir. Bioavailability is poor for penciclovir, and an orally administered prodrug has been developed. Famciclovir is a prodrug of penciclovir with a higher bioavailability and elimination rate. The members of this series of acyclovir derivatives are all effective for HSV-1, HSV-2, and VZV, with a relatively high elimination rate of more than 90% through urine.

RIBAVIRIN

When ribavirin was first synthesized, it was thought to be a promising antiviral agent, since the drug showed a wide spectrum of antiviral activity for both DNA and RNA viruses in cell culture and in experimental animals. Ribavirin resembles guanosine in its structure, but the mode of action has not been precisely defined. It appears that ribavirin functions at multiple stages of cellular process. In cells, ribavirin is phosphorylated by cellular kinase and converted to ribavirin monophosphate. Ribavirin monophosphate inhibits inosine monophosphate dehydrogenase, an enzyme essential for the synthesis of GTP. GTP is an essential component for DNA synthesis, and its inhibition results in the decrease of the cellular pool of GTP, preventing DNA synthesis. Ribavirin also inhibits the capping process of the 5' end of messenger RNA. In eukaryotic cells, 5' capping of mRNA mediates translation initiation, and thus its inhibition blocks protein synthesis. Ribavirin also directly inhibits the RNA-dependent RNA polymerase of influenza virus.

Clinical Application of Nucleoside Analogs

Idoxuridine has been successfully used in horses infected with herpesvirus. Foals suffering from equine herpesvirus type 2 (EHV-2) keratopathy and conjunctivitis with nodular corneal opacity infection were successfully treated with ophthalmic medication containing 0.5% idoxuridine during an outbreak on a large breeding farm (Collinson et al., 1994). Trifluridine and idoxuridine have been also tested for feline herpesvirus type 1 (FHV-1) infection, which causes acute respiratory disease, keratitis, and conjunctivitis in cats. Both trifluridine and idoxuridine as 0.1% ophthalmic solution are effective for FHV-1 conjunctivitis. Trifluridine had better corneal penetration than idoxuridine. Trifluridine eyedrops may be applied 6 times daily for 2–3 weeks. However, idoxuridine was ineffective for treatment of systemic canine herpesvirus (CHV) infection. In contrast, pups given vidarabine survived CHV infection.

A major toxic effect of ribavirin is anemia. The phosphorylated ribavirin diffuses into erythrocytes and accumulates in the erythrocytes without further processing. The erythrocytes become damaged and are subsequently eliminated from the circulation, causing anemia. Although the side effect is reversible, the half-life of ribavirin in erythrocytes is 40 days in humans, and thus the side effect is prolonged. In infants with respiratory syncytial virus, ribavirin has some effects of reducing the severity and duration of illness. Ribavirin has been shown to possess therapeutic effects for bunyaviruses, especially human hantavirus infection, arenaviruses, and reoviruses to some extent and especially when given at an early stage of illness. Ribavirin is an expensive drug; the cost of treatment may be more than $400 per day.

Ribavirin has been shown to be effective against feline infectious peritonitis virus (FIPV) in vitro and in vivo. Ribavirin treatment of cats infected with FIPV, combined with human interferon alpha (IFN-α), increases survival time and reduces clinical signs of the disease. Although interferon is well tolerated in cats, ribavirin is toxic at a normal dosage of 10 mg/kg. A much lower dosage of ribavirin (5 mg/kg), combined with interferon, is recommended for better therapeutic effects for FIPV infection. For feline calicivirus (FeCV) infection in cats, ribavirin treatment did not modify the disease clinically, nor did it reduce the duration of virus shedding even when the treatment started within 1 day of exposure. Toxic effects of ribavirin are severe in cats with depression of red blood cell and white blood cell counts and thrombocytopenia (Povey, 1978). In ferrets, ribavirin has significant therapeutic effects on influenza A virus infection.

Acyclovir treatment as a 3% ointment is used to treat chronic FHV-1 conjunctivitis, although results are variable (Greene, 1998). The cat may feel irritation in the eyes upon application of the acyclovir ointment. Acyclovir has been tested for systemic treatment of FHV-1 infection, but its efficacy is apparently far less (80 times) in cats than in humans. Cats treated with valaciclovir for FHV-1 infection became more lethargic and dehydrated. Total WBC and neutrophil counts were significantly decreased, and even high doses did not suppress FHV-1 replication in acutely infected cats (Nasisse et al., 1997). Valaciclovir was ineffective against systemic FHV-1 infection in cats, and moreover, cats are very sensitive to its toxic effects.

Acyclovir has been also used in horses in an attempt to treat foals affected with equine herpesvirus (EHV-1) during an outbreak on a breeding farm. Of 5 foals with obvious morbidity with EHV-1 infection, 3 foals were given 16 mg/kg of acyclovir. Two foals survived the infection, suggesting that acyclovir might have influenced the clinical outcome (Murray et al., 1998). Acyclovir is effective in vitro for other herpesviruses such as turkey herpesvirus and Marek's disease virus (MDV). Acyclovir suppresses the development of tumors in birds infected with MDV (Samoreksalamonowicz and Wijaszka, 1987).

Pyrophosphate Analog

Foscarnet is a pyrophosphate analog that directly inhibits both DNA polymerase and RNA polymerase. Foscarnet is chemically distinct from nucleoside analogs and does not incorporate into the DNA or RNA chain but inhibits the synthesis of nucleic acids. By oral administration, the bioavailability of foscarnet is poor—10% in dogs and 35% in cats—and thus the drug is given by IV injection. Although foscarnet is rapidly eliminated from plasma in young cats, clearance is slower in older cats, and approximately 5–10% of the administered foscarnet accumulates in bones (Swenson et al., 1990). Foscarnet is strongly nephrotoxic, and accordingly renal dysfunction is evident upon foscarnet administration.

Inhibitors of Reverse Transcription

Retroviruses are RNA viruses, the RNA genome of which requires conversion to DNA to proceed to further replication. For this process, retroviruses encode reverse transcriptase, which is the major target for antiviral chemotherapy for retrovirus infections, since the process is unique and essential for virus replication. The first antiretroviral compound licensed for human use is a thymidine analog, zidovudine (AZT, azidothymidine). In virus-infected cells, AZT is phosphorylated by cellular kinases and is subsequently converted to AZT triphosphate (AZT-PPP) (Fig. 18.3).

AZT-PPP then competes with thymidine triphosphate (TTP) for the synthesis of the DNA strand. However, the affinity of AZT-PPP for reverse transcriptase is 100 times its affinity for the cellular DNA polymerase. Thus, AZT-PPP is preferably incorporated into the growing chain of viral DNA by the reverse transcriptase, leading to the premature termination of viral DNA. It is important to note that since the retrovirus genome is integrated into the host chromosome indefinitely, AZT will only suppress active virus replication. Therefore, in individuals already infected, it is not possible to eliminate the integrated viral genome from the body by any chemotherapeutic treatment. Several other drugs as a nucleoside analog have been licensed for treating AIDS in humans; dideoxyinosine (ddI, didanosine), dideoxycytidine (ddC, zalcitabine), d4T (stavudine), and 3TC (lamivudine). These analogs are all chain terminators that inhibit viral DNA synthesis.

Zidovudine has been used to treat cats infected with feline leukemia virus (FeLV) and feline immunodeficiency virus (FIV). Up to 50 mg/kg of

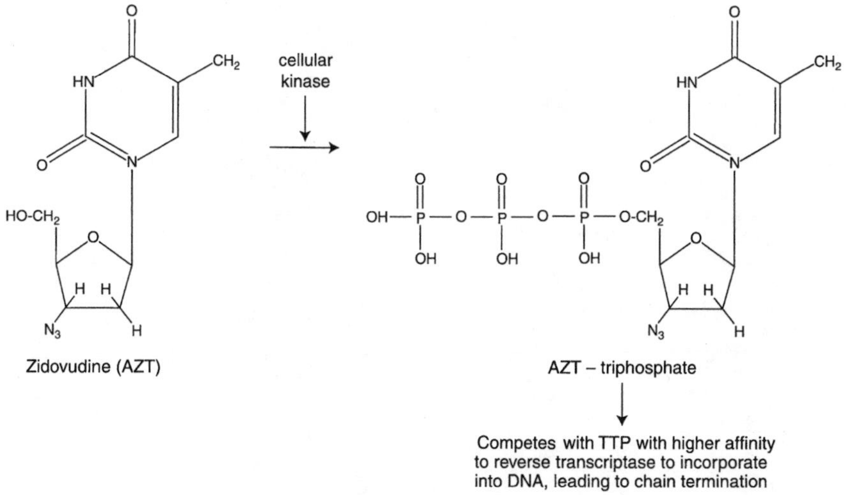

Fig. 18.3. Mechanism of metabolism of zidovudine in the cell to produce the active drug.

zidovudine given as prophylactic treatment for FIV did not prevent cats from developing viremia and lymphadenopathy, although the onset of immunodeficiency was delayed at the highest dose (Smyth et al., 1994a). High doses of zidovudine caused severe anemia. Zidovudine was therefore much less effective in cats than expected from the results of in vitro studies. Other nucleoside analogs, including dideoxyinositol (ddI), dideoxycytosine (ddC), and dideoxyadenine (ddA), have all been shown to have antiviral activity to FIV in cell culture (Smyth et al., 1994b), but their clinical effects are unknown. For FeLV, the time for administration after infection is crucial for therapeutic effects. When administered immediately following infection, AZT abrogates virus replication at 10 mg/kg. However, if therapy is initiated 4 weeks after infection, when cats have already developed viremia, AZT therapy does not prevent progression of infection even at high doses (Tavares et al., 1987).

Inhibitors of mRNA Translation
Antisense Oligonucleotides as Selective Inhibitors
The sequence of a nucleotide chain that contains the information for protein synthesis is called the sense sequence. The nucleotide strand that is complementary to the sense sequence is its antisense sequence. Antisense drugs recognize and bind to the nucleotide sense sequence of specific mRNA molecules, thereby preventing the synthesis of specific proteins and leading to destruction of the mRNA molecules by ribonucleases

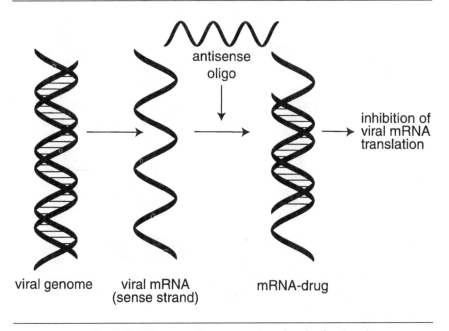

Fig. 18.4. Diagrammatic representation of mode of action of antisense-based antiviral drugs.

in the cell (Fig. 18.4). Antisense approaches have been commercially used to interfere with expression of plant genes, such as interference with fruit softening during the ripening process of genetically engineered tomatoes. The first antisense-based antiviral agent, fomivirsen, for use in humans was recently approved in the United States (Fox, 1998). Fomivirsen is licensed to treat retinitis caused by cytomegalovirus infection in patients with AIDS. Fomivirsen is an antisense oligonucleotide, binding to the complementary strand of the cytomegalovirus gene and blocking the regular function of the viral messenger RNA to synthesize the protein. The product is administered locally into the eye by intravitreal injection. This drug appears to be safe and effective, with minimal side effects, since it is highly selective for viral mRNA. Fomivirsen is significantly more effective in CMV retinitis than the conventional antiviral drugs, ganciclovir and foscarnet.

Interferons

Interferons (IFNs) are cytokines, a large family of cellular proteins that regulate immune responses by coordinating the activities of various types of immune cells. IFNs play a major role in host defenses against viral infection. IFNs of humans are divided into type 1 (IFN-α and IFN-β) and type 2 (IFN-γ). IFN-α and IFN-β are produced from leukocytes and fibroblasts, respectively, in response to virus infections, especially by RNA viruses, whereas IFN-γ is released from T-lymphocytes by antigen or mitogen stimulation. Based on its cellular origin, IFN-γ is classified as a lymphokine. There are 13 subtypes of IFN-α, from IFN-α1 to IFN-α21, whereas there is only a single type for IFN-β and IFN-γ.

The principal activity for IFN-α and IFN-β is antiviral action, whereas IFN-γ possesses immunomodulatory and antiproliferative effects (Vilcék and Sen, 1996). IFN-α and IFN-β share common receptors on their target cells and are rapidly internalized after binding to cell membrane receptors. IFNs increase antibody production and natural killer cell activity, as well as the expression of class I major histocompatibility complex antigen on the cell surface, thus enhancing recognition of virally infected cells by the immune system. The antiviral activity of these IFNs is rather indirect, altering host cell metabolism to impair the protein synthesis and thereby suppressing assembly of viral components. The antiviral effects of IFNs result from induction of several proteins in the exposed cells. These proteins are involved in protecting cells from a range of viral infections. For example, the 2',5'-oligoadenylate synthetase causes breakdown of mRNAs, and the protein kinase that is activated by double-stranded RNA blocks protein translation.

IFN-γ has distinct immunomodulating effects, inducing expression of class II major histocompatibility complex antigen in macrophages (Vilcék and Sen, 1996). IFN-γ has a central role in activating macrophages and thus has considerable potential clinical use in enhancing resistance to intracellular pathogens. Its use for this purpose against specific infections is under active investigation, inspired in part by the variety of opportunist, intracellular infections in human patients with AIDS.

IFN-α and IFN-β are active against a broad range of viruses, while IFN-γ has additional activity against intracellular pathogens, as described. The immunomodulatory effects of IFN-γ may have clinical effects that cannot be predicted by current theoretical considerations; thus experimental and clinical study is required before IFN-γ can be recommended for specific purposes.

CLINICAL APPLICATION

Recombinant DNA technology has resulted in the production of large quantities of human, bovine, and feline IFNs for assessment of their clinical potential. Other species-specific IFNs may also be produced. Although IFNs are produced in most animal species, they, especially IFN-β and IFN-γ, tend to be active mainly in the species in which they are induced. However, there is no viral specificity, so that the interferon produced by one virus is effective against other viruses. The clinical role of

IFNs in prophylaxis and treatment of viral infections is of considerable interest in human and veterinary medicine. IFN-α can be administered SC, IM, IV, or locally. IFNs are generally administered IM and have serum half-lives of 3–8 hours. Continued use of human IFNs in animals is eventually accompanied by development of neutralizing antibodies (Zeidner et al., 1990). Synergism with other antiviral drugs has sometimes been described (Weiss, 1989). Synergism of IFN-γ with azithromycin against experimental toxoplasmosis was described (Aranjo and Remington, 1991).

Among potential uses of IFNs in human medicine are intranasal application of IFN-α in prevention of rhinovirus infections, an effect also described in cattle (Rosenquist and Allen, 1990); the treatment of chronic viral hepatitis; the intralesional treatment of some papillomavirus infections; and the treatment of herpes simplex infections. The suggestion is currently being explored that IFN might have an adjunctive role in managing certain neoplasms and might provide effective therapy in rabies and hemorrhagic fevers. The adverse effects of IFNs suggest that these drugs will generally be reserved for severe infections in humans and animals or for local use.

In cattle, IM or intranasal treatment of calves with human IFN-α reduced morbidity caused by bovine herpesvirus 1 and *Pasteurella haemolytica*, possibly due to the immunomodulatory activity of the drug (Babiuk et al., 1987). No antiviral effect was observed in calves infected with respiratory syncytial virus (Dennis et al., 1991). Calves treated with bovine IFN-α were protected against experimental vaccinia infection (Schwerset al., 1989). Recombinant bovine IFN-γ administered by the intramammary route considerably reduced the severity of experimentally induced acute *E. coli* mastitis in cattle (Sordillo and Babiuk, 1991), as well as enhancing mammary phagocyte function (Fox et al., 1990). In cats, oral dosage with bovine beta or human IFN-α resulted in favorable resolution of nonregenerative anemia after feline leukemia virus infection (Steed, 1987). Treatment with high doses of human IFN-α temporarily suppressed disease signs and increased survival time in experimentally induced feline infectious peritonitis (Weiss et al., 1990). Recombinant feline IFN-α produced in silkworms has been shown to have antiviral effects in vitro against feline herpesvirus, feline calicivirus, feline leukemia virus, feline infectious peritonitis virus, and feline immunodeficiency virus (Yamamoto et al., 1990). Feline IFN-α was especially effective in reducing clinical symptoms caused by FHV and FCV in cats when administered at 5×10^6 units/kg.

Persistent fatigue and acute flu-like illness (fever, chills, myalgia) always accompany IFN therapy in humans, although this may decline with continued administration of IFN-α and IFN-β, but not IFN-γ. Peripheral neuropathy and neuropsychiatric symptoms may also occur. Mild, reversible neutropenia is common. Fever and neutropenia were reported in calves treated with IFN-α (Dennis et al., 1991). Transient anorexia and weight loss have been described in cats (Zeidner et al., 1990). Adverse effects are dose related and substantial.

Inhibitors of Posttranslation Modification
Proteolytic Cleavage Inhibitors

Many viral proteins undergo further processing after being translated, and cleavage of the precursor proteins is required to activate enzymatic function, fusion, and maturation of virion. During the replication of retrovirus, viral genome is translated to produce two major polyproteins, gag and gag-pol. A portion of the gag-pol polyprotein is a virus-coded protease enzyme, and by this enzyme activity, the gag and gag-pol polyproteins are self-cleaved to yield various functional proteins essential for the replication cycle. Inhibition of the protease enzyme, therefore, can block cleavage of the viral polyprotein, leading to the prevention of virus replication. In human immunodeficiency virus (HIV), the viral protease is a member of the aspartic protease family. The HIV protease is structurally different from other cellular aspartic proteases such as renin, pepsin, and gastricsin, and thus the viral protease can be a selective target for antiviral agents.

A series of protease inhibitors has been recently licensed to treat HIV infections in AIDS patients. The protease inhibitors act directly on the target enzyme and do not require metabolic activation. Clinical studies suggest that the protease inhibitors are generally superior to the established nucleoside analogs for HIV treatment. Ritonavir has a selectivity more than 500 times higher for the HIV protease than for other cellular aspartic proteases and suppresses HIV replication effectively, increasing CD4+ cell counts. The oral bioavailability of ritonavir is as high as 70%, the highest among the approved retrovirus-specific protease inhibitors. Saquinavir is another type of HIV protease inhibitor. It has a poor bioavailability of only 4% but has shown durable antiviral activity in vivo with 50,000-fold lower affinity for cellular protease. Reported toxicities of the protease inhibitors include loose stools or diarrhea and elevated transaminases. Protease inhibitors are metabolized in liver, and this may be the cause of liver enzyme elevation. Protease inhibitors are exclusively used to treat AIDS patients and have not been evaluated yet for veterinary practice.

Glycosylation Inhibitors

2-Deoxy-D-glucose (2-dG) is a glucose analog that interferes with the synthesis of oligosaccharides of the viral surface glycoproteins. 2-dG inhibits a wide range of enveloped DNA and RNA viruses, especially orthomyxoviruses, paramyxoviruses, and herpesviruses. Viruses containing glycoproteins decorated with abnormal sugar moiety have decreased infectivity because of their inability to recognize specific cell receptors or to penetrate into cells. Clinical benefit has been claimed for topical application to initial lesions of genital herpes in women. This has not been confirmed in controlled trials.

Calves administered 20 mg/kg daily IV had no protection against experimentally induced respiratory infectious bovine rhinotracheitis (IBR) infection, but ocular instillation markedly reduced the severity of experimental keratoconjunctivitis (Mohanty et al., 1980). For respiratory syncytial virus infection, a dosage of 10 mg/kg daily IV apparently protected calves against the mild clinical signs without any toxicity. The drug had no effect once clinical signs developed (Mohanty et al., 1981) or against a more severe respiratory tract illness like bovine herpesvirus infection. The drug has potential application in the prophylaxis of canine distemper, equine influenza, and parainfluenza infections.

Sources and Potential Clinical Applications for Antiviral Drugs

Sources and potential application of antiviral drugs in veterinary medicine are shown in Tables 18.1–18.3.

Future Prospects for Antiviral Chemotherapy

Even though viruses do not carry mechanisms per se for developing resistance to antiviral agents, viruses can undergo mutations to introduce changes in the viral enzymes or structural components. Resistant viruses are generally less virulent and poor in their transmission. However, in immunosuppressed conditions, mutant viruses may proliferate favorably under the selective pressure of antiviral drugs. Rimantadine-resistant influenza A virus is as readily transmissible and as virulent in ferrets and in humans as wild-type virus. Viruses resistant to nucleoside analogs may have developed mutations on the viral DNA polymerase and the reverse transcriptase, and similarly resistance to protease inhibitors may arise from mutations at the drug-binding sites. Resistance to one drug is usually accompanied by reduced susceptibility to the drugs in the same class, but different classes of drugs may still retain antiviral effects to the resistant virus. In this regard, combination drug therapy has become an effective approach to some viral infections. Combination therapy has several advantages. First, it delivers the most efficient individual drugs simultaneously and may provide synergistic effects. Second, combination of two

TABLE 18.1.   Commercially available antiviral drugs

Generic Name	Trade Name	Manufacturer and Formula
Acyclovir	Zovirax	Glaxo Wellcome, 5% ointment for ophthalmic application, 200 mg/capsule, 400 mg/tablet or 800 mg tablet, 200 mg/5 ml of syrup in 1 pint, 500 mg/vial for IV
Amantadine	Symmetrel	Du Pont Pharma, 100 mg/tablet, 50 mg/5 ml of syrup
Amantadine	Symadine	Solvay, 100 mg/tablet
2-Deoxy-D-glucose	2-dG	ICN Pharmaceuticals, powder, 1 g, 5 g, 25 g
Famciclovir	Famvir	SmithKlein Beecham, 500 mg/tablet
Fomivirsen	Vitravene	CIBA Vision, 0.25-ml solution for ophthalmic application
Foscarnet	Foscavir	Astra, 24 mg/ml in 250 ml or 500 ml for IV use
Ganciclovir	Cytovene	Hoffmann–La Roche, 1,000 mg capsule
Idoxuridine	Herplex	Allergan, 0.1% solution
Interferon-α2a	Roferon-A	Roche, 3, 6, 36 × 10^6 IU/vial, IV
Interferon-αN3	Alferon N	Purdue Frederick, 5 × 10^6 U/vial, IV
Interferon-β	Betaseron	Berlex, 0.3 mg/vial, IV
Interferon-γ1b	Actimmune	Genentech, 3 × 10^6 U/0.5 ml, IV
Lamivudine	Epivir	Glaxo Wellcome, 150 mg/tablet
Ribavirin	Virazole	ICN Pharmaceuticals, 6 g/vial for reconstitution for aerosol
Rimantadine	Flumadine	Forest Laboratories, 50 mg/5 ml of syrup
Ritonavir	Norvir	Abbott Laboratories, 100 mg/capsule, 80 mg/240 ml oral solution
Saquinavir	Invirase	Hoffman–La Roche, 200 mg/capsule
Trifluridine	Viroptic	Burroughs Wellcome, 1% solution
Valaciclovir	Valtrex	Glaxo Wellcome, 500 mg/capsule, zoster and genital herpes
Vidarabine	Vira-A	Parke-Davis, 3% ointment, FHV-1
Zalcitabine (ddC)	Hivid	Hoffmann–La Roche, 0.375 mg/tablet, 0.750 mg/tablet
Zidovudine (AZT)	Retrovir	Glaxo Wellcome, 100 mg/oral capsule, 50 mg/5 ml of syrup, 10 mg/ml solution for IV

or more drugs may allow the dosage of individual drugs to be reduced, and thus dosage-dependent cytotoxicity may be minimized. Third, combination therapy may prevent emergence of drug resistance by using different antiviral drugs that have different mechanisms of action. A study using AZT, ddI, and a protease inhibitor in combination in AIDS clinical trials suggests that there is no interference in the kinetics among the individual drugs (Vanhove et al., 1997). AZT and IFN-α combination showed a favorable effect on CD4+ cell counts in symptomatic AIDS patients (Jos Frissen et al., 1994). A synergistic effect was also observed for feline infectious peritonitis virus (FIPV) when 10 × 10^6 units of IFN-α was combined with variable amounts of ribavirin. The combination produced an 80-to-200-fold increase in the effects of the individual drug alone (Weiss and Oostrom-Ram, 1989). When the same combination was tested for feline herpesvirus, at an 8-fold reduction of the acyclovir dosage, the maximum inhibitory effect against the virus replication was still maintained (Weiss, 1989).

TABLE 18.2. **Topical antiviral drugs used in humans and their potential veterinary use**

Drug	Human Use	Potential Veterinary Use
Acyclovir	First genital herpes infections in otherwise healthy persons; limited mucocutaneous infections in immunocompromised patients; herpes zoster	Local herpes infections: bovine herpes mammillitis, equine coital exanthema, feline rhinotracheitis, viral keratoconjunctivitis
2-Deoxy-D-glucose	Not approved	Local herpes infections (above); bovine vulvovaginitis and keratoconjunctivitis
Fomivirsen	Cytomegalovirus retinitis (intravitreal)	Cytomegalovirus
Foscarnet	Genital herpes	Same as 2-deoxy-D-glucose
Idoxuridine	Herpes simplex keratitis	Same as 2-deoxy-D-glucose; feline herpesvirus keratitis
Methisazone	Not used topically	Bovine vaccinia or pseudocowpox teat lesions
Ribavirin	Aerosol in animal model; for influenza and respiratory syncytial virus	Local herpes infections (not feline); vaccinia teat lesions
Trifluridine	Herpetic keratitis	Same as 2-deoxy-D-glucose (drug of choice for feline herpesvirus keratitis)
Vidarabine	Herpes keratitis	Local bovine herpes or vaccinia teat lesions

Antiviral agents may have an antiproliferative influence on cells, which may lead to suppression of host immune responses. A study indicates that AZT, ganciclovir, and ribavirin decrease mitogenesis, whereas acyclovir and ddI have no inhibitory effects on peripheral blood mononuclear cells in humans (Heagy et al., 1991). Another study suggests that AZT, ddI, and ddC have no inhibitory effects on the polymorphonuclear leukocytes (Rollides et al., 1990). Further studies are required to identify immunosuppressive properties of the antiviral agents.

Protease inhibitors and antisense oligonucleotides are the "new generation" antiviral agents. These agents are highly selective and thus reduce undesirable cytotoxicity significantly. The development of highly specific antiviral drugs requires in-depth understanding of the replication cycles and of the molecular biology of viruses. The three-dimensional structure of viral proteins is elucidated by X-ray crystallographic studies, and drugs may be designed by computer simulation to delineate interactions of the proteins with other molecules. Chemical compounds may then be synthesized based on this information. Design of antisense oligonucleotides as antiviral drugs also requires two-dimensional analy-

TABLE 18.3. Systemic antiviral agents in human clinical use and experimental drugs under investigation in human medicine with suggested veterinary use

Drug	Human Use (Administration)	Suggested Veterinary Use
Acyclovir	Systemic herpes infections prophylaxis; varicella eye infection	Animal herpesviruses generally not very susceptible; equine herpes in foals
Amantadine	Influenza A prophylaxis and treatment (PO); chronic hepatitis C	Equine influenza A prophylaxis
Foscarnet	Herpes simplex encephalitis (IM); cytomegalovirus retinitis	Infectious bovine rhinotracheitis; feline rhinotracheitis; Aujeszky's disease prophylaxis; retrovirus infections
Ganciclovir	Herpesvirus infections, especially cytomegalovirus retinitis	Cytomegalovirus infections
Interferon	Papillomavirus warts; chronic hepatitis B, chronic hepatitis C (IM, SC)	Feline herpes, feline leukemia (FeLV), feline infectious peritonitis, feline immunodeficiency virus (FIV)
Ribavirin	Influenza A and B; measles; hepatitis A; Lassa fever (IV); respiratory syncytial virus (PO, aerosol); hepatitis C (PO); hantavirus (IV)	Influenza; parainfluenza; bovine herpesvirus; canine distemper; bluetongue; rotavirus; Marek's disease; feline infectious peritonitis virus; feline calicivirus
Ritonavir, saquinavir	Human immunodeficiency virus (PO)	Potentially for FIV, FeLV
Vidarabine	Disseminated herpes simplex, herpes zoster; herpes simplex encephalitis (IV)	Canine herpesvirus; and same as foscarnet
Zidovudine (AZT)	Retrovirus, human immunodeficiency virus (PO)	Retrovirus FeLV, equine infectious anemia, FIV

sis of targeted mRNA structure. Poliomyelitis virus, influenza virus, and hepatitis C virus are among the targeted viruses for such sophisticated approaches. Antiviral chemotherapy is still in its infancy relative to the development of other antimicrobial chemotherapies. Nonetheless, progress is being made rapidly and will eventually lead to the discovery of safe, specific, and effective antiviral drugs.

Bibliography

Aranjo FG, Remington JS. 1991. Synergistic activity of azithromycin and gamma interferon in murine toxoplasmosis. Antimicrob Agents Chemother 35:1672.
Babiuk LA, et al. 1987. Use of recombinant bovine IFN-α1 in reducing respiratory disease induced by bovine herpesvirus type 1. Antimicrob Agents Chemother 31:752.
Collinson PN, et al. 1994. Isolation of equine herpesvirus type 2 (equine gammaherpesvirus 2) from foals with keratoconjunctivitis. J Am Vet Med Assoc 205:329.

Dennis MJ, et al. 1991. Effects of recombinant human alpha A interferon in gnotobiotic calves challenged with respiratory syncytial virus. Res Vet Sci 50:222.

Fox JL. 1998. FDA approves first antisense drug for CMV retinitis. ASM News 64:679.

Fox LK, et al. 1990. The effect of interferon-gamma intramammary administration on mammary phagocyte function. J Vet Med 37B:28.

Greene CE. 1998. Ocular infections. In: Greene CE, ed. Infectious Diseases of the Dog and Cat, 2nd ed. Philadelphia: WB Saunders, p658.

Heagy W, et al. 1991. Inhibition of immune functions by antiviral drugs. J Clin Invest 87:1916.

Jos Frissen PH, et al. 1994. Zidovudine and interferon-α combination therapy versus zidovudine monotherapy in subjects with symptomatic human immunodeficiency virus type 1 infection. J Infect Dis 169:1351.

Lee JB, et al. 1995. Immunological response to recombinant VP8* subunit protein of bovine rotavirus in pregnant cattle. J Gen Virol 76:2477.

Mohanty SB, et al. 1980. Chemotherapeutic value of 2-deoxy-D-glucose in infectious rhinotracheitis viral infection in calves. Am J Vet Res 41:1049.

Mohanty SB, et al. 1981. Chemotherapeutic effect of 2-deoxy-D-glucose against respiratory syncytial viral infection in calves. Am J Vet Res 42:336.

Murray MJ, et al. 1998. Neonatal equine herpesvirus type 1 infection on a Thoroughbred breeding farm. J Vet Intern Med 12:36.

Nasisse MP, et al. 1997. Effects of valaciclovir in cats infected with feline herpesvirus 1. Am J Vet Res 58:1141.

Pennington JE. 1990. Newer uses of intravenous immunoglobulin as anti-infective agents. Antimicrob Agents Chemother 34:1463.

Povey C. 1978. Effect of orally administered ribavirin on experimental feline calicivirus infection in cats. Am J Vet Res 39:1337.

Rees WA, et al. 1997. Amantadine and equine influenza: pharmacology, pharmacokinetics, and neurological effects in the horse. Equine Vet J 29:104.

Rollides E, et al. 1990. Effects of antiretroviral dideoxynucleosides on polymorphonuclear leukocyte function. Antimicrob Agents Chemother 34:1672.

Rosenquist BD, Allen GA. 1990. Effect of bovine fibroblast interferon on rhinovirus infection in calves. Am J Vet Res 51:870.

Rueckert RR. 1996. Picornaviridae: the viruses and their replication. In: Fields BN, et al., eds. Fields Virology, 3rd ed. New York: Lippincott-Raven, p609.

Samorek-salamonowicz A, Wijaszka T. 1987. Effect of acyclovir of the replication of turkey herpesvirus and Marek's disease virus. Res Vet Sci 42:334.

Schwerset A, et al. 1989. Protection of cattle from infection with vaccinia virus by bovine interferon alpha C. Vet Rec 12 5:15.

Smyth NR, et al. 1994a. Effect of 3'-azido-2',3'-deoxythymidine in domestic cats. Res Vet Sci 57:220.

Smyth NR, et al. 1994b. Susceptibility in cell culture of feline immunodeficiency virus to eighteen antiviral agents. J Antimicrob Chemother 34:589.

Sordillo LM, Babiuk LA. 1991. Controlling acute Escherichia coli mastitis during the periparturient period with recombinant bovine interferon gamma. Vet Microbiol 28:189.

Steed VP. 1987. Improved survival of four cats infected with feline leukemia virus after oral administration of interferon. Feline Pract 17(3):24.

Swenson CL, et al. 1990. Age related differences in pharmacokinetics of phosphonoformate in cats. Antimicrob Agents Chemother 34:871.

Tavares L, et al. 1987. 3'-Azio-3'-deoxythymidine in feline leukemia virus–infected cats: a model for therapy and prophylaxis of AIDS. Cancer Res 47:3190.

Vanhove GF, et al. 1997. Pharmacokinetics of saquinavir, zidovudine, and zalcitabine in combination therapy. Antimicrob Agents Chemother 41:2428.

Vilcék J, Sen GC. 1996. Interferons and other cytokines. In: Fields BN, et al., eds. Fields Virology, 3rd ed. New York: Lippincott-Raven, p375.

Weiss RC. 1989. Synergistic antiviral activities of acyclovir and recombinant human leukocyte (alpha) interferon on feline herpesvirus replication. Am J Vet Res 50:1672.

415

Weiss RC, Oostrom-Ram T. 1989. Inhibitory effects of ribavirin alone or combined with human alpha interferon on feline infectious peritonitis virus replication in vitro. Vet Microbiol 20:255.

Weiss RC, et al. 1990. Effect of interferon or *Propionibacterium acnes* on the course of experimentally induced feline infectious peritonitis in specific-pathogen-free and random-source cats. Am J Vet Res 51:726.

Yamamoto JK, et al. 1990. Antifeline herpesvirus and calicivirus effects of feline interferon. J Interferon Res 10:S114.

Zeidner NS, et al. 1990. Alpha interferon (2b) in combination with zidovudine for the treatment of presymptomatic feline leukemia virus–induced immunodeficiency syndrome. Antimicrob Agents Chemother 34:1749.

19 | Special Considerations

This chapter discusses special considerations required when treating infections of selected organ systems (bones and joints, eyes, nervous system, urinary tract, and the prostate), dose modification in the very young and in animals with kidney failure, and drug selection in pregnancy, as well as treatment of selected bacterial infections (anaerobic, atypical mycobacterial, *Brucella*, mycoplasma, *Nocardia*, and leptospirosis).

SELECTED ORGAN SYSTEMS

Infections in Bones and Joints

J. F. PRESCOTT

Osteomyelitis
The important features of the treatment of osteomyelitis are the need for early, aggressive, and prolonged treatment that achieves adequate, pharmacodynamically appropriate local concentrations of bactericidal drugs, particularly in chronic infections where bacteria may be present in necrotic bone. Apart from antimicrobial therapy, the cornerstones of osteomyelitis treatment include debridement and sequestrectomy, open wound drainage, fracture stabilization, and grafting of bone deficits (Johnson, 1994). Necrotic bone must be removed surgically.

Acute hematogenous osteomyelitis is a disease of young animals that usually involves the metaphyses of the long bones. The disease may spread through lymphatics to involve the periosteum and may also cause thrombophlebitis of intraosseous vasculature, resulting in ischemic necrosis and chronic infection, including formation of sequestra. Agents involved are the common opportunist pathogens of individual animal species. Osteomyelitis secondary to spread of infection from a local source occurs following open reduction of fractures and involves common opportunist pathogens, including *Pseudomonas aeruginosa*. A microbiologic diagnosis based on isolation of infecting organisms is an essential guide to treatment and can be obtained from samples taken during surgical debridement or by biopsy. Parenteral treatment, started as soon as culture specimens are taken, should, in acute osteomyelitis, be administered in high doses for at least 3 weeks and changed if necessary, depending on susceptibility test results. Oral antibiotic treatment is then continued for a further 3 weeks; bactericidal antibiotics are required. The treatment of chronic osteomyelitis is by surgical removal of sequestra, often following 10–14 days of parenteral antibiotic therapy. Parenteral antibiotics should be administered after surgery and replaced after 3–4 weeks by oral antibiotics, which should be continued for a further 1–2 months. Fluoroquinolones are promising bactericidal drugs for oral treatment of Gram-negative bacterial osteomyelitis. One interesting development helps reduce infection in treating chronic osteomyelitis, since bone debridement leads to production of dead space. Acrylic beads impregnated with antibiotics are used to pack areas where bone has been removed temporarily prior to bone grafts. This ensures high local concentration of drugs, usually aminoglycosides or cephalosporins, at the site of infection. The beads are removed within 2–4 weeks and usually replaced by a cancellous bone graft.

Septic Arthritis

Infectious, septic arthritis is inflammation of the joint space caused by a variety of opportunist pathogens that reach the joint hematogenously, by puncture, or by extension from adjacent infection. It is important that septic arthritis be treated as soon as possible to prevent chronic joint damage. A precise microbiological diagnosis is critical, and treatment can be started on the basis of Gram stain from joint aspirates, until culture results are available. Therapy should be with bactericidal drugs (a beta-lactam is preferred), administered parenterally for 2 weeks with subsequent orally administered drugs for a further 2–4 weeks. Drainage of the joint is essential to remove bacteria, debris, and inflammatory products that cause cartilage damage, as well as to reduce intra-articular pressure that may cause ischemic necrosis. Repeated closed-needle aspiration (q24 or q12 hours for 7–10 days) can be recommended. Joint aspiration may be adequate in early stages of septic arthritis, but repeated distension irrigation or joint lavage is recommended if clinical improvement does not occur within 24–48 hours (Martens et al., 1986).

Intra-articular injection of antimicrobial drugs is not generally recommended, since it may provoke a chemical synovitis. Irrigation with isotonic, balanced electrolyte solutions, administered by closed syringes, hastens removal of inflammatory products. Antibiotic-impregnated absorbable collagen sponges have been used in the effective treatment of infectious arthritis in animals (Hirsbrunner and Steiner, 1998); they have the advantage over antibiotic-impregnated polymethylmethacrylate beads that do not need to be subsequently removed.

Bibliography

Budsberg SC, Kemp DT. 1990. Antimicrobial distribution and therapeutics in bone. Compend Contin Educ Pract Vet 12:1758.

Cimmino MA. 1997. Recognition and management of bacterial arthritis. Drugs 54:50.

Hirsbrunner G, Steiner A. 1998. Treatment of infectious arthritis of the radiocarpal joint of cattle with gentamicin-impregnated collagen sponges. Vet Rec 142:399.

Johnson KA. 1994. Osteomyelitis in dogs and cats. J Am Vet Med Assoc 205:1882.

Mader JT, et al. 1997. A practical guide to the diagnosis and management of bone and joint infection. Drugs 54:253.

Martens RJ, et al. 1986. Equine pediatrics: septic arthritis and osteomyelitis. J Am Vet Med Assoc 188:582.

Smith JA, et al. 1989. Drug therapy for arthritis in food-producing animals. Compend Contin Educ Pract Vet 11:87.

Stoneham SJ. 1997. Septic arthritis in the foal: practical considerations on diagnosis and treatment. Equine Vet Ed 9:25.

Tobias KMS, et al. 1996. Use of antimicrobial-impregnated polymethyl methacrylate. J Am Vet Med Assoc 208:841.

Trostle SS, et al. 1996. Use of antimicrobial-impregnated polymethyl methacrylate beads for treatment of chronic, refractory septic arthritis and osteomyelitis of the digit in a bull. J Am Vet Med Assoc 208:404.

Infections of the Eyes: Conjunctivitis, Keratitis, and Endophthalmitis

J. F. PRESCOTT

The treatment of serious infections of the eyes requires clinical expertise beyond the scope of this book. This section briefly describes some principles of treatment of the more common infections of the eyes.

Infectious Agents

In dogs and cats, the common agents of conjunctivitis and keratitis are the opportunistic bacteria that normally inhabit the conjunctivae and adjacent skin. In dogs these are predominantly *Staphylococcus aureus,* followed in decreasing frequency by beta-hemolytic streptococci, *Proteus* species, and *Escherichia coli*. In cats, *Chlamydia* and to a lesser extent *Mycoplasma felis* cause contagious conjunctivitis. In horses the bacteria involved are generally Gram-negative (*Pseudomonas aeruginosa*, Enterobacteriaceae), but fungi (*Aspergillus, Alternaria, Penicillium*) are more important as causes of ulcerative keratitis than in species such as dogs and cats, in which mycotic infection is usually a sequel to the use of corticosteroid eye ointments. The cause of infectious keratoconjunctivitis in cattle is *Moraxella bovis*, and in sheep, the rickettsial agent *Colesiota conjunctivae*. Laboratory diagnosis of infectious keratitis or conjunctivitis is important because of the variety of causative agents involved.

Routes of Antibiotic Administration

Antibiotics can be administered topically, by subconjunctival or intraocular injection, or systemically. The choice depends on the site and severity of the infection.

Topical application gives high local concentrations and is the route of choice for superficial infections of the eyes. Ointments persist longer than drops. The ability of antimicrobial agents to penetrate across conjunctival and corneal epithelia depends on the molecular weight and lipophilic characteristics. Subconjunctival injection of most antibiotics (but not tetracyclines), in volumes of up to 1 ml, results in high local concentrations in conjunctival secretions, the cornea, and the aqueous and to a lesser extent vitreous humors (Table 19.1). It is thus the preferred route in the treatment of serious suppurative keratitis and, combined with parenterally administered agents, in endophthalmitis, as well as in animals in which repeated handling is a problem. Therapeutic concentrations of subconjunctivally injected antibiotics persist for up to 48 hours.

The blood supply to the eyes lacks capillary pores, so that penetration by drugs takes place by nonionic diffusion. Lipid-soluble, low-molecular-weight, nonionized, and non-protein-bound drugs therefore penetrate

TABLE 19.1. **Intraocular penetration of antibiotics in normal eyes**

Drug	Systemic	Topical	Subconjunctival
		Route of Administration	
Ampicillin	+	+	+++
Chloramphenicol	+++	+++	++++
Enrofloxacin	++	++	+++
Erythromycin	+	+	++
Gentamicin	+	+	++
Neomycin	+	++	++
Penicillin G	+	++	+++
Polymyxin	+	++	+++
Tetracyclines	++	++	+

Note: +, poor; ++, fair; +++, good; ++++, excellent. These data represent general estimations only, because of limited investigations in animals.

best, both after topical application and after systemic administration. Inflammation increases penetration of antimicrobial agents; corneal ulceration also increases the ability of topically applied agents to penetrate into the aqueous humor. Most antibiotics, except tetracyclines, penetrate the inflamed eye at least moderately. Systemic administration of antibiotics gives lower, often subtherapeutic, vitreous humor concentrations than subconjunctival injection. Direct injection of antimicrobial agents into the vitreous is the approach of choice in treating serious endophthalmitis.

Antimicrobial Agents of Choice
Several antibiotic preparations are available for local ophthalmic use, often as a 0.5% (weight by volume) ointment or 1% drops. More concentrated solutions are probably unnecessary, given the choice of agents available and the ability to administer them frequently. The initial choice of antibiotic is best guided by a Gram or Giemsa stain. Many clinicians use broad-spectrum bactericidal antibiotics or combinations as first-line drugs. The use of corticosteroids should generally be avoided. Drugs of first choice for Gram-positive infections are erythromycin, cephalothin, or chloramphenicol; gentamicin is suitable for Gram-negative infections. Suitable first-choice combinations include neomycin-polymyxin (-bacitracin) and cephalosporins-aminoglycosides.

Clinical Applications
INFECTIOUS CONJUNCTIVITIS
Conjunctivitis is treated with eye drops or ointment every 8 hours, with more frequent administration in the early stages. In cats, tetracyclines and macrolides are used to treat *Chlamydia* or mycoplasma conjunctivitis. Treatment of acute disease should last 5 days, and clinical response should be observed within 48 hours of starting treatment. If no response occurs, the agent should be changed according to results of culture and susceptibility tests.

ULCERATIVE KERATITIS
Bacterial ulcerative keratitis is treated by the application of antimicrobial drops every 30 minutes or every hour for 24–48 hours. This is reduced to 6 times daily and, in serious disease, subconjunctival injections of antibiotic are included (Table 19.2). Topical or local subconjunctival anesthetic (0.2 ml 2% lidocaine) can be administered before injection. A broad-spectrum bactericidal drug is used while waiting for culture and susceptibility results. Giemsa staining for fungal hyphae should be done, particularly in horses.

For ulcerative keratitis caused by *Pseudomonas aeruginosa*, treatment with gentamicin (0.3–1.5%) or tobramycin (0.3–1%) is appropriate while

TABLE 19.2. **Suggested dosages in the treatment of infections of the eyes in humans**

Drug	Route of Administration	
	Topical (mg/ml)	Subconjunctival (mg)
Penicillin G	3	300–600
Ampicillin	10	100
Cefazolin	50	100
Cefuroxime	50	100
Chloramphenicol	10	10
Tetracycline	5–10	—[a]
Erythromycin	5–10	50
Gentamicin	3–15	40
Polymyxin	5–10	5–10

[a]Irritant.

waiting results of susceptibility tests. Gentamicin-resistant *P. aeruginosa* may be treated with amikacin (2.5%), piperacillin (5%), ceftazidime (5%), or ciprofloxacin (0.3%).

Fungal keratitis in horses and other species can be treated with miconazole (1%) or natamycin (5%) instilled onto the cornea every hour for the first 48 hours, reducing to 6 or 8 times daily thereafter. Itraconazole may be a better choice because of its greater and broader antifungal activity. In horses, topically applied 1% itraconazole with 30% DMSO ointment gave considerably higher corneal concentrations than the drug without DMSO (Ball et al., 1997a); applied every 4 hours for a median of 35 days, it was effective in resolving keratomycosis in the majority of cases (Ball et al., 1997b).

Topical antiviral drugs (acyclovir, idoxuridine, vidarabine) used in treatment of herpetic keratitis are described in Chapter 18.

Systemic antimicrobial treatment of ulcerative keratitis is not generally recommended. Exceptions are ovine rickettsial keratoconjunctivitis, in which a single IM injection of long-acting oxytetracycline or spiramycin, repeated at 5 and 10 days, appears to give excellent results. For *Moraxella bovis* infection, the usual treatment is IM injection of long-acting tetracyclines administered twice q72 hours, with topical application of tetracycline ointment at the time of treatment with long-acting tetracycline, or subconjunctival injection of ampicillin or penicillin.

BACTERIAL ENDOPHTHALMITIS

Bacterial endophthalmitis usually results in loss of the eye. It should be treated with topical, systemic, and intravitreal bactericidal antibiotics. Preventing such infections by administering prophylactic antibiotics during eye surgery is recommended.

Bibliography

Ball MA, et al. 1997a. Corneal concentrations and preliminary toxicological evaluation of an itraconazole/dimethyl sulphoxide ophthalmic ointment. J Vet Pharmacol Ther 20:100.

Ball MA, et al. 1997b. Evaluation of itraconazole–dimethyl sulfoxide ointment for treatment of keratomycosis in nine horses. J Am Vet Med Assoc 211:199.

Brooks DE, et al. 1998. Antimicrobial susceptibility patterns of fungi isolated from horses with ulcerative keratomycosis. Am J Vet Res 59:138.

Dowling PM, Grahn BH. 1998. Antimicrobial therapy of ocular infections. Can Vet J 39:121.

Piercy DWT. 1985. Factors influencing the penetration of therapeutic substances into the eye following topical application. Vet Rec 116:99.

Sansom J. 1988. Antibacterials in the treatment of ocular infections. J Small Anim Pract 29:487.

Sweeney CR, Irby NL. Topical treatment of *Pseudomonas* sp.–infected corneal ulcers in horses: 70 cases (1977–1994). J Am Vet Med Assoc 209:954.

Infections of the Nervous System: Meningitis and Encephalitis

J. F. PRESCOTT

Meningitis occurs most commonly in neonatal farm animals that have not received sufficient colostral antibodies. The causes are commonly Enterobacteriaceae in ruminants, Enterobacteriaceae and beta-hemolytic streptococci in foals, and beta-hemolytic streptococci in piglets. In other than the neonatal period, the most common cause of infectious meningitis in pigs is *Streptococcus suis* type 2. In adult cattle and sheep, meningoencephalomyelitis is caused by *Haemophilus somnus* and encephalitis by *Listeria monocytogenes*. Meningitis is uncommon in adult dogs and cats but may occur because of penetrating wounds or foreign bodies. Abscesses in the central nervous system (CNS) are uncommon in animals; one of the most frequent types is the pituitary abscess in cattle caused by *Arcanobacterium pyogenes* and associated anaerobic bacteria.

Infections of the CNS are associated with high mortality. Treatment is hampered by the poor phagocytic activity within the CNS because of the absence of complement and immunoglobulins, by the lack of drainage, and by the poor penetration of many antibiotics. There are two distinct barriers to the passage of drugs into the CNS—the blood–cerebrospinal fluid (CSF) barrier and the blood-brain barrier. The former consists of the epithelial cells lining the choroid plexus and is important in the treatment of meningitis. The latter consists of end capillaries in brain tissue, with their surrounding glial cells; it is an important consideration in treating encephalitis and brain abscesses. Drugs that best penetrate the blood-CSF barrier are lipid soluble, nonionized at physiologic pH, not extensively bound to plasma proteins, and of low molecular weight. Drugs that meet these criteria include amphotericin B, chloramphenicol, doxycycline, many fluoroquinolones, metronidazole, rifampin, sulfonamides, and trimethoprim. The most important factor in enhancing penetration is the presence of inflammation, which markedly enhances CSF concentrations of penicillin and cephalosporins, most of which normally penetrate poorly. Aminoglycosides do not penetrate CSF even in the presence of inflammation.

Treatment of Meningitis

The critical therapeutic implication of the poor host defenses of CSF is that only antibiotics that achieve bactericidal concentrations within the CSF should be used. In bacterial meningitis, antibiotic concentrations that are 10–30 times minimum bactericidal concentration (MBC) are required to sterilize the CSF. Bacteriostatic antibiotics and bactericidal antibiotics that achieve only MIC concentrations are unlikely to be effective. Recent evidence suggests that peak concentrations of drugs are important, because of the importance of exceeding MBC for a period. In an experimental study of ampicillin treatment of streptococcal meningitis in rabbits, Tauber et al. (1989) found that peak concentration of drug in CSF that exceeded the minimum bactericidal concentration by 10 times was the single most important factor determining the favorable outcome of treatment. The time that ampicillin exceeded bacterial MIC and the interval between doses was less important. Whether these findings can be extrapolated to other infections and agents is not known, but in the absence of additional information, bactericidal drugs must attain high serum and CSF concentrations, which usually requires administration by IV bolus injection. Drugs should be given frequently, but it is not necessary that concentrations in CSF continually exceed MBC. The critical factor appears to be that peak CSF drug concentration exceeds MBC by 10 times for even a short period. The size of the dose should be the maximum that is nontoxic. It is generally recommended that duration of therapy be 10–14 days, but shorter times may be sufficient with antibiotics that rapidly sterilize the CSF, such as the newer cephalosporins.

Two questions that arise in the treatment of bacterial meningitis are the use of combinations of drugs and intrathecal administration. Both are therapeutic approaches that are no longer regarded as significant in human medicine because of the widespread use of newer cephalosporins in treating meningitis caused by Enterobacteriaceae. The combination of trimethoprim with sulfamethoxazole or sulfadiazine may have special place in the treatment of Gram-negative meningitis in farm animals because of its bactericidal nature and relatively low cost. Local intrathecal administration of drugs has been advocated as a means of achieving adequate CSF concentrations against Enterobacteriaceae. This has been done most commonly with aminoglycosides, but results from controlled clinical trials in human medicine have not established the value of the procedure. Such a procedure is probably a gesture of despair.

ANTIBIOTICS OF CHOICE IN MENINGITIS

Beta-lactam antibiotics for bacterial meningitis are standard therapy that has been revolutionized by the newer ("third-generation") cephalosporins, because of their high bactericidal activity against Enterobacteriaceae. Antibiotics of choice in meningitis and the recommended dosages are summarized in Table 19.3. Beta-lactam antibiotics penetrate noninflamed CSF poorly, but in meningitis they attain adequate MBC concentrations against highly susceptible bacteria. Because enteric bacteria are often resistant to ampicillin, this drug cannot be recommended in the treatment of meningitis in farm animals. The value of beta-lactamase inhibitors (clavulanate, sulbactam) with aminopenicillins or carboxypenicillins in the treatment of meningitis caused by beta-lactamase-producing bacteria remains to be defined, since the evidence from beta-lactamase inhibitors' use in treatment of experimentally induced infections is conflicting. Chloramphenicol, because of its bacteriostatic action, is not a suitable choice for the treatment of bacterial meningitis in neonatal farm animals. Its use in treatment of meningitis in humans results from its bactericidal action against *Neisseria meningitidis*.

Trimethoprim-sulfamethoxazole penetrates uninflamed CSF well and has been used with clinical success in humans in treating meningitis caused by Enterobacteriaceae. This combination administered IV is sec-

TABLE 19.3. **Drugs of choice and recommended dosages in the treatment of bacterial meningitis in animals**

Organism	Standard Treatment	Alternative Treatments
Enterobacteriaceae	Newer cephalosporin, cefotaxime,[a] ceftriaxone[b]	Group 5 ureidopenicillin plus aminoglycoside;[c] ticarcillin-clavulanate;[d] fluoroquinolones;[e] trimethoprim-sulfamethoxazole[f]
Haemophilus parasuis, H. somnus	Penicillin[g] or ampicillin[h]	Trimethoprim-sulfamethoxazole[f]
Listeria monocytogenes	Ampicillin[h] or penicillin G[g]	Trimethoprim-sulfamethoxazole[f]
Pseudomonas aeruginosa	Ceftazidime[i]	Group 5 ureidopenicillin plus aminoglycoside[c]
Staphylococcus aureus	Oxacillin,[j] nafcillin	Trimethoprim-sulfamethoxazole;[f] fluoroquinolone[e]
Beta-hemolytic streptococcus, *S. suis*	Penicillin G[g] or ampicillin[h] (± aminoglycoside)	Newer cephalosporin[a,b]

[a]50 mg/kg IV q6 hours.
[b]50 mg/kg IV q8 hours.
[c]50–75 mg/kg IV q8 hours with gentamicin 3 mg/kg IM and IV.
[d]50 mg/kg IV q8 hours.
[e]5–10 mg/kg q8 hours.
[f]24 mg (combined)/kg IV q6–8 hours.
[g]40,000 IU/kg IV q4–6 hours.
[h]50 mg/kg IV q4–6 hours.
[i]50 mg/kg IV q8 hours.
[j]50 mg/kg IV q8 hours.

ond place to newer cephalosporins as a treatment of choice for coliform meningitis in farm animals. Its effectiveness in *Streptococcus suis* type 2 meningitis in pigs is well established. Fluoroquinolones penetrate well into CSF during meningitis (20–50% of plasma concentrations) and are potentially of use in meningitis in patients with resistant Gram-negative bacteria that do not respond to beta-lactam drugs. Aminoglycosides should be administered only as an adjunct to trimethoprim-sulfamethoxazole or ampicillin because of poor penetration of even inflamed CSF by the aminoglycoside. First- and second-generation cephalosporins penetrate the CSF poorly and have relatively high MBCs against many Gram-negative pathogens.

Adjunct therapy of meningitis with anti-inflammatory drugs, particularly methylprednisolone or dexamethasone, appears to reduce brain edema, CSF pressure, and neurologic sequelae in recovered human patients, but the use of these drugs for this purpose has not been fully accepted (Meric, 1990; Tunkel et al., 1990). Since tissue damage in meningitis is the result of the intense inflammatory response rather than the microorganisms themselves, methods of neutralizing this response are important, given that microorganisms can be eliminated using the powerful bactericidal drugs available. In particular, lysis of bacteria by these antibiotics may contribute to inflammation by the associated release of endotoxin. This effect can be blocked by dexamethasone.

PENETRATION OF ANTIBIOTICS INTO BRAIN TISSUE, INCLUDING ABSCESSES

The poor penetration of most antibiotics into brain tissue results from factors similar to those that determine entry into cerebrospinal fluid; lipid solubility is of greater importance. Low-molecular-weight, poorly protein-bound, highly lipid-soluble drugs such as chloramphenicol and metronidazole penetrate easily into brain tissue and brain abscesses. Aminoglycosides and older cephalosporins penetrate poorly. Metronidazole and chloramphenicol appear to concentrate in the brain. It seems that bacteriostatic drugs are adequate (but not ideal) for the treatment of encephalitis or brain abscess. Third-generation cephalosporins have been used successfully in human medicine in the treatment of brain abscesses.

Haemophilus somnus is highly susceptible to many antibiotics; infection in cattle can be treated with penicillin and probably with erythromycin, sulfonamides, and tetracyclines. Failure to respond is more likely the result of late treatment relative to the extent of the CNS lesions than of bacterial resistance to the antimicrobial agent. Listeriosis in ruminants is traditionally treated with tetracycline, although the drug of choice in humans is ampicillin or trimethoprim-sulfamethoxazole. There is a need for a clinical comparison of tetracycline, penicillin G, ampicillin, and trimethoprim-sulfamethoxazole in the treatment of listeriosis in ruminants.

Brain abscesses in humans often involve mixed anaerobic and aerobic bacteria. Many physicians treat with a combination of penicillin G and chloramphenicol, sometimes combined with metronidazole, until culture and susceptibility results become available. Increasingly, penicillin G and chloramphenicol are being replaced by newer cephalosporins in combination with metronidazole and an aminoglycoside.

Bibliography

Decazes JM, et al. 1987. Bactericidal activity against *Haemophilus influenzae* of cerebrospinal fluid of patients given amoxicillin-clavulanic acid. Antimicrob Agents Chemother 31:2018.
Lebel MH, et al. 1988. Dexamethasone therapy for bacterial meningitis: results of two double-blind placebo-controlled trials. N Engl J Med 319:964.
Meric SM. 1990. Corticosteroid therapy for bacterial meningitis in dogs. Cornell Vet 80:3.
Tarlow MJ. 1991. Adjunct therapy in bacterial meningitis. J Antimicrob Chemother 28:329.
Tauber MG, et al. 1989. Influence of antibiotic dose, dosing interval, and duration of therapy on outcome in experimental pneumococcal meningitis in rabbits. Antimicrob Agents Chemother 33:418.
Tunkel AR, et al. 1990. Bacterial meningitis: recent advances in pathophysiology and treatment. Ann Intern Med 112:610.

Urinary Tract Infections

N. RINKARDT AND S. KRUTH

Bacterial urinary tract infections are the most common cause of urinary tract disease in dogs. Approximately 14% of all dogs will acquire a bacterial urinary tract infection (UTI) during their lifetimes and approximately 10% of dogs presented to the veterinarian for other problems will have a concurrent bacterial UTI (Ling, 1984, 1993). Studies of feline lower urinary tract disease suggest that the prevalence of bacterial UTI is less than 5% in cats presenting with an initial episode of signs related to urinary tract disease (Lees, 1984; Kruger et al., 1991; Buffington et al., 1997). One retrospective study evaluating the prevalence of bacterial UTI in cats that were referred to a teaching hospital found that 25% of feline urine samples were infected. These findings suggest that the prevalence of bacterial UTI in cats may not be as low as previously reported. The mean age of cats in the study was 8.2 years, and it was hypothesized that older cats may be more susceptible to bacterial UTI because of diminished host defenses secondary to aging or concomitant disease (diabetes mellitus, renal failure, hyperthyroidism) (Davison et al., 1992).

The consequences of bacterial UTI in dogs and cats can be significant if the infection goes undiagnosed and untreated. Because many cats and dogs with UTI do not display clinical signs or have detectable bacteruria or pyuria, diagnosis may be incidental in some cases. Colonization of any part of the urinary tract with bacteria makes the animal susceptible to infection in other parts of the urinary tract and body. Some consequences of undiagnosed UTI include infertility, urinary incontinence, discospondylitis, pyelonephritis, and renal failure. Septicemia can occur as a consequence of pyelonephritis in immunosuppressed patients. In intact male dogs, bacterial UTI often extends to the prostate and occasionally to the spermatic cords and/or testicles. Bacterial prostatitis can cause infertility, abscess formation, and recurrent UTI. In dogs, infection of the urine with urea-splitting bacteria *(Staphylococcus intermedius* and *Proteus mirabilis)* is often associated with the formation of struvite uroliths.

Pathogenesis

The establishment of bacterial UTI in dogs and cats is primarily dependent upon the interaction between host defenses and virulence factors of the bacteria. Studies in cats and dogs have shown that when the host defenses are altered by catheterization, surgery, or other diseases of the urinary tract (eg, idiopathic cystitis, urolithiasis, neoplasia), the incidence of bacterial UTI is high (Barsanti et al., 1985; Barsanti et al., 1992; Griffin and Gregory, 1992). Abnormalities of host defenses are thought to be the most important factor in the pathogenesis of UTI (Osborne et al., 1979) and the persistence of complicated UTI. Defense mechanisms of the host can be found in all areas of the urinary tract, including the urethra, bladder, ureters, kidneys, and urine itself.

The most common route of infection in dogs and cats is through ascent of microorganisms within the urethra. Normal bacterial flora of the distal urethra are thought to compete with invading uropathogenic bacteria through bacterial interference (Osborne et al., 1979; Senior, 1985). In the normal urethra, the resident flora may consume essential nutrients, interfere with bacterial adhesion to the uroepithelium, or secrete bacteriocins, thus preventing the uropathogen from colonizing the urethra. In addition, the surface of the urethra has intrinsic properties that prevent bacterial colonization. Scanning electron microscopy of the urethra in female dogs reveals that the urothelium of the distal urethra and vagina has surface microvilli that allow for the attachment of resident bacteria. In contrast, the surfaces of the proximal urethra and bladder have microplicae, folds present when the lumen of the urethra is contracted. These folds flatten when the lumen of the urethra is distended during the act of micturition, thus making it difficult for bacteria to adhere. Such structural differences between epithelia may be associated with resistance to bacterial colonization. Another host defense of the urethra involves the production of secretory IgA, which prevents bacterial adherence and colonization.

Intrinsic properties of the urethra such as urethral peristalsis and a functional high-pressure zone in the mid-urethra also act to prevent bacterial colonization.

Micturition is an important defense against bacterial colonization of the lower urinary tract. Abnormal bacterial flora that gain access to the urethra are washed out by frequent voiding of adequate amounts of urine. In addition, the flattening of urethral folds may dislodge adherent bacteria during voiding. The production of fresh urine dilutes bacterial counts in urine and complete voiding empties the bladder of bacteria. Some diseases of the urinary tract such as bladder atony, urolithiasis, and prolonged urine retention predispose to infection because of the presence of residual urine.

The antibacterial properties of urine have been studied extensively in humans, dogs, rabbits and cats (Mullholland et al., 1969; Lees et al., 1979a,b; Senior, 1985; Measley and Levinson, 1991). Although urine supports bacterial growth, there are components of the urine that are antibacterial, including a very acidic or alkaline pH, a high concentration of urea, a high osmolality. and some weak organic acids (hippuric, benzoic, and quinic acids). Urine oligosaccharides and Tamm-Horsfall mucoproteins entrap bacteria and prevent bacterial colonization (Jarvinen and Sandholm, 1980; Orskov et al., 1980). Changes in the urine composition predispose some patients to urinary tract infection. For example, diuresis decreases the osmolality of urine and may decrease the antibacterial properties of urine. Urine dilution as well as an impaired immune response may contribute to the development of UTI in dogs receiving corticosteroids (Ihrke et al., 1985). In addition, excessive amounts of glucose in the urine inhibit phagocytosis and may predispose to bacterial colonization of the uroepithelium (Chernew and Braude, 1962).

The anatomy and function of the ureters provide a mechanism of defense against bacterial invasion of the kidneys. The distal ureter courses through the bladder wall at an angle that forms a one-way flap, thus preventing regurgitation of urine from the bladder (vesicoureteral reflux). Peristalsis of the ureters promotes unidirectional flow of urine from the kidneys to the bladder and is an important defense against the migration of bacteria that are able to ascend the ureters independent of vesicoureteral reflux.

Renal defenses are limited and rely mostly on local and systemic immune responses in preventing the development of pyelonephritis. The renal cortex has been shown to be much less susceptible to infection than the medulla, possibly due to increased blood flow in this area (Osborne et al., 1979; Measley and Levinson, 1991). Several factors, including decreased blood flow, high ammonia concentrations, and increased osmolality, prevent adequate local immune responses in the medulla, thus making it more susceptible to infection.

In the normal host, there is resistance to the development of bacterial urinary tract infection for the reasons discussed. In addition to a disruption of the normal host defenses, certain bacterial virulence factors enhance colonization of the urinary epithelium and allow the development of UTI. Bacterial adhesion to the uroepithelium is thought to be the most important virulence factor of uropathogenic organisms. *E. coli* and *Proteus mirabilis* both have specific types of fimbriae that enhance bacterial adherence to the epithelial surface of the urinary tract (Westerlund et al., 1987; Senior et al., 1992; Gaastra et al., 1996). Many of the common uropathogens, including *E. coli*, *Proteus* spp., *Staphylococcus* spp., and *Pseudomonas* spp. carry R plasmids, which confer bacterial resistance to antimicrobial agents, enhancing their pathogenicity. Other virulence factors include capsules that surround the bacterium to increase the inflammatory response of the host and to prevent phagocytosis, antibody coating, and opsonization. In addition, *E. coli* produce factors that promote bacterial growth, such as hemolysin and aerobactin (Wilson et al., 1988).

Routes of Infection

The most common route of infection in dogs and cats is the ascending migration of bacteria through the urethra. In humans and dogs, the normal flora of the genital, rectal, and perineal areas have been shown to be the primary reservoirs of infection (Low et al., 1988). The normal flora of the prepuce and vagina have been previously reported (Ling and Ruby, 1978). The most frequently isolated bacterium from dogs with UTI is *E. coli*, followed by *Staphylococcus* spp., *Proteus* spp., *Streptococcus* spp., *Klebsiella* spp., and *Pseudomonas* spp. *Mycoplasma* was isolated as a single agent in 68% of dogs presented for signs of UTI in one study, suggesting that *Mycoplasma* spp. may be an important uropathogen in some cases (Jang et al., 1984). In cats, *E. coli* is the most frequently isolated organism and is found in up to 50% of infected urine samples. *Staphylococcus* spp. and *Streptococcus* spp. are the second most frequently isolated, followed infrequently by other opportunistic pathogens.

Clinical Manifestations

Clinical signs associated with bacterial urinary tract infections in dogs and cats are variable and depend upon the site of infection, the duration of infection, the number and virulence of the bacteria, and the response of the host to the invading organism. In animals that are immunosuppressed or have chronic disease, bacterial UTI may be asymptomatic. History and physical examination findings assist in localizing disease to the urinary tract but are not specific for bacterial UTI. Historical findings associated with UTI of the lower urinary tract include dysuria, pollakiuria, incontinence, hematuria, and abnormal urine odor or color. As a singular problem, infection confined to the lower urinary tract will not cause systemic signs of disease. Historical findings associated with infection of the upper urinary tract usually include polyuria and polydipsia due to bacterial-derived toxins that act in the distal tubule to inhibit antidiuretic hormone (ADH) activity. Signs of systemic disease may or may not be present. Physical examination of the dog or cat with an upper or lower urinary tract infection may reveal no abnormal findings. Infection of the lower urinary tract may be associated with a small, firm, thickened, and painful bladder on palpation. Infection of the upper urinary tract may reveal fever, abdominal pain (localized to the kidney), and palpably enlarged or normal-sized kidneys.

Diagnosis
URINALYSIS

Infection of the urinary tract is confirmed by examination and culture of the bladder urine. Knowledge of the method of urine collection and sample handling is crucial in diagnostic evaluation of the urine. All specimens from normal dogs collected by antepubic cystocentesis are bacteriologically sterile. Urine samples from normal dogs collected by catheterization and voided specimens had 26% and 85% bacterial growth, respectively (Comer and Ling, 1981). Patients that are immunosuppressed may be at greater risk for iatrogenic UTI if urinary catheterization is performed. White blood cells and protein as well as bacteria that are normally present at the external urethral orifice can contaminate specimens collected by means other than cystocentesis, making interpretation of bacteriuria, pyuria, and proteinuria in these samples difficult. Cystocentesis is a well-described method of urine collection, has low morbidity, and is the only method that yields a specimen free of contaminants (Ling, 1976; Osborne, 1977).

Samples collected for urinalysis should be processed within 15 minutes or refrigerated immediately. Specimens for quantitative culture can be refrigerated for up to 6 hours without significant increases in bacterial numbers (Padilla et al., 1981). Refrigeration and prolonged storage can alter the morphology of crystals in the urine, can alter urine pH, and may kill some fastidious uropathogens.

Urine sediment should be evaluated for the presence of white blood cells, red blood cells, and bacteria, findings consistent with inflammation and possibly infection. Samples collected by cystocentesis that have evidence of inflammation localize the disease to the bladder, ureters, or kidneys. Normal urine collected by cystocentesis should have less than 3 white blood cells per high power field (WBC/hpf). Evidence of pyuria may indicate either infection or inflammation that is not associated with bacteria. Patients that are immunosuppressed (hyperadrenocorticism, diabetes mellitus, or immunosuppressive therapy) may have no evidence of inflammation, because of an inability to mount an adequate immune response. Ihrke et al. (1985) found that only 54% of dogs receiving corticosteroids for the treatment of chronic skin disease had more than 3 WBC/hpf in infected urine. Evaluating white blood cells using the dipstick method alone is unreliable (Vail et al., 1986). Hematuria is diagnosed when a urine sample collected by cystocentesis has greater than 3 RBC/hpf. Hematuria in the absence of pyuria may be iatrogenic (due to cystocentesis) or may be due to renal or bladder wall hemorrhage that is unrelated to inflammation or infection. The visualization of bacteria in uncontaminated urine collected by cystocentesis is diagnostic for a bacterial UTI; however, the absence of bacteria does not rule out a UTI. Rod-shaped bacteria may not be visualized during examination of urine sediment if they are at a concentration of ≤10,000/ml; cocci may not be visualized if they are at a concentration of ≤100,000/ml. If the urine is dilute (<1.013), bacteria may not be visualized and white blood cell counts may not be elevated.

Infection of the urine with urea-splitting bacteria such as *Proteus* spp. or *Staphyloccus* spp. may result in an increase in the urine pH (>7.5), predisposing the patient to the development of struvite urolithiasis. The visualization of struvite crystals together with an alkaline pH and evidence of urinary tract inflammation are significant findings and should be pursued further with a urine culture and radiography or ultrasound to evaluate for the presence of urolithiasis. Fungal elements are rarely visualized during microsopic evaluation of urine sediment but may be indicative of systemic mycotic infection. *Candida* spp., normally present on the external genital mucosa, may become opportunistic pathogens in immunosuppressed patients.

URINE CULTURE

Urine culture is the "gold standard" for the diagnosis of urinary tract infection. Indications for performing urine culture include the visualization of bacteria during urine sediment examination, evidence of pyuria, dilute urine (<1.013), and possible immunosuppression. Urine should be collected for culture prior to the institution of antibiotic therapy. Qualitative urine culture will identify the species of bacteria; however, it will not determine the number of bacteria. Urine culture results must be interpreted in light of the method of collection, as previously discussed. Quantitative urine culture determines the number of bacteria/unit volume, identifies the bacterial species, and is the preferred method of culture for urine collected by any method. Techniques of urine culture have been previously reported (Ling, 1993; Osborne, 1995b). In general, urine may be sent to a diagnostic laboratory for this service or may be cultured in-house. Urine for culture should be processed within 15 minutes but can be refrigerated for up to 6 hours without affecting bacterial growth. Susceptibility testing should be considered with complicated or recurrent cases of UTI, immunosuppressed patients, patients that have been recently catheterized, or patients treated with antimicrobials within the preceding 3 weeks (due to selection for resistance). In addition, culture and susceptibility testing should be performed in cases that do not respond within 7 days of therapy for UTI or cases that are associated with multiple pathogens.

Treatment

A detailed history will aid the clinician in determining whether the UTI is simple or complicated. A simple urinary tract infection is usually due to a transient and reversible abnormality in the host defenses, responds quickly to appropriate therapy, and does not recur. A complicated UTI is usually due to an underlying abnormality in the urinary tract or host defenses. Immunosuppression caused by high doses of glucocorticoids or other immunosuppressive drugs, hyperadrenocorticism, renal failure, or diabetes mellitus may be a cause of complicated UTI. In addition, conditions that damage the urothelium such as urolithiasis, neoplasia, catheterization, surgery, or cystitis caused by cyclophosphamide or idiopathic causes can predispose to the development of complicated UTI. Other causes of complicated UTI include anatomic defects (ectopic ureters, urachal diverticula), interference of normal micturition (urinary obstruction; damaged nervous innervation, causing bladder atony) or changes in urine concentration or composition (glucosuria). If such an abnormality exists, UTI may relapse or recur. A relapse (recurrent infection caused by the same bacterial organism) indicates that previous therapy failed. Reinfection is defined as a UTI that is recurrent but caused by a different bacterial organism than that previously isolated. Patients that experience a relapse or reinfection warrant further evaluation. Before treatment for UTI is undertaken, the UTI should be classified as simple or complicated. Treatment for a simple UTI may be empirical, based upon knowledge of the commonly isolated organisms and their susceptibility to antimicrobial agents; however, empirical therapy often fails and is not recommended (Ling, 1993). To effectively treat and eliminate a complicated UTI, further diagnostics should be considered to identify the underlying problem.

The choice of an antimicrobial to treat any infection should be based upon the ability of the drug to reach the site of infection, knowledge of side effects and adverse reactions, route of elimination, ease of administration, and cost. Urine concentrations of antimicrobials are more important than serum levels during the treatment of UTI (Stamey, 1974) and have been previously published. In general, concentrations of antibiotics in urine will exceed those in serum if the antimicrobial is excreted in an

TABLE 19.4. Bacteria isolated from dogs and cats with urinary tract infections and suggested antimicrobial drugs of choice

Pathogen	Dogs (%)	Cats (%)	Suggested Antibiotics
Escherichia coli	43	47	Amoxicillin-clavulanate; trimethoprim-sulfa; cephalexin
Staphylococcus spp.	20	18	Amoxicillin-clavulanate; ampicillin; cephalexin
Streptococcus spp.	11	13	Ampicillin; amoxicillin-clavulanate
Proteus spp.	13	4	Ampicillin; amoxicillin-clavulanate
Klebsiella spp.	4	4	Cephalexin; trimethoprim-sulfa; amoxicillin-clavulanate
Enterobacter spp.	3	1	Trimethoprim-sulfa; amoxicillin-clavulanate
Pseudomonas aeruginosa	2	1 (*Pseudomonas* spp.)	Enrofloxacin; tetracycline
Pasteurella spp.	—	2	Ampicillin
Mycoplasma spp.	—	1	Tetracycline; enrofloxacin

active form in the urine. If the urine concentration of an antibiotic is 4 times (or greater) than the MIC, it will most likely be effective for treatment of UTI caused by that pathogen (90% effective) (Ling, 1993). Knowledge of the specific bacterial species, the MIC, and anticipated urine concentration of the antibiotic allow the clinician to make an appropriate decision regarding antimicrobial therapy for UTI (Table 19.4). For example, since the MIC of virtually all urinary *Streptococcus* spp. and *Staphyloccus* spp. is ≤ 10 μg/ml, and 8-hour urine concentration of oral ampicillin and amoxicillin is about 300 μg/ml at recommended doses, these drugs will be effective in the treatment of these infections, despite MICs that would be interpreted as resistant if the infections were in other sites in the body. For the same reason, oral tetracycline has been used successfully in the treatment of urinary tract infections caused by *Pseudomonas aeruginosa*, and cephalexin in the successful treatment of *Klebsiella* urinary tract infections, despite apparent resistance assessed in vitro, using usual interpretive criteria (Ling, 1993).

The dosage and drug interval determined to treat UTI should be those recommended by the manufacturer. Ideally, 3 equal doses of antibiotic per day should be given except when administering trimethoprim-sulfa or enrofloxacin (Lees and Rogers, 1986). Most antimicrobials used to treat UTI have relatively short half-lives and may not maintain high concentrations in the urine. Therefore, client compliance during therapy for UTI is imperative (see Chapter 22). In addition, some dogs void frequently during the day and may not maintain high urine concentrations of antibiotics. It is also recommended that dogs void just prior to receiving a dose of antibiotic, especially if a long period of confinement (overnight) is anticipated. Because many drugs are excreted by the kidneys and some are nephrotoxic, patients with renal failure or insufficiency should have the dosage and interval of the chosen antibiotic adjusted (see Renal Impairment, below).

In general, the duration of therapy for UTI is based upon whether the infection is simple or complicated. Studies have shown that single-dose therapy and three-day therapy are not effective for the treatment of experimentally induced UTI in female and male dogs, respectively (Turnwald et al., 1986; Rogers et al., 1988). Although clinical studies evaluating the optimum duration of therapy have not been done, most patients with simple UTI will require a course of antibiotics 10–14 days in duration. This length of treatment allows host defenses to recover and ensures that the urine is sterile. Patients with complicated UTI usually require a longer course of therapy. If an underlying problem such as neoplasia or urolithiasis is diagnosed, antimicrobial therapy is administered in conjunction with treatment of the primary problem. Many chronic, complicated cases of UTI, pyelonephritis, and prostatitis are treated with antimicrobials for 4–6 weeks. In many cases, it is ideal to culture the urine (via cystocentesis) 1 week after therapy begins and 1 week after therapy ends (urinalysis is not required) to document resolution of UTI. In patients that have frequent recurrences of UTI without an underlying problem, prophylactic low-dose therapy can be instituted. In these patients, conventional therapy for UTI should be administered (simple or complicated), the urine should culture negative near the end of therapy, and the patient should be put on a dose that is one-half to one-third of the total daily dose. This dose should be administered once daily, prior to a period of confinement (overnight). This treatment regime should be continued for 6 months, with monthly urine cultures collected via cystocentesis. If the cultures are negative for 6 months, therapy can be discontinued; however, the urine should be cultured periodically (every 3–4 months) to monitor for recurrence of UTI. Disadvantages of this form of therapy include the possible toxicity associated with certain antimicrobials (eg, chloramphenicol, trimethoprim-sulfa), cost, and the risk of inducing antimicrobial resistance.

Treatment failures may be due to poor owner compliance, inappropriate choice of antimicrobial, inappropriate dose or duration of treatment, antimicrobial resistance, superinfection, or an underlying predisposing cause (eg, urolithiasis, neoplasia, urachal diverticula). If treatment for a simple or complicated UTI fails, a complete urinalysis should be performed, including culture and susceptibility, with urine collected via cystocentesis. Plain radiographs and contrast studies, as well as ultrasound, may be indicated in these cases. In addition, a complete blood count and biochemical profile should be performed to rule out systemic disease.

Measures to prevent iatrogenic UTI include using urinary catheters only if absolutely necessary and using a closed-collection technique for indwelling urinary catheters. Immunosuppressed patients should be considered at increased risk for iatrogenic UTI during urinary catheterization.

Prostatitis

Prostatitis, defined as inflammation of the prostate, is usually caused by the ascent of normal distal urethral flora in the intact dog. This condition is rare in neutered dogs; however, an infection present prior to castration may persist postoperatively. Prostatitis may manifest as an acute or a chronic problem. The clinical signs of acute bacterial prostatitis may include depression, fever, vomiting, inappetence, urethral discharge (possibly bloody), and pain on rectal palpation of the prostate. Dogs with prostatitis may have a stiff gait and a hunched appearance. The prostate may be symmetrical and of normal size in some cases. Chronic prostatitis may be difficult to diagnose, as dogs with chronic prostatitis often do not display clinical signs other than mild inappetence and lethargy. The prostate may not be enlarged on rectal palpation, and a mild urethral discharge may or may not be present. Chronic prostatitis may be a cause or a result of chronic UTI and may lead to abscessation of the prostate.

Laboratory evaluation in the dog with acute prostatitis will often reveal a neutrophilia with a left shift and a urinalysis consistent with inflammation. Patients with chronic prostatitis may or may not have changes indicative of infection on routine blood work. A urinalysis will again reveal inflammation. Further diagnostic evaluation, including radiography and ultrasonography, are often useful in assisting the diagnosis of benign prostatic hypertrophy, prostatitis, prostatic cysts/abscessation, or neoplasia. Prostatic fluid evaluation is not routinely performed in the dog with suspected prostatitis.

Treatment of prostatitis should be approached in a similar manner as for a complicated UTI. Urine culture (obtained by cystocentesis or fine needle aspiration of the prostate) and sensitivity are essential in formulating a therapeutic plan. The choice of antimicrobial drug should be based upon sensitivity results and the ability of the antibiotic to cross the blood-prostate barrier. In cases of acute inflammation, most antibiotics are effective; however, as the infection becomes chronic, only antimicrobials that are lipid soluble, have a basic pH, and are not highly protein bound will cross the prostatic epithelium. Trimethoprim-sulfa and the fluoroquinolones are recommended for treatment of prostatitis. The duration of treatment should be 4 weeks for acute infections and 6 weeks for chronic infections. The urine should be cultured during therapy and recultured (by cystocentesis) 1 week after therapy is completed, to ensure resolution of the infection. Castration may be beneficial in resolving prostatitis and preventing recurrence. If recurrence does occur, low-dose, once-daily antimicrobial therapy, as previously discussed, may be initiated. Prostatic abscesses may develop as a consequence of prostatitis, are difficult to treat medically, and should be managed surgically.

Bibliography

Allen TA, et al. 1987. Microbiologic evaluation of canine urine: direct microscopic examination and preservation of specimen quality for culture. J Am Vet Med Assoc 190:1289.
Barsanti JA, et al. 1985. Urinary tract infection due to indwelling bladder catheters in dogs and cats. J Am Vet Med Assoc 187:384.
Barsanti JA, et al. 1992. Effect of therapy on susceptibility to urinary tract infection in male cats with indwelling urethral catheters. J Vet Int Med 6:64.
Buffington CAT, et al. 1997. Clinical evaluation of cats with nonobstructive urinary tract diseases. J Am Vet Med Assoc 210:46.
Chernew I, Braude AL. 1962. Depression of phagocytosis by solutes in concentration found in the kidney and urine. J Clin Invest 41:1945.
Comer KM, Ling GV. 1981. Results of urinalysis and bacterial culture of canine urine obtained by antepubic cystocentesis, catheterization, and midstream voided methods. J Am Vet Med Assoc 179:891.
Davison AP, et al. 1992. Urinary tract infections in cats: a retrospective study, 1977–1989. Calif Vet 46:32.
Gaastra W, et al. 1996. Isolation and characterization of dog uropathogenic *Proteus mirabilis* strains. Vet Microbiol 48:57.
Griffin DW, Gregory CR. 1992. Prevalence of bacterial urinary tract infection after perineal urethrostomy in cats. J Am Vet Med Assoc 200:681.
Ihrke PJ, et al. 1985. Urinary tract infection associated with long-term corticosteroid administration in dogs with chronic skin diseases. J Am Vet Med Assoc 186:43.
Jang SS, et al. 1984. Mycoplasma as a cause of canine urinary tract infections. J Am Vet Med Assoc 185:45.
Jarvinen AK, Sandholm M. 1980. Urinary oligosaccharides inhibit adhesion of E. coli onto canine urinary tract epithelium. Invest Urol 17:443.
Kruger JM, et al. 1991. Clinical evaluation of cats with lower urinary tract disease. J Am Vet Med Assoc 199:211.
Lees GE. 1984. Epidemiology of naturally occurring feline bacterial urinary tract infection. Vet Clin North Am Small Anim Pract 14:471.
Lees GE, Osborne CA. 1979. Antibacterial properties of urine: a comparative review. J Am Anim Hosp Assoc 15:125.
Lees GE, Rogers KS. 1986. Treatment of urinary tract infections in dogs and cats. J Am Vet Med Assoc 189:648.
Lees GE, et al. 1979a. Antibacterial properties of urine: studies of feline urine specific gravity, osmolality, and pH. J Am Anim Hosp Assoc 15:135.
Lees GE, et al. 1979b. Urine: a medium for bacterial growth. Vet Clin North Am Small Anim Pract 9:611.
Ling GV. 1976. Antepubic cystocentesis in the dog: an aseptic technique for routine collection of urine. Calif Vet 30:50.
Ling GV. 1984. Therapeutic strategies involving antimicrobial treatment of the canine urinary tract. J Am Vet Med Assoc 185:1162.
Ling GV. 1993. Urinary tract infections. In: Prescott JF, Baggot JD, eds. Antimicrobial Therapy in Veterinary Medicine, 2nd ed. Ames: Iowa State Univ Press, p349.
Ling GV, Ruby AL. 1978. Aerobic bacterial flora of the prepuce, urethra, and vagina of normal dogs. Am J Vet Res 39:695.
Low DA, et al. 1988. Isolation and comparison of E. coli strains from canine and human patients with urinary tract infection. Infect Immun 56:2601.

Measley RE, Levinson ME. 1991. Host defense mechanisms in the pathogenesis of urinary tract infection. Med Clin North Am 75:275.

Mooney JK, Hinman F. 1974. Surface differences in cells of proximal and distal canine urethra. J Urol 111:495.

Mulholland SG, et al. 1969. The antibacterial properties of urine. Invest Urol 6:569.

Orskov I, et al. 1980. Tamm-Horsfall protein or uromucoid is the normal urinary slime that traps type 1 fimbriated *E. coli*. Lancet 1:887.

Osborne CA. 1977. Cystocentesis: indications, contraindications, technique, and complications. Minn Vet 17:9.

Osborne CA. 1995a. Chronic Renal Failure. In: Ettinger SJ, Feldman EC, eds. Textbook of Veterinary Internal Medicine, 3rd ed. Philadelphia: WB Saunders, p1746.

Osborne CA. 1995b. Three steps to effective management of bacterial urinary tract infections: diagnosis, diagnosis, and diagnosis. Compend Contin Educ Pract Vet 17:1233.

Osborne CA, et al. 1979. Urinary tract infections: normal and abnormal host defense mechanisms. Vet Clin North Am Sm Anim Pract 9:587.

Padilla J, et al. 1981. Effects of storage time and temperature on quantitative culture of canine urine. J Am Vet Med Assoc 178:1077.

Rogers KS, et al. 1988. Effects of single-dose and three-day trimethoprim-sulfadiazine and amikacin treatment of induced *Escherichia coli* urinary tract infections in dogs. Am J Vet Res 49:345.

Senior DF. 1985. Bacterial urinary tract infections: invasion, host defenses, and new approaches to prevention. Compend Contin Educ Pract Vet 7:334.

Senior DF, et al. 1992. Serotype, hemolysin production, and adherence characteristics of strains of *E. coli* causing urinary tract infection in dogs. Am J Vet Res 53:4.

Stamey TA. 1974. Serum versus urinary antimicrobial concentrations in cure of urinary tract infections. N Engl J Med 291:1159.

Turnwald GH, et al. 1986. Comparison of single-dose and conventional trimethoprim-sulfadiazine therapy in experimental *Staphylococcus intermedius* cystitis in the female dog. Am J Vet Res 47:2621.

Vail DM, et al. 1986. Applicability of leukocyte esterase test strip in detection of canine pyuria. J Am Vet Med Assoc 189:1451.

Westerlund B, et al. 1987. Characterisation of *E. coli* strains associated with canine urinary tract infections. Res Vet Sci 42:404.

Wilson RA, et al. 1988. Strains of *E. coli* associated with urogenital disease in dogs and cats. Am J Vet Res 49:743.

DOSE MODIFICATION

Drug Disposition and Dosage in Neonatal Animals

J. D. BAGGOT

Differences between neonatal and adult animals in the intensity and duration of the effects produced by a drug when given at usual (adult) dosage can generally be attributed to altered pharmacokinetics during the neonatal period. The alterations affect the plasma drug concentration profile and the concentrations attained at the site of infection. They account for the clinical observation that neonatal animals are often more "sensitive" to the pharmacologic effects of drugs, particularly drugs that act on the central nervous system. Some characteristics of the neonatal period include better absorption from the gastrointestinal tract, lower binding to plasma proteins, lower ratio of body fat to fluids, increased volume of distribution of drugs that distribute in extracellular fluid or total body water, increased permeability of the blood-brain barrier, and slower elimination (longer half-life) of most drugs. It is conceivable that the altered absorption and disposition (distribution and elimination) processes could be accommodated by adjusting the usual (adult) dosing rate. The meager information available on drug bioavailability and disposition in neonatal animals limits the recommendations that can be made on dosage adjustment. The situation is further complicated by interspecies variation in the rate at which the physiological processes affecting drug absorption and disposition mature (Short, 1983; Baggot and Short, 1984). The neonatal period, which is generally considered to be the first month of postnatal life, varies among species. It appears to be 1–2 weeks in foals; about 8 weeks in calves, kids, lambs and piglets; and 10–12 weeks in puppies. However, the most profound adaptive changes in physiological variables occur during the first 24 hours after birth in all species. This coincides with the time that the pharmacokinetic behavior of drugs is most "unusual."

Absorption

Colostral antibodies (macromolecules) are absorbed from the gastrointestinal tract during the first 24 hours after birth. This suggests that the intestinal epithelium is more permeable during the first 24–36 hours. The systemic availability of orally administered absorbable antimicrobial agents is higher in neonatal than in adult animals, and repeated dosage of drugs that are poorly absorbed (such as neomycin) could give rise to systemic toxic effects from accumulation, due to both increased absorption and impaired elimination. The relatively less acidic pH in the stomach and upper small intestine and the nature of the ingesta (mainly milk) influence the extent of drug absorption (systemic availability). Antimicrobial agents, such as penicillins, that are poorly absorbed and cause digestive disturbances in older foals (over 4 months of age) and adult horses can be administered orally to neonatal and young foals (up to 4 months of age) for the treatment of systemic bacterial infections caused by susceptible microorganisms. Oral administration of amoxicillin trihydrate (30 mg/kg), as a 5% oral suspension, to 5-to-10-day-old foals produced serum amoxicillin concentrations above 1 mg/ml for 6 hours (Love et al., 1981). Systemic availability of amoxicillin was 30–50% in the foals, in contrast to 5–15% in adult horses (Baggot et al., 1988). Pivampicillin, a prodrug of ampicillin, has systemic availability (ampicillin) of 40–53% in foals between 11 days and 4 months of age (Ensink et al., 1994). In adult horses, the systemic availability of ampicillin administered as pivampi-cillin is within the range of 31–36%. The half-life of aminobenzylpeni-cillins is approximately 2-fold longer following oral administration than following intravenous administration. It may be because of their moder-ate extent of absorption that the detrimental effect of oral penicillins, which is due to severe disturbance of the balance among the commensal bacterial flora in the colon of adult horses, is avoided in neonatal and young foals. There is no need to adjust the dosage interval in neonatal foals, because penicillins in the systemic circulation have a wide margin of safety. Penicillin V, the phenoxymethyl analog of penicillin G, does not have a place (due to low systemic availability and the production of digestive disturbances) in the treatment of bacterial infections in foals or adult horses (Baggot et al., 1990).

The systemic availability of cefadroxil (5% oral suspension) decreases progressively from 68% in 1-month-old foals to 14.5% in foals 5 months of age (Duffee et al., 1997). The half-life of the drug remains unchanged over this age range. Cephradine, another first-generation oral cephalosporin, administered in sucrose syrup to 10-to-14-day-old foals has an average systemic availability of 64% and a half-life of 1.1 hours (Henry et al., 1992).

Erythromycin estolate is used in conjunction with rifampin for the treatment of *Rhodococcus equi* pneumonia in foals between 6 and 16 weeks of age but, in common with other macrolide antibiotics and lincosamides, would produce gastrointestinal disturbance in older foals and in matur-ing and adult horses.

Since the rumen takes 4–8 weeks to develop and become functional, the bioavailability (rate and extent of absorption) of drugs administered orally to preruminant calves resembles that in monogastric species rather than in cattle. Although chloramphenicol is not approved for use in food-producing animals, a comparison between preruminant calves and neonatal foals is informative. Chloramphenicol, administered as an oral solution, is well absorbed in preruminant calves, and oral dosage (25 mg/kg at 12-hour dosage intervals) will maintain therapeutically effective plasma concentrations (>5 µg/ml) of the antibiotic (Huffman et al., 1981). In ruminant calves and adult cattle, orally administered chlor-amphenicol fails to provide effective plasma concentrations because the antibiotic is inactivated (reductive reaction) in the rumen. A single oral dose (50 mg/kg) of chloramphenicol solution administered to foals between 3 and 8 weeks of age produced an average peak plasma/serum concentration of 6 µg/ml, which was lower than the peak concentration produced in adult horses (18 µg/ml) given the drug at the same dose level (Buonpane et al., 1988). Changes in the disposition kinetics of chloram-phenicol (administered as a single IV dose) are age related, and the pat-tern of the change differs among species; a marked increase in the rate of

TABLE 19.5. **Age-related changes in the disposition kinetics of chlorampenicol in calves (50 mg/kg, IV) and foals (25 mg/kg, IV)**

Age	$V_{d(ss)}$ (ml/kg)	Cl_B (ml/kg/min)	$t_{1/2}$ (h)
Calves ($n = 5$)			
1 day	$1,130 \pm 50$	1.1 ± 0.24	11.7 ± 1.7
7 days	$1,180 \pm 70$	1.9 ± 0.03	7.5 ± 0.9
10–12 weeks	$1,230 \pm 60$	3.1 ± 0.63	4.9 ± 0.7
Foals ($n = 6$)			
1 day	992 ± 269	2.25 ± 0.67	6.19 ± 2.43
3 days	543 ± 173	6.24 ± 2.22	1.48 ± 0.51
7 days	310 ± 67	8.86 ± 1.90	0.64 ± 0.14

chloramphenicol elimination (hepatic metabolism) during the first week after birth is a consistent finding (Table 19.5). Assuming that chloramphenicol is mainly eliminated by glucuronide conjugation, it would appear that this microsomal-associated metabolic pathway develops far more rapidly in foals (within 1 week) (Adamson et al., 1991) than in calves (8–12 weeks) (Reiche et al., 1980). This finding is consistent with the shorter neonatal period in foals than in calves.

Antimicrobial agents that undergo extensive first-pass metabolism by hepatic microsomal oxidative reactions would be expected to have higher systemic availability in neonatal animals. This applies to trimethoprim, which has far higher systemic availability in newborn kids than in older kids and adult goats. In addition to lower hepatic microsomal oxidative activity, the ruminal microflora have not developed in neonatal ruminant species. Hydrolysis of pivampicillin to ampicillin, which takes place in the intestinal mucosa, is well developed in young foals.

Distribution

Body composition may largely account for species variations or age-related differences in the distribution pattern and extent of distribution of drugs. Total body water may constitute 75% of the body weight in neonatal animals, where as it is 50–60% in adults. It is the extracellular fluid volume that is considerably larger (almost doubled) in the neonate and that decreases with age. This accounts for the larger apparent volumes of distribution in neonates of drugs that are highly ionized or relatively polar (eg, penicillins, aminoglycosides). Although usual doses will provide lower plasma concentrations, because of increased extravascular distribution, the concentrations attained at drug receptors (pharmacological agents) or sites of bacterial infection (antimicrobial agents) may be higher.

The ratio of body fat to fluids, which is lower in newborn animals, contributes to the smaller apparent volumes of distribution of lipophilic drugs (eg, macrolides, fluoroquinolones) in newborns. The age-related change in body fat content is considerably smaller in horses than in other species. Total body fat normally constitutes 2–3% of body weight in neonatal foals and 5% in adult horses.

Drugs reversibly bind in varying degrees to plasma proteins. Since only the unbound fraction can diffuse into tissues, extensive (>80%) binding of a drug to plasma proteins influences the total (bound plus unbound) concentration in the plasma, the extent of distribution, and the availability of the drug for elimination (metabolism and excretion). Examples of antimicrobial agents that bind extensively to plasma proteins include cloxacillin, cefoperazone, clindamycin, and ketoconazole. Acidic drugs (penicillins, cephalosporins, sulfonamides) bind to plasma albumin, whereas some basic drugs (macrolides, lincosamides) bind to other plasma proteins (α_1-acid glycoprotein). In the case of extensively bound drugs, a small change in the concentration of drug-binding protein, or displacement of an acidic drug by another with higher affinity for albumin binding, can significantly affect the amount of drug available for extravascular distribution and elimination. During neonatal development, albumin concentrations in plasma are a function of hepatocyte maturity. Relative hypoalbuminemia is characteristic of neonatal animals, apart from foals; it is most pronounced in piglets at birth. The lower binding of acidic drugs to plasma albumin contributes to the increased extravascular distribution of these drugs, particularly in piglets under 2 weeks of age. The plasma concentration of α_1-acid glycoprotein is highest in piglets at birth and, conversely to plasma albumin, decreases during the first 2 weeks of postnatal life. The declining concentration of α_1-acid glycoprotein significantly decreases the binding of organic bases (erythromycin, lincomycin and trimethoprim) to plasma proteins and increases their extravascular distribution and availability for elimination by the liver (Tagawa et al., 1994; Kinoshita et al., 1995).

Since disposition refers to the simultaneous effects of distribution and elimination, it is necessary to consider both components of the process when interpreting changes that occur during the neonatal period or in the presence of a disease state. Enrofloxacin is converted by N-dealkylation, a hepatic microsomal oxidative reaction, to ciprofloxacin. Both enrofloxacin and ciprofloxacin are active antimicrobially. Comparison of the disposition kinetics of enrofloxacin (2.5 mg/kg administered IV) in 1-day-old and 1-week-old calves shows that the volume of distribution at steady state is smaller and the systemic clearance of the drug is lower in the 1-day-old calves, whereas the half-life does not differ significantly between the 1-day-old and 1-week-old calves (Table 19.6). The changes in the disposition kinetics of enrofloxacin that occur during the first week of postnatal life in calves could be attributed to differences in

TABLE 19.6. **Disposition kinetics of enrofloxacin and formation of ciprofloxacin in newborn and 1-week-old Finnish Ayrshire calves**

Pharmacokinetic Parameter	Age of Calves		Statistical Significance
	1 Day	1 Week	
Enrofloxacin			
$V_{d(ss)}$ (l/kg)	1.81 ± 0.10	2.28 ± 0.14	$p = 0.035$
	(1.54 – 2.01)	(1.88 – 2.52)	
Cl_B (l/h × kg)	0.19 ± 0.03	0.39 ± 0.06	$p = 0.021$
	(0.14 – 0.28)	(0.31 – 0.56)	
$t_{1/2}$ (h)	6.61 ± 1.12	4.87 ± 0.68	Not significant
	(4.28 – 9.36)	(3.13 – 6.43)	
Ciprofloxacin			
t_{max} (h)	15.0 ± 3.0	2.8 ± 0.8	$p = 0.007$
	(12 – 24)	(1 – 4)	
C_{max} (mg/l)	0.087 ± 0.017	0.142 ± 0.005	$p = 0.023$
	(0.07 – 0.14)	(0.13 – 0.15)	

Note: A single dose (2.5 mg/kg) of enrofloxacin was administered by intravenous injection to the calves ($n = 4$ in each age group). Results are expressed as mean ± SEM and (range).

plasma protein binding of enrofloxacin and in the ratio of body fat to fluids, since fluoroquinolones are lipid-soluble drugs. Newborn calves metabolize enrofloxacin to ciprofloxacin, but the rate of formation of the active metabolite is slower and the peak serum concentration (C_{max}) is lower than in the 1-week-old calves; mean t_{max} is about 5 times longer in newborn calves (Fig. 19.1) (Kaartinen et al., 1997). Since the content of cytochrome P-450 has been shown to double during the first week of postnatal life in calves (Shoaf et al., 1987), it can be concluded that the rate of conversion of enrofloxacin to ciprofloxacin is age related. Following IV administration of a single dose (2.5 mg/kg) of enrofloxacin, the sum of enrofloxacin and ciprofloxacin concentrations in plasma/serum was above 0.1 µg/ml at 30 hours and 24 hours in 1-day-old and 1-week-old calves, respectively. The MIC_{90} for the majority of susceptible *E. coli* strains isolated from calves is 0.25 µg/ml.

The blood-brain barrier restricts (although to a lesser extent in the presence of fever) the passage of drugs, particularly those that are poorly diffusible (eg, penicillins, most cephalosporins, aminoglycosides), from the systemic circulation into the central nervous system. This barrier is, in effect, a less porous capillary structure than that present in skeletal muscle and soft tissue organs. Passage across the blood-brain barrier is limited to free (unbound) drug in the plasma that is of sufficient lipid solubility to passively diffuse through both the capillary endothelium and the astrocytic sheath. Since this morphological barrier is only partially developed at birth, drugs of low lipid solubility and certain endogenous substances

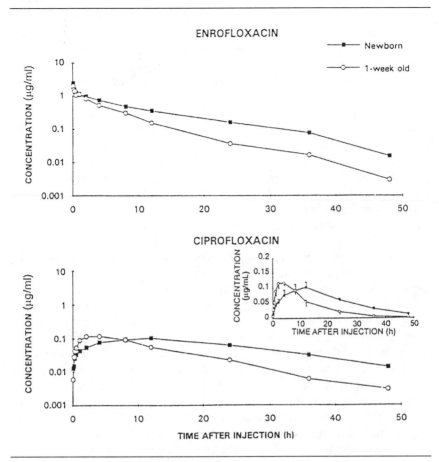

Fig. 19.1. Mean concentration-time curves of enrofloxacin and its metabolite ciprofloxacin in newborn and 1-week-old calves (4 calves per group). Enrofloxacin was administered IV at a dosage of 2.5 mg/kg. Drug concentrations were analyzed using a high-pressure liquid chromatography (HPLC) method. The insert in the lower panel shows the mean ciprofloxacin concentrations and standard errors of mean on a nonlogarithmic scale.

(eg, bilirubin) that cannot normally enter the extracellular fluid of the brain gain access during the early neonatal period. The presence of fever enhances the capacity of penicillins and cephalosporins, but not aminoglycosides, to penetrate the blood-brain barrier.

Metabolism

Metabolism (biotransformation) converts most lipid-soluble drugs into polar metabolites that are far less widely distributed and are readily excreted mainly in the urine, while some metabolites (in particular glucuronide conjugates) are also excreted in bile. A minority of antimicrobial agents are initially converted to active metabolites that possess antimicrobial activity at least equal to that of the parent drug; some examples include enrofloxacin, ceftiofur, and rifampin. Pivampicillin, a prodrug, is activated by hydrolysis to ampicillin. The liver is the principal organ of drug metabolism, although drugs and other foreign chemical substances (xenobiotics) can be metabolized, at least by some pathways, in other organs (lungs and kidneys) and tissues (intestinal mucosa and blood plasma). Ruminal microorganisms can metabolize some antimicrobial agents by reductive and hydrolytic reactions, whereas intestinal microorganisms can hydrolyze glucuronide conjugates excreted in bile, thereby liberating the metabolite or the parent drug. Antimicrobial agents that are mainly eliminated by metabolism include most sulfonamides, trimethoprim, fluoroquinolones, chloramphenicol, clindamycin, metronidazole, rifampin, ceftiofur (unique among the cephalosporins in this regard), and ketoconazole (but not fluconazole, which is eliminated by renal excretion).

Although there are species differences in the degree to which some drug metabolic pathways are deficient in neonatal animals, a relative lack of development of hepatic smooth-surfaced endoplasmic reticulum and its associated drug metabolizing enzyme systems (oxidative reactions and glucuronide conjugation) appears to be a characteristic of the neonatal period in all mammalian species. Because of the low activity of most metabolic pathways, the half-lives of drugs that undergo extensive hepatic metabolism are prolonged in neonatal animals, particularly during the first 24 hours after birth. The maturation of the various metabolic pathways could be related to hormonal influence on postnatal enzyme induction. In the majority of species (ruminant animals, pigs, dogs, and presumably cats), the hepatic microsomal-associated metabolic pathways develop rapidly during the first 3–4 weeks after birth, and at 8–12 weeks of age they have developed activity approaching that of adult animals (Short and Davis, 1970; Nielsen and Rasmussen, 1976; Reiche et al., 1980; Reiche, 1983). The foal appears to be an exception in at least the rate of development of glucuronide synthesis, which develops very rapidly during the first week after birth (Adamson et al., 1991). Although a long dosage interval should be applied during the first 3 days after birth, it can gradually be decreased, depending on the animal species, as the neonate matures.

Conversion of ceftiofur to desfuroylceftiofur, a third-generation cephalosporin, is catalyzed by an esterase, which is most active in the kidneys and next most active in the liver (Olson et al., 1998). Desfuroylceftiofur has antibacterial activity similar to that of the parent drug, and the active metabolite rapidly becomes reversibly bound to proteins in plasma

445

and tissues and forms conjugates with glutathione and cysteine. The high-performance liquid chromatographic (HPLC) assay method measures the combined plasma concentration of ceftiofur and desfuroylceftiofur conjugates as a single derivative, desfuroylceftiofur acetamide, which is expressed as mg ceftiofur free acid equivalents per ml (Jaglan et al., 1990). In a study of the influence of age on the disposition kinetics of ceftiofur, administered IV as ceftiofur sodium at a dose of 2.2 mg ceftiofur free acid equivalents per kg body weight, in Holstein bull calves, the volume of distribution at steady state ($V_{d(ss)}$) decreased, and systemic clearance (Cl_B) increased during the first 3 months after birth (Brown et al., 1996). The progressive decrease in volume of distribution of ceftiofur and desfuroylceftiofur conjugates could be attributed to the age-related decrease in extracellular fluid volume. The lower clearance in the 7-day-old and 1-month-old calves than in the older calves is probably due to maturation of the processes of elimination for ceftiofur and desfuroylceftiofur metabolites. Because the decreases in volume of distribution were proportionally less than the increases in clearance in calves 1 month of age and older, the half-life decreased more or less in accordance with the increased clearance (Table 19.7). Plasma concentrations of ceftiofur and its metabolites (measured as a single derivative) remained above the limit of quantification (LOQ, 0.15 mg/ml) of the assay method for the entire 72-hour blood sampling period in 7-day-old and 1-month-old calves, but it decreased to below the LOQ within 48 hours of drug administration to 6- and 9-month-old calves.

From studies of antipyrine, a marker substance used to indicate hepatic microsomal oxidative activity (Depelchin et al., 1988; Delpechin, pers. comm., 1988), it could be concluded that hepatic microsomal oxidative activity develops rapidly in calves during the first 2 weeks after birth, more slowly between 2 and 6 weeks of age, and gradually reaches activity (probably at about 3 months of age) similar to that in adult cattle. The

TABLE 19.7. **Comparison of pharmacokinetic values derived from plasma concentrations of ceftiofur and metabolites after IV injection of ceftiofur sodium in Holstein bull calves of various ages**

Age	$V_{d(ss)}$ (ml/kg)	Cl_B (ml/kg/h)	$t_{1/2}$ (h)
1 week	345 ± 62	17.8 ± 3.2	16.1 ± 1.5
1 month	335 ± 92	16.7 ± 3.1	17.2 ± 3.1
3 months	284 ± 49	30.3 ± 4.6	8.2 ± 2.8
6 months	258 ± 72	39.8 ± 14.9	5.95 ± 1.2

Note: Plasma concentrations of ceftiofur and metabolites were measured as desfuroylceftiofur acetamide by HPLC. Dosage of ceftiofur sodium was 2.2 ceftiofur free acid equivalents per kilogram.

half-life of trimethoprim, which is mainly metabolized by hepatic micro-somal oxidation, is 4–5 times longer in newborn kids than in adult goats (Nielsen and Rasmussen, 1976). In kids, a period of about 8 weeks would appear to be required for the half-life of trimethoprim to approach the value found in adult goats. This would roughly coincide with the period taken for development of hepatic microsomal oxidative activity.

Since adult cats have a relative deficiency in microsomal glucuronyl transferase activity, glucuronide conjugates of drugs and endogenous substances (such as bilirubin) are slowly synthesized in cats. Immaturity of this metabolic pathway would render neonatal kittens particularly sus-ceptible to toxicity with drugs that undergo glucuronide conjugation.

Renal Excretion

Renal excretion is the principal elimination process for drugs that are predominantly ionized at physiological pH (eg, penicillins, cephalo-sporins), for polar drugs (aminoglycosides, spectinomycin), and for mol-ecules with limited lipid solubility (tetracyclines, except doxycycline and minocycline). Exceptions among the beta-lactam antibiotics include naf-cillin, cefoperazone, and ceftriaxone, which (like erythromycin) are excreted in bile, and cephalothin and cefotaxime, which are deacetylated prior to excretion in urine. Even though fluoroquinolones, trimethoprim, and sulfonamides are mainly eliminated by hepatic metabolism, a frac-tion of the dose is excreted unchanged in urine.

The renal excretion mechanisms (glomerular filtration and active, carrier-mediated tubular secretion) are incompletely developed at birth in all mammalian species. During the neonatal period, renal excretion mech-anisms mature independently at rates that are species related. Glomeru-lar filtration rate (GFR), based on inulin clearance, attains adult values at 2 days in calves and 2–4 days in lambs, kids, and piglets, and it may take at least 14 days in puppies. Proximal tubular secretion, based on clearance of para-aminohippurate, matures within 2 weeks after birth in the rumi-nant species and pigs but may take up to 6 weeks in dogs. Indirect evi-dence, provided by pharmacokinetic studies of some antimicrobial agents, suggests that renal function develops rapidly in foals at a rate sim-ilar to that in ruminant species. In a recently published study of the mat-uration of renal function in full-term pony foals during the first 10 days postpartum, it was shown (using the single injection technique) that the glomerular filtration rate and effective renal plasma flow remain rela-tively constant throughout the postnatal period (Holdstock et al., 1998). This implies that the neonatal foal, like the calf, has relatively mature renal function compared with neonates of most other species. The hydra-tion state of newborn animals would affect renal function (GFR). Even though renal function is immature in neonatal, particularly newborn, animals, it has the capacity adequate to meet physiological requirements. However, when lipid-soluble drugs are administered to neonatal animals, the combined effect of slow hepatic microsomal-associated metabolic reactions (oxidation and glucuronide conjugation) and relatively inefficient renal excretion mechanisms considerably decreases the rate of elimination of the parent drugs and their polar metabolites. Urinary pH is acidic in neonates of all species; this would favor renal tubular reabsorption and extend the half-life of drugs that are weak organic acids and are of sufficient lipid solubility to be reabsorbed by passive diffusion (eg, most sulfonamides).

The pharmacokinetic parameters describing the disposition of gentamicin (4 mg/kg, IV) were determined in foals of various ages (12–24 hours, 5, 10, 15 and 30 days) and in mares (Cummings et al., 1990). The apparent volume of distribution of the aminoglycoside did not change significantly with age of the foals but was approximately 2-fold larger than in mares. Since the distribution of gentamicin is virtually restricted to the extracellular fluid (ECF), it could be concluded that ECF volume is larger in young foals than in adult horses. Gentamicin is eliminated solely by glomerular filtration. The systemic clearance of gentamicin in 1-day-old foals is similar to that in adult horses; this indicates that glomerular filtration is well developed in newborn foals. Because of the larger volume of distribution and unchanged systemic clearance, the half-life of gentamicin in newborn foals is twice as long as in adult horses, while in foals between 5–15 days of age, it is approximately 1.5 times the half-life in adult horses. The pattern of age-related changes in the disposition of gentamicin in calves (Clarke et al., 1985) is similar to that in foals (Table 19.8).

The disposition of gentamicin differs significantly between newborn (4–12 hours of age at the time of dosing) and 42-day-old piglets (Giroux et

TABLE 19.8. Age-related changes in the disposition of gentamicin in foals and calves

Age (days)	$V_{d(ss)}$ (ml/kg)	Cl_B (ml/kg/min)	$t_{1/2}$ (min)
Foals			
1	307 ± 30	1.75 ± 0.47	127 ± 23
5	350 ± 66	2.98 ± 1.48	90 ± 32
10	344 ± 95	2.60 ± 0.96	101 ± 33
15	325 ± 48	2.40 ± 0.87	106 ± 33
Mares	156 ± 22	1.69 ± 0.65	65 ± 55
Calves			
1	376 ± 41	1.92 ± 0.43	149 ± 38
5	385 ± 44	2.44 ± 0.34	119 ± 20
10	323 ± 20	2.02 ± 0.27	118 ± 13
15	311 ± 29	2.10 ± 0.32	111 ± 8.5
Cows	129 ± 17	1.29 ± 0.26	76 ± 11

al., 1995). The age-related pattern of changes in piglets is consistent with that in foals and calves. As the neonate matures, the apparent volume of distribution decreases, systemic clearance increases, and the half-life of gentamicin becomes shorter. The average half-life of gentamicin is 5.2 hours in newborn piglets and 3.8, 3.5, and 2.7 hours in 4-, 6-, and 10-week-old piglets, respectively. In a study of the pharmacokinetics of amikacin in critically ill full-term foals ranging in age from 2 to 12 days, the systemic clearance of the aminoglycoside was lower and the half-life was considerably prolonged in uremic compared with nonuremic foals (Adland-Davenport et al., 1990). Renal excretion mechanisms appear to mature within the first 2 weeks after birth in ruminant species (Friis, 1983), horses, and pigs (Short, 1983), while their maturation in dogs may take 4–6 weeks.

Oxytetracycline is eliminated by glomerular filtration, but because it undergoes enterohepatic circulation, the half-life of oxytetracycline is longer than that of aminoglycoside antibiotics and varies among animal species. The apparent volume of distribution and the half-life of oxytetracycline decrease with age in calves between 3 and 14 weeks old and further in adult cattle (Nouws et al., 1983). The changes could be attributed to the decrease in total body water volume and the progressive development of the rumen. Even though the volume of distribution of oxytetracycline is larger in 4-to-5-day-old foals than in adult horses, the half-life of the drug does not appear to be extended in foals (Papich et al., 1995). The half-life of ceftriaxone—a third-generation cephalosporin that distributes widely in body fluids, penetrates the blood-brain barrier, and is eliminated by biliary rather than renal excretion—is twice as long in 2-to-12-day-old foals (Ringger et al., 1998) as in adult horses (Ringger et al., 1996). The longer half-life of the drug could be attributed to the larger volume of extracellular fluid in the neonatal foals. The average half-life of erythromycin, administered IV as erythromycin gluceptate, in Shetland-cross foals of various ages (from 1 to 12 weeks old) is the same (1 hour) as in mares (Prescott et al., 1983). It is likely that biliary and renal excretion mechanisms mature at the same rate in neonatal animals of any species, while hepatic formation of conjugates controls the rate of their excretion in bile and/or urine.

Drug Selection and Administration

The immunodeficient state of the neonatal (especially newborn) animal, combined with the decreased ability to eliminate (metabolize and excrete) drugs, makes it preferable to select antimicrobial agents that have a bactericidal action and a wide margin of safety. Such drugs include penicillins, amoxicillin, or ticarcillin combined with clavulanic acid, trimethoprim-sulfonamide combinations, and most of the cephalosporins. To offset the variation associated with drug absorption, a parenteral preparation can be administered by IV infusion or slow IV injection to avoid circulatory overload. For some antimicrobial agents (eg, penicillins, cefotaxime, ceftriaxone, and aminoglycosides) intraosseous administration may be a useful alternative to IV injection in neonatal foals (Fig. 19.2) (Golenz et al., 1994) and puppies (Lavy et al., 1995) in cases in which a vein cannot be raised. Whether the IV or intraosseous route of administration is used, the usual dose (mg/kg) recommended for parenteral therapy in adult animals can generally be used, but the dosage interval should be increased (extended) in neonatal animals. Age-related species variations in development of the various elimination processes (hepatic metabolic pathways and renal excretion mechanisms) make prediction of appropriate dosage intervals uncertain. Because of individual variation in the plasma/serum concentrations of aminoglycosides

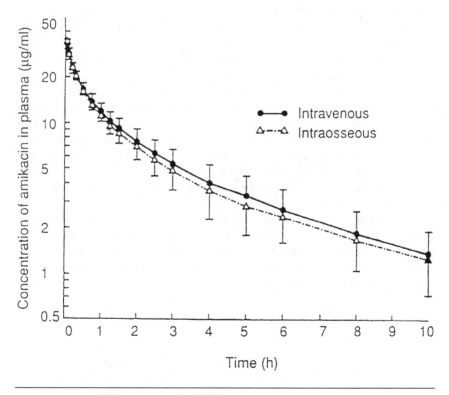

Fig. 19.2. Concentrations (mean ±SD) of amikacin in plasma after intravenous and intraosseous administration of amikacin sulfate (7 mg/kg) to 6 foals at 3–5 days of age.

attained in neonatal foals and the risk of producing nephrotoxicity, maintenance dosage should be based on measured peak and trough concentrations. Absorption from IM sites largely depends on regional blood flow, which can vary with the site of injection and is influenced by the formulation of the parenteral dosage form and by the presence of disease states (such as dehydration). The sum of these variables not only influences the plasma concentration profile that will be obtained but also may affect the response to therapy. In mild to moderate infections, the oral route may be used for maintenance therapy with aminobenzylpenicillins (use pivampicillin in foals), cefadroxil, trimethoprim-sulfonamide combinations, and fluoroquinolones (in calves and piglets). Since fluoroquinolones can cause damage to articular cartilage of weight-bearing joints in rapidly growing animals, their use in neonates should be limited. The absorption pattern of drugs in neonatal ruminants more closely resembles that in monogastric species than in mature ruminant animals. The systemic availability of orally administered drugs is higher in neonates, and elimination, regardless of the route of administration, is slower, particularly when hepatic metabolism is involved. Throughout the neonatal period, systemic availability decreases and the rate of drug elimination increases to gradually approach pharmacokinetic behavior of the drug in adult animals.

In the case of infections caused by microorganisms of unpredictable susceptibility, the choice of antimicrobial agent and its dosing rate should be based upon susceptibility, preferably MIC, determined in vitro. The relatively larger extracellular fluid volume in neonatal animals may require a higher dose to be administered of antimicrobials that mainly distribute in extracellular fluid (aminoglycosides, penicillins, and most cephalosporins). Even though the apparent volume of distribution of enrofloxacin in newborn calves is smaller than in 1-week-old calves, the same dose can be used in both age groups, since metabolic conversion of enrofloxacin to ciprofloxacin takes place more slowly in the newborns. The dosage interval should be increased in neonatal animals for all antimicrobial agents, particularly those that are mainly eliminated by hepatic metabolism (fluoroquinolones, trimethoprim, sulfonamides).

Bibliography

Adamson PJW, et al. 1991. Influence of age on the disposition kinetics of chloramphenicol in equine neonates. Am J Vet Res 52:426.

Adland-Davenport P, et al. 1990. Pharmacokinetics of amikacin in critically ill neonatal foals treated for presumed or confirmed sepsis. Equine Vet J 22:18.

Baggot JD, Short CR. 1984. Drug disposition in neonatal animals, with particular reference to the foal. Equine Vet J 16:364.

Baggot JD, et al. 1988. Bioavailability and disposition kinetics of amoxicillin in neonatal foals. Equine Vet J 20:125.

Baggot JD, et al. 1990. Oral dosage of penicillin V in adult horses and foals. Equine Vet J 22:290.

Brown SA, et al. 1996. Effects of age on the pharmacokinetics of single dose ceftiofur sodium administered intramuscularly or intravenously to cattle. J Vet Pharmacol Ther 19:32.

Buonpane NA, et al. 1988. Serum concentrations and pharmacokinetics of chloramphenicol in foals after a single oral dose. Equine Vet J 20:59.

Clarke CR, et al. 1985. Pharmacokinetics of gentamicin in the calf: developmental changes. Am J Vet Res 46:2461.

Cummings LE, et al. 1990. Pharmacokinetics of gentamicin in newborn to 30-day-old foals. Am J Vet Res 51:1988.

Depelchin BO, et al. 1988. Effects of age, sex, and breed on antipyrine disposition in calves. Res Vet Sci 44:135.

Duffee NE, et al. 1997. The pharmacokinetics of cefadroxil over a range of oral doses and animal ages in the foal. J Vet Pharmacol Ther 20:427.

Ensink JM, et al. 1994. Oral bioavailability of pivampicillin in foals at different ages. Vet Q 16:S113.

Friis, C. 1983. Postnatal development of renal function in goats. In: Ruckebusch Y, et al., eds. Veterinary Pharmacology and Toxicology. Lancaster, England: MTP Press, p57.

Giroux D, et al. 1995. Gentamicin pharmacokinetics in newborn and 42-day-old male piglets. J Vet Pharmacol Ther 18:407.

Golenz MR, et al. 1994. Effect of route of administration and age on the pharmacokinetics of amikacin administered by the intravenous and intraosseous routes to 3- and 5-day-old foals. Equine Vet J 26:367.

Henry MM, et al. 1992. Pharmacokinetics of cephradine in neonatal foals after single oral dosing. Equine Vet J 24:242.

Holdstock NB, et al. 1998. Glomerular filtration rate, effective renal plasma flow, blood pressure, and pulse rate in the equine neonate during the first 10 days *post partum*. Equine Vet J 30:335.

Huffman EM, et al. 1981. Serum chloramphenicol concentrations in preruminant calves: a comparison of two formulations dosed orally. J Vet Pharmacol Ther 4:225.

Jaglan PS, et al. 1990. Liquid chromatographic determination of desfuroylceftiofur metabolite of ceftiofur as residue in cattle plasma. J Assoc Off Anal Chem 73:26.

Kaartinen L, et al. 1997. Pharmacokinetics of enrofloxacin in newborn and one-week-old calves. J Vet Pharmacol Ther 20:479.

Kinoshita T, et al. 1995. Impact of age-related alteration of plasma α_1-acid glycoprotein concentration on erythromycin pharmacokinetics in pigs. Am J Vet Res 56:362.

Lavy E, et al. 1995. Disposition kinetics of ampicillin administered intravenously and intraosseously to canine puppies. J Vet Pharmacol Ther 18:379.

Love DN, et al. 1981. Serum levels of amoxicillin following its oral administration to Thoroughbred foals. Equine Vet J 13:53.

Nielsen P, Rasmussen F. 1976. Influence of age on half-life of trimethoprim and sulphadoxine in goats. Acta Pharm Toxicol 38:113.

Nouws JFM, et al. 1983. Age-dependent pharmacokinetics of oxytetracycline in ruminants. J Vet Pharmacol Ther 6:59.

Olson SC, et al. 1998. In vitro metabolism of ceftiofur in bovine tissues. J Vet Pharmacol Ther 21:112.

Papich MG, et al. 1995. Pharmacokinetics of oxytetracycline administered intravenously to 4- to 5-day-old foals. J Vet Pharmacol Ther 18:375.

Prescott JF, et al. 1983. Pharmacokinetics of erythromycin in foals and in adult horses. J Vet Pharmacol Ther 6:67.

Reiche R. 1983. Drug disposition in the newborn. In: Ruckebusch Y, et al., ed. Veterinary Pharmacology and Toxicology. Lancaster, England: MTP Press, p49.

Reiche R, et al. 1980. Pharmacokinetics of chloramphenicol in calves during the first weeks of life. J Vet Pharmacol Ther 3:95.

Ringger NC, et al. 1996. Pharmacokinetics of ceftriaxone in healthy horses. Equine Vet J 28:476.

Ringger NC, et al. 1998. Pharmacokinetics of ceftriaxone in neonatal foals. Equine Vet J 30:163.
Shoaf SE, et al. 1987. The development of hepatic drug-metabolizing enzyme activity in the neonatal calf and its effect on drug disposition. Drug Metab Dispos 15:676.
Short CR. 1983. Developmental patterns of penicillin G excretion. In: Ruckenbusch Y, et al., eds. Veterinary Pharmacology and Toxicology. Lancaster, England: MTP Press, p63.
Short CR, Davis LE. 1970. Perinatal development of drug-metabolizing enzyme activity in swine. J Pharm Exp Ther 174:185.
Tagawa Y, et al. 1994. α_1-Acid glycoprotein-binding as a factor in age-related changes in the pharmacokinetics of trimethoprim in piglets. Vet Q 16:13.
Wilcke JR, et al. 1993. Pharmacokinetics of phenylbutazone in neonatal foals. Am J Vet Res 54:2064.

Antimicrobials and Anthelmintics in Pregnancy

J. D. BAGGOT

Physiological adaptations that occur during pregnancy and could influence the oral bioavailability and disposition of drugs include an increase in gastric pH, an increase in the circulating blood (plasma) volume and in renal blood flow, an alteration in body fluid compartments, and hormonal-induced change in hepatic microsomal enzyme activity. A major concern in the use of drugs during pregnancy is the potential for adverse effects on the fetus, since all drugs administered to the mother cross the placental barrier, although at different rates, and the fetus is ill equipped to eliminate drugs.

Placental drug transfer by passive diffusion is similar to passage across any epithelial barrier, and in many respects it resembles passage from the systemic circulation into milk of lactating animals. Since the pH of arterial blood in the fetus (7.27) is only slightly lower than in the mother (7.37), the ion-trapping effect whereby lipophilic organic bases attain higher concentrations in the milk does not apply to the fetal circulation. Drug diffusion across the placenta from mother to fetus is favored by lipid solubility, a large concentration gradient of unbound drug between the maternal and fetal circulations, and maintenance of drug in the nonionized form in the maternal circulation. Conversely, molecules that are ionized (penicillins, cephalosporins), hydrophilic (aminoglycosides), and present in low free drug concentrations (doxycycline, macrolides, and lincosamines) have restricted access to the fetus. Differences in the extent of plasma protein binding by the mother and fetus (in which it is lower) affect the total plasma drug concentrations in the maternal and fetal circulations.

Because toxic effects could be produced in the fetus, caution should be exercised with the use of a wide variety of antimicrobial agents in pregnant animals (Table 19.9), while some others (fluoroquinolones, tetracyclines, griseofulvin) are contraindicated.

Some benzimidazole carbamates, in particular albendazole and presumably netobimin (which is metabolically converted by ruminal

TABLE 19.9. Suggested cautions or contraindications of potentially toxic antimicrobial drugs in pregnant animals

Drug	Toxicity	Recommended Use Caution[a]	Contraindicated
Antibacterial			
Aminoglycosides	Auditory nerve toxicity?	+	
Chloramphenicol	Gray syndrome in newborn	+	
Fluoroquinolones	Arthropathy in immature animals	+	+
Metronidazole	Carcinogenic in rodents?	+	At term
Nitrofurantoin	Hemolytic anemia in newborn	+	
Sulfonamides	Increased risk of neonatal jaundice; teratogenic in some studies	+	
Tetracyclines	Tooth discoloration; inhibited bone growth in fetus; hepatic toxicity in pregnant animals with impaired renal function		+
Trimethoprim	Folate antagonist may cause congenital anomalies	+	
Antifungal			
Azoles	Teratogenic	+	
Griseofulvin	Teratogenic		+

[a]*Caution:* Do not use if suitable alternative is available.

microorganisms and hepatic microsomes to albendazole), are known to cause teratogenesis in animals. Albendazole or netobimin should not be administered during the first 5 weeks of pregnancy in ewes or the first 7 weeks of pregnancy in cows. The use of mebendazole is contraindicated during the first 4 months of pregnancy in donkeys treated for *Dictyocaulus*. Haloxon, an organophosporus compound, should not be administered to mares during the first 2 months of pregnancy. The exercise of caution is advisable when considering the use of dichlorophen (a phenol derivative that acts by uncoupling oxidative phosphorylation) either alone or combined with piperazine in pregnant bitches or queens. Praziquantel-pyrantel embonate combination is contraindicated in pregnant queens.

When selecting an antimicrobial or anthelmintic drug for administration to a pregnant animal, due consideration must be given to the potential of many of these drugs to produce adverse effects on the fetus.

Renal Impairment

J. E. RIVIERE

Many antimicrobial drugs used in veterinary medicine are eliminated from the body primarily by the kidney. When routine dosage regimens designed for healthy animals are used in animals with renal dysfunction, accumulation may occur. If the drug is toxic, this could result in serious complications. If this situation occurs in a food-producing animal, violative tissue residues could occur. The purpose of this section is to briefly overview the pharmacokinetic and pharmacodynamic effects of renal dysfunction on antimicrobials and to suggest dosage modifications that may minimize the risk of adverse complications. Other references can be consulted for further details (Riviere and Davis, 1984; Riviere et al., 1991).

Renal Pathophysiology Pertinent to Antimicrobial Dosimetry

The primary pathophysiologic sequelae of pertinence to antimicrobial dosing in renal dysfunction is a decreased glomerular filtration rate (GFR), which results in a decreased clearance of drugs eliminated by the kidney. Because of the large renal functional reserve, 75% of GFR must generally be lost before signs of clinical disease are readily evident. Adjustments to dosage regimens generally account only for decreased GFR, and unless therapeutic drug monitoring (TDM) is employed, other changes seen in severe renal dysfunction will not be accounted for. When renal disease is severe, electrolyte and fluid homeostasis is often disrupted; this may alter a drug's volume of distribution by altering fluid spaces or decreasing protein binding via conformational changes in albumin. The accumulation of endogenous metabolic products normally eliminated through the kidney may compete with the antimicrobial agent for protein binding, also resulting in an increased volume of distribution secondary to decreased binding. This is primarily seen with acidic drugs such as some beta-lactams and sulfonamides. The hepatic biotransformation of drugs has also been documented to be affected by renal disease, although these changes are drug and species specific. Decreased biotransformation in human uremics has been observed with cefonicid, cefotaxime, cilastatin, imipenem, and moxalactam (Matzke and Keane, 1989).

In cases of severe uremia, administration of antimicrobials containing sodium or potassium could result in electrolyte overload. The antianabolic activity of some tetracyclines may also exacerbate the uremic state.

Construction of Modified Dosage Regimens

The construction of modified dosage regimens in renal failure assumes that renal drug clearance directly correlates with clinical estimates of GFR (eg, creatinine clearance, or 1/serum creatinine); the intact nephron hypothesis holds true and relative glomerular-tubular balance is present. In these cases, an antimicrobial's renal clearance is a linear function of GFR, independent of whether the drug is filtered, secreted, and/or absorbed in the kidney. In addition, the volume of distribution of the drug is assumed to be unchanged.

When TDM is available, both a drug's clearance and volume of distribution may be directly determined in an individual pharmacokinetic study. The resulting individualized dosing regimen thus accounts for the renal insufficiency present. However, even in this scenario, as is true for other approaches, the shape of the serum concentration-time profile in an animal with renal failure cannot be made to precisely duplicate that in a healthy animal since the drug's clearance is reduced and half-life is prolonged (Frazier and Riviere, 1987). In general, TDM is employed only for toxic antimicrobials whose accumulation would adversely affect the animal's health. Thus a great deal of effort, both in veterinary and human medicine, has been spent on the nephrotoxic aminoglycoside antibiotics. The effort is further necessitated by the great variability often seen in aminoglycoside pharmacokinetics in diseased animals where both creatinine clearance (Cl_{cr}) and fluid status (V_d) are often changed (Frazier et al., 1988), necessitating close monitoring to avoid drug-induced nephrotoxicity.

The initial loading dose of the drug should be the same as in the normal animal. Dose reduction schemes attempt to decrease the subsequent maintenance doses or increase the dosing interval, both in proportion to decreased Cl. Table 19.10 lists the antimicrobial agents commonly used in veterinary medicine for which modified dosage regimens can be formulated on the basis of existing data. Extrapolation from human studies is often necessary because of a lack of such work in animals. For drugs eliminated primarily by hepatic mechanisms (eg, chloramphenicol) or drugs with wide safety indices (eg, penicillins), dosage modification is often unnecessary. In cases in which such antimicrobials would be efficacious, the drugs that are cleared by hepatic mechanisms are preferred. When modification based on Cl_{cr} is indicated, the following two methods are suggested.

Interval extension: Administer normal maintenance dose

$$\text{Interval} = \text{Normal interval} \times \frac{(\text{Normal } Cl_{cr})}{(\text{Patient } Cl_{cr})}$$

Dose reduction: Administer at the normal dose interval

$$\text{Dose} = \text{Normal dose} \times \frac{(\text{Patient } Cl_{cr})}{(\text{Normal } Cl_{cr})}$$

In severe renal failure, use of the interval extension method may result in excessively prolonged periods of subinhibitory drug concentrations. In this case, one-half or one-third of the dose should be given at one-half or one-third, respectively, of the calculated intervals.

TABLE 19.10. **Drug dosage adjustments in the presence of renal failure**

Drug	Route of Elimination	Dosage Adjustment
Aminoglycosides		
Amikacin	Renal	Interval extension[a]
Gentamicin	Renal	Interval extension[a]
Kanamycin	Renal	Interval extension[a]
Sisomicin	Renal	Interval extension[a]
Tobramycin	Renal	Interval extension[a]
Streptomycin	Renal	2–3 × interval with severe renal failure
Neomycin	Renal	Contraindicated
Cephalosporins		
Cefazolin	Renal	Interval extension
Cephalexin	Renal	Interval extension
Cefachlor	Hepatic	No change
Cefamandole	Renal, hepatic	½ dose with severe renal failure
Cephalothin	Renal, hepatic	2 × interval with severe renal failure
Penicillins		
Cloxacillin	Hepatic	No change
Nafcillin	Hepatic	No change
Oxacillin	Hepatic	No change
Amoxicillin	Renal, hepatic	½ dose or 2 × interval in severe renal failure
Ampicillin	Renal, hepatic	½ dose or 2 × interval in severe renal failure
Carbenicillin	Renal, hepatic	½ dose or 2 × interval in severe renal failure
Methicillin	Renal, hepatic	½ dose or 2 × interval in severe renal failure
Penicillin G and V	Renal, hepatic	½ dose or 2 × interval in severe renal failure
Ticarcillin	Renal, hepatic	½ dose or 2 × interval in severe renal failure
Clavulanic acid	Renal, hepatic	½ dose or 2 × interval in severe renal failure
Imipenem/cilastatin	Renal, hepatic	½ dose or 2 × interval in severe renal failure
Sulfonamides		
Sulfisoxazole	Renal, hepatic	2–3 × interval with severe renal failure
Trimethoprim-sulfamethoxazole	Renal, hepatic	No change, but do not use in severe renal failure
Tetracyclines	Renal, hepatic	Contraindicated except for doxycycline
Doxycycline	GI mucosa	No change
Miscellaneous agents		
Amphotericin	Hepatic	½ dose in severe renal failure
Chloramphenicol	Hepatic	No change, but avoid in severe renal failure
Clindamycin	Hepatic	No change
Erythromycin	Hepatic, renal	No change
Lincomycin	Hepatic, renal	3 × interval with severe renal failure
Methenamine mandelate		Contraindicated
Metronidazole	Hepatic, renal	Unknown
Nalidixic acid		Contraindicated
Nitrofurantoin		Contraindicated
Polymyxin B		Contraindicated
Fluoroquinolones		
Ciprofloxacin	Renal	Dosage reduction
Enrofloxacin	Renal	Dosage reduction
Norfloxacin	Renal	Dosage reduction
Tylosin	Hepatic, renal	No change
Vancomycin	Renal	Interval extension

[a]Individual therapeutic drug monitoring should be used when available because of variability in disposition.

If Cl_{cr} is not available, some researchers have suggested that 1/SCR (serum creatinine) or 1/BUN (blood urea nitrogen) be substituted. However, in severe renal failure, this may not be accurate.

A great deal of effort has been expended trying to define how a dosage regimen in a diseased individual can be constructed to maintain efficacy and avoid toxicity. This may be an impossible goal suggesting that trade-offs must be made. Close clinical monitoring is required to ensure antimicrobial efficacy and no drug-induced toxicity. The latter is especially difficult when detection of aminoglycoside-induced nephrotoxicity is confounded by the underlying renal dysfunction. For aminoglycosides, interval extension has been shown to produce less toxicity than dose reduction. The data are not as clear for other drugs. Serial monitoring of renal function tests (SCR, BUN), urinary enzymes, or TDM is the only approach that may be used.

Finally, it must be stressed that if renal disease is present in food-producing animals, the decreased GFR would be expected to result in a prolonged elimination half-life, possibly necessitating a prolonged withdrawal time. Guidelines have not been established in veterinary medicine to address this problem, other than using drugs not eliminated by the kidney or using drugs with very short half-lives so that prolonged withdrawal times would suffice. Again, aminoglycosides, characterized by prolonged tissue half-lives, would be contraindicated. On-site urine monitoring could also be employed to reduce the chance of residues.

Conclusions

The specific recommendations listed in Table 19.10 should provide the basis for initial dosage adjustment. Depending on the underlying cause of the renal disease process, renal function may rapidly change, necessitating close monitoring. Paradoxically, some clinicians at North Carolina State University actually use the pharmacokinetic parameters of gentamicin obtained from TDM studies in patients with renal failure to monitor changes in GFR (Cl_B) and V_d.

The efficacy of an antimicrobial may also be affected in severe renal disease associated with very low GFR. For example, in treating urinary tract infections with renally excreted drugs, renal clearance may be so low that little drug actually reaches the urine. In polyuric renal disease states, dilution secondary to increased urine flow coupled with decreased GFR may result in therapeutic failure in cases with urinary tract infections. Similar situations exist in treating intrarenal infections such as pyelonephritis.

If dialysis is employed to treat the uremic patient, drug clearance from the body may be increased through drug removal by dialysis. In general, hemodialysis and hemofiltration are more efficient than peritoneal dialysis. Specific guidelines may be found in nephrology texts.

In conclusion, because of the limited systemic toxicity of most approved veterinary antimicrobial agents and their wide therapeutic index, precise dosage adjustment is not required. For example, even if penicillin clearance is drastically reduced, administration of normal dosages will result in drug accumulation but not increased toxicity in nonallergic patients. In fact, the elevated serum concentrations of drugs may actually potentiate antimicrobial efficacy. In contrast, aminoglycoside accumulation may kill the patient. In severe Gram-negative infections in uremic patients, newer quinolone antibiotics (eg, norfloxacin) might now be selected where aminoglycosides were the only choice in the past. Although quinolones will accumulate in renal disease, their lack of systemic toxicity promotes their use in renal disease. Alternatively, drugs eliminated by hepatic or nonrenal mechanisms such as chloramphenicol, macrolides, doxycycline, and some cephalosporins may be selected and the question of dosage adjustment avoided.

Bibliography

Frazier DL, Riviere JE. 1987. Gentamicin dosing strategies for dogs with subclinical renal dysfunction. Antimicrob Agents Chemother 31:1929.

Frazier DL, et al. 1988. Gentamicin pharmacokinetics and nephrotoxicity in naturally acquired and experimentally induced disease in dogs. J Am Vet Med Assoc 192:57.

Matzke GR, Keane WF. 1989. Drug dosing in patients with impaired renal function. In: DiPiro JT, et al., eds. Pharmacotherapy: A Pathophysiologic Approach. New York: Elsevier.

Riviere JE, Davis LE. 1984. Renal handling of drugs in renal failure. In: Bovee KC, ed. Canine Nephrology. Media, PA: Harwal Publishers.

Riviere JE, et al. 1991. Handbook of Comparative Pharmacokinetics and Residues of Veterinary Antimicrobials. Boca Raton, FL: CRC Press.

SELECTED BACTERIAL INFECTIONS

Anaerobes

D. C. HIRSH

Bacteria that are unable to grow in the presence of molecular oxygen are defined as obligate anaerobes, or simply anaerobes. They can be Gram-negative or Gram-positive, rods or cocci. They include a significant proportion of bacterial populations that comprise the normal flora on all mucosal surfaces that harbor bacteria. Rather few of the several hundred different species produce primary disease. The exceptions include members of the genera *Clostridium* (eg, *C. difficile, C. perfringens*), enterotoxigenic *Bacteroides fragilis,* and the pathogenic anaerobic spirochetes (eg, *Serpulina*) (Myers et al., 1984; Twedt, 1993; Struble et al., 1994; Madewell et al., 1995; Ter Huurne and Gaastra, 1995; Trott et al., 1996). These microorganisms produce disease, but most are always (except with some foals affected with *C. difficile*) preceded by a "trigger event"—eg, diarrhea associated with *C. difficile* following administration of an antimicrobial agent (Jones et al., 1988; Bartlett, 1994). The most commonly encountered infectious processes involving anaerobes, however, are those stemming from infection of a normally sterile site by a member of the relatively pathogenic species of the genera of normal flora (eg, *Actinomyces, Bacteroides, Clostridium, Eubacterium, Peptostreptococcus, Porphyromonas*) occupying the mucosal surface contiguous to the compromised site (Prescott, 1979; Hirsh et al., 1985).

Resistance

All anaerobes are naturally resistant to the aminoglycosides, since these antibiotics require an oxygen-dependent transport system to get into the bacterial cell. Likewise, anaerobes are inherently resistant to the earlier fluoroquinolones, though there are some fluoroquinolones in development that have some activity against some anaerobes (eg, levofloxacin, trovafloxacin) (Goldstein, 1996). Some anaerobes are resistant to cell-wall–active antimicrobials: the penicillins and the first-generation cephalosporins (Appelbaum et al., 1990; Stark et al., 1993), because of possession of beta-lactamases that break down these drugs (Sebald, 1994). The most commonly encountered is a cephalosporinase active on the first-generation cephalosporins (eg, cephalexin, cefazolin), the penicillins (ie, penicillin G, ampicillin, amoxicillin, ticarcillin), and some third-generation cephalosporins (notably ceftiofur) (Livermore, 1995; Samitz et al., 1996). Members of the *Bacteroides fragilis* group *(B. distasonis, B. eggerthii, B. fragilis, B. sterocoralis, B. ovatus,* and *B. uniformis)* more often than not contain the gene encoding this enzyme. Resistance to the tetracyclines is unpredictable. The effectiveness of trimethoprim-sulfonamides is unpredictable for the treatment of infectious processes involving anaerobes. The reason is that some anaerobes (and there is no way to predict which ones—hence the unpredictability) are able to scavenge thymidine from necrotic material and thereby bypass the block in the production of this chemical by trimethoprim-sulfonamides (Indiveri and Hirsh, 1992). So even though in vitro tests (done under controlled thymidine-less conditions) may predict effectiveness, trimethoprim-sulfonamides are not recommended for treatment of infectious processes involving anaerobes.

Susceptibility

Chloramphenicol and presumably florfenicol, the macrolides, metronidazole, clindamycin, and some second-generation (cefoxitin) and third-generation cephalosporins (ceftizoxime) are effective in the treatment of anaerobic infections (Jang and Hirsh, 1991a; Jang et al., 1997a). Penicillins (penicillin G, amoxicillin, ampicillin, and ticarcillin) are effective against most anaerobes except members of the *Bacteroides fragilis* group and occasionally other Gram-negative species, but when combined with clavulanic acid, which irreversibly binds the cephalosporinase produced by resistant strains, they are effective against all (Appelbaum et al., 1990).

Resistance to metronidazole and to clindamycin is uncommon; thus these are often drugs of choice for treating anaerobic infections (Jang and Hirsh, 1991a; Jang et al., 1997a). Clinically significant metronidazole resistance has been reported only for *Clostridium difficile*–associated diarrhea affecting horses (Jang et al., 1997b).

Clinical Application

Infectious processes involving normally sterile sites are usually a mixture of anaerobes and aerobes (facultative as well as obligate species) (Jang and Hirsh, 1991b; Jang and Hirsh, 1994; Jang et al., 1997a). Empiric treatment (usually the case since susceptibility test results of aerobic organisms are unavailable for at least 48 hours, and of anaerobic species, at least 5 days) of such conditions is relatively straightforward. Examples include an antibiotic effective against the aerobic component (eg, an aminoglycoside or a fluoroquinolone if retrospective data indicate that the most often encountered aerobe is susceptible to these particular drugs) and the anaerobic component (eg, a cell-wall–active antibiotic— which one is dictated by the amount of coverage desired; retrospective data from our institution show that approximately 80% of anaerobes are inhibited by penicillins and cephalosporins, but 100% are inhibited by a penicillin combined with clavulanic acid) (Jang and Hirsh, 1991a; Jang et al., 1997a). A combination of enrofloxacin and amoxicillin-clavulanic acid are commonly used to empirically treat such infectious processes.

Treatment of anaerobe-associated conditions involving sites that contain a microbial flora is more problematic. All such cases involve the intestinal tract: *Clostridium perfringens, C. difficile, Serpulina pilosicoli, S. hyodysenteriae*, and enterotoxigenic *Bacteroides fragilis*. Diarrhea associated with *C. perfringens* responds to treatment with ampicillin (amoxicillin), tylosin, or metronidazole (Twedt, 1993). Diarrhea associated with *C. difficile* responds to metronidazole or to vancomycin (horses may be affected with metronidazole resistant strains) (Jang et al., 1997b; Magdesian et al., 1997). Treatment of *S. pilosicoli* and enterotoxigenic *B. fragilis*–associated diarrhea is with metronidazole. Treatment of disease produced by *S. hyodysenteriae* is discussed in Chapter 25.

461

Bibliography

Appelbaum PC, et al. 1990. Beta-lactamase production and susceptibilities to amoxicillin, amoxicillin-clavulanate, ticarcillin, ticarcillin-clavulanate, cefoxitin, imipenem, and metronidazole of 320 non–*Bacteroides fragilis Bacteroides* isolates and 129 *Fusobacterium* from 28 U.S. centers. Antimicrob Agents Chemother 34:1546.

Bartlett JG. 1994. *Clostridium difficile:* History of its role as an enteric pathogen and the current state of knowledge about the organism. Clin Infect Dis 18:S265.

Goldstein EJC. 1996. Possible role for the new fluoroquinolones (levofloxacin, grepafloxacin, trovafloxacin, sparfloxacin, and DU-6859a) in the treatment of anaerobic infections: review of current information on efficacy and safety. Clin Infect Dis 23:S25.

Hirsh DC, et al. 1985. Changes in prevalence and susceptibility of obligate anaerobes in clinical veterinary practice. J Am Vet Med Assoc 186:1086.

Indiveri MC, Hirsh DC. 1992. Tissues and exudates contain sufficient thymidine for growth of anaerobic bacteria in the presence of inhibitory levels of trimethoprim-sulfamethoxazole. Vet Microbiol 32:235.

Jang SS, Hirsh DC. 1991a. Broth-disk elution determination of antimicrobial susceptibility of selected anaerobes isolated from animals. J Vet Diagn Invest 3:82.

Jang SS, Hirsh DC. 1991b. Identity of *Bacteroides* isolates and previously named *Bacteroides* spp. in clinical specimens of animal origin. Am J Vet Res 52:738.

Jang SS, Hirsh DC. 1994. Characterization, distribution, and microbiological associations of *Fusobacterium* spp. in clinical specimens of animal origin. J Clin Microbiol 32:384.

Jang SS, et al. 1997a. Organisms isolated from dogs and cats with anaerobic infections and susceptibility to selected antimicrobial agents. J Am Vet Med Assoc 210:1610.

Jang SS, et al. 1997b. Antimicrobial susceptibilities of equine isolates of *Clostridium difficile* and molecular characterization of metronidazole-resistant strains. Clin Infect Dis 25 (Suppl 2):S266.

Jones RL, et al. 1988. Hemorrhagic necrotizing enterocolitis associated with *Clostridium difficile* infection in four foals. J Am Vet Med Assoc 193:76.

Livermore DM. 1995. Beta-lactamases in laboratory and clinical resistance. Clin Microbiol Rev 8:557.

Madewell BR, et al. 1995. Apparent outbreak of *Clostridium difficile*–associated diarrhea in horses in a veterinary medical teaching hospital. J Vet Diagn Invest 7:343.

Magdesian KG, et al. 1997. *Clostridium difficile* and horses: a review. Rev Med Microbiol 8:S46.

Myers LL, et al. 1984. *Bacteroides fragilis:* a possible cause of acute diarrheal disease in newborn lambs. Infect Immun 44:241.

Prescott JF. 1979. Identification of some anaerobic bacteria in nonspecific anaerobic infections in animals. Can J Comp Med 43:194.

Samitz EM, et al. 1996. In vitro susceptibilities of selected obligate anaerobic bacteria obtained from bovine and equine sources to ceftiofur. J Vet Diagn Invest 8:121.

Sebald M. 1994. Genetic basis for antibiotic resistance in anaerobes. Clin Infect Dis 18:S297.

Stark CA, et al. 1993. Antimicrobial resistance in human oral and intestinal anaerobic microfloras. Antimicrob Agents Chemother 37:1665.

Struble AL, et al. 1994. Fecal shedding of *Clostridium difficile* in dogs: a period prevalence survey in a veterinary medical teaching hospital. J Vet Diagn Invest 6:342.

Ter Huurne AAHM, Gaastra W. 1995. Swine dysentery: more unknown than known. Vet Microbiol 46:347.

Trott DJ, et al. 1996. *Serpulina pilosicoli* sp. nov., the agent of porcine intestinal spirochetosis. Int J Syst Bacteriol 46:206.

Twedt DC. 1993. *Clostridium perfringens* associated diarrhea in dogs. Proc 11th Ann ACVIM Forum, p121.

Brucella

D. C. HIRSH

Brucellosis is the disease produced by members of the genus *Brucella*. The genus contains six species: *B. abortus, B. canis, B. melitensis, B. neotomae, B. ovis*, and *B. suis*. Treatment of brucellosis is usually restricted to affected companion animals—ie, dogs and horses—because this disease in food-producing livestock is usually controlled by various nationally administered eradication programs. Treatment strategies are expensive and typically involve long-term administration of antibiotics that may not be approved for use in food producing animals. Brucellae are facultative intracellular parasites that survive within the phagolysosome of phagocytic cells (macrophages). It is important that this fact be kept in mind when predicting in vivo efficacy based on the results of standard in vitro susceptibility tests. Therapy with two antimicrobials is indicated because of recurrence of disease otherwise after cessation of therapy (Solera et al., 1997). Experimental evidence and clinical experience treating human patients have shown that at least one of the antibiotics has intracellular distribution (Solera et al., 1997).

Resistance

Though very susceptible in vitro, relapses are common with monotherapy with the tetracyclines, rifampins, and trimethoprim-sulfonamides (Solera et al., 1997). Brucellae are also very susceptible in vitro to the fluoroquinolones, yet clinical data show that treatment of human patients with members of this class of drug (ciprofloxacin) is ineffectual (García-Rodriguez et al., 1991). Fluoroquinolones are less active at the pH (<5) of the phagolysosome (García-Rodriguez et al., 1991).

Susceptibility

The treatments that have been found to control brucellosis in human patients involve the use of two agents: doxycycline plus an aminoglycoside (gentamicin or netilmicin), which is a synergistic combination; or doxycycline plus rifampin (Richardson and Holt, 1962; Solera et al., 1997). For children (and probably younger animals), rifampin plus trimethoprim-sulfonamide or rifampin plus an aminoglycoside is a recommended alternative (Solera et al., 1997). Therapies showing promise (effective in rodent models of brucellosis) include the newer macrolides, clarithromycin, or azithromycin, and liposomal formulations containing an aminoglycoside (gentamicin) (Hernández-Caselles et al., 1989; Lang et al., 1994). In the latter case, high intracellular concentrations of this class of drug are attained.

Clinical Application

The most common presentation of brucellosis in horses is fistulous withers *(Brucella abortus)*, and in dogs, abortion, discospondylitis, arthritis, involvement of accessory sex organs and glands, and other manifestations of a septicemic process (Zicker, 1996; Carmichael and Greene, 1998). Though culture is the definitive diagnostic criteria, serology is usually used to make the diagnosis. Since brucellae have zoonotic potential, careful consideration should be given to the appropriateness of treatment. It is important to remove niduses of infection (uterus, testes, other areas that give rise to organisms in the blood). Recommended treatment regimes also include a tetracycline for 4 weeks and an aminoglycoside during weeks 1 and 4 (Carmichael and Greene, 1998). There are no current published recommendations for a tetracycline and rifampin for animal patients with brucellosis, but clinical data acquired from human experience indicate that tetracycline plus rifampin should be given together for at least a 4-week period.

Bibliography

Carmichael LE, Greene CE . 1998. Canine Brucellosis. In: Greene CE, ed. Infectious Diseases of the Dog and Cat, 2nd ed. Philadelphia: WB Saunders, p248.

García-Rodriguez JA, et al. 1991. Lack of effective bactericidal activity of new quinolones against *Brucella* spp. Antimicrob Agents Chemother 35:756.

Hernández-Caselles T, et al. 1989. Treatment of *Brucella melitensis* infection in mice by use of liposome-encapsulated gentamicin. Am J Vet Res 50:1486.

Lang R, et al. 1994. Therapeutic effects of roxithromycin and azithromycin in experimental murine brucellosis. Chemother 40:252.

Richardson M, Holt JN. 1962. Synergistic action of streptomycin with other antibiotics on intracellular *Brucella abortus* in vitro. J Bacteriol 84:638.

Solera J, et al. 1997. Recognition and optimum treatment of brucellosis. Drugs 53:245.

Zicker SC. 1996. Fistulous withers. In: Smith BP, ed. Large Animal Internal Medicine. St. Louis: Mosby-Year Book, p1320.

Atypical Mycobacteria

D. C. HIRSH

For convenience, members of the genus *Mycobacterium* are categorized into those that produce tuberculosis *(M. tuberculosis, M. bovis)*, leprosy *(M. leprae)*, and the atypical mycobacteria. The atypical mycobacteria are those species that are so-called slow growers (taking weeks to months to form visible colonies in vitro: eg, *M. avium* complex; *M. genavense; M. gordonae; M. kansasii; M. marinum; M. simiae; M. szulgai; M. ulcerans; M. xenopi)* and those that are called rapid growers (taking days to weeks to form visible colonies in vitro: eg, *M. chelonae; M. fortuitum; M. phlei;*

M. smegmatis; M. vaccae) (Wolinsky, 1979). The distinction between rapid growers and slow growers is sometimes important when trying to formulate a treatment strategy, since there are differences in susceptibility between members of these two groups (García-Rodriguez and García, 1993).

Members of the *M. avium* complex are the main atypical mycobacteria affecting human patients with acquired immunodeficiency syndrome (AIDS), in birds (second to *M. genavense* in pet birds), swine, and rarely in horses and sheep (Grange et al., 1990; Hoop et al., 1996). Dogs and cats are highly resistant to disease caused by members of the *M. avium* complex (though disseminated disease has been described in previously normal cats), being affected most often by other atypical strains, such as *M. chelonae, M. fortuitum, M. lepraemurium* (cats), *M. phlei, M. smegmatis,* and *M. xenopi* (Tomasovic et al., 1976; Dewevre et al., 1977; McIntosh, 1982; Wilkinson et al., 1982; White et al., 1983; Grange et al., 1990; Studdert and Hughes, 1992; Jordan et al., 1994). Almost all of the atypical mycobacteria are environmental dwellers, and as such the environment is the major source of infection, rather than an infected patient (Heifets, 1996). However, since some form of immunosuppression is usually (but not always) a prerequisite for disease, the infected patient may be an added "environmental" source of atypical mycobacteria for the immunosuppressed individual.

Numerous trials involving human patients have demonstrated that monotherapy leads to the development of resistance to the drug being used (Heifets, 1996; Alangaden and Lerner, 1997). Consequently, most regimens recommended for the treatment of atypical mycobacteriosis involve the use of at least two antibiotics. In addition, mycobacteria are facultative intracellular parasites, able to survive within the phagolysosome. Thus, it is important when choosing an antibiotic that attention be paid to its intracellular distribution.

Resistance

Mycobacteria are naturally resistant to all of the antibiotics that affect the cell wall (penicillins and cephalosporins), probably because of the nature of the mycobacterial cell wall, which is high in lipid. Resistance rapidly occurs subsequent to use of a single antimicrobial to which the bacterium was originally susceptible. Though mycobacteria contain numerous plasmids, genes encoding resistance have not been found on them (Grange et al., 1990). Thus, resistance results from mutations in the gene encoding the target of the antibiotic. However, sulfonamide resistance has been found on a transposable element in an isolate of *M. fortuitum,* the only example of this type of occurrence (Zhang and Young, 1994).

Susceptibility

There are no firm rules for treating infectious processes that involve atypical mycobacteria. The following recommendations have been taken in part from recommendations for treating human patients and from the few successful attempts at treating nonhuman animals. In general, the antibiotics used to treat typical mycobacterial infections (caused by *M. bovis* or *M. tuberculosis*) are ineffective for infectious processes involving atypical mycobacteria (Davis et al., 1987). Most strains of atypical mycobacteria are susceptible to clarithromycin (and azithromycin). Drugs that have shown effectiveness as added partners to clarithromycin include clofazimine; fluoroquinolones (members of the *M. avium* complex are unpredictable; most human isolates are susceptible; most animal isolates are resistant; *M. chelonae* is resistant); ethambutol (*M. fortuitum* is resistant); rifampin (*M. fortuitum* is resistant); amikacin (most predictably active against rapid growers) (Byrne et al., 1990; Khardori et al., 1994; Kaufman et al., 1995; Heifets, 1996; Yajko et al., 1996; Alangaden and Lerner, 1997; Watt, 1997).

Clinical Application

The first clues that an atypical mycobacterium may be involved is the presence of chronically occurring lesions that include draining tracts, lack of response to a variety of antimicrobial agents, and the lack of growth on media after 24–48 hours of incubation. In addition to historical clues, if portions of the affected area are stained with either a Romanowsky-type stain (Giemsa; Wright's) or with Gram's, atypical mycobacterial cells have characteristic properties. In the former, the bacterial cells may appear as "ghosts," and in the latter, they may appear as rods with "speckles." Such clues should prompt the use of the acid-fast stain, as well as the inoculation of appropriate media to be incubated for a suitable length of time. If an acid-fast bacterium is present, then appropriate antibiotic therapy should be started. A combination of clarithromycin and a fluoroquinolone (and/or rifampin and/or ethambutol and/or clofazimine) is a possible starting regimen. If an isolate is obtained, it should be sent to an appropriate reference laboratory for susceptibility testing (in the United States such a location is the National Jewish Hospital and Research Center, 3800 East Colfax Avenue, Denver CO 80206, USA).

Bibliography

Alangaden GJ, Lerner SA. 1997. The clinical use of fluoroquinolones for the treatment of mycobacterial diseases. Clin Infect Dis 25:1213.

Byrne SK, et al. 1990. Comparison of in vitro antimicrobial susceptibilities of *Mycobacterium avium–M. intracellulare* strains from patients with acquired immunodeficiency syndrome (AIDS), patients without AIDS, and animal sources. Antimicrob Agents Chemother 34:1390.

Davis CE, et al. 1987. In vitro susceptibility of *Mycobacterium avium* complex to antibacterial agents. Diagn Microbiol Infect Dis 8:149.

Dewevre PJ, et al. 1977. *Mycobacterium fortuitum* infection in a cat. J Am Anim Hosp Assoc 13:68.

García-Rodriguez JA, García ACG. 1993. In-vitro activities of quinolones against mycobacteria. J Antimicrob Chemother 32:797.

Grange JM, et al. 1990. The avian tubercle bacillus and its relatives. J Appl Bacteriol 68:411.

Heifets L. 1996. Susceptibility testing of *Mycobacterium avium* complex isolates. Antimicrob Agents Chemother 40:1759.

Hoop RK, et al. 1996. Etiological agents of mycobacteriosis in pet birds between 1986 and 1995. J Clin Microbiol 34:991.

Jordan HL, et al. 1994. Disseminated *Mycobacterium avium* complex infection in three Siamese cats. J Am Vet Med Assoc 204:90.

Kaufman AC, et al. 1995. Treatment of localized *Mycobacterium avium* complex infection with clofazimine and doxycycline in a cat. J Am Vet Med Assoc 207:457.

Khardori N, et al. 1994. In vitro susceptibilities of rapidly growing mycobacteria to newer antimicrobial agents. Antimicrob Agents Chemother 38:134.

McIntosh DW. 1982. Feline leprosy: a review of forty-four cases from Western Canada. Can Vet J 23:291.

Studdert V, Hughes KL. 1992. Treatment of opportunistic mycobacterial infections with enrofloxacin in cats. J Am Vet Med Assoc 201:1388.

Tomasovic AA, et al. 1976. *Mycobacterium xenopi* in a skin lesion of a cat. Aust Vet J 52:103.

Watt B. 1997. In vitro sensitivities and treatment of less common mycobacteria. J Antimicrob Chemother 39:567.

White SD, et al. 1983. Cutaneous atypical mycobacteriosis in cats. J Am Vet Med Assoc 182:1218.

Wilkinson GT, et al. 1982. Pyogranulomatous panniculitis in cats due to *Mycobacterium smegmatis*. Aust Vet J 58:77.

Wolinsky E. 1979. Nontuberculous mycobacteria and associated diseases. Am Rev Respir Dis 119:107.

Yajko DM, et al. 1996. In vitro activities of rifabutin, azithromycin, ciprofloxacin, clarithromycin, clofazimine, ethambutol, and amikacin in combination of two, three, and four drugs against *Mycobacterium avium*. Antimicrob Agents Chemother 40:743.

Zhang Y, Young D. 1994. Molecular genetics of drug resistance in *Mycobacterium tuberculosis*. J Antimicrob Chemother 34:313.

Mycoplasmas

D. C. HIRSH

The term *Mycoplasma* is used to denote a member of the order Mycoplasmatales and class Mollicutes. Six genera are recognized: *Acholeplasma, Anaeroplasma, Asteroplasma, Mycoplasma, Spiroplasma,* and *Ureaplasma;* members of the genera *Mycoplasma* and *Ureaplasma* are important in veterinary medicine. Mycoplasmas are associated with the respiratory tract, arthritis, mastitis, septicemia, and the urogenital tract of many animal species.

Resistance

Because of their inability to synthesize a cell wall, all mycoplasmas are resistant to all cell-wall–active antibiotics (eg, penicillins, cephalosporins, glycopeptides). In addition, mycoplasmas are resistant to rifampin. Some strains of *M. hominis* are resistant to the tetracyclines because of the acquisition of the *tet*(M) gene, a gene found also in some members of the genus *Streptococcus*, suggesting transfer between these two genera or from a common ancestor (Roberts et al., 1985). Acquisition of tetracycline resistance by this mechanism may explain in part why susceptibility of some bovine isolates of mycoplasma (*M. bovis, M. dispar, U. diversum*) is unpredictable with respect to susceptibility to chlortetracycline and oxytetracycline (Ter Laak et al., 1993). In Denmark, the progressive development of resistance to tylosin over two decades by *M. hyopneumoniae* was linked to the extensive use of this drug in swine during this period (Aarestrup and Friis, 1998).

Susceptibility

It is difficult to easily ascertain susceptibility since in vitro testing of isolates is extremely difficult and is usually not performed except by specialized laboratories. In general, however, the macrolides (in particular erythromycin, clarithromycin, azithromycin, tylosin, and tiamulin) and the fluoroquinolones appear to be the most active (Kenny et al., 1989; Arai et al., 1992; Ter Laak et al., 1993; Kobayashi et al., 1996; Musser et al., 1996; Hannan et al., 1997). Mycoplasmas are also usually susceptible in vitro to aminoglycosides, chloramphenicol, lincosamides, and tetracyclines. In poultry, injection of eggs with aminoglycosides is effective in eliminating mycoplasmas (McCapes et al., 1975). Ketolides are highly active against mycoplasmas. With the possible exception of the fluoroquinolones, mycoplasma-active antibiotics have a bacteriostatic activity and may be another factor that makes mycoplasma infections often only slowly responsive to treatment.

Clinical Application

Mycoplasmas are often both hard to isolate and slow growing. As a consequence, treatment of mycoplasma infections is, more often than not, empirical rather than based on in vitro–determined antibiotic susceptibility. Elimination from tissues is, however, often slow, since most antibiotics have only a bacteriostatic effect against mycoplasmas. In addition, there is increasing evidence that some mycoplasmas may become intracellular (Taylor-Robinson and Bebear, 1997). For both these reasons, despite excellent susceptibility in vitro, treatment of established mycoplasma infections in animals has sometimes been disappointing (Jasper, 1982; Ross and Cox, 1988), perhaps because effective treatment may require a 2-to-3-week course rather than a shorter course. There is a paucity of data on the clinical efficacy of treatment of many mycoplasma infections in animals, which contrasts with the proven efficacy in human medicine of tetracycline or macrolide treatment of mycoplasma pneumonia (Taylor-Robinson and Bebear, 1997). The guiding general principle required for effective treatment of a mycoplasma infection is therefore to choose an antibiotic (fluoroquinolone, lincosamide, macrolide, tetracycline) that penetrates cells well and to administer the drug for 2–3 weeks, with isolation and in vitro susceptibility testing in cases of failure of clinical response.

Bibliography

Aarestrup FM, Friis NF. 1998. Antimicrobial susceptibility testing of *Mycoplasma hyosynoviae* isolated from pigs during 1968 to 1971 and during 1995 and 1996. Vet Microbiol 61:33.

Arai S, et al. 1992. Antimycoplasmal activities of new quinolones, tetracyclines, and macrolides against *Mycoplasma pneumoniae*. Antimicrob Agents Chemother 36:1322.

Ball HJ, et al. 1995. Antibiotic susceptibility of *Mycoplasma bovis* strains isolated in Northern Ireland. Irish Vet J 48:316.

Hannan PCT, et al. 1997. Comparative susceptibilities of various animal-pathogenic mycoplasmas to fluoroquinolones. Antimicrob Agents Chemother 41:2037.

Jasper DE. 1982. The role of *Mycoplasma* in bovine mastitis. J Am Vet Med Assoc 181:158.

Kenny GE, et al. 1989. Susceptibilities of genital mycoplasmas to the newer quinolones as determined by the agar dilution method. Antimicrob Agents Chemother 33:103.

Kobayashi H, et al. 1996. Macrolide susceptibility of *Mycoplasma hyorhinis* isolated from piglets. Antimicrob Agents Chemother 40:1030.

McCapes RH, et al. 1975. Injecting antibiotics into turkey hatching eggs to eliminate *Mycoplasma meleagridis* infection. Avian Dis 19:506.

Musser J, et al. 1996. Comparison of tilmicosin with long-acting oxytetracycline for treatment of respiratory tract disease in calves. J Am Vet Med Assoc 208:102.

Roberts MC, et al. 1985. Tetracycline-resistant *Mycoplasma hominis* contain streptococcal *tetM* sequences. Antimicrob Agents Chemother 28:141.

Ross RF, Cox DF. 1988. Evaluation of tiamulin for treatment of mycoplasmal pneumonia in swine. J Am Vet Med Assoc 193:441.

Taylor-Robinson D, Bebear C. 1997. Antibiotic susceptibilities of mycoplasmas and treatment of mycoplasmal infections. J Antimicrob Chemother 40:622.

Ter Laak EA, et al. 1993. Susceptibilities of *Mycoplasma bovis, Mycoplasma dispar,* and *Ureaplasma diversum* strains to antimicrobial agents in vitro. Antimicrob Agents Chemother 37:317.

Nocardia

D. C. HIRSH

Nocardiosis has been reported to occur in a variety of animal species, but of the domesticated variety, cattle, horses, dogs, and cats are most commonly affected (Beaman and Beaman, 1994). *Nocardia asteroides* is reported to be the species found most frequently from affected domestic animals. This species is heterogeneous, being composed of *N. asteroides* sensu stricto, *N. farcinica,* and *N. nova* (Yano et al., 1990; Wallace et al., 1991). The distinguishing characteristics used to differentiate among these three species are the types of cell wall mycolic acids and the susceptibility to antimicrobial agents. In our experience, N. *nova* is the species most often isolated from dogs and cats (localized lesions most often associated with an extremity), while N. *asteroides* sensu stricto is most often isolated from cattle (mastitis) and horses (Arabian foals; horses with Cushing's disease secondary to pituitary adenomas) (Bushnell et al., 1979; Biberstein et al., 1985).

Resistance and Susceptibility

Though N. *asteroides* sensu stricto and N. *nova* remain susceptible to the sulfonamides (trimethoprim-sulfas are most commonly used), long-term treatment with this class of antimicrobial is sometimes associated with undesirable side effects (Werner and Bright, 1983) (see Chapter 14). Alternative treatment includes the tetracyclines (minocycline, doxycycline), some cephalosporins, and imipenem (Table 19.11). However, if the use of other antibiotics is contemplated, then it may make a great deal of difference whether an animal is affected with N. *asteroides* sensu stricto (often resistant to the macrolides and to the penicillins), or N. *nova* (often susceptible to the macrolides and sometimes to the penicillins) (Lerner, 1996).

Clinical Application

The diagnosis of nocardiosis can be made by observation of moderately acid-fast branching filaments in a sample collected from the affected site, or by culture. Trimethoprim-sulfa drugs are the antimicrobial of choice, though other choices may be available, depending upon animal species (see above and Table 19.11).

TABLE 19.11. **Comparison of the susceptibilities of *Nocardia asteroides* sensu stricto and *N. nova***

Antimicrobial Drug	*Nocardia asteroides* sensu stricto (% susceptible)	*Nocardia nova* (% susceptible)
Ampicillin	27	44
Amoxicillin-clavulanate	67	6
Cefuroxime, cefotaxime, ceftriaxone	94–98	Cefuroxime, 100; other third generation, 83–94
Ciprofloxacin	38	0
Dapsone	92	94
Doxycycline	88	94
Minocycline	94	100
Amikacin	90–95	100
Erythromycin	60	100
Clarithromycin	—	100
Trimethoprim-sulfa	100	89
Imipenem	77	100
Tobramycin	—	33

Source: Data abstracted from Lerner (1996); clarithromycin data unpubl.

Bibliography

Beaman BL, Beaman L. 1994. *Nocardia* species: Host parasite relationships. Clin Microbiol Rev 7:213.

Biberstein EL, et al. 1985. *Nocardia asteroides* infection in horses: a review. J Am Vet Med Assoc 186:273.

Bushnell RB, et al. 1979. Clinical and diagnostic aspects of herd problems with nocardial and mycobacterial mastitis. Proc Am Assoc Lab Diagn 22:1.

Lerner PI. 1996. Nocardiosis. Clin Infect Dis 22:891.

Wallace RJ, et al. 1991. Clinical and laboratory features of *Nocardia nova*. J Clin Microbiol 29:2407.

Werner LL, JM Bright. 1983. Drug-induced hypersensitivity disorders in two dogs treated with trimethoprim sulfadiazine. J Am Anim Hosp Assoc 19:783.

Yano I, et al. 1990. Characterization of *Nocardia nova*. Int J Syst Bacteriol 40:170.

Leptospira

J. F. PRESCOTT

MIC determinations show leptospires to be susceptible to a wide variety of antimicrobial drugs. They are highly susceptible in vitro to penicillin G, ampicillin, amoxicillin, cefotaxime, erythromycin, and fluoroquinolones; susceptibility to streptomycin, tylosin, tiamulin, and tetracyclines is good; and they are relatively resistant to cephalothin, chloramphenicol, and sulfonamides. Penicillin G has weak bactericidal activity. Acquired resistance has not been reported. Experimental infections with laboratory animals have established the value of penicillin G, erythromycin, streptomycin, and tetracyclines in treatment of leptospirosis. Cephalexin, cefadroxil, and cefoperazone had little activity, although cefotaxime was effective. First- and second-generation cephalosporins should not be used for treatment. Treatment of human patients has established the value of penicillin G and doxycycline therapy in leptospirosis. In acute leptospirosis, recommended treatments in animals include ampicillin or amoxicillin, penicillin G, streptomycin, doxycycline or other tetracyclines, and erythromycin. Amoxicillin is the drug of choice. Treatment should probably last 7 days. One advantage of streptomycin, which can be combined with amoxicillin treatment, is that the persistence of this antibiotic in the kidney after even a single injection assists in the removal of the kidney carrier state. Chronic leptospirosis is characterized by abortion and stillbirth, recurrent iridocyclitis, repeat breeding in pigs and possibly cattle, and subclinical meningeal infection, depending on the serovar involved and the animal species affected. Many studies of *Leptospira pomona* infection in swine and cattle have established the value of a single IM injection of 25 mg/kg of dihydrostreptomycin or streptomycin in removing the kidney carrier state. It did not, however, remove *Lep-*

tospira borgpetersenii serovar *hardjo* from the genital tract and kidney of bovine carriers in one study (Ellis et al., 1985). Oral treatment of swine with tetracyclines (800 g/ton for 8–11 days) will control leptospirosis but cannot be relied on to remove renal carriage, possibly because of their bacteriostatic action. In outbreaks of leptospiral abortion in cattle, the usual recommendation is to vaccinate after treating once with streptomycin. Since streptomycin is now prohibited in some countries for use in food animals, attempts have been made to find alternatives. Injection of 1 or 2 doses (q48 hours) of 15 mg/kg of amoxicillin was found to remove the kidney carrier state of serovar *hardjo* in cattle (Smith et al., 1997). Tylosin (44 mg/kg 5 days), erythromycin (25 mg/kg 5 days), and tetracycline (40 mg/kg for 3 or 5 days) all given IM q24 hours effectively removed kidney carriage of serovar *pomona* in swine; ceftiofur or ampicillin at standard dosage for 3–5 days was not effective (Alt and Bolin, 1996). The effective drugs listed above can all be recommended during outbreaks of abortion. Further studies are needed to determine whether and which antimicrobial treatments are effective in therapy of periodic ophthalmia of horses.

Bibliography

Alt DP, Bolin CA. 1996. Preliminary evaluation of antimicrobial agents for treatment of *Leptospira interrogans* serovar *pomona* infection in hamsters and swine. Am J Vet Res 57:59.

Ellis WA, et al. 1985. Dihydrostreptomycin treatment of bovine carriers of *Leptospira interrogans* serovar *hardjo*. Res Vet Sci 39:292.

Prescott JF. 1991. Treatment of leptospirosis. Cornell Vet 81:7.

Smith CR, et al. 1997. Amoxycillin as an alternative to dihydrostreptomycin sulphate for treating cattle infected with *Leptospira borgpetersenii* serovar *hardjo*. Aust Vet J 75:818.

INFECTIONS ASSOCIATED WITH NEUTROPENIA IN THE DOG AND CAT

A. C. G. ABRAMS-OGG AND S. A. KRUTH

Neutropenic animals are at increased risk of developing bacterial and fungal infections, and established infections in neutropenic patients are more difficult to eradicate with appropriate antimicrobial therapy. Such infections may be due either to organisms that are normally considered to be pathogenic or to opportunistic pathogens, organisms that rarely cause disease in animals with normal defense mechanisms. This section on the management of infection in the neutropenic dog and cat focuses on neutropenia resulting principally from impaired granulopoiesis and the attendant risk of opportunistic bacterial and fungal infection. Considerable attention has been given recently to the use of granulocyte colony-stimulating factor to increase neutrophil production, but antimicrobial therapy remains the cornerstone of managing neutropenia. A number of factors influence the risk and outcome of infection during neutropenia, but in most cases prompt therapy with familiar antibiotics will result in successful patient outcome. In cases of prolonged severe neutropenia, patient management strategies must be extrapolated from the therapy of human neutropenic patients.

Causes of Neutropenia

Neutropenia may occur as a primary or secondary disorder, as an isolated hematologic abnormality, or as a feature of pancytopenia (Hawkins, 1990; Weiss, 1995). Cyclic hematopoiesis of Gray Collies is a well-characterized primary disorder, though unlikely to be encountered in clinical practice. Idiopathic neutropenia is occasionally seen in both dogs and cats. In some cases this is probably a result of immune-mediated mechanisms. Neutropenia may also occur secondary to infectious diseases. Canine parvovirus-2 (CPV-2) and *Ehrlichia canis* are the principal infectious causes of neutropenia in the dog. Feline panleukopenia virus (FPL), feline leukemia virus (FeLV), and feline immunodeficiency virus (FIV) are the principal infectious causes of neutropenia in the cat.

Neutropenia may result from primary bone marrow neoplasia or from bone marrow involvement in metastatic disease. In either case there is likely to be concurrent anemia and thrombocytopenia. Cytotoxic chemotherapy and radiation therapy for neoplastic and immune-mediated diseases predictably cause myelosuppression. The degree of resulting neutropenia varies with the agent and the dose administered. Other drugs with a known risk for causing neutropenia include estrogen and phenylbutazone in dogs and chloramphenicol, griseofulvin, propylthiouracil, and methimazole in cats. Theoretically, any drug may be associated with an idiosyncratic reaction resulting in neutropenia. Such reactions have been described with cephalosporins (dogs and cats), sulfonamides (dogs), angiotensin-converting enzyme inhibitors (dogs), and, most recently, phenobarbital in dogs (Jacobs et al., 1998).

Overwhelming bacterial infection may cause neutropenia in animals with normal granulopoiesis, by exhausting marrow granulocyte reserve. Neutrophil consumption exacerbates neutropenia in animals with impaired granulopoiesis.

Infectious Complications of Neutropenia
RISK FACTORS

Factors important in determining the probability of acquiring infection during neutropenia, and the severity and outcome of an established infection, include the severity and duration of neutropenia, disruption of natural barriers, defects in specific defenses, organisms involved, site of infection, type of tumor and its biological stage, and host species (Feld, 1989; Wade, 1994). The risk of infection is directly related to the degree of neutropenia. The risk of opportunistic infection occurs when the neutrophil count falls below $2.0 \times 10^9/1$ (mild neutropenia). Below $1.0 \times 10^9/1$ (moderate neutropenia) the risk increases. Animals with neutrophil counts below $0.5 \times 10^9/1$ (severe neutropenia) have a high risk of infection; below $0.2 \times 10^9/1$ the risk of infection is very high. Below $0.2 \times 10^9/1$ there is still a relationship between worsening myelosuppression and adverse clinical consequences, but this is not reflected in the peripheral blood, since any neutrophils released from the bone marrow immediately migrate into tissues. For a given degree of neutropenia, a higher risk of infection is associated with a falling, rather than a stable, neutrophil count. These figures are based upon a classic study of humans with leukemia (Bodey et al., 1966). No such studies have been conducted with dogs or cats, but based upon experimental studies with total body irradiation and clinical experience with veterinary cancer patients, these figures appear to be applicable to the dog and the cat (Couto, 1990; Abrams-Ogg et al., 1993).

The duration of neutropenia is also important. Humans with neutropenia of short duration (<7 days) are unlikely to have severe infections that cannot be controlled with appropriate antimicrobial therapy. Infections accompanying neutropenia of moderate duration (7–14 days) are more difficult to manage. Infections in patients with prolonged neutropenia (>14 days) are even more difficult to manage, especially if the neutrophil count is less than $0.2 \times 10^9/1$ (Feld, 1989). This difficulty is because antimicrobial agents act in concert with host defenses in eradicating infections.

Disruption of natural physical barriers and suppression of humoral and cell-mediated immunity increase the risk of infection during neutropenia. Natural barriers are disrupted, for example, with gastrointestinal damage during parvoviral infections and with anticancer chemotherapy, facilitating invasion by enteric bacteria. IV catheterization and percutaneous biopsy procedures increase the risk of infection with cutaneous organisms. Immunosuppression may accompany myelosuppression, because of the primary disease, anticancer therapy, and malnutrition. The risk of infection in neutropenic humans is greater if there is concurrent lymphopenia and monocytopenia. The type of tumor and its stage appear to be important factors in humans and animals with malignancies (Hirsh, 1986). Infections are more likely to be severe with (1) acute rather than chronic hematologic malignancies; (2) hematologic malignancies in relapse relative to those in remission; and (3) patients with hematologic malignancies relative to those with solid tumors.

The site of infection is important in determining outcome. Bacteremia and pneumonia are more difficult to treat than soft tissue, gastrointestinal, or urinary tract infections. The severity of infection is also affected by the type of organism. Infections with Gram-positive organisms tend to be more easily managed than infections with Gram-negative organisms. Finally, host species is probably important. Neutropenic cats appear to be less susceptible than dogs to opportunistic infections during neutropenia.

MICROBIOLOGY

Infections in neutropenic animals may occur with exogenous or endogenous organisms. Exogenous organisms are acquired from the environment. Nosocomial organisms are an important source of exogenous infections in human hospitals (Wade, 1994) and probably represent a risk to neutropenic animals in veterinary hospitals. Endogenous infections occur with organisms from the host's own flora. The most important source is the intestinal tract. Other sources of endogenous infections include the oral cavity, skin, upper respiratory tract, and lower urogenital tract. Exogenous and endogenous pathogens do not represent two entirely distinct groups of organisms, and the same organism may act as both an endogenous and exogenous pathogen for different individual animals.

The majority of data characterizing infection in neutropenic small animals has been reported for myelosuppression secondary to cytotoxic therapy in the dog. The most frequently reported sites of infection are the bloodstream (bacteremia) and the lung. Local cellulitis may occur, manifested as edema of one or more limbs. Other possible sites of infection include the oral cavity, gastrointestinal tract, genitourinary tract, heart, and central nervous system.

Bacteremia is most often of intestinal origin and corresponds to the pattern of bacterial translocation in healthy dogs (Dahlinger et al., 1997). Members of the Enterobacteriaceae, especially *E. coli* and *Klebsiella* spp., are commonly isolated (Couto, 1990). *Pseudomonas* spp. are less frequently isolated but have historically been associated with the most severe infections, because a number of the antibiotics effective against this organism have only recently become available. Although the majority of bacteria in the intestinal tract are obligate anaerobes, they are not commonly the first invaders in opportunistic infection during neutropenia. Gram-positive bacteremia, usually with *Staphylococcus* spp. and *Streptococcus* spp., is less common than Gram-negative bacteremia but more common than anaerobic bacteremia. Gram-positive bacteremia can arise from the skin, the intestinal tract, or the oral cavity. Urinary tract infections are a possible source of bacteremia (Barsanti and Finco, 1986).

Pneumonia occurs as an opportunistic infection with upper respiratory flora or from translocation of intestinal bacteria. The same organisms

475

are implicated as in bacteremia. Neutropenic dogs should probably also be considered at risk for *Bordetella bronchiseptica* pneumonia. Cats are likely at risk for pneumonia with *B. bronchiseptica* and *Pasteurella multocida*.

Fewer data are available characterizing opportunistic infection during neutropenia due to causes other than cytotoxic therapy. With respect to parvoviral infections, Gram-negative organisms are the principal cause of sepsis. Bacteremia and pneumonia may occur. *Klebsiella oxytoca* and *Enterobacter cloacae* were isolated on blood culture from a severely neutropenic puppy with CPV-2 infection (Kreeger et al., 1984). *Escherichia coli* was isolated from postmortem tissues of 88 of 98 dogs with CPV-2 infection (Turk et al., 1990). *Escherichia coli* is also the most common isolate from postmortem tissues of cats dying from FPL (Scott, 1987); in one study of experimental FPL virus infection, 10 of 30 blood cultures were positive (Hammon and Enders, 1939). Isolates included *Pasteurella* spp., Gram-negative bacilli, *Streptococcus* spp., and *Staphylococcus* spp. *Bacillus* sp. was isolated in one culture, along with a staphylococcus. It is widely assumed, but not proven, that anaerobic bacteria contribute to bacteremia during parvoviral infections. It has been documented that *Clostridium perfringens* proliferates in the intestinal tract of dogs with CPV-2 infection (Turk et al., 1992), but the role of the organism in sepsis is not known.

Local and systemic infections with *Candida* spp. and *Aspergillus* spp. are an important cause of disease in neutropenic humans (Wade, 1994). Risk factors for fungal infections are the same as those for bacterial infections. In addition, the risk of fungal infection increases with the duration of antibacterial therapy. Invasive fungal infections are not as common in neutropenic dogs and cats. This may be due in part to the use of less aggressive cytotoxic therapy for cancer. However, the risk for fungal infection is comparatively low even in experimental dogs with prolonged, severe neutropenia. Systemic candidiasis has been reported in a pup with CPV-2 infection (Rodriguez et al., 1998). Pneumonia due to *Aspergillus* spp. has been reported in a dog following autologous bone marrow transplantation for treatment of lymphoma (Rosenthal, 1988) and in a cat with FPL infection (Holzworth, 1987). Intestinal candidiasis associated with intensive antibiotic therapy occurred in 3 of 6 dogs with severe neutropenia induced by cytotoxic therapy (Abrams-Ogg et al., 1993). Intestinal candidiasis has also been reported as a complication of CPV-2 infection (Anderson and Pidgeon, 1987), and intestinal candidiasis and aspergillosis have been reported as complications of FPL infection (Holzworth, 1987).

PATIENT MANAGEMENT

The majority of neutropenia that is managed in small animal medicine is of short duration (<7 days) and/or of mild to moderate severity. Animals with prolonged neutropenia usually have only mildly depressed counts. This reflects a tendency on the part of veterinarians to reduce or discontinue cytotoxic therapy when neutropenia develops and to euthanize animals with severe pancytopenia that have a poor prognosis for prompt recovery. As veterinarians continue to employ more-aggressive cytotoxic protocols and to manage dogs and cats with complex hematologic problems, the management of severe and prolonged neutropenia may be more frequently required.

The risk of acquiring an exogenous infection is reduced by isolation. Neutropenic animals that do not require critical supportive care should be maintained at home. Cats should be kept indoors and dogs confined to the house and yard. In the hospital, contact with the general hospital population should be avoided. Hands should be thoroughly washed and laboratory coats changed before handling a neutropenic animal, and barrier nursing procedures, such as wearing gloves, gowns, and isolation boots, should be considered for severe cases. The thermometer used for the neutropenic animal should not be used for other patients. Human patients with severe neutropenia are provided with a "low microbial diet" (Wade, 1994). The role of dietary pathogens has not been evaluated in neutropenic pet animals, but it is reasonable to recommend that only canned foods be offered and table scraps avoided in dogs and cats with severe neutropenia.

Antimicrobial therapy for neutropenic animals may be divided into three categories: (1) prophylactic therapy; (2) empirical treatment during febrile episodes; and (3) treatment of documented infection. Optimal protocols have not been defined for the management of infections in human neutropenic patients and much less so for veterinary patients.

PROPHYLAXIS

Prophylactic therapy is directed at the intestinal flora. The principal objective is "selective intestinal decontamination" (Van der Waaij, 1988). This refers to reduction of the aerobic Gram-negative organisms most often responsible for infections. The anaerobic population is left relatively undisturbed, since it contributes to resistance to fungal overgrowth and colonization by exogenous organisms. A second objective of prophylactic therapy is to provide sufficient blood and tissue antimicrobial concentrations to contain an incipient bacterial infection.

Choices for prophylactic therapy are presented in Table 19.12. Neomycin and polymyxin B were first used but have been replaced by sulfonamides and fluoroquinolone antibiotics (Vriesendorp et al., 1981; Klastersky, 1989). Prophylactic therapy for human neutropenic patients has been reviewed (Wade, 1994; Donnelly, 1997). Its use is controversial. The benefits are not clear, both with respect to reducing infection rates and with respect to reducing mortality rates. In general, prophylactic therapy

TABLE 19.12. **Prophylactic oral antimicrobial therapy for the neutropenic dog and cat**

Antimicrobial	Doses	Comment
Sulfonamides		
Trimethoprim-sulfamethoxazole	**15 mg/kg (combined dose) q12 hours**	Inexpensive
	30 mg/kg (combined dose) q12–24 hours	No prophylaxis against *Pseudomonas* spp. Risk for keratoconjunctivitis sicca with prolonged use May retard marrow recovery following severe myelosuppression
Trimethoprim-sulfadiazine	15 mg/kg (combined dose) q12 hours	As for trimethoprim-sulfamethoxazole but more expensive
Ormetoprim-sulfadimethoxine	30 mg/kg (combined dose) q12–24 hours 55 mg/kg on first day, then 27.5 mg/kg q24 hours	As for trimethoprim-sulfamethoxazole but more expensive
Fluoroquinolones		
Enrofloxacin	**5–15 mg/kg q12 hours**	Expensive
	10–20 mg/kg q24 hours	Lower dose effective for selective intestinal decontamination >10 mg/kg needed to achieve tissue levels effective against *Pseudomonas* spp.
Ciprofloxacin	**5–15 mg/kg q12 hours**	As for enrofloxacin
	10–30 mg/kg q24 hours	Tablet strength restricts use to dogs
Orbifloxacin	5 mg/kg q12–24 hours	Expensive Less well evaluated than enrofloxacin or ciprofloxacin
Marbofloxacin	2–4 mg/kg q12–24 hours	As for orbifloxacin
Difloxacin	5–10 mg/kg q24 hours	As for orbifloxacin; approved for use in dogs only
β-lactam antibiotics		
Cephalexin	**30 mg/kg q12 hours**	Expensive No prophylaxis against *Pseudomonas* spp.
Amoxicillin	10–20 mg/kg q12 hours	Inexpensive No prophylaxis against *Pseudomonas* spp. Not first choice, used mostly in cats not tolerating other choices Ampicillin causes more intestinal disturbance than amoxicillin
Amoxicillin-clavulanate	12.5–25 mg/kg q12 hours	As for amoxicillin; increased activity against *Staphylococcus* spp., *Klebsiella* spp., *Escherichia coli*, and *Bacteroides* spp. relative to amoxicillin activity
Combinations		
Fluroquinolone + β-lactam	As given for individual agents above	Reserved for animals with severe neutropenia

Sources: Doses adapted from Allen (1998), and Greene (1998).
Notes: Drugs and dosages presented in bolded text are those most commonly used by the authors. Use of certain drugs for prophylaxis during neutropenia may be extralabel usage. Flexible labeling specifies once- or twice-daily use of most fluoroquinolones in dogs and cats, depending upon the clinical situation. Once-daily use at the lower dose in the dose range probably results in selective intestinal decontamination, although this has not been established with all drugs. Flexible dosing specifies twice-daily use of most fluoroquinolones when treating systemic infections and is more appropriate than once-daily use if the goal of antimicrobial prophylaxis is also to provide tissue drug levels to treat incipient bacterial infections. The authors usually use enrofloxacin or ciprofloxacin at 5–10 mg/kg q12 hours.

appears to be more beneficial in reducing infection rates in humans with neutropenia of greater severity and duration than in humans with mild to moderate neutropenia. In a study of veterinary cancer patients receiving vincristine-doxorubicin-cyclophosphamide chemotherapy, which resulted in neutropenic episodes of short duration with a median neutrophil count of $0.8 \times 10^9/l$, trimethoprim-sulfonamide prophylaxis reduced the number of antibiotic-responsive febrile episodes, presumably of infectious etiology, from 40% to 20% (Couto, 1990). The potential advantages of prophylactic therapy include a reduction in infection rate, a reduction in the time to onset of infection, and a reduction in the speed in which an incipient infection develops into overwhelming sepsis. These benefits may facilitate home management of neutropenic animals and improve quality of life. Potential disadvantages include shifts in the host's flora, development of resistant organisms, adverse drug reactions, and expense (Wade, 1994), although preventing sepsis is less expensive than treating it.

Antimicrobial prophylaxis in the asymptomatic patient should be considered whenever a neutrophil count of $0.5–1.0 \times 10^9/l$ is present or anticipated. We do not recommend routine prophylactic therapy during anticancer chemotherapy if the owner can closely observe the animal for signs of infection and if the anticipated neutropenia is of short duration, such as occurs with many commonly used protocols. Prophylactic therapy is specifically discouraged in cats, because they have a better tolerance of neutropenia than dogs and are more susceptible to antibiotic-induced gastrointestinal disorders (Kunkle et al., 1995). Prophylaxis is, however, initiated in the asymptomatic animal when a neutrophil count $<0.5–1.0 \times 10^9/l$ is noted or anticipated during pretreatment evaluation. The chemotherapy treatment is not given, and antimicrobial prophylaxis is continued until the animal is returned for its next chemotherapy treatment 4–7 days later, at which point the neutrophil count has usually recovered. If the neutrophil count has not recovered sufficiently to administer the next chemotherapy treatment, antimicrobial prophylaxis is discontinued if the neutrophil count is $>1.0–2.0 \times 10^9/l$.

If an animal has had a previous episode of chemotherapy-induced sepsis, then antimicrobial prophylaxis is given following the next treatment with the offending agent, but prophylaxis may be restricted to the period of 5–10 days posttreatment, ie, the period when most postchemotherapy neutrophil nadirs occur.

Antimicrobial prophylaxis is also recommended if severe and prolonged neutropenia is anticipated, such as with pancytopenia caused by estrogen or phenylbutazone toxicity. Prolonged neutropenia may also occur during the chronic phase of ehrlichiosis in dogs. Ehrlichiosis is usually treated with tetracyclines. Doxycycline is less likely than tetracycline to disturb resistance to colonization by exogenous bacteria and may be a superior choice in dogs with chronic neutropenia due to ehrlichiosis. Therapy with tetracyclines may also reduce the risk of secondary bacterial infections, since such therapy was beneficial in controlling infections in early studies of severe radiation-induced neutropenia (Sorensen et al., 1960).

Antifungal prophylaxis using topical decontamination with amphotericin B, nystatin, and clotrimazole has been practiced widely for many years in neutropenic humans. Despite these measures the incidence of invasive fungal infections is increasing as anticancer therapy becomes more aggressive. This has led to the use of itraconazole and fluconazole for systemic antifungal prophylaxis (Glasmacher et al., 1996). Routine antifungal prophylaxis is not recommended in veterinary medicine but should be considered in experimental bone marrow transplantation.

EMPIRICAL TREATMENT OF FEBRILE NEUTROPENIC PATIENTS

Neutropenia itself does not cause clinical signs; these result from the underlying disease and infection. Most septic neutropenic animals will develop a fever, because macrophages, rather than neutrophils, are largely responsible for the production of interleukin-1 and other endogenous pyrogens. Occasionally inactivity, inappetence, and tachycardia are the only signs of sepsis. This occurs mostly in older animals and in animals receiving corticosteroids, which may have blunted febrile responses. Septic animals may also present with vomiting, diarrhea, or septic shock. Local signs of inflammation are subtle or absent if granulopoiesis is impaired, and the site of infection may be difficult to determine. In many cases it is not possible to document a suspected infection. Approximately 50% of fevers in human neutropenic patients are unexplained (Hughes et al., 1997).

Body temperature should be monitored in the asymptomatic neutropenic animal and in the animal at risk for neutropenia. Depending upon perceived risk, this may vary from recording temperature when the animal shows signs of lethargy or 2–4 times a day. Axillary temperature measurements facilitate home monitoring and minimize rectal trauma; they measure 0.5–1° C lower than rectal temperature measurements. The definition of pyrexia depends to some extent on baseline body temperatures obtained for an individual animal. In general, a rectal temperature >39.0° C in dogs and 39.2° C in cats should be regarded with suspicion, and either the animal should be treated for sepsis or the temperature rechecked in several hours to detect progressive elevation. A temperature above 39.5° C in most cases represents true fever.

A febrile episode or unexplained depression or inappetence in a neutropenic animal should be considered bacterial in origin until proven otherwise, and antimicrobial therapy should be initiated promptly. The animal should be closely examined for any signs of inflammation, and an appropriate specimen cultured. If there is no obvious site of infection, blood cultures should be considered. Our protocol is to obtain two simultaneous samples for culture from different veins (Reller, 1994). Blood cultures are expensive, and results take 2–7 days to report and are often negative or do not alter initial therapy. For these reasons blood cultures are not always performed during anticancer chemotherapy when the anticipated duration of neutropenia and fever is short, nor are they routinely performed in animals with parvoviral infections. Blood cultures are always recommended if the cause of neutropenia is not known or if the animal is very sick.

Additional tests may be performed in an effort to localize infection and determine the severity of illness. Recommended baseline measurements in hospitalized animals include serum glucose, urea, and electrolyte levels and urine specific gravity. Thoracic radiographs may be considered as part of the minimum database and should always be obtained if the animal is coughing, is dyspneic, or has nasal discharge. Culture of airway (transtracheal or bronchoalveolar) lavage samples should be performed if there are radiographic signs of pneumonia. Normal thoracic radiographs, however, do not rule out pneumonia, and airway lavage cultures should be considered if the animal has signs of respiratory tract disease, is severely ill without localizing signs, or does not respond to antimicrobial therapy.

Urinalysis and urine culture are recommended if there are any signs of urinary tract disease, but therapy should not be delayed more than 1–2 hours—or less, depending upon the clinical status of the animal—while awaiting adequate urine production for collection. This recommendation applies to obtaining other cultures as well. Catheterization should be avoided because of the risk of introducing infection. If cystocentesis cannot be performed because of thrombocytopenia ($<50 \times 10^9$/l), a free catch sample submitted for quantitative culture will suffice. A serum chemistry profile, abdominal radiographs, and/or abdominal ultrasound examination are recommended if the animal is vomiting or has abdominal pain. All the preceding tests may be needed to characterize the illness if the cause of neutropenia is not known, if the animal is severely ill, or if there is no response to antimicrobial therapy.

Because the likelihood is that pyrexia is due to infection, untreated infection may be rapidly fatal, and because neutropenic animals have died of sepsis with negative antemortem cultures, the recommendation is to initiate empirical antimicrobial therapy while awaiting culture results and, in most cases, to continue therapy in spite of negative results (Hughes et al., 1997). Antimicrobial selection may be assisted by previous culture results (eg, in a dog with a history of recurrent urinary tract infection), localizing signs, Gram stain of body fluid (eg, airway wash), and the antibiogram of a suspected nosocomial pathogen. If there is a history of prophylactic therapy with a fluoroquinolone, a febrile episode is most likely due to a Gram-positive organism. Cultures of feces, the oral cavity, and the skin of an animal without clinical signs prior to the induction of neutropenia are not likely to yield useful information.

In many cases the choice of antimicrobial agents must be empirical. Numerous trials with various antibiotic combinations have been conducted in humans (Chanock and Pizzo, 1996; De Lalla, 1997; Hughes et al., 1997). Veterinary experience is much more limited. The antibiotics chosen should be bactericidal, should have limited toxicity to the bone marrow, should be given parenterally, and should be active against Enterobacteriaceae, *Pseudomonas*, and Gram-positive cocci. Standard recommended drug doses are employed. A representative selection of antibiotics is presented in Table 19.13. These protocols provide some activity against anaerobic organisms (except for imipenem-cilastatin, which has broad-spectrum antianaerobe activity). More-complete therapy against anaerobic organisms is not recommended for initial therapy, because anaerobic infections are not common and such therapy may disturb colonization resistance. Combination therapy has historically been preferred over therapy with a single agent in order to increase the antibacterial spectrum, to take advantage of additive and synergistic effects while minimizing toxicity, and possibly to reduce the development of resistance. Most approaches have combined an aminoglycoside antibiotic with a beta-lactam antibiotic. Combination therapy with beta-lactam antibiotics has been used in order to avoid aminoglycoside nephrotoxicity. This may also be accomplished by substituting a fluoroquinolone for an aminoglycoside. Although fluoroquinolones are considered broad-spectrum antibiotics, in neutropenic patients they have limited activity against Gram-positive organisms. Fluoroquinolones are similar in spectrum to aminoglycosides, with excellent activity against Enterobacteriaceae and *Pseudomonas* and limited activity against anaerobes. Single-agent therapy with ceftazidime or imipenem-cilastatin is being increasingly used in humans (Klastersky, 1997). For infections complicating the mild to moderate episodes of neutropenia usually encountered by veterinarians, the various protocols are probably of near equivalent efficacy. The authors generally use enrofloxacin plus cefazolin in cancer patients and gentamicin plus ampicillin, or cefoxitin, in patients with parvoviral infections. Imipenem-cilastatin is our preferred choice for initial therapy in animals with sepsis associated with neutropenia of unknown cause.

TABLE 19.13. **Parenteral empirical antimicrobial therapy for the febrile neutropenic dog or cat**

Drug(s)	Comments
Combinations	
Aminoglycoside + cefazolin or cephalothin (first-generation cephalosporin)	Commonly used in veterinary medicine for cancer patients
	Once commonly used in human medicine
	Relatively inexpensive
	Spectrum may not cover *Pseudomonas*
	Cephalosporin may increase risk of nephrotoxicity
Aminoglycoside + ampicillin (aminopenicillin)	Commonly used in veterinary medicine for patients with parvoviral infections
	Relatively inexpensive
	Spectrum may not cover *Pseudomonas* or *Staphylococcus*
	Increased activity against anaerobes over aminoglycoside + first-generation cephalosporin
	More likely to disturb colonization resistance
	Can prevent beta-lactamase activity by using ampicillin-sulbactam (parenteral substitute for amoxicillin-clavulanate), but it is expensive
Aminoglycoside + antipseudomonal penicillin or ceftazidime (third-generation cephalosporin)	Commonly used in human medicine for cancer patients
	More expensive than above combinations
	Synergy against *Pseudomonas* and Enterobacteriaceae
	Less activity against Gram-positive organisms
	Can prevent beta-lactamase activity by using ticarcillin-clavulanate or piperacillin-tazobactam
Fluoroquinolone substituted for aminoglycoside in above combinations	Less well evaluated than aminoglycoside combinations
	More expensive than aminoglycoside
	Combinations more likely to be additive than synergistic
	Avoids aminoglycoside nephrotoxicity
Combination of two beta-lactam antibiotics[a]	Avoids aminoglycoside nephrotoxicity
	Potential antagonism
	Resistance more likely to develop?
	Prolongation of neutropenia?

Single agents	
Cefoxitin (second-generation cephalosorin [cefamycin])	Substitute for aminoglycoside + ampicillin No activity against *Pseudomonas* Activity against anaerobes More likely to disturb colonization resistance
Ceftazidime (third-generation cephalosporin)	Less well evaluated in veterinary medicine Commonly used in human medicine for cancer patients Expensive Less activity against Gram-positive organisms than combination therapy
Imipenem-cilastatin (carbapenem)	Commonly used in human medicine and, to a lesser extent, in veterinary medicine, for cancer patients Expensive Active against complete antimicrobial spectrum

Sources: Doses adapted from Allen (1998) and Greene (1998).

Note: Optimal doses in recommended dose ranges are not known. IV routes of administration are preferred, and all intravenous injections are given over 15–20 minutes unless indicated otherwise. *Aminoglycosides:* Amikacin, 5–10 mg/kg q8 hours or 15–20 mg/kg q24 hours, IV, IM, SC; gentamicin, 2–3 mg/kg q8 hours or 7–10 mg/kg q24 hours, IV, IM, SC; netilmycin, 2–3 mg/kg q8 hours or 6 mg/kg q24 hours, IV; tobramycin, 2 mg/kg q8 hours or 6 mg/kg q24 hours, IV, IM, SC. In order to reduce the risks of nephrotoxicity due to aminoglycoside antibiotics, we prefer the lower doses and once-daily administration, and, avoid their use in dehydrated animals and in animals receiving furosemide. *Fluoroquinolones:* Ciprofloxacin, 5–10 mg/kg q12–24 hours, IV (1-hour infusion); enrofloxacin, 5–10 mg/kg q12–24 hours IV, IM. The authors' initial dose is usually 5 mg/kg q12 hours. Enrofloxacin is approved for IM use only, but the solution is irritating to tissues, and the authors prefer IV administration. For IV injection, the solution should be injected over 20–60 minutes; some recommend dilution of 1 part parenteral solution with 9 parts sterile water for injection. We do not recommend injecting the parenteral solution SC. Reduction in the frequency of administration and/or dose may be necessary in animals at risk for seizure activity (see text). *Aminopenicillins:* Ampicillin, 20–40 mg/kg q6–8 hours, IV, IM, SC; ampicillin-sulbactam, 50 mg/kg q6–8 hours, IV, IM. *Anti-pseudomonal penicillins:* Piperacillin, 25–50 mg/kg q6–8 hours, IV, IM; piperacillin-tazobactam, 25–50 mg/kg q6–8 hours, IV, IM; ticarcillin, 40–75 mg/kg q6–8 hours, IV, IM; ticarcillin-clavulanate, 30–50 mg/kg q6–8 hours IV, IM. *Cephalosporins:* Cefazolin, 20–30 mg/kg q6–8 hours, IV, IM, SC; cephalothin, 25–40 mg/kg q6–8 hours, IV, IM, SC; cefoxitin, 20–30 mg/kg q6–8 hours, IV, IM, SC; ceftazidime, 25–30 mg/kg q8 hours, IV, IM, SC. We usually dose these cephalosporins at 30 mg/kg q8 hours, IV. *Carbapenems:* Imipenem-cilastatin, 2–10 mg/kg q6–8, IV (1-hour infusion), IM (reconstitute with 1% lidocaine without epinephrine). We usually use 5 mg/kg q8 hours IV.

[a]For example, first-generation cephalosporin + antipseudomonal penicillin; first-generation cephalosporin + third-generation cephalosporin; third-generation cephalosporin + antipseudomonal penicillin.

IV administration is preferred, to ensure rapid drug distribution, to minimize tissue trauma and patient discomfort, and to minimize bleeding in thrombocytopenic animals. IV catheterization is preferred over repetitive venipuncture and is necessary for fluid therapy. However, there must be strict adherence to aseptic procedure during catheter placement. Povidone-iodine or chlorhexidine ointment from single-use packages should be placed on the skin entry site, and the site bandaged. Injection ports should be cleansed with alcohol and allowed to dry before injection. The catheter should be removed promptly and cultured if signs of phlebitis occur.

Drug toxicity should be considered during therapy. Animals receiving aminoglycosides should be monitored for evidence of nephrotoxicity (eg, urinary casts, glucosuria, azotemia), especially when the duration of therapy is >5 days. The order of aminoglycosides with respect to increasing nephrotoxicity (and decreasing cost) is netilmicin, amikacin, tobramycin, gentamicin. Fluoroquinolones should be avoided in animals less than 6 months old, because of the possibility of inducing cartilage defects, although the risks for such defects following short courses of treatment at standard doses is not known. Fluoroquinolones may cause seizures and other neurologic signs at higher doses, especially with repetitive administration. Geriatric animals, animals with hypoalbuminemia, and animals with a history of seizures are at increased risk. Antibiotics may inhibit platelet function (Catalfamo and Dodds, 1988). This effect is clinically most relevant with penicillins, and animals so treated should be observed for bleeding if there is concurrent thrombocytopenia, especially if the platelet count is $<20 \times 10^9/l$. Profound thrombocytopenia is not a contraindication to the use of penicillins but may increase transfusion requirements. Fluoroquinolones have minimal effects on platelet function; cefazolin does not alter platelet function in normal dogs (Wilkens et al., 1995).

Reduction of fever is expected within 72 hours after starting antimicrobial therapy, and the animal should be more alert. Increasing depression coinciding with a falling temperature may be a sign of septic shock. In many cases improvement is noted after the first dose. The duration of antibacterial therapy once pyrexia has resolved is controversial. Prolonged therapy increases expense, hospitalization, side effects, and risk of fungal infection. Therapy should be continued for 1–7 days beyond achievement of a neutrophil count of $1.0 \times 10^9/l$. Changing from intravenous therapy to oral therapy (see Table 19.12) during this period facilitates discharge from the hospital and reduces expense. For cancer patients without a documented site of infection, we stop intravenous antimicrobial drugs the day after recovery of the neutrophil count to $1.0 \times 10^9/l$ and resolution of pyrexia. We continue oral antimicrobial prophylaxis in those patients that were receiving it and give oral antimicrobials for 7 days in those that were not. We do not usually continue with oral antimicrobials in patients recovering from parvoviral infections. In animals with pancytopenia with prolonged neutropenia, intravenous or oral antimicrobial therapy is continued for a minimum of 10 days beyond resolution of fever. At that time, withdrawal of antimicrobial therapy may be attempted.

Pyrexia may not resolve if (1) it is not bacterial in origin (and this should be reconsidered); (2) the organism is not sensitive to the antimicrobial drug(s); (3) drug doses are too low (although this does not commonly occur); or (4) there is such a severe compromise of host defenses that the infection and associated fever will not respond to any antimicrobial agent. The latter occurs with prolonged, severe neutropenia. This is infrequently encountered in veterinary medicine but has been observed during marrow transplantation studies. Initial culture results may assist therapeutic decision making with unresponsive fever. If a resistant organism is documented, antimicrobial therapy may be changed, based upon susceptibility testing. However, the organism involved may be sensitive to the current medication, or an infectious cause of the fever may not be documented, in which case another empirical judgment will be necessary. If the animal is clinically stable, the current medication may be continued until resolution of fever and achievement of a neutrophil count of $1.0 \times 10^9/l$. The dose(s) may be increased within recommended ranges, although this does not often result in clinical improvement. If the animal's clinical status is becoming worse, new antimicrobial agents should be employed. These should also be considered if there is rapid deterioration of the patient during the first 72 hours of treatment. The new drugs are usually given in addition to, rather than as a substitute for, existing therapy. The choice of additional drugs depends on which antibiotics were used for initial therapy. Classically, failure of response to empirical therapy with cefoxitin or an aminoglycoside and first-generation cephalosporin, would prompt additional therapy against *Pseudomonas* with an antipseudomonal penicillin. Ceftazidime and imipenem-cilastatin could also be used to intensify activity against *Pseudomonas*. If a resistant Gramnegative organism is suspected (eg, if there are signs of intestinal damage or respiratory signs), choices for additional therapy include an aminoglycoside, fluoroquinolone, cefoxitin, ceftazidime, and other third-generation cephalosporins, and imipenem-cilastatin. Aztreonam is also used in humans to intensify therapy against Gram-negative organisms and *Pseudomonas*, but there is limited veterinary experience with this drug. Resistant Gram-positive organisms are increasingly responsible for infections in neutropenic humans, for which vancomycin and teicoplanin are the drugs of choice (Hughes et al., 1997). Veterinary experience with these drugs is limited. If a resistant Gram-positive organism is suspected (eg, if there are signs of phlebitis, injury to the skin or oral cavity, or respiratory signs), the drug of choice in animals is clindamycin, 10 mg/kg q12 hours IV, SC, although it is bacteriostatic. Imipenem-cilastatin could also be used, although its activity against *Streptococcus* spp. is not complete.

A nonresponding fever may also be due to a resistant anaerobic infection. Additional therapy could include metronidazole (10–15 mg/kg q8 hours IV [1-hour infusion]), clindamycin, cefoxitin, ampicillin-sulbactam, and imipenem-cilastatin. The latter is suitable as a means of increasing broad-spectrum antibacterial activity. Although imipenem-cilastatin is expensive, it is less expensive than combined administration of an aminoglycoside or fluoroquinolone, first-generation cephalosporin, and metronidazole and in some cases is substituted for such combinations. If multiple antimicrobial agents are being used, then selective withdrawal of agents may be considered once there is clinical improvement.

The preceding recommendations are appropriate for most cases but may not be feasible due to cost restrictions and to inability or unwillingness of the owner to return the animal to the hospital. In such cases, initial use of oral antimicrobial agents may be used if the animal is clinically stable. In addition, oral antimicrobial agents may be sufficient for initial treatment of neutropenic animals that have been febrile and clinically stable for several days. For animals with mild neutropenia and mild pyrexia, therapy with trimethoprim-sulfonamide, a fluoroquinolone, amoxicillin, or amoxicillin-clavulanate is recommended. For animals with moderate to severe neutropenia or pyrexia, a fluoroquinolone plus cephalexin, amoxicillin, or amoxicillin-clavulanate is recommended. Doses may be increased within standard recommendations above those given in Table 19.12. Therapy with tetracyclines or doxycycline for ehrlichiosis may also control secondary infections. In all cases, the animal should be closely observed for clinical deterioration and arrangements made to initiate parenteral therapy. Oral antimicrobial therapy should not be used when the animal is hypovolemic or vomiting or when there is disruption of the intestinal mucosa.

With human neutropenic patients, if there is no response to multiple antibacterial agents after approximately 5–7 days of therapy, then empirical antifungal therapy may be initiated with amphotericin B (Hughes et al., 1997). This situation is not commonly encountered in veterinary medicine. Antifungal therapy is not recommended in the dog or cat unless a fungal infection is documented. If neutropenia and antibacterial therapy persist beyond 10 days, then stools should be monitored by culture or cytologic studies for candidal overgrowth and prophylaxis with nystatin, ketoconazole, or itraconazole considered, especially if antibacterial agents are being used that disturb colonization resistance (eg, ampicillin, cefoxitin, metronidazole, imipenem-cilastatin).

THERAPY OF DOCUMENTED INFECTIONS

An infection is considered documented in strict terms when the site of infection and infecting organism are both known. In broader terms an infection is also considered documented if only the site of infection is known (eg, radiographic evidence of pneumonia). Therapy of documented bacterial infections should consist of bactericidal antibiotics, with the choice based upon susceptibility testing. The guidelines for choosing parenteral or oral routes of administration are the same as those previously discussed. In most situations empirical therapy will have already been started. The guidelines for duration of therapy with documented bacteremia but no localization into other organs are also as previously discussed. Treatment for documented pneumonia and urinary tract and soft tissue infections should be continued to a minimum of 7 days beyond recovery of the neutrophil count to $1.0 \times 10^9/1$ and resolution of clinical and radiographic signs. The infection may transiently appear to become worse as neutrophil recovery occurs, because of increased inflammation. However, fever should be decreasing if the antimicrobial therapy is appropriate. The guidelines for intensifying therapy if fever and clinical signs are progressing are similar to those previously discussed, with drug selection aided by susceptibility test results.

Documented fungal infections should be treated with antimycotic drugs used at standard recommended doses (Allen, 1998; Greene, 1998). Amphotericin B is the therapy of choice for *Aspergillus* sp. infection. The risk of nephrotoxicity can be reduced by using liposome-encapsulated amphotericin B, but the drug is considerably more expensive. Some cases of topical and systemic aspergillosis can also be treated successfully with itraconazole. Amphotericin B is also used for treatment of systemic candidiasis, but therapy with ketoconazole or itraconazole may suffice (Weber et al., 1985). Intestinal candidiasis can be treated with nystatin, ketoconazole, or itraconazole. Fluconazole is the drug of choice for urinary candidiasis, but its use may be cost-prohibitive.

Bibliography

Abrams-Ogg ACG, et al. 1993. Clinical and pathologic findings in dogs following supralethal total body irradiation with and without infusion of autologous long-term marrow culture cells. Can J Vet Res 57:79.

Allen DG. 1998. Handbook of Veterinary Drugs, 2nd ed. Philadelphia: Lippincott-Raven.

Anderson PG, Pidgeon G. 1987. Candidiasis in a dog with parvoviral enteritis. J Am Anim Hosp Assoc 23:27.

Barsanti JA, Finco DR. 1986. Bacteremia of urinary tract origin (urosepsis). In: Kirk RW, ed. Current Veterinary Therapy IX: Small Animal Practice. Philadelphia: WB Saunders, 1986.

Bodey GP, et al. 1966. Quantitative relationship between circulating leukocytes and infections in patients with acute leukemia. Ann Int Med 64:328.

Catalfamo JL, Dodds WJ. 1988. Hereditary and acquired thrombopathias. Vet Clin North Am Small Anim Pract 18:185.

Chanock SJ, Pizzo PA. 1996. Fever in the neutropenic host. Infect Dis Clin North Am 10:777.

Couto CG. 1990. Management of complications of cancer chemotherapy. Vet Clin North Am Small Anim Pract 20:1037.

Dahlinger J, et al. 1997. Prevalence and identity of translocating bacteria in healthy dogs. J Vet Intern Med 11:319.

De Lalla, F. 1997. Antibiotic treatment of febrile episodes in neutropenic cancer patients: clinical and economic considerations. Drugs 53:789.

Donnelly JP. 1997. Is there a rationale for the use of antimicrobial prophylaxis in neutropenic patients? J Intern Med 242 (Suppl 740):79.

Feld R. 1989. The compromised host. Eur J Cancer Clin Oncol 25 (Suppl 2):S1.

Glasmacher A, et al. 1996. Antifungal prophylaxis with itraconazole in neutropenic patients: pharmacological, microbiological, and clinical aspects. Mycoses 39:249.

Greene CE. 1998. Infectious Diseases of the Dog and Cat. Philadelphia: WB Saunders.

Hammon WD, Enders JF. 1939. A virus disease of cats, principally characterized by aleucocytosis, enteric lesions, and the presence of intranuclear inclusion bodies. J Exp Med 67:327.

Hawkins EC. 1990. Investigation and management of neutropenia. In: August JR, ed. Consultations in Feline Internal Medicine. Philadelphia: WB Saunders.

Hirsh DC. 1986. Infectious complications of cancer. In: Kirk RW, ed. Current Veterinary Therapy IX: Small Animal Practice. Philadelphia: WB Saunders.

Holzworth J. 1987. Mycotic diseases. In: Holzworth J, ed. Diseases of the Cat: Medicine andSurgery. Philadelphia: WB Saunders.

Hughes WT, et al. 1997. 1997 guidelines for the use of antimicrobial agents in neutropenic patients with unexplained fever. Clin Infect Dis 25:551.

Jacobs G, et al. 1998. Neutropenia and thrombocytopenia in three dogs treated with anticonvulsants. J Am Vet Med Assoc 212:681.

Klastersky J. 1989. Infections in compromised hosts: considerations on prevention. Eur J Cancer Clin Oncol 25 (Suppl 2):S53.

Klastersky J. 1997. Treatment of neutropenic infection: trend towards monotherapy? Support Care Cancer 5:365–370.

Kreeger TJ, et al. 1984. Bacteremia concomitant with parvovirus infection in a pup. J Am Vet Med Assoc 184:196.

Kunkle GA, et al. 1995. Adverse effects of oral antibacterial therapy in dogs and cats: an epidemiologic study of pet owners' observations. J Am Anim Hosp Assoc 31:46.

Reller LB. 1994. What the practicing physician should know about blood cultures. In: Koontz F, ed. Blood Culture Controversies—Revisited. Iowa City, IA: American Society of Microbiology.

Rodriguez F, et al. 1998. Acute disseminated candidiasis in a puppy associated with parvoviral infection. Vet Rec 142:434.

Rosenthal RC. 1988. Autologous bone marrow transplantation for lymphoma. Proc 6th Annu Vet Med Forum Am Coll Vet Intern Med 397.

Scott FW. 1987. Viral diseases. In: Holzworth J, ed. Diseases of the Cat. Philadelphia: WB Saunders.

Sorensen DK, et al. 1960. An effective therapeutic regimen for the hemopoietic phase of the acute radiation syndrome in dogs. Radiat Res 13:669.

Turk J, et al. 1990. Coliform septicemia and pulmonary disease associated with canine parvoviral enteritis: 88 cases (1987–1988). J Am Vet Med Assoc 196:771.

Turk J, et al. 1992. Enteric Clostridium perfringens infection associated with parvoviral enteritis in dogs: 74 cases (1987–1990). J Am Vet Med Assoc 200:991.

Van Der Waaij D. 1988. Selective decontamination of the digestive tract: general principles. Eur J Cancer Clin Oncol 24 (Suppl 1):S1.

Vriesendorp HM, et al. 1981. Gastrointestinal decontamination of dogs treated with total body irradiation and bone marrow transplantation. Exp Hematol 9:904.

Wade JC. 1994. Epidemiology and prevention of infection in the compromised host. In: Rubin RH, Young LS, eds. Clinical Approach to Infection in the Compromised Host, 3rd ed. New York: Plenum.

Weber MJ, et al. 1985. Treatment of systemic candidiasis in neutropenic dogs with ketoconazole. Exp Hematol 13:791.

Weiss DJ. 1995. Leukocyte disorders and their treatment. In: Bonagura JD, ed. Kirk's Current Veterinary Therapy XII: Small Animal Practice. Philadelphia: WB Saunders, 1995.

Wilkens B, et al. 1995. Effects of cephalothin, cefazolin, and cefmetazole on the hemostatic mechanism in normal dogs: implications for the surgical patient. Vet Surg 24:25.

20 | Anthelmintic Chemotherapy

R. S. REW and E. MCKENZIE

A review of anthelmintics in a short chapter by necessity omits much of the detailed information on these products. The goal of the authors in this chapter is to give the highlights of information (as up-to-date as possible) and to refer to more in-depth reviews or books for a more complete picture. This chapter will be organized artificially by discussing products in three activity groups: endectocides, broad-spectrum anthelmintics, and narrow-spectrum anthelmintics. This approach is designed to be a practical method that follows the reader's thought process through the scope of the parasite problem from diagnosis to treatment. The aim is to help the reader select appropriate compounds for the breadth of the problem encountered. The activity groupings will be subdivided into chemical groups for each species of host. As much safety and efficacy information as can be reasonably placed into tabular form by host species will be presented for easy access. Discussion of the chemical groups will include chemical structure, mode of action, comments on efficacy, safety, formulation, and parasite resistance.

Anthelmintic activity results from delivery of a chemical to a helminth receptor that interrupts a life-requiring function in a concentration/time-dependent manner. The helminth receptor must either be distinct from the host or be more sensitive to the chemical than the host receptor to permit selective toxicity. Therefore, parasite receptor, host pharmacodynamics, and parasite location are all a part of anthelmintic activity.

Anthelmintics for use in nonlactating cattle, sheep and goats, swine, horses, dogs, and cats are shown in Tables 20.1 to 20.6, respectively. These tables describe dose range, formulations, safety, and efficacy of anthelmintic drugs against particular classes of parasite.

490

TABLE 20.1. **Anthelmintics used in nonlactating cattle**

| Class/Compound | Dose Range (mg/kg) | Formulations[a] | Safety | Relative Efficacy[b] | | | | | |
| | | | | Nematodes | | | Trematodes | | Cestodes |
				GI[c]	EL4	Lung	Liver Fluke	Other[d]	Moniezia
Avermectins[e]	0.2–(0.5T)	O, T, I	4 mg/kg	A	A	A	N	N	N
Milbemycin/moxidectin	0.2–(0.5T)	O, T, I	1 mg/kg	A	A	A	N	A[h]	N
Benzimidazole thiazoles/ thiabendazole	66–110	O	700 mg/kg	A	N	N	N	N	N
Benzimidazole carbamates[f]	4.5–30	O	>10 × use level	A	B	A	A (adults)	N	A
Imidazothiazole/ levamisole	8	O, T, I	4–12 × use level	A	A–D	A	N	N	C
Tetrahydropyrimidines/ morantel	8.8	O	200 mg/kg	A	N	N	N	N	A
Organophosphates[g]	Variable	O, T	Variable	A–C	C	N	N	A[di]	N
Salicylanilides/ closantel, rafoxanide (R)	3–7.5	O, I	>58 mg/kg (R)	C	N	N	A (adults) C (imm.)	B–C[dh, i, j]	N
Thiobenzimidazole/ triclabendazole	12	O	>200 mg/kg	N	N	N	A (adults) A (imm.)	N	N
Disulfonamide/ clorsulon	7	O, I	>100 mg/kg	N	N	N	A (adults) D (imm.)	N	N
Isoquinoline/praziquantel	2.5–20	O, I	>100 mg/kg	N	N	N	N	A[di]	A

Note: Products approved for lactating cattle are one organophosphate (coumaphos); one tetrahydropyrimidine (morantel), two benzimidazoles (thiabendazole and fenbendazole), and one avermectin (eprinomectin).

[a]O, oral, including feed, tube, drench, and bolus; T, topical; L, injectable.

[b]A, 90–100%; B, 75–90%; C, 50–75%; D, <50%; N, no activity.

[c]GI = Adult and non-tissue–dwelling forms of gastrointestinal nematodes, including *Haemonchus, Ostertagia, Trichostrongylus, Oesophagostomum, Cooperia, Nematodirus, Bunostomum, Trichuris.* Not all products have label claims for each genus included here; thus each label should be examined.

[d]Other trematodes include [h]immature paramphistomes, [i]*Schistosoma,* and [j]*Dicrocoelium.*

[e]Compounds include ivermectin, doramectin, and eprinomectin. Each product should be studied individually for details.

[f]Compounds include thiophanate, parbendazole, fenbendazole, albendazole, oxfendazole, oxibendazole. Each compound should be studied individually for details.

[g]Compounds include coumaphos, trichlorfon, crufomate, and haloxon. Each product should be studied individually for details.

TABLE 20.2. **Anthelmintics used in sheep and goats**

Class/Compound	Dose Range (mg/kg)[a]	Formulations[b]	Safety	Relative Efficacy[c]						
				Nematodes			Trematodes		Cestodes[d]	
				GI	EL4	Lung	Liver Fluke	Other[e]	Echino.	Other
Avermectins[f]	0.2	O, I	1 mg/kg	A	A	A	N	N	N	N
Milbemycin/ moxidectin	0.2	O	1 mg/kg	A	A	A	N	N	N	N
Benzimidazole thiazoles/ thiabendazole	44	O	80–100 mg/kg	A	A/C	N	N	N	N	N
Benzimidazole carbamates[g]	Variable	O	>10 × use level	A	A	A	A (adults)	N	N	A
Imidazothiazole/ levamisole	8	O	4–12 × use level	A	A/B	A	N	N	N	N
Tetrahydropyrimidines/ morantel	10	O	>40 mg/kg per day	A	?	N	N	N	N	N
Organophosphates[h]	Variable	T, O	Variable	A	N	N	N	N	N	N
Salicylanilides/ closantel, rafoxanide	7.5–10	O	40–45 mg/kg	A	N	N	A (adults) C (imm.)	B–C	N	N
Thiobenzimidazole/ triclabendazole	10	O	200 mg/kg	N	N	N	A (adults) A (imm.)	N	N	N
Disulfonamide/ clorsulon	20	O	>100 mg/kg	N	N	N	A (adults) C (imm.)	N	N	N
Isoquinoline/ praziquantel	5–15	O, I	>100 mg/kg	N	N	N	N	A (Schistosoma)	A	A

[a]Goats generally have more rapid depletion of compound than sheep, but the same dose is recommended for both species.
[b]O, oral, either drench, tube, feed, or bolus; I, injectable; T, topical.
[c]A, 90–100%; B, 75–90%; C, 50–75%; N, no activity.
[d]Echino., *Echinococcus granulosa* or *E. multilocularis;* other, *Moniezia, Stilesia,* or *Avitellina.*
[e]*Dicrocoelium,* paramphistomes, or *Schistosoma.*
[f]Avermectins include ivermectin, doramectin, and eprinomectin.
[g]Second-generation benzimidazoles include parbendazole, oxibendazole, mebendazole, fenbendazole, oxfendazole, albendazole, and thiophanate. Each compound should be studied individually for details.
[h]Organophosphates include coumaphos, trichlorfon, and haloxon. Each compound should be studied individually before a definitive recommendation can be made.

TABLE 20.3.   Anthelmintics used in swine

Class/Compound	Dose Range (mg/kg)	Formulations[a]	Safety	Relative Efficacy[b]					
				As[c]	H	Oe	T	S	M
Avermectins[d]	0.3, 0.1 × 7 days	I, O	15 mg/kg	A/A[f]	A/A	B/B	C	A	A
Benzimidazole thiazoles/ thiabendazole	50	O	>70 mg/kg 2× per day	D/D	A/C	A/C	D/D	A	N
Benzimidazole carbamates[e]	5–100	O	Variable	A/B	A/A	A/B	A/D	D–N	A
Imidazothiazole/ levamisole	7.5	I, O	4–12 × use level	A/A	A/B	B/B	B/B	A	A
Tetrahydropyrimidines/ pyrantel	22	O	Unknown	A/A	A	A	N	N	N
Organophosphates/ dichlorvos	11.2–21.6	O	50–300 (unformulated)	A	A	A	A/A	C–N	N
Hygromycin B	12 g/900 kg feed	O	Do not feed continuously	A	N	A	A	N	N
Piperazine	110	O	5 × use level	A	N	D	N	N	N

[a] I, injectable; O, oral, including feed.

[b] A, 90–100%; B, 75–90%; C = 50–75%; D, < 50%; N, no activity.

[c] As, Ascaris; H, Hyostrongylus; Oe, Oesophagostomum; T, Trichuris; S, Strongyloides; M, Metastrongylus.

[d] Avermectins include ivermectin and doramectin.

[e] Compounds include flubendazole, thiophanate, parbendazole, cambendazole, fenbendazole, oxibendazole. Each compound should be studied individually for details.

[f] Letters on left side of slash indicate efficacy against adults; letters on right side indicate efficacy against immatures.

TABLE 20.4. Anthelmintics used in horses

Class/Compound	Dose Range (mg/kg)	Formulations[a]	Safety	Nematodes[b]						Cestodes
				LS	SS	SW	P	As	L	
Avermectin/ivermectin	0.2	O	2 mg/kg	A[f]	A	A	A	A	A	N
Milbemycin/moxidectin	0.4	O	1.2 mg/kg	A	A	A	A	A	A	N
Benzimidazole thiazole[c]	Variable	O	>20× use level	A	A	A	A	B (adults) C (imm.)	—	N
Benzimidazole carbamates[d]	Variable	O	Variable	A	A	A	A	A	A	N
Imidazothiazole/levamisole	7.5–15(O)	O, I	>20 mg/kg	B–D	B–D	N	N	A	A	N
Tetrahydropyrimidines/pyrantel	6.6 (15–20 for A; 20 for L)	O	>20× use level	A/B	A	N	B	A (adults) A (imm.)	A	A
Organophosphates[e]	Variable	O	Variable	A	A	N	A	A	N	N

[a] O, oral, I, injectable.
[b] LS, large strongyles; SS, small strongyles; SW, *Strongyloides westeri*; P, pinworms; As, ascarids; L, lungworms.
[c] Compounds include thiabendazole (44mg/kg; 88mg/kg for ascarids) and cambendazole (20 mg/kg).
[d] Compounds include mebendazole, oxibendazole, and fenbendazole. Each compound should be studied individually for details.
[e] Compounds include haloxon, trichlorfon, and dichlorvos. Each compound should be studied individually for details.
[f] A, 90–100%; B, 75–90%; C, 50–75%; D, <50%; N, no activity.

TABLE 20.5. **Anthelmintics used in dogs**

Class/Compound	Dose Range (mg/kg)[a]	Formulations[b]	Safety	Relative Efficacy[c] Nematodes[d] Ascarids	Hook	Whip	Heart	Strong	Cestodes[e] E	T	D
Avermectin/ ivermectin	0.006	O	2.0 mg/kg (not for collie)	N	N	N	A (prevent)	N	N	N	N
Milbemycin	0.003–0.5 (GI nemat.)	O		A	A	A	A (prevent)	N	N	N	N
Benzimidazole carbamates[f]	Variable	O	10 × use level	A	A	A	N	N	N	A–B	N
Imidazothiazole/ levamisole	10	O	>20 × use level	A	A	N	A (mf)	N	N	N	N
Butamisole HCl	2.4	I	4 × use level	N	A	A	A	N	N	N	N
Tetrahydropyrimidines/ pyrantel	5–10	O	7 × use level	A	A	?	N	N	N	N	N
Organophosphates/ dichlorvos	27–33	O	182–384	A	A	A–B	N	N	N	N	N
Quaternary ammonium/ thenium closylate[g]	125–500	O	1 × use level	B–C	A	D	N	N	N	N	N
Cyanine/ dithiazinine iodide	3.3; 6.6–11	O	12–20 mg/kg	A–B	A–B	N	A (mf)	A	N	N	N
Piperazine/ diethylcarbamazine	2.75–6.6	O	(Chronic) 55–110	B	N	N	A (prevent)	A	N	N	N
Arsenical/ thiacetarsamide sodium	2.2	I	1 × use level	N	N	N	A (adult)	A	N	N	N
Isoquinolone/ praziquantel, epsiprantel	2–10	O, I	>200 mg/kg	N	N	N	N	A	A	A	A
Salicylanilide/ niclosamide	100–157	O	2 × use level	N	N	N	N	N	N	B	C–D
Chlorinated HCH/ bunamidine HCl	25–50	O	1 × use level	N	N	N	N	N	A–B	A	B–C

[a]Dosing regimens are often complicated and are not explained or implied by the figures given. The figures here reflect the amount of compound in the particular formulation per dose.
[b]O, oral, including tablets, syrup, paste, and feed; I, injectable.
[c]A, 90–100%; B, 75–90%; C, 50–75%; D, <50%; N, no activity.
[d]Ascarids = *Toxocara* and *Toxascaris*; Hook, *Ancylostoma* and *Uncinaria*; Whip, *Trichuris*; Heart, *Dirofilaria*; mf = microfilaria; Strong = *Strongyloides*.
[e]E, *Echinococcus*; T, *Taenia*; D, *Diplidium*.
[f]Includes fenbendazole and mebendazole. Specific product details should be determined before decisions are made.
[g]Dosage is determined based on one 500-mg tablet for all dogs heavier than 10 lb and 125 mg b.i.d. for dogs 5–10 lb. The product is greatly enhanced when combined with piperazine salts. Contraindicated for collies and Airedales.

TABLE 20.6. **Anthelmintics for cats**

| Class/Compound | Dose Range (mg/kg)[a] | Formulations[b] | Safety | Relative Efficacy[c] | | | |
| | | | | Nematodes | | Cestodes | |
				Ascarids	Hookworm	Taenia	Dipylium
Benzimidazole carbamates	Variable	O	Variable	A	A	A	N
Chlorinated HCH:phenol/ n-butyl chloride	Variable	O	1 × use level	A	C	N	N
Toluene dichlorophene	0.22 ml/kg	O	1 ×–5 × use level	A	A–B	B–C	B–C
Disophenol	10	I	3 × use level	N	A	N	N
Salicylanilide/ niclosamide	100–157	O	>2 × use level	N	N	A	B–D
Isoquinoline/ praziquantel	5	O	?	N	N	A	A
Tetrahydropyrimidine/ levamisole	8	O	1 × use level	A	A	N	N
Organophosphate/ dichlorvos	11	O	55 mg/kg	A	A	N	N

[a]Dosing regimens are often complicated; thus careful attention must be paid to product specifications on the label.
[b]O, oral, including tablets and liquids; I, injectable.
[c]A, 90–100%; B, 75–90%; C, 50–75%; D, <50%; N, no activity.

Controlled (continuous or pulsatile)-release anthelmintic drug delivery systems (ruminal boluses) have been developed for use in cattle and sheep. Recently developed controlled-release oral products include the Paratect bolus (contains morantel tartrate), the Ivomec bolus (which uses the ALZET 2 ML mini-osmotic pump for intraruminal delivery of ivermectin), and the Romensin RDD bolus (contains monensin sodium). These oral dosage forms release drug continuously at a constant rate over a prolonged period (90–135 days). Autoworm and Multidose 130 release pulse doses of the anthelmintic oxfendazole at approximately 3-week intervals. It is significant that this time span roughly coincides with the prepatent period of the major gastrointestinal trichostrongylids of cattle. After releasing their drug content, these delivery systems remain permanently in the reticulorumen. The controlled-release systems, unlike sustained-release boluses, are depleted of drug at the end of the stated delivery period. This is important in food-producing animals, since tissue residues are unwanted.

Endectocides

In 1981 with the launch of ivermectin (dihydroavermectin $B_{1a} > 80\%$, $B_{1b} < 20\%$) onto the animal health market, a new word—endectocide— and a new concept in parasite control was initiated. Endectocides are effective against both arthropod and nematode parasites. These two phylogenetic groups of organisms include the major, economically important ectoparasites and endoparasites of domestic animals. Endectocides are not active against fluke and tapeworm parasites, but these parasite classes are of less economic importance.

The endectocides, whether they be avermectins or milbemycins, are fermentation-based products that may or may not be derived chemically. The marketed avermectins (ivermectin, abamectin, doramectin, and eprinomectin) and the milbemycins (moxidectin, milbemycin D, and milbemycin oxime) are macrocyclic lactone fermentation products of the actinomycete *Streptomyces*. The avermectins are characterized as macrocyclic lactones with an L-oleandrose sugar at position 13. The milbemycins are quite similar in structure but are without the sugar side chain. The natural fermentation precursor for moxidectin, nemadectin, has little or no ectoparasite activity. The synthesis of the methoxime at position 23 appears to bring the ectoparasite activity to this precursor.

The primary mode of action of the avermectins and most likely the milbemycins is in their interaction with gamma-amino-butyric acid (GABA)-related and non-GABA-related chloride (Cl^-) channels. The avermectins appear to bind irreversibly with *Caenorhabditis elegans* Cl^- channels that are not GABA related (most likely glutamate related) with a very high affinity constant ($K_D = 2.6 \times 10^{-10}$ M). This binding opens the channel, allowing Cl^- flux and creating an ion imbalance that is eventually lethal. The same action is seen on GABA-related Cl^- channels, but it is reversible and has a $K_D = 3.7 \times 10^{-8}$ M; that is, it is 100 times less avid. The effect of this second interaction is a reversible paralysis of the organism. These receptors have not been demonstrated in protozoa or flatworms such as flukes and tapeworms and is the likely explanation for the lack of activity.

The toxicity of avermectins and milbemycins is related to their GABA-receptor binding in the central nervous system (CNS) of the mammalian host. Selective toxicity is based upon receptor binding affinity and the impermeability of the blood-brain barrier in mammals, since the GABA-related neurons are restricted to the CNS. The idiosyncratic toxicity in a subpopulation of collies and Murray Gray cattle may be related to a breed-related, compromised blood-brain barrier. Recently reported toxicity of abamectin and moxidectin in calves weighing less than 100 kg may be related to an age-dependent permeability of the blood-brain barrier.

Ivermectin has been formulated for cattle, swine, and sheep as an injectable or oral product in propylene glycol:glycerol formal (60:40) carrier and has been formulated for cattle as a topical product in isopropanol:crodamol (75:25) and as an in-feed premix for swine. It has also been formulated in tablets for dogs and as an oral paste for horses. Doramectin has been formulated for cattle, swine, and sheep as an injectable sesame oil:ethyl oleate product and formulated for cattle as a pour-on with isopropanol: cetearyl octanoate. Eprinomectin has been formulated in an oil-based carrier as a topical product for cattle. Moxidectin, a milbemycin, has been formulated as an aqueous-based injectable preparation and as an oil-based pour-on for cattle, as well as an oral paste for horses. Milbemycin oxime and milbemycin D have been formulated as tablets for dogs to prevent heartworm (*Dirofilaria immitis*) infection. Milbemycin oxime has additional claims for gastrointestinal roundworms because it can be given safely at a dose rate effective for heartworm prophylaxis and gastrointestinal roundworm therapy.

The plasma and tissue pharmacokinetics of injectable ivermectin, doramectin, and moxidectin were recently published (Lanusse et al., 1997; Lifschitz et al., 1998). The maximum plasma concentrations (C_{max}) of the molecules were similar following subcutaneous administration of 200 mg/kg. The time to maximum plasma concentration (T_{max}) was significantly shorter for moxidectin (8 hours) than for doramectin and ivermectin (4–6 days). The area under the curve (AUC) for the 80 sampling days was significantly greater for doramectin (627 ng × day/ml) than for ivermectin (459 ng × day/ml) and cydectin (217 ng × day/ml). Similarly, AUCs for doramectin tissue levels were significantly greater after treatment than for ivermectin and moxidectin, respectively (abomasal mucosa, 1,292, 959, 371 ng × day/g; intestinal mucosa, 942, 736, 228 ng × day/g;

skin, 657, 412, 387 ng × day/g). At day 48 posttreatment, doramectin and moxidectin plasma concentrations had dropped to 1 ng/ml, both higher than those of ivermectin. After 48 days posttreatment, moxidectin plasma concentrations were the highest.

Pharmacokinetics of pour-on doramectin and ivermectin adminis-tered at 500 mg/kg demonstrated a similar C_{max} and T_{max} with a signifi-cantly greater AUC for doramectin (168 ng × day/ml) than ivermectin (116 ng × day/ml) (Gayrard et al., 1999). It is noteworthy that topical administration of these products at 2.5 times greater dose gave plasma C_{max} levels and AUCs 60–70% less than their injectable counterpart.

The pharmacokinetic profile of avermectins and milbemycins pro-vide a basis for persistent activity in cattle against gastrointestinal round-worms from 7 to 35 days posttreatment, depending upon the species of nematode and the product used. The persistent activity allows pasture larval cleanup, and thus reduced reinfection rates under grazing condi-tions. In conditions of high stocking densities with warm, moist weather conditions, recommended 2- or 3-dose programmed use of these products at 5-to-8-week intervals for gastrointestinal parasite control has been very effective in the prevention of parasitic gastroenteritis.

A unique anthelmintic feature of the endectocides is their consis-tently excellent efficacy against inhibited (hypobiotic) larvae of *Osterta-gia* in cattle and sheep. Another feature is the sensitivity of nematodes to very low dosages. Nearly all species of economically important nematodes in domestic animals are sensitive to 200 mg/kg or 300 mg/kg in swine. *Dirofilaria immitis* (dog heartworm) fourth-stage larvae are effectively killed by 6 mg/kg of ivermectin given once per month. The approved dose-limiting nematode species appears to be *Cooperia* and *Nematodirus* in cattle and sheep, *Trichuris* in swine, *Toxas-caris* in dogs, and *Parascaris* in horses. Recently, activity of moxidectin has been registered for immature paramphistomes, a stomach fluke of cattle. Confirmation of this activity against paramphistomes has not been obtained.

Resistance to ivermectin has been documented in several isolates of *Haemonchus contortus* in sheep and goats in South Africa, Uruguay, Brazil, New Zealand, Australia, and the United States (one isolate). As might be expected, the isolates that were resistant to ivermectin were resistant to doramectin (Echevarria et al., 1997) and by regression analysis also resis-tant to moxidectin (Shoop et al., 1993). As with other classes of anthelmintics, resistance is also seen in small strongyles of horses but is essentially unrecorded in cattle, swine, or dog parasites. Whether this host restriction is due to genetic plasticity of the parasites, treatment fre-quency, host metabolism, management methods, or a combination of these variables is still unknown.

Broad-spectrum Anthelmintics

The classes of compounds in the broad-spectrum group have efficacy against a wide variety of parasitic nematodes. Some of these compounds also act against tapeworms and/or flukes.

Benzimidazoles

Benzimidazole (BZ) anthelmintics can be grouped chemically into two subclasses, the thiazoles and the carbamates. The first of this group, thiabendazole (TBZ), was marketed in 1961. TBZ has a thiazole ring at the 2 position and no substitution at the (5) 6 position. The activity site of this class is related to the group at position 2, while metabolism by the cytochrome P-450 system is related to the (5) 6 position. Cambendazole (CBZ) has a thiazole at the 2 position but has an isopropoxy:carbonylamino group at the (5) 6 position. This reduces the dose rate from 50–100 mg/kg for TBZ to 20–25 mg/kg for CBZ, because of a decreased rate of metabolism of CBZ.

The second-generation BZs evolved when the group at the 2 position was changed to a carbamate. The result of this modification was an enhanced fit to the parasite receptor, with a subsequent decrease in dosage to 5–10 mg/kg against nematodes and added activity against adult tapeworms. Interestingly, replacement of the oxygen bridge at the (5) 6 position with a sulfur, as was done with albendazole and fenbendazole, added activity against liver flukes.

Enhanced receptor binding and decreased metabolic inactivation increased the spectrum of activity and reduced the required dosage from the BZ-thiazoles to the BZ-carbamates. In addition, these chemical changes resulted in tissue-stage larval activity. Certain nematode species go into a suspended or inhibited larval state in tissues. Apparently during "deep" inhibition, the metabolism of the larvae is so retarded that the BZ-carbamates are only marginally active. However, during the transition from inhibited to active state, BZ-carbamate products are very effective (Miller, 1994). BZs also have antimitotic activity in helminth eggs, which provides some reproductive control following treatment.

In vivo activity also relates to other pharmacodynamic properties. Solubility of benzimidazoles increases as pH decreases. This characteristic accounts for the reservoir effect of a benzimidazole suspension in the rumen or reticulum, where the pH is 5.5–6.5, and the absorption in the abomasum, where the pH is approximately 2. Subsequently, we see transport from bloodstream back into the abomasum and conjugation in the liver, with secretion into the intestine via the bile, reexposing gastrointestinal parasites to the drug. Factors such as increase in the pH in the abomasum caused by parasitosis or diet and binding of drug to fibrous dietary materials also affect pharmacodynamic properties and related efficacy (Hennessey et al., 1995).

Persistent activity of the BZs lasts for only a few days after treatment. Therefore, programmed use recommendations are for 3-week intervals between doses, since many economically important nematode life cycles take 3 weeks to complete.

The mode of action of these groups relates primarily to binding to parasite tubulin, the subunit protein of microtubules. Several mechanisms have been proposed for this group, but recent information has indicated that all proposed metabolic and transport functions interrupted by BZs are related to the primary action on the microtubule. Selective toxicity is based upon the binding-affinity differential between mammalian and helminth tubulin. Binding of antimitotic and anticancer mammalian microtubule inhibitors such as colchicine or vinblastine are essentially irreversible in mammalian systems and quite reversible in helminth systems. Binding of benzimidazoles is exactly the opposite, since binding is essentially irreversible in helminth tubulin and quite reversible in mammals. The maximum concentration of BZ that will bind (B_{max}) to helminth tubulin is significantly reduced in tubulin isolated from BZ-resistant nematodes as compared with tubulin from a BZ-sensitive nematode. Several resistance detection systems are based on decreased hatchability of ova or inhibition of larval development; such resistance results from interruption of microtubular-based functions.

Toxicity of the benzimidazoles, especially parbendazole, is generally related to teratogenic effects. This is consistent with interference in proper functioning of microtubules of mitotic spindles during early development. Other less common effects such as hepatotoxicity may well be related to interference with bile transport, another microtubular-related event.

Benzimidazoles are generally called the "white" drenches, which refers to their insolubility in water. Common formulations are emulsions or suspensions in nonclear carriers and are administered orally. Recently, a report on using oxfendazole as a pour-on indicates that a pour-on benzimidazole may become available (Leathwick et al., 1998). Pro-benzimidazoles such as netobimin, febantel, and thiophanate are generally much more water soluble and may in fact be formulated as injectable products. Activation of these pro-benzimidazoles requires passage through the liver for ring closure before the drugs are efficacious.

Benzimidazoles can also be split-dosed or formulated as continuous or intermittent boluses or in-feed formulations. These delivery systems provide prophylactic activity against third-stage larvae, decrease the amount of drug in the system and so decrease toxicity, increase the efficacy, and provide long-term activity. A partial, naturally controlled release of BZs occurs in ruminants (because of the rumen) and, to a much lesser extent, in horses (probably because of the colon). By increasing residence time in the gastrointestinal tract, single-dose BZs are more effective in these hosts.

Resistance to the BZs is quite extensive in sheep trichostrongyles, such as *Trichostrongylus, Ostertagia,* and *Haemonchus*. BZ resistance is also seen quite extensively in small strongyles of horses. Combination products are being recommended, as well as rotational use of the product groups, to combat resistance. Few reports of resistance have been documented in cattle, swine, or dog parasites (Conder and Campbell, 1995).

Imidazothiazoles, Tetrahydropyrimidines, and Pyridines

The imidazothiazoles, tetrahydropyrimidines, and pyridines are generally grouped together for discussion of properties other than chemistry because they share common properties, including mode of action. All of these chemical classes are referred to as the "clear" drenches, since the oral formulations are true solutions. The imidazothiazole levamisole has been formulated as an injectable or topical product, as well as the more usual oral formulation generally found in this broad-spectrum activity group.

The mode of action of the clear drench group is, like the macrocyclic lactones, expressed through the nervous system, but in this case it is through the cholinergic receptors. Levamisole appears to bind to ganglionic acetylcholine receptors of nematodes, specifically those blocked by nicotine, and stimulates nerve depolarization. This action results in a contracted paralysis of the worm, which is reversible. A contracted paralysis impairs the ability of the parasite to maintain its site in the gastrointestinal tract, so when the worm "wakes up," the host is gone. Levamisole, morantel, thenium, bephenium, and pyrantel have been shown to have similar paralytic action on nematodes, and cross-resistance has been seen in the field. However, certain isolates of levamisole-resistant nematodes are not cross-resistant to morantel, indicating some slight binding difference, as might be expected from such different chemistry. Pyrantel tends to be poorly absorbed and consequently has little if any activity on tissue nematodes or larval stages embedded in the tissues. Morantel is absorbed but rapidly metabolized by the liver (first-pass effect) and thus has a similar activity limitation. Both drugs are effective against infective larvae (L3) as they enter the host. This property has been exploited via development of continuous-release bolus formulations or in-feed formulations and provides prophylactic activity against cattle and swine nematode infections.

Levamisole is absorbed and is active against tissue larval stages and lungworms but not against inhibited larvae. Toxicity of levamisole when overdosed is expressed through neurological symptoms.

Following oral administration to ruminant species, levamisole has an apparent plasma half-life of a few hours, much shorter than the 8.3 days for ivermectin injectable and 2–3 days for oral BZ-carbamates (Short et al., 1987). This short duration does not provide persistent activity with single-dose treatments. Because the therapeutic index of levamisole is low in animals, particularly in horses and dogs, and alternative drugs are available, the use of levamisole in these species is not recommended.

Organophosphates

The broad-spectrum antinematodal properties of organophosphates (OPs) are seen when administered as drenches or when oral formulations are delivered by continuous release, such as dichlorvos, or delivered in feed as crumbles or top-dressing in swine, cattle, and horses. Organophosphates are also active orally against arthropods such as nasal bots in sheep and stomach bots in horses; such effectiveness gives them endectocidal activity. Organophosphates are, of course, a primary class of compounds used for ectoparasite control via topical application (eg, dips, dust bags, sprays, or ear tags).

Organophosphates delivered orally have also been used for narrow-spectrum activity against *Haemonchus contortus* in sheep, primarily on BZ-resistant properties. OPs also have blood fluke activity and have been used for treatment of human schistosomiasis.

The mode of action of OPs is inhibition of acetylcholinesterase (AChE); that is, it inhibits the enzyme that inactivates acetylcholine after it has been released from the presynaptic side of a cholinergic synapse that has bound to the postsynaptic acetylcholine receptor. As a result, acetylcholine builds up in the synapse, causing a continuous stimulation that is manifested as a contracted paralysis in nematodes and arthropods. Interestingly, this paralysis is flaccid in flukes, because acetylcholine is an inhibitory neurotransmitter rather than stimulatory in these parasites. Differential toxicity between parasite and host lies in the quantitative difference between the concentrations required to inhibit mammalian AChE and nematode AChE. Fifty percent inhibition of the mammalian enzyme requires 10^{-5} to 10^{-6} M OP. Similar inhibition of the nematode enzyme requires 10^{-13} M in *Haemonchus* and 10^{-5} M in *Bunostomum*.

Toxicity is well documented with OP overdosage. Neurological symptoms develop rapidly in acute poisoning and are manifested as lack of coordination, hypersalivation, hyperventilation, and death. Chronic exposure is often initially diagnosed by a decrease in activity of serum cholinesterase and may result in transitory inappetence, salivation, lacrimation, and restlessness. OPs are sensitive to hydrolysis in the presence of water, especially at an alkaline pH, which is the primary mechanism of detoxification. Some OPs are quite volatile. Therefore, OPs must be either formulated in oil or in some way protected from water through encapsulation, resin embedment, or delivery in dry feed.

Orally administered OPs tend to have reduced activity against nematodes as they move farther through the digestive tract. To compensate for this loss of activity, continuous multiple doses at safe dose levels may deliver sufficient active drug to the large intestine.

Resistance to OPs is well documented in ectoparasites such as ticks and flies. Resistance in nematodes has been recorded very rarely; in fact, OPs have been used in combination with BZs to overcome small strongyle resistance in horses.

Narrow-spectrum Anthelmintics

Compounds may have a narrow spectrum because of a unique mode of action, some pharmacodynamic property that does not allow sufficient concentration or contact time for a target parasite, or the inherent host toxicity that limits their dose rate. However, narrow spectrum may simply mean that the compound is active against only a few economically important parasites such as flukes or tapeworms that are represented by few genera.

Chlorinated Hydrocarbons and Phenols

n-Butyl chloride, disophenol, and toluene are membrane-active drugs that are active against a narrow spectrum of nematodes in the gastrointestinal tract of dogs and cats. These drugs have a very narrow safety index and rely upon poor absorption in the host following oral administration for their differential toxicity.

This class of compounds is active against hookworms. Their mode of action is to uncouple electron-transport-associated phosphorylation, which occurs both in parasite and host-isolated mitochondria at similar concentrations. Therefore, even though substrate metabolism in the cell continues at an accelerated rate, no energy is generated and the cell dies.

Direct exposure of helminths to these compounds in vitro provides an array of visible effects because of the general membrane activity. Paralysis and membrane disruption result from generalized ionophore-type effects on nerve and surface membranes.

Host toxicity is generally expressed through hepatotoxic symptoms. More-acute symptoms are seen when ulceration of the digestive tract allows abnormal uptake into the bloodstream.

Salicylanilides

Rafoxanide, closantel, clioxanide, and niclosamide are similar in their mode of action to the substituted phenols but are less toxic. Drugs in this class are readily absorbed and avidly bind to serum albumin. This binding prevents high concentrations of free drug but keeps the drug circulating for long periods, providing broader spectrum and persistence of activity. Blood-ingesting nematodes (*Haemonchus*, hookworms), larval flies (nasal and stomach bots), ticks, and adult liver flukes are all within the spectrum of this class. Direct exposure in the gastrointestinal tract following oral administration provides additional activity against adult tapeworms.

Nitroxynil is the one exception to the orally administered salicylanilides. This subcutaneously administered product is active against adult liver flukes.

Piperazine

Two distinctly different, narrow-spectrum products are in the piperazine chemical group: piperazine and diethylcarbamazine (DEC). Piperazine is superbly active against intestinal-dwelling ascarids of swine and horses. The diethyl analog is active against L4 (fourth-stage larvae) of the filarial heartworm of dogs (*Dirofilaria immitis*). The mode of action of piperazine involves the hyperpolarization of the nematode muscle as a result of direct binding of the drug on the muscle membrane, causing an influx of chloride ions across the muscle cell. The resultant effect of the influx is to induce a reversible flaccid paralysis of the affected worm. Once the nematode is paralyzed, gastrointestinal motility removes the worm from the host.

DEC, on the other hand, does not appear to act directly on the parasite, but rather it "opsonizes" the larval (L3/L4) heartworms to be cleared by the immune system by immune-competent hosts. The exact method of opsonization is not clear, but lack of action in nonimmune hosts confirms this immune-related action. DEC toxicity is seen in occult heartworm infections. When microfilariae (L1) are absent from a blood smear, daily DEC therapy may begin. If microfilariae are sequestered and treatment with DEC begins, they are killed and a large dose of foreign protein can be released into the system, resulting in an anaphylactic shock reaction. Recently introduced diagnostic kits help identify these occult infections, so that arsenical treatment (for slow adult and microfilaria removal) or concomitant steroid therapy can obviate this problem.

Benzenedisulfonamide

Clorsulon is active specifically against the adult liver fluke, *Fasciola hepatica*, at an oral dose of 7 mg/kg or injectable dose of 2 mg/kg. The mechanism of action appears to be at the triose level of glucose metabolism by inhibition of two enzymes, phosphoglyceromutase and phosphoglycerate kinase. This inhibition effectively stops energy generation in the fluke. Because this drug binds tightly to carbonic anhydrase in the red blood cell, the pharmacodynamics may favor concentration in the fluke-ingesting red blood cells. This drug has a very wide margin of safety.

Clorsulon is available in combination with ivermectin as a product effective against nematodes, arthropods, and flukes.

Thiobenzimidazole

Triclabendazole, a thiobenzimidazole, chemically resembles the combination of a benzimidazole and a chlorinated phenol and seems to have action mechanisms similar to both classes. When administered orally, it is effective against all stages of liver flukes in sheep and cattle from day 1 postinfection through adults.

Phenothiazine

Phenothiazine (PZ) could be considered the first (or precursor) of the broad-spectrum anthelmintics. Phenothiazine appears to have a mode of action like a weakly binding BZ. It is partially effective against adult nematode parasites and decreases eggs being shed in the feces of treated animals. PZ-salt blocks have been used to reduce pasture contamination or to clean up pastures. Treated animals can show photosensitive reactions. The problem that resulted from use of PZ appears to have been a predisposition of certain isolates to BZ resistance even before these products were discovered. Presently, PZ is primarily used in combination products for efficacy against horse strongyles.

Cyanine Dyes

Cyanine dyes such as pyrvinium and dithiazanine are orally active products used primarily in dogs and rely on poor absorption by the host to prevent toxicity. These compounds appear to act by inhibition of glucose transport in anaerobic nematodes such as *Trichuris* and of electron-transport-associated oxidative metabolism in aerobic nematodes such as *Litomosoides*.

Arsenicals

Thiacetarsamide is still the drug of choice for adult heartworm in spite of its narrow margin of safety. This product kills adult worms slowly, so that a large, foreign protein load is not suddenly released on the immune system, thus avoiding an anaphylactic shock reaction. The mechanism of action of this drug is multifaceted, in that arsenical compounds bind to sulfhydryl (—SH) groups on protein. Many of these groups are key to the active site of enzymes in carbohydrate and folate metabolic pathways, glutathione reductase, and glucose transport. Which one is the primary site is impossible to determine; however, the ultimate mechanism and sites of host toxicity may involve many sites.

Isoquinolines

Praziquantel and epsiprantel are active against adult and larval tapeworms. In addition, praziquantel is active as an injectable and has activity against the blood flukes, *Schistosoma* spp., found in humans and cattle. The mode of action centers around ion flux across the surface membranes. In flukes exposed to praziquantel in vitro, calcium is taken up rapidly and results in a rapid, contracted paralysis. In adult cestodes, drug exposure results in the release of Ca^{2+} from muscle cell stores (calcareous corpuscles). In both cases, membrane integrity is compromised by these ionic effects, resulting in surface swellings and lesions. Host immune factors are activated by the damage and aid in the ultimate removal of the parasites. This class of drugs is chemically related to the benzodiazepines, which are psychoactive drugs in mammalian systems. Adverse side effects are generally mild and transitory in humans, with such symptoms as abdominal pain, headache, and nausea.

Conclusions

With the widespread use of anthelmintics, especially where domestic animals are raised in dense populations, anthelmintic resistance will continue to become a more important problem. Intelligent programs of drug class and pasture rotation combined with appropriate epidemiological timing have become absolute necessities in using the existing classes of compounds to their maximum benefit.

One area of parasite control that has received little attention has been the control of free-living larval development. Molt inhibitors such as invertebrate-specific steroid analogs, chitin synthesis inhibitors, and *Bacillus thuringiensis* endotoxins have been used successfully for control of arthropod larval development. Sufficient similarities exist between arthropod development and helminth development that they may warrant a similar approach.

A new direction in free-living larval control is the use of the nematophagous fungi such as *Duddingtonia flagrans*. Feed-through formulations of the digestion-resistant spores provide fungal hyphae in the fecal pat when parasitic nematode eggs hatch. These hyphae then paralyze and feed on the newly hatched larvae. The result is a much reduced pasture larval contamination, culminating in lowered reinfection rates (Faedo et al., 1998).

A second area of helminth parasitic control still not realized is control by immunization. Ever since successful vaccination of cattle with an attenuated larval lungworm vaccine, high hopes have been held for immunization. Recent molecular biological techniques and a more thorough understanding of helminth and host immune interactions may lead to future successes, but many difficulties still block this path. Until such time, continued searches for novel chemical classes that are nontoxic to the host will remain the approach adopted for helminth control.

Bibliography

Bennett JL, Kohler P. 1987. *Fasciola hepatica:* Action in vitro of triclabendazole on immature and adult stages. Exp Parasit 63:49.

Campbell WC. 1989. Ivermectin and Abamectin. New York: Springer-Verlag.

Campbell WC, Rew RS. 1986. Chemotherapy of Parasitic Disease. New York: Plenum.

Conder GA, Campbell WC. 1995. Chemotherapy of nematode infections of veterinary importance with special reference to drug resistance. Adv Parasitol 35:1.

Echevarria F, et al. 1997. Comparative study among moxidectin, ivermectin, and doramectin against ivermectin resistant *Haemonchus contortus* strain in artificially infected sheep in Brazil. Proc WAAVP, p24.

Faedo M, et al. 1998. The potential of nematophagous fungi to control the free-living stages of nematode parasites of sheep: pasture plot study with *Duddingtonia flagrans*. Vet Parasitol 76:129.

Gayrard V, et al. 1999. Comparison of pharmacokinetic profiles of doramectin and ivermectin pour-on formulations in cattle. Vet Parasitol 81:47.

Harnett W. 1988. The anthelmintic action of praziquantel. Parasit Today 4:144.

Hennessey DR, et al. 1995. The effect of short-term reduction in feed on the pharmacokinetics and efficacy of albendazole in sheep. Aust Vet J 72:29.

Lanusse C, et al. 1997. Comparative plasma disposition kinetics of ivermectin, moxidectin, and doramectin in cattle. J Vet Pharmacol Ther 20:91.

Leathwick DM, et al. 1998. Comparative efficacy of a new oxfendazole pour-on in cattle. Vet Rec 142:463.

Lifschitz A, et al. 1998. Distribution of endectocide compounds to target tissues in cattle. AAVP abstract, Baltimore, p59.

McKellar QA, Scott EW. 1990. The benzimidazole anthelmintic agents—a review. J Vet Pharmacol Ther 13:233.

Miller, J. 1994. Variable efficacy of benzimidazole anthelmintics against inhibited larvae of *Ostertagia ostertagi*. 26th Am Assoc Bovine Pract Proc, pp150.

Rew RS. 1978. Mode of action of common anthelmintics. J Vet Pharmacol Ther 1:183.

Shoop WL, et al. 1993. Mutual resistance to avermectins and milbemycins: oral activity of ivermectin and moxidectin against ivermectin-resistant and susceptible nematodes. Vet Rec 133:445.

Short CR, et al. 1987. Disposition of fenbendazole in cattle. Am J Vet Res 48:958.

21 | Antimicrobial Drug Use in Horses

S. GIGUERE and C. R. SWEENEY

Rational drug therapy has been defined as the selection of the proper drug to be administered according to a dosage regimen appropriate to the patient after due appraisal of potential benefits and risks of the therapy (Davis, 1982). The first step in this decision-making process is to determine whether an infectious agent is the likely cause of the disease, and if so, that the animal is unlikely to eliminate the infection efficiently without antibiotic therapy. In choosing the appropriate antimicrobial agent, the veterinarian must consider (1) the identity of the infecting microorganism(s); (2) the in vitro antimicrobial susceptibility pattern or the clinical response in equine patients infected with the same pathogen(s); (3) the nature and site of the infectious disease process; (4) the pharmacokinetic characteristics of the chosen antimicrobial agent in horses, such as bioavailability, tissue distribution, and rate of elimination; (5) the pharmacodynamic properties of the antimicrobial agent selected; (6) its safety in horses; and (7) the cost of therapy.

Because the identity and in vitro susceptibility of an infecting microorganism are rarely known when therapy is begun, initial therapy is usually empirical and is based on knowledge of the agents likely to be present and their historical susceptibility (see Tables 21.1 and 21.2). In some cases, the most likely etiologic agent can be highly suspected simply based on the clinical presentation and the horse's history. For example, abscessation of the submandibular and retropharyngeal lymph nodes is most likely caused by *Streptococcus equi* subsp. *equi*. On the other hand, pleuropneumonia in an adult horse may be caused by any one or combinations of a number of bacteria and thus requires bacteriologic culture of a tracheobronchial aspirate and pleural fluid to determine the etiologic

509

agent(s). A Gram stain of properly collected material is a simple, rapid, and inexpensive means of identifying the presence and morphological features of microorganisms in body fluids that are normally sterile. A negative Gram stain is, however, not sufficient to confirm the absence of microorganisms. Although visualization of bacteria on a Gram stain rarely reveals their identity, it can provide useful information regarding therapy while awaiting bacterial culture and antimicrobial susceptibility testing. For example, Gram-positive cocci in chains suggest *Streptococcus* spp., and *Streptococcus* spp. isolated from a purulent lesion in a horse are likely group C streptococci, which are usually susceptible to penicillin. On the other hand, the presence of both Gram-positive and Gram-negative bacteria indicate a mixed infection, which will require broad-spectrum antimicrobial agents at least until bacterial culture reveals the etiologic agents and their in vitro susceptibility pattern.

Once the etiological agent has been identified, the next step is to select an appropriate antibiotic. Susceptibility testing is not necessary for all clinical isolates. For example, most hemolytic *Streptococcus* pathogens isolated from horses are susceptible to penicillin G, as are most anaerobes except some *Bacteroides* spp. In contrast, most *Staphylococcus* and Gram-negative pathogens isolated from horses have variable antimicrobial susceptibility patterns (Table 21.1). While the etiologic agent may be susceptible to several antimicrobial agents, not all such agents may reach therapeutic concentrations at the site of infection. The rate and extent of penetration of a drug into sites outside the vascular space are determined by the drug's concentration in plasma, molecular charge and size, lipid solubility, and extent of plasma protein binding (see Chapters 4 and 5). It can also be affected by specific uptake by cells, cellular barriers (eg, blood-brain barrier), and tissue blood flow. Thus, the goal of antimicrobial therapy is to select an antibiotic that, in addition to exhibiting good antimicrobial activity against the infecting microorganism, will achieve therapeutic concentrations in the infected area.

Determination of the appropriate dose and dosing interval of an antimicrobial agent requires knowledge and integration of both its pharmacokinetics and pharmacodynamic properties. The pharmacokinetic properties of a drug describes its disposition within the body and includes the process of drug absorption, distribution, metabolism, and excretion (see Chapter 4). On the other hand, pharmacodynamic properties of a drug address the relationship between drug concentration and antimicrobial activity. The most significant factor determining the efficacy of beta-lactams, macrolides, tetracyclines, trimethoprim-sulfonamide combinations, chloramphenicol, and glycopeptides is the length of time that serum levels exceed the MIC of the pathogen. Increasing the concentration of the drug several-fold above the MIC does not significantly

TABLE 21.1. In vitro antimicrobial susceptibility of aerobic bacterial isolates from horses

Organisms	Number of Isolates	Antimicrobials[a]																
		ENR	AMI	GEN	PEN	AMP	OXA	CEF	CEP	TIC	TIM	CHL	ERY	RIF	TET	SUL	TMS	VAN
Gram-negative																		
Escherichia coli	380	98[b]	96	83	1	65	0	86	44	66	78	78	0	1	55	2	59	0
Pseudomonas aeruginosa	168	50	90	71	2	1	3	1	1	84	86	5	1	1	7	1	16	0
Actinobacillus equuli	98	99	99	97	59	74	89	96	95	86	98	93	12	95	93	60	74	7
Pasteurella/Actinobacillus spp.	59	100	88	100	92	93	78	100	100	97	100	100	44	96	92	48	95	12
Proteus spp.	40	98	93	70	8	23	0	88	45	55	88	55	20	0	8	5	40	0
Klebsiella spp.	115	95	96	81	3	5	2	92	79	5	75	79	1	1	69	1	70	1
Salmonella spp.	136	95	99	27	0	22	0	88	53	23	36	43	0	0	23	2	21	2
Enterobacter agglomerans	55	97	98	96	3	55	0	85	56	55	93	91	0	3	96	7	85	0
Enterobacter spp. (all other)	89	98	76	63	1	18	0	70	8	48	55	51	0	0	57	0	52	0
Gram-positive																		
Staphylococcus spp. (coagulase+)	166	95	96	71	27	42	83	76[c]	86	50	84	94	84	94	73	30	78	100
β-Hemolytic *Streptococcus* (group C)	122	75	26	68	93	97	100	97	99	98	97	95	94	96	61	28	81	98
α Hemolytic *Streptococcus* (not *Enterococcus*)	57	60	56	74	72	91	76	86	93	95	95	98	82	74	65	26	88	91
Enterococcus spp.	151	30	22	25	22	34	8	10	20	70	68	69	25	40	42	2	68	98
Rhodococcus equi	96	31	92	97	11	22	18	44	15	54	58	81	90	94	67	65	71	100

Sources: Data from clinical microbiology laboratories, University of Pennsylvania and University of Guelph (1993–1997).

[a] ENR, enrofloxacin; AMI, amikacin; GEN, gentamicin; PEN, penicillin; AMP, ampicillin; OXA, oxacillin; CEF, ceftiofur; CEP, cephalothin; TIC, ticarcillin; TIM, ticarcillin-clavulanic acid (Timentin); CHL, chloramphenicol; ERY, erythromycin; RIF, rifampin; TET, tetracycline; SUL, sulfadimethoxine; TMS, trimethoprim-sulfonamide; VAN, vancomycin.

[b] % of susceptible isolates [(number of susceptible isolates/number of isolates tested) × 100].

[c] In vivo, ceftiofur is rapidly metabolized to desfuroylceftiofur. Desfuroylceftiofur is as effective as ceftiofur against most bacterial pathogens but most coagulase-positive *Staphylococcus* spp. are resistant. Therefore, despite in vitro susceptibility, ceftiofur is not the ideal choice for the treatment of staphylococcal infections.

increase the rate of microbial killing. Rather, it is the length of time that bacteria are exposed to concentrations of these drugs above the MIC that dictates the rate of killing. Optimal dosing of such antimicrobial agents involves frequent administration. Other antimicrobial agents such as the aminoglycosides and fluoroquinolones exert concentration-dependent killing characteristics. Their rate of killing increases as the drug concentration increases above the MIC for the pathogen, and it is not necessary or even beneficial to maintain drug levels above the MIC between doses. Thus, optimal dosing of aminoglycosides and fluoroquinolones involves administration of high doses with long dosing intervals.

The route of administration and the antimicrobial preparations available also greatly influence the choice of an antimicrobial agent for use in the horse. Intravenous medication is usually restricted to hospitalized horses or those under the direct care of a veterinarian. Maintenance of an intravenous catheter in the field, while certainly possible, is not considered a routine practice. Intramuscular administration of antibiotics to the horse is restricted by duration of treatment and volume of the preparation (total dose) to be administered. Repeated injection of large volumes of medication results in local muscle necrosis and pain. Even well-behaved horses object to repeated injections. Novice horse owners can rarely use the IM site of injection in the rump and thus are limited to rotation of injection sites on both sides of the neck. For this reason, oral administration of antibiotics is the most popular route of administration to horses.

Unfortunately, several antimicrobial agents commonly used orally in other monogastric species, such as penicillin G, amoxicillin, cefadroxil, and ciprofloxacin, are poorly absorbed, particularly in adult horses, and therefore cannot be used orally. The large bowel of the horse makes this species particularly susceptible to antimicrobial-induced enterocolitis secondary to disruption of the normal colonic microflora and overgrowth of pathogenic microorganisms, most likely *Clostridium* spp., including *C. difficile*. The onset of acute and sometimes fatal diarrhea in the horse has been anecdotally associated with the use of almost every oral and parenteral antimicrobial agent. However, orally administered antimicrobials with low bioavailability and good activity against anaerobes are most likely to induce diarrhea. For this reason, oral beta-lactam antimicrobials should be used with caution in the horse. Antimicrobials that are partially excreted in the bile after parenteral administration should also be used with caution. Certain antibiotics such as lincomycin and clindamycin are associated with well-recognized enterocolitis syndromes, and their use must be avoided in horses. Other antibiotics such as oral trimethoprim-sulfonamide combinations, erythromycin, chloramphenicol and metronidazole, and parenteral oxytetracycline and cephalosporins have been occasionally linked to enterocolitis in horses. In one study, administration of oxytetracycline to horses was associated with the proliferation of *Clostridium perfringens* type A and possible toxin production (White and Prior, 1982). Anecdotally, in some parts of the world some antibiotics are known to induce diarrhea, whereas they are used extensively in other parts of the world without evidence of such side effect. This marked geographic variation in the incidence of antibiotic-induced diarrhea likely results from differences in colonic microflora. Foals seem less susceptible to antibiotic-induced enterocolitis than adult horses.

Many of the diseases involving the neonatal foal are the sequelae of septicemia. These diseases include pneumonia, peritonitis, meningitis, osteomyelitis, septic arthritis, and omphalophlebitis. Although specific recommendations have been made for each of the sites of infection, there are general recommendations for therapy of such bacterial infections. Pending culture results, a broad-spectrum bactericidal antibiotic combination should be used. If blood or other cultures are positive, antibiotic therapy can then be adjusted according to the susceptibility test results. If the animal is septicemic, a minimum of 2 weeks of antibiotic therapy is recommended; if the infection is well established in an organ, such as the lung, joints, or bones, then antibiotics should be provided on a long-term basis (Koterba, 1990). For other nonsepticemic bacterial infections, duration of treatment should continue for at least 72 hours after return to clinical normality and should be considerably longer in the case of life-threatening infections such as pleuropneumonia, pulmonary or abdominal abscess, peritonitis, osteomyelitis, and endocarditis. In addition to a thorough physical examination, other diagnostic tests such as hematology, serum biochemistry, radiographs, and/or ultrasonographic examination may be useful, depending on the disease process, to determine when it is appropriate to discontinue therapy.

The remainder of this chapter outlines major infectious diseases of horses by organ system and provides recommendations for initial selection of antimicrobial agents while awaiting culture and sensitivity results (Table 21.2). Suggested drug dosages are shown in Tables 21.3 and 21.4. Once an antimicrobial agent has been selected, the reader should consult the appropriate chapter for potential toxicities and specific contraindications. Very few of the antimicrobial agents mentioned in this chapter have been approved for use in horses. Those that have been approved are often recommended at higher dosages or to treat a disease other than that for which the compound is approved. Therefore, for most antibiotics, controlled safety studies involving administration of the drug to a large number of horses have not been performed. It must also be remembered that, although this chapter deals strictly with antimicrobial therapy, supportive, local, or surgical therapy may in some cases be as important as the antibiotic in resolution of the infection.

Bibliography

Beard LA. 1998. Principles of antimicrobial therapy. In: Reed SM, Baily WM, eds. Equine Internal Medicine. Philadelphia: WB Saunders.

Brumbaugh GW. 1987. Rational selection of antimicrobial drugs for treatment of infections of horses. Vet Clin Equine Pract 3(1):191.

Caprile KA, Short CR. 1987. Pharmacologic consideration in drug therapy in foals. Vet Clin Equine Pract 3(1):123.

Davis LE. 1982. Rational therapeutics. In: Mansmann RA, et al., eds. Equine Medicine and Surgery, 3rd ed. Santa Barbara, CA: American Veterinary Publications.

Ensink JM, et al. 1993. In-vitro susceptibility to antimicrobial drugs of bacterial isolates from horses in the Netherlands. Equine Vet J 25:309.

Hirsh DC. 1987. Antimicrobic susceptibility of bacterial pathogens from horses. Vet Clin Equine Pract 3(1):181.

Hyatt JM, et al. 1995. The importance of pharmacokinetic/pharmacodynamic surrogate markers of outcome. Clin Pharmacokinet 28:143.

Koterba AM. 1990. Antibiotic therapy. In: Koterba AM, et al., eds. Equine Clinical Neonatology. Philadelphia: Lea and Febiger.

Moore RM, et al. 1992. Antimicrobial susceptibility of bacterial isolates from 233 horses with musculoskeletal infection during 1979-1989. Equine Vet J 24:450.

Walker RD. 1997. New perspectives on antimicrobial chemotherapy. In: Robinson NE, ed. Current Therapy in Equine Medicine, 4th ed. Philadelphia: WB Saunders.

White G, Prior SD. 1982. Comparative effects of oral administration of trimethoprim/sulphadiazine or oxytetracycline on the faecal flora of horses. Vet Rec 111:316.

TABLE 21.2. **Antimicrobial drug selection in infection of horses**

Site	Diagnosis	Common Infecting Organism(s)	Comments	Suggested Drug(s)	Alternative Drug(s)
Upper respiratory tract	Strangles	*Streptococcus equi*	Treatment of a horse with strangles depends on the stage of the disease. Although the organism is sensitive to penicillin, parenteral antibiotics given after abscess formation may prolong the disease. Horses with severe systemic signs require antibiotics.	Penicillin G[a]	Ceftiofur; trimethoprim-sulfonamide[b]
	Gutteral pouch empyema	*Streptococcus* spp.	Local irrigation with saline is the treatment of choice. Lowering the horse's head facilitates drainage and reduces the risks of aspiration. Systemic antimicrobials rarely indicated unless infection is spreading.	Penicillin G[a]	Ceftiofur; trimethoprim-sulfonamide[b]
	Gutteral pouch mycosis	*Aspergillus nidulans*, *A. fumigatus*, other opportunistic fungi	Surgical therapy is the treatment of choice. Even when	Topical natamycin; systemic antifungal	Topical enilconazole

TABLE 21.2. *Continued*

Site	Diagnosis	Common Infecting Organism(s)	Comments	Suggested Drug(s)	Alternative Drug(s)
			successful, medical therapy is too slow to prevent several bouts of hemorrhage.	agents usually not required	
	Fungal rhinitis	Aspergillus spp., other opportunistic fungi	Surgical removal of the mycotic plaque and associated necrotic tissue, combined with topical antifungal therapy.	Topical natamycin	Topical enilconazole
	Sinusitis, primary	Streptococcus zooepidemicus, S. equi	Treatment may consist of a daily lavage of sinus with saline (± antiseptics or antimicrobial agents) combined with systemic antimicrobial agents. Nonresponsive cases may require sinusotomy.	Penicillin G[a]	Ceftiofur; trimethoprim-sulfonamide[b]
	Sinusitis, secondary	Mixed opportunistic aerobic[c] and anaerobic[d] infection	Usually requires treatment of primary problem, ie, removal of diseased tooth.	Penicillin G[a]	Trimethoprim-sulfonamide[b] and metronidazole; chloramphenicol

System	Condition	Organism(s)	Comments	First choice	Alternative
Lung	Bacterial pneumonia or lung abscesses; adults	S. zooepidemicus, opportunistic aerobic pathogens,[c] S. pneumoniae	S. zooepidemicus is most commonly isolated.	Penicillin G[a] is drug of choice initially if streptococcal infection suspected. If mixed infection, broad-spectrum antibiotics[e] are required.	Ceftiofur; trimethoprim-sulfonamide;[b] erythromycin ± rifampin for S. zooepidemicus abscesses
		Mycoplasma spp.		Oxytetracycline	Enrofloxacin,[f] erythromycin; chloramphenicol
	Bacterial pneumonia or lung abscesses; older foals	S. zooepidemicus	Most common cause of pneumonia/bronchitis in older foals.	Penicillin G[a]	Ceftiofur; trimethoprim-sulfonamide;[b] erythromycin ± rifampin for S. zooepidemicus abscesses
		Opportunistic aerobic[c]		Broad-spectrum antibiotics[e]	Third-generation cephalosporins; ticarcillin–clavulanic acid
		Rhodococcus equi	Treatment must be a minimum of 3–4 weeks.	Rifampin and erythromycin	Chloramphenicol ± rifampin; trimethoprim-sulfonamide ± rifampin
		Pneumocystis carinii	May be found in immunocompromised foals or in association with R. equi.	Trimethoprim-sulfonamide	
	Bacterial pneumonia; neonatal foals	Opportunistic aerobic pathogens[c]	Neonatal pneumonia often a part of a generalized infection affecting many different organ systems.	Broad-spectrum antibiotics[e] (amikacin preferred over gentamicin)	Third-generation cephalosporins; ticarcillin–clavulanic acid

TABLE 21.2. *Continued*

Site	Diagnosis	Common Infecting Organism(s)	Comments	Suggested Drug(s)	Alternative Drug(s)
	Pleuropneumonia	Opportunistic aerobic[c] and anaerobic pathogens[d]	Although systemic antimicrobial agents are most essential treatment for bacterial pleuropneumonia, thoracic drainage and nursing care are important.	Broad-spectrum antibiotics[e] ± metronidazole	Ceftiofur ± metronidazole; trimethoprim-sulfonamide and metronidazole; penicillinG[a] and enrofloxacin[f] ± metronidazole
		Mycoplasma felis		Oxytetracycline	Enrofloxacin;[f] erythromycin; chloramphenicol
	Fungal pneumonia	Opportunistic fungi: *Aspergillus* spp., *Candida* spp., *Mucor* spp., *Cryptococcus* spp.	If fungal pneumonia is secondary to severe primary disease (ie, liver failure, enterocolitis, peritonitis, etc.), treatment is difficult and prognosis is poor. If fungal pneumonia is secondary to aggressive antibiotic therapy (ie, neonatal foal), then prognosis is guarded.	Amphotericin B	Itraconazole

System	Disease	Organism	Comments	Drug of Choice	Alternative
Gastro-intestinal	Tuberculosis	*Mycobacterium*	Treatment is not usually attempted. Public health concern. Reportable disease.	See Chapter 19	
	Oral, gastric candidiasis	*Candida* spp.	Seen in immuno-suppressed animals or animals on long-term antibiotic therapy. May just require discontinu-ation of antibiotic therapy.	Fluconazole	Amphotericin B; itraconazole
	Acute enterocolitis; salmonellosis	*Salmonella typhimurium*, other serovars	Systemic antimicrobials indicated in animals showing signs of or at risk for septicemia (foals, immunocompro-mised animals, aged animals). Treatment with antibiotic is not thought to alter the course of the disease.	Broad-spectrum antibiotics;[e] susceptibility variable	Third-generation cephalosporins; susceptibility variable
	Acute enterocolitis; clostridiosis	*Clostridium difficile*, C. perfringens type A; C. perfringens type C	The first approach in therapy is to stop the precipitating antimicrobial agent when applicable.	Metronidazole	Oral bacitracin (22 mg/kg PO BID day 1, then SID); oral vancomycin[g]
	Potomac horse fever (equine ehrlichial colitis)	*Ehrlichia risticii*		Oxytetracycline	Rifampin and erythromycin; oral doxycycline[h]
	Proliferative enteropathy	*Lawsonia intracellularis*	Proliferative illeitis and diarrhea in foals.	Erythromycin ± rifampin	Oxytetracycline

TABLE 21.2. *Continued*

Site Diagnosis	Common Infecting Organism(s)	Comments	Suggested Drug(s)	Alternative Drug(s)
Abdominal abscess	*Streptococcus equi,* *S. zooepidemicus,* *Corynebacterium* *pseudotuberculosis*	Most commonly a complication of strangles. Long-term treatment frequently required.	Penicillin G[a]	Erythromycin ± rifampin; chloramphenicol; trimethoprim-sulfonamide[b]
	R. equi (foals)	Abdominal abscess(es) and ulcerative enterocolitis. Peritonitis may be present. Pneumonia, diarrhea, septic physitis or arthritis may occur concurrently.	Rifampin and erythromycin	Chloramphenicol ± rifampin; trimethoprim-sulfonamide ± rifampin
Peritonitis	Mixed opportunistic aerobic[c] and anaerobic[d] pathogens, *Actinobacillus equuli*	Obtaining culture and sensitivity of peritoneal fluid highly recommended. Peritoneal lavage may be beneficial in some cases.	Broad-spectrum antibiotics[e] and metronidazole	Third-generation cephalosporin and metronidazole; penicillin G[a] + enrofloxacin + metronidazole
Tyzzer's disease	*Clostridium piliforme*	Treatment is usually not successful.	Erythromycin ± rifampin; penicillin G[a] and aminoglycoside	Oxytetracycline
Liver abscess	Beta-hemolytic streptococci, *Corynebacterium pseudotuberculosis*, opportunistic aerobic[c] or anaerobic[d] pathogens	Ultrasound may be helpful in diagnosis. May occur concurrently with other abdominal abscess(es). Long-term treatment required.	Broad-spectrum antibiotics[e] in combination with rifampin or metronidazole	

Cholangiohepatitis	Gram-negative enteric organisms	May be difficult to identify the offending organism(s). Long-term therapy required. Prognosis is poor when several obstructing calculi are present. For obstructing stones, choledo-cholithotomy may be indicated.	Trimethoprim-sulfonamide	Ceftiofur; enrofloxacin
Soft tissue				
Candidiasis	Candida spp.	Infection of multiple systems may occur. Fungemia, although uncommon, has been seen in immunocompromised foals on aggressive, broad-spectrum antibiotic therapy.	Fluconazole	Amphotericin B; itraconazole
Bacterial septicemia	E. coli, opportunistic aerobic[c] pathogens (mostly Gram-negatives)	Neonate is most commonly affected. Parental administration of antibiotics recommended, at least initially. Treatment required for a minimum of 2 weeks.	Broad-spectrum antibiotics[e] (amikacin preferred over gentamicin)	Third-generation cephalosporins; ticarcillin–clavulanic acid

TABLE 21.2. *Continued*

Site	Diagnosis	Common Infecting Organism(s)	Comments	Suggested Drug(s)	Alternative Drug(s)
	Omphalaphlebitis	Opportunistic aerobic[c] pathogens	Diagnostic ultrasound is useful when external signs of infection are not apparent. Surgical resection may be the treatment of choice in some cases.	Broad-spectrum antibiotic[e] (amikacin preferred over gentamicin)	Third-generatioan cephalosporins; ticarcillin–clavulanic acid
	Fistulous withers	*Brucella abortus, Actinomyces bovis*	Public health concern with brucellosis. Treatment regimen using killed *Brucella* vaccine may be effective.	Oxytetracycline and streptomycin or gentamicin	Oral doxycycline[h] or trimethoprim-sulfonamid and gentamicin or rifampin
		Opportunistic aerobic[c] and anaerobic[d] pathogens		Broad-spectrum antibiotics[e]	Ceftiofur; trimethoprim-sulfonamide
	Traumatic and contaminated wounds	Opportunistic aerobic[c] and anaerobic[d] pathogens	Exploration, lavage, debridement, and local therapy are more important than systemic antimicrobial agents.	Trimethoprim-sulfonamide (superficial wound); broad-spectrum antibiotics[e] (deep contaminated wound)	Ceftiofur
	Ulcerative lymphangitis, subcutaneous abscesses	*C. pseudotuberculosis*	Drainage of *C. pseudotuberculosis* abscesses is preferred over antibiotic therapy. Systemic antibiotics required for ulcerative	Penicillin G[a]	Erythromycin ± rifampin; trimethoprim-sulfonamide; chloramphenicol

Disease	Organisms	Comments	Antibiotic of choice	Alternative antibiotics
Subcutaneous abscesses	Beta-hemolytic *Streptococcus* spp.	lymphangitis, for internal abscesses, or in horses with signs of systemic illness. Drainage of abscesses preferred over antibiotic therapy. Systemic antibiotics required for internal abscesses or in horses with signs of systemic illness.	Penicillin G[a]	Erythromycin ± rifampin; chloramphenicol; trimethoprim-sulfonamide[b]
Burns	*Pseudomonas aeruginosa*, *Staphylococcus aureus*, other opportunistic aerobic[c] pathogens	Care of burn wounds includes thorough cleansing, surgical debridement, daily hydrotherapy, and topical antimicrobials. Systemic antibiotics are not effective in preventing local burn wound infections and may permit the growth of resistant bacteria. Systemic antibiotics only if signs of systemic infection.	Topical: silver sulfadiazine cream. Systemic: broad-spectrum antibiotics[e]	Ticarcillin–clavulanic acid; third-generation cephalosporins
Clostridial myonecrosis	*Clostridium perfringens*, *C. septicum*, *C. chauvoei*, other spp.	Surgical debridement, including fasciotomy, and supportive care are essential. Poor prognosis.	Penicillin G (IV every 2–4 hours)	Metronidazole; chloramphenicol

TABLE 21.2. *Continued*

Site	Diagnosis	Common Infecting Organism(s)	Comments	Suggested Drug(s)	Alternative Drug(s)
Bone and joint	Osteomyelitis; septic arthritis (neonates)	Opportunistic aerobic[c] pathogens *R. equi*, *Salmonella* spp.	In foals, osteomyelitis and septic arthritis are seen secondary to septicemia. Antibiotics and surgical debridement are required for osteomyelitis. Antibiotics and joint lavage are required for septic arthritis. Intra-articular antibiotics (eg, amikacin 125 mg) may be beneficial.	Broad-spectrum antibiotics[e] (amikacin preferred over gentamicin); rifampin and erythromycin for *R. equi*	Third-generation cephalosporins; ticarcillin–clavulanic acid
	Osteomyelitis (adults)	Opportunistic aerobic[c] pathogens	Usually secondary to traumatic and contaminated wounds. Antibiotics and surgical debridement are required.	Broad-spectrum antibiotics[e]	Third-generation cephalosporins; trimethoprim-sulfa
	Septic arthritis or tenosynovitis (adults)	*Staphylococcus* spp., opportunistic aerobic[c] pathogens	In adults, septic arthritis is usually associated with intra-articular injection or wounds. Joint/tendon sheath drainage and lavage are highly recommended. Intra-articular antibiotics (eg, amikacin 125 mg) may be beneficial. In vitro susceptibility testing highly recommended.	First-generation cephalosporin and amikacin or gentamicin	Broad-spectrum antibiotics;[e] trimethoprim-sulfonamide

	Disease	Organism	Comments		
Skin	Lyme disease	*Borrelia burgdorferi*	Definitive diagnosis is difficult. Presence of serum antibody does not indicate disease.	Oxytetracycline	Oral doxycycline;[h] ceftriaxone; ceftiofur
	Dermatophilosis (streptothricosis, rain rot)	*Dermatophilus congolensis*	Systemic therapy often unnecessary and generally reserved for severe or generalized cases. Infected animals should be groomed and bathed daily with providone-iodine shampoo or chlorhexidine solution (Novalsan 2%). If treatment is systemic, a short course of antibiotics is often effective (3–5 days).	Procaine penicillin G	Ampicillin
	Folliculitis/furunculosis	*Staphylococcus* spp., *Streptococcus* spp., *Corynebacterium pseudotuberculosis*	Same as dermatophilosis. Antibiotics, if required, should be based on culture/sensitivity.	Trimethoprim-sulfonamide	Broad-spectrum antibiotics[e]
	Staphylococcal cellulitis	*Staphylococcus aureus, S. intermedius*	Requires aggressive systemic antibiotics.	First-generation cephalosporin and gentamicin or (amikacin preferred)	Broad-spectrum antibiotics;[e] trimethoprim-sulfonamide; erythromycin

TABLE 21.2. *Continued*

Site	Diagnosis	Common Infecting Organism(s)	Comments	Suggested Drug(s)	Alternative Drug(s)
	Dermatophytosis	*Trichophyton equinum, T. mentagrophytes, Microsporum gypseum, M. equinum,* etc.	Disease may spontaneously regress, but therapy may shorten the recovery period and may decrease the spread of the disease. Topical therapy is sufficient. Treat the whole body of all contact animals.	5% lime sulfur or 0.5% sodium hypochloride solution or providone-iodine topically daily for 3–5 days and reapply weekly until resolution of infection	Topical natamycin; topical enilconazole; topical miconazole
	Sporotrichosis	*Sporothrix schenckii*	Treatment is often effective. Continue treatment for several weeks after lesions disappear, or relapse will occur. Systemic iodides may cause abortion in pregnant mares.	Sodium iodide (40 mg/kg of 20% solution IV for 2–5 days), followed by oral potassium iodide (2 mg/kg SID PO until lesions regress)	Fluconazole; itraconazole
	Pythiosis (phycomycosis, swamp cancer, Florida horse leech, Bursatti, Gulf Coast fungus)	*Pythium insidiosum*	Immediate radical surgical removal of all infected tissues is essential for effective treatment. Early immunotherapy with soluble *Pythium* antigens[i] is effective, especially when combined with surgical removal.	Topical or intralesional amphotericin B	Systemic amphotericin B; systemic sodium iodide (see Sporotrichosis)

System	Disease	Pathogens	Comments	Drug of choice	Alternative
Renal	Cystitis	Opportunistic aerobic[c] bacteria, *Candida* spp.	Cystitis is usually secondary to urolithiasis, bladder neoplasia, or bladder paralysis. Treat for 7–10 days, and reculture urine.	Trimethoprim-sulfonamide; fluconazole for *Candida* spp.	Ceftiofur; broad-spectrum antibiotics[e]
	Pyelonephritis	Opportunistic aerobic[c] bacteria	Same predisposing factors as cystitis. Usually chronic and insidious, may be difficult to treat. Use aminoglycosides cautiously in face of renal disease. Treat a minimum of 2–3 weeks; duration required is variable and may be longer.	Trimethoprim-sulfonamide; third-generation cephalosporin	Broad-spectrum antibiotics;[e] penicillin G[a] and enrofloxacin[f]
Cardiovascular	Bacterial endocarditis	*Streptococcus* spp., opportunistic aerobic[c] pathogens	Prognosis is poor to grave. Long-term treatment is required (several months). Antibiotic choice should be based on blood culture.	Broad-spectrum antibiotics[e] ± rifampin	Third-generation cephalosporin
	Bacterial pericarditis	*Streptococcus* spp., mixed opportunistic aerobic[c] and anaerobic[d] pathogens	Prognosis is guarded. Culture of pericardial fluid is recommended. Drainage and lavage of the pericardial sac are also recommended.	Broad-spectrum antibiotics[e]	Third-generation cephalosporin

TABLE 21.2. *Continued*

Site	Diagnosis	Common Infecting Organism(s)	Comments	Suggested Drug(s)	Alternative Drug(s)
	Thrombophlebitis	Mixed opportunistic aerobic and anaerobic pathogens	Blood culture recommended.	Broad-spectrum antibiotics[e] ± metronidazole	Ceftiofur; trimethoprim-sulfonamide
Nervous	Bacterial meningitis or spinal abscess	Opportunistic aerobic[c] pathogens	Most often associated with neonatal septicemia. Prognosis is poor.	Third-generation cephalosporin[i] ± aminoglycoside (amikacin preferred)	Broad-spectrum antibiotics;[e] trimethoprim-sulfonamide
	Mycotic meningitis/encephalitis	*Cryptococcus neoformans, Aspergillus* spp.	Prognosis is grave.	Amphotericin B	Fluconazole
	Brain abscess	*Streptococcus equi, Streptococcus* spp.	Prognosis grave.	Penicillin G[a]	Third-generation cephalosporin;[j] trimethoprim-sulfonamide
	Tetanus	*Clostridium tetani*	Antibiotics to eliminate the infection, but tetanus antitoxin to neutralize the unbound toxin.	Penicillin G[a]	Ampicillin
	Botulism	*Clostridium botulinum*	Antitoxin to neutralize unbound toxin. Antibiotics if suspected wound contamination or to prevent complications such as aspiration pneumonia.	Penicillin G[a]	Ampicillin

528

	Condition	Organisms	Comments	Treatment	
	Otitis media/interna	*Actinobacillus* spp. *Staphylococcus* spp., *Streptococcus* spp., opportunistic aerobic[c] pathogens		Trimethoprim-sulfonamide	Chloramphenicol; third-generation cephalosporin
	Equine protozoal myeloencephalitis	*Sarcocystis neurona*	Cause vestibulocochlear and/or facial nerve dysfunction, as well as head shaking. Treatment may stop progression of disease and occasionally reverse clinical signs. Long-term therapy required (3–5 months).	Sulfadiazine (24 mg/kg PO SID or BID) and pyrimethamine (1 mg/kg PO SID)	Diclazuril (5 mg/kg PO SID)
Ophthalmic	Bacterial keratitis; mild corneal ulceration	Gram-negative or Gram-positive opportunistic bacteria	Topical (or subconjunctival when appropriate) application (see Chapter 19)	Topical bacitracin-neomycin-polymixin B combinations	Topical gentamicin
	Bacterial keratitis; severe melting keratitis	*Pseudomonas aeruginosa*	Topical (or subconjunctival when appropriate) application (see Chapter 19)	Topical tobramycin; topical amikacin	Topical ciprofloxacin
	Fungal keratitis	*Aspergillus* spp., *Alternaria* spp. *Mucor* spp., *Fusarium* spp., *Candida* spp.	Topical application.	Natamycin	Miconazole; silver sulfadiazine; itraconazole-DMSO ointment
	Foreign body penetration	Gram-negative or Gram-positive bacteria, fungal agents	Topical broad-spectrum coverage. Systemic antimicrobials indicated if anterior chamber penetrated and/or if periorbital tissues are infected.	Topical gentamicin; systemic broad-spectrum antibiotics[e]	Topical tobramycin; systemic trimethoprim-sulfonamide; penicillin G[a] and enrofloxacin[f]

TABLE 21.2. *Continued*

Site	Diagnosis	Common Infecting Organism(s)	Comments	Suggested Drug(s)	Alternative Drug(s)
	Manifestation of systemic disease	Bacterial: *Actinobacillus equuli*, leptospirosis, *R. equi, Streptococcus equi* Fungal: *Cryptococcus* spp., *Histoplasma* spp., *Aspergillus* spp.	Ocular signs are often immune mediated. Primary treatment is aimed at systemic disease. Often associated with optic neuritis, chorioretinitis, anterior uveitis, blepharitis, purulent conjunctivitis.	See specific infection See Chapter 19	
Reproductive tract	Retained placenta	*S. zooepidemicus*, coliforms	Bacterial infections are commonly associated with prolonged (>6–8 hours) retention of membranes. Systemic antimicrobials recommended if early treatment with oxytocin fails.	Broad-spectrum antibiotics[e]	Trimethoprim-sulfonamide; third-generation cephalosporin
	Endometritis, metritis, and pyometra	*S. zooepidemicus*, *E. coli, P. aeruginosa*, *Klebsiella pneumoniae*	Control of pneumo-vagina (Caslick's) is indicated in most cases. Urovagina and peritoneal lacerations also predispose to infection. Anti-septics used by the	Intrauterine therapy daily for 4–6 days during estrus or early diestrus (see Table 21.4); choice of agent based on culture and sensitivity	

Condition	Organisms	Comments	Treatment	
		intrauterine route may induce a chemical irritation. Uterine lavage and hormonal therapy (eg, oxytocin, PGF_2) are adjunct treatments. Systemic antibiotics are indicated primarily when endometrial biopsy suggests a deep endometrial infection or in cases of septic metritis with systemic clinical signs. Therapy based on in vitro susceptibility testing.		
Fungal endometritis	*Candida* spp., *Aspergillus* spp.	Systemic antifungal agents are usually not warranted.	Intrauterine: clotrimazole (cream or suspension 500 mg daily for 7 days) Trimethoprim-sulfonamide	Intrauterine: nystatin (500,000 IU); amphotericin B (50–100 mg) Broad-spectrum antibiotics[e]
Placentitis	Highly variable. *S. zooepidemicus, E. coli, Klebsiella* spp., are most common	Culture and sensitivity of discharge are highly recommended because organism(s) involved is unpredictable. It may be difficult to obtain effective antibiotic levels at site of infection, and resolution of infection may not be possible until after paturition.		

TABLE 21.2. *Continued*

Site	Diagnosis	Common Infecting Organism(s)	Comments	Suggested Drug(s)	Alternative Drug(s)
	Contagious equine metritis	*Taylorella equigenitalis*	Mares may become carriers once infected. Stallions are asymptomatic carriers. Reportable disease.	Mares: intrauterine potassium penicillin, cleansing of vulva and clitoral fossa with 4 chlorexidine solution, followed with packing of the clitoral fossa with chlorexidine or nitrofurazone ointment. Stallions: potassium penicillin G 2000 IU/ml of semen extender. Wash penis daily with chlorhexidine solution and pack with nitrofurazone ointment.	
	Mastitis	*S. zooepidemicus*, *Staphylococcus* spp., other opportunistic aerobic[c] pathogens, *Mycoplasma* spp.	Systemic antimicrobial therapy is recommended. Intramammary preparations for cows may also be used.	Trimethoprim-sulfonamide; oxytetracycline for *Mycoplasma* spp.	Broad-spectrum antibiotics[e]
	Balanoposthitis	*Streptococcus zooepidemicus*, *Pseudomonas* spp., *Klebsiella* spp.	Bacterial balanoposthitis as a clinical problem is uncommon. Antimicrobial therapy is directed at infected semen or the recipient mare	Potassium penicillin G 1000 IU and amikacin 1000 g per ml of semen extender	Ticarcillin 1000 g per ml of semen extender

		through the use of antimicrobials in semen extender. Recipient is infused with treated extender immediately prior to natural service. Washing of penis and prepuce with a mild soap is recommended. Disinfectant or topical antibiotics should not be used routinely because recolonization may occur and this treatment may displace commensals and allow pathogens to become established.	
Seminal vesiculitis	*P. aeruginosa, K. pneumoniae, Streptococcus* spp., *Staphylococcus* spp.	Systemic antibiotics based on in vitro susceptibility testing. Antibiotics can also be deposited in the seminal vesicle, using a flexible endoscope. If infection cannot be eradicated, appropriate semen extender must be used for breeding (see recommendations for balanoposthitis).	Broad-spectrum antibiotics[e]
			Ticarcillin–clavulanic acid; penicillin G[a] and ciprofloxacin[f] or enrofloxacin[f]

TABLE 21.2. *Continued*

Site	Diagnosis	Common Infecting Organism(s)	Comments	Suggested Drug(s)	Alternative Drug(s)
	Orchitis, epididymitis	*Streptococcus zooepidemicus, K. pneumoniae*	In vitro susceptibility testing is recommended.	Broad-spectrum antibiotics[e]	Third-generation cephalosporins; trimethoprim-sulfonamide
Systemic diseases	Leptospirosis	*Leptospira interrogans* serovar *bratislava, pomona,* and others	Uveitis, nephritis, abortions, pyrexia, liver dysfunction.	Ampicillin or penicillin G	Oxytetracycline; streptomycin
	Equine ehrlichiosis	*Ehrlichia equi*	Fever, limb edema, petechiation, ataxia, anemia, leukopenia, thrombocytopenia.	Oxytetracycline	Oral doxycycline[h]

[a] Penicillin G (potassium, sodium, procaine).

[b] Some streptococci may be resistant to trimethoprim-sulfonamide.

[c] Includes *E. coli, Pasteurella* spp., *Actinobacillus* spp., *Klebsiella* spp., *Pseudomonas aeruginosa, Enterobacter* spp., *Proteus* spp., *Staphylococcus aureus,* and *Streptococcus zooepidemicus.*

[d] Includes *Bacteroides* spp., *Fusobacterium* spp., *Clostridium* spp., *Peptostreptococcus* spp., and others.

[e] Combination of a beta-lactam (penicillin G or ceftiofur or ampicillin) and an aminoglycoside (gentamicin or amikacin).

[f] Should not be used in young growing horses because of the risk of arthropathy.

[g] The use of vancomycin should be restricted for severely ill cases with confirmed *Clostridium* sp. infection resistant to conventional antimicrobials.

[h] Administer orally only. Intravenous doxycycline has resulted in severe cardiovascular effects, including collapse and death in some horses.

[i] Biomedical services, Austin, Texas, USA.

[j] As opposed to most other third-generation cephalosporins, ceftiofur does not cross the normal blood-brain barrier.

TABLE 21.3. **Common antimicrobial drug dosage in horses**

Drug Preparation	Dose	Dose Interval (h)	Route of Administration
Beta-lactams			
Benzyl penicillins			
Penicillin G (Na, K)	20,000–40,000 IU/kg	6	IV
Penicillin G (procaine)	20,000 IU/kg	12	IM
Penicillin V	110,000 IU/kg	8	PO
Aminobenzylpenicillins			
Ampicillin sodium	20–30 mg/kg	6–8	IV or IM
Ampicillin trihydrate	20 mg/kg	12	IM
	20 mg/kg	8	PO (foals only)
Amoxicillin trihydrate	30 mg/kg	8	PO (foals only)
Bacampicillin	25 mg/kg	12	PO
Pivampicillin	25 mg/kg	12	PO
Antistaphylococcal penicillins			
Oxacillin	25 mg/kg	8–12	IM
	25–35 mg/kg	6	IV
Antipseudomonal penicillins			
Ticarcillin	50 mg/kg	6	IV
Ticarcillin–clavulanic acid	50 mg/kg	6	IV
Piperacillin	30 mg/kg	6	IV
First-generation cephalosporins			
Cefazolin	20 mg/kg	8	IM
	20 mg/kg	6	IV
Cephalothin	20 mg/kg	8	IM
	20–30 mg/kg	6	IV
Cephapirin	20 mg/kg	8	IM
	20–30 mg/kg	6	IV
Cephradine	25 mg/kg	6	IV
	25 mg/kg	6–8	PO (foals only)
Cefadroxil	20–40 mg/kg	8	PO (foals only)
Second-generation cephalosporins			
Cefoxitin	20 mg/kg	8	IV or IM
Third-generation cephalosporins			
Cefepime	2.2 mg/kg	8	IV or IM
Cefoperazone	30 mg/kg	6–8	IV or IM
Cefotaxime	40 mg/kg	6	IV
Ceftiofur	2.2–5 mg/kg	12	IM
Ceftriaxone	25 mg/kg	12	IV or IM
Aminoglycosides			
Amikacin	21 mg/kg	24	IV or IM
Gentamicin	6.6 mg/kg	24	IV or IM
Streptomycin	10 mg/kg	12	IM
Fluoroquinolones			
Ciprofloxacin[a]	5.5 mg/kg	12–24	IV
Enrofloxacin[a]	5.5 mg/kg	24	IV
	7.5 mg/kg	24	PO
Tetracyclines			
Oxytetracycline	5 mg/kg	12	IV[b]
Doxycycline	10 mg/kg	12	PO[c]
Macrolides			
Erythromycin (phosphate, stearate, ethylsuccinate, estolate)	25 mg/kg	6–8	PO
Erythromycin (lactobionate, gluceptate)	5 mg/kg	4–6	IV[b]

TABLE **21.3.** *Continued*

Drug Preparation	Dose	Dose Interval (h)	Route of Administration
Other			
Chloramphenicol (palmitate or base)	50 mg/kg	6 or 12[d]	PO
Chloramphenicol (sodium succinate)	25–50 mg/kg	6 or 12[d]	IV
Metronidazole	15 mg/kg	12	PO
	25 mg/kg	6	Per rectum
Rifampin	5 mg/kg	12	PO (foals)
	10 mg/kg	12	PO (adults)
Sulfadiazine	24 mg/kg	12–24	PO
Trimethoprim-sulfonamide	5 mg/kg (of trimethoprim)	12	PO or IV
Pyrimethamine	1 mg/kg	24	PO
Vancomycin[e]	4.5–7.5 mg/kg	8	IV[f]
Sodium iodide (20% solution)	20–40 mg/kg	24	IV[g]
Potassium iodide	2 mg/kg	24	PO[g]
Antifungal agents			
Amphotericin B	0.3–0.7 mg/kg	24	IV[i]
Fluconazole	4 mg/kg[h]	24	PO
Itraconazole	5 mg/kg[h]	12	PO
Ketoconazole	30 mg/kg (in 0.2N HCl)	12	Intra-gastric[j]

Note: Pharmakokinetics data are available for horses but in most cases safety studies have not been performed in the equine species.

[a] Should not be used in young growing horses because of the risk of arthropathy.

[b] Dilute and give by slow IV infusion.

[c] Administer orally only. Intravenous doxycycline has resulted in severe cardiovascular effects including collapse and death in some horses.

[d] Administer BID in foals less than 7 days of age and QID thereafter.

[e] Should be used only for the treatment of serious bacterial infections caused by microorganism resistant to all other antimicrobial agents.

[f] Dilute and administer over 1 hour.

[g] May cause abortion in pregnant mares.

[h] Pharmacokinetic studies are not available. Empirical dose based on human dose, measurement of serum levels in clinical cases and observation of positive clinical response in equine patients.

[i] Dilute in 5% dextrose and give over 2–4 hours. Start with lower dose and increase by 0.1 mg/kg every other day until the higher dose is reached.

[j] Administer by nasogastric tube to prevent irritation by 0.2N HCl.

TABLE **21.4.** **Suggested doses for intrauterine antimicrobial therapy in mares**

Drug	Spectrum	Dose[a]
Amikacin sulfate	Excellent Gram-negative coverage (including most *Pseudomonas aeruginosa*)	2 g[b]
Gentamicin sulfate	Gram-negative	2 g[b]
Ticarcillin	Broad spectrum (not effective against *Klebsiella*)	6 g
Ticarcillin–clavulanic acid	Broad spectrum	6 g
Penicillin G (potassium)	Gram-positive	5×10^6 IU
Ceftiofur	Broad spectrum (not effective against *P. aeruginosa*)	1 g

[a] Administer daily for 4–6 days. The volume infused is determined by the size of the uterus (35–150 ml is usually sufficient).

[b] Buffered with equal volume of 7.5% bicarbonate.

22 | Antimicrobial Drug Use in Dogs and Cats

A. D. J. WATSON and E. ROSIN

Veterinarians treating dogs and cats have some advantages over colleagues treating larger animals. The generally stronger economic basis of small animal practice may better support appropriate laboratory investigations, choice of more expensive drugs when necessary, and closer patient monitoring. However, there is evidence of some laxity in drug use in small animal practice, especially for difficult cases where diagnostic uncertainty and pressure from the owner can lead to inappropriate use of antimicrobials as if they were placebos or antipyretic agents. This can increase costs and risks to the patient and also create a false sense of security that may delay more appropriate investigation and therapy.

Debate continues about whether veterinary use of antimicrobial drugs results in development of resistance in human pathogens, but there is little evidence that therapeutic use in companion animals poses a threat to human health. Nevertheless, there is likely to be increasing pressure on veterinarians in small animal practice to ensure that their use of antimicrobial drugs is prudent. A concerted effort toward more judicious (selective and restricted) use is advisable, to avoid potential criticism and consequent enforced restrictions on use. Antimicrobials are a precious resource requiring conservation. There is little doubt that widespread inappropriate use could reduce overall efficacy and create problems with infections that are more difficult and expensive to treat. This has been demonstrated by outbreaks of nosocomial infections in human and veterinary hospitals, often attributable in part to selection pressure applied by continued overuse of antimicrobial drugs, especially for prophylaxis in surgical and nonsurgical patients.

537

Antimicrobial Prophylaxis

Antimicrobial Prophylaxis in Surgery

There is remarkably little information documenting the effectiveness of antimicrobial chemoprophylaxis in domestic animals. However, human studies have provided considerable information justifying use of these agents prophylactically in surgical procedures that have a high risk of infection and where the consequences of infection seriously endanger the patient or the success of surgery. These observations and supporting experimental studies have shown that effective prophylaxis requires high concentrations of a suitable drug to be present in tissues at the time contamination occurs, as discussed in Chapter 5. It must be emphasized that antimicrobials are no substitute for asepsis, gentle handling of tissues, judicious use of suture materials, and accurate apposition of tissue without obstructing blood supply. As others have said, prophylactic antimicrobials may make a second-rate surgeon out of a third-rate one but will never make a second-rate surgeon first-rate.

There are few situations warranting prophylactic administration of antimicrobials in small animal surgery; some potential indications are listed in Table 22.1. Drugs selected for perioperative prophylaxis must be effective against microbes most likely to cause postoperative wound infections in dogs and cats, namely coagulase-positive *Staphylococcus* spp. and *Escherichia coli*. Cefazolin has excellent activity against these pathogens and low toxicity. Intravenous administration of cefazolin at 20 mg/kg at the beginning of surgery in dogs produces drug concentrations at the surgical site sufficient to protect against most staphylococci for at least 6 hours; repeating the dose subcutaneously at 6 hours extends protection beyond 12 hours (Rosin et al., 1993a). Cefazolin is less effective against *E. coli*, and if the risk from this pathogen is very high or surgery lasts more than 2 hours, a second dose of cefazolin may be advisable 3 hours after the first. Cefazolin is active against many obligately anaerobic pathogens, but cefoxitin or cefotetan (both cephamycins and more

TABLE 22.1. **Surgical procedures that may warrant antimicrobial prophylaxis**

Alimentary tract	Dental procedures combined with other surgery; biliary surgery if infection present; resection of esophagus, stomach in gastric dilation/volvulus, intestine in obstruction, colon; rectal and anal surgery
Orthopedic	Extensive internal fracture fixation, open fracture repair, total hip prosthesis
Other procedures	Perineal herniorrhaphy, hernia repairs with nonabsorbable mesh, pacemaker implantation, lobectomy in infection, extensive neurosurgery, prolonged (>2 hours) surgery with much tissue manipulation

Source: Modified with permission from Rosin et al. (1993b).

expensive) may be preferred if anaerobes are of particular concern, as with colonic and rectal surgery. Where available, injectable amoxicillin-clavulanate preparations provide an economical alternative to cephalosporins for prophylaxis: a dose of 15–25 mg (combined)/kg is suggested, the solution given IV when surgery begins, or the suspension IM 1 hour beforehand. Injectable ampicillin-sulbactam could be used similarly, dosage being based on the ampicillin content.

Human studies have generally shown that single doses of antimicrobial drugs provide effective perioperative antimicrobial prophylaxis, with no additional benefit from continued administration after surgery unless infection is present or surgery exceeded 6 hours.

Antimicrobial Prophylaxis in Nonsurgical Patients

Prophylactic use of antimicrobial drugs in nonsurgical patients is controversial, and veterinary data are limited. There are undoubtedly individuals who have a high risk of disease because they are exposed episodically to an acute transmissible infection or have local or systemic defense mechanisms severely compromised by disease, investigative procedures, or therapy. Antimicrobial prophylaxis may sometimes benefit these individuals and has been recommended, for example, in human patients threatened by rheumatic fever, meningitis, tuberculosis, or bacterial endocarditis. Trials have also shown satisfactory results in preventing travelers' diarrhea, *Pneumocystis* pneumonia in cancer patients, and recurrent urinary tract infections in women. Analogous situations in dogs and cats seem uncommon.

Chemoprophylaxis has been generally more effective when the period of unusual risk is short, as occurs with episodic exposure to a pathogen, or with brief impairment of local defenses by minor trauma, catheterization, or other procedures. It has proven less satisfactory with prolonged impairment of antimicrobial defense mechanisms, as in patients with primary immunodeficiencies, immunodeficiencies secondary to systemic disease or drug treatment, or prolonged local risk factors like catheters and drainage tubes. An unfortunate outcome of routine chemoprophylaxis in these settings may be an infection caused by an unusual drug-resistant pathogen.

Observations suggest that antimicrobial drugs can protect against infection when the period of risk is brief (a few hours to a few days) or the target is a single drug-susceptible species that is unlikely to become resistant. However, attempts at long-term chemoprophylaxis in patients continually at risk are liable to failure. A better approach is to watch these individuals carefully for signs of infection and to treat promptly and appropriately if infection occurs.

Antimicrobial Chemotherapy

The principles governing selection and therapeutic use of antimicrobial drugs described in Chapter 5 apply also in treating dogs and cats. Of prime importance in deciding whether and how to treat is an adequate clinical assessment. This should identify the system or systems involved and the pathogens likely to be responsible. Although there is a tendency for the inexperienced to assume that an increased rectal temperature indicates an infection, this is not always so. Increased temperatures also occur in other pathologic conditions (neoplasms, drug reactions, immune-mediated disorders, other nonspecific inflammations) and some physiologic states (exercise, excitement, high ambient temperature and humidity). Likewise, leukocytosis is not pathognomonic for infection and can occur with nonspecific inflammatory processes, hemolysis, neoplasms, trauma, excitement, stress, and glucocorticoid administration.

When a bacterial infection is suspected, identification of involved pathogens can be facilitated by examining smears of exudates or aspirates from the infected site treated with Gram stain and/or a Romanowsky method (Giemsa, Diff-Quik). In vitro culture and susceptibility testing will provide more-precise information but may not be feasible because of added costs, delays, or lack of facilities. However, these procedures are advisable for patients with very serious, recurrent, or nonresponding infections.

If other information is lacking, drug selection can be based on knowledge of the site of infection and the pathogens more frequently implicated therein, coupled with the likely susceptibility of these organisms. Compilations of such data are shown in Table 22.2 for dogs and Table 22.3 for cats.

In many routine or less serious infections, treatment on this basis will prove satisfactory, without the need for additional investigation. If microbiological tests are undertaken, one could withhold therapy for 1–2 days, pending results, provided the delay is unlikely to be harmful. If the infection is serious or life threatening, treatment should commence immediately, with the option of changing the medication when results become available. During the selection process, it may be necessary to decide between several drugs likely to be effective against the pathogen. All other things being equal, the drug with the narrowest antimicrobial spectrum is preferred, to reduce effects on untargeted microflora. Costs, routes of administration, and toxic potential should be considered. It may be necessary to modify drug selection in renal failure, liver failure, pregnancy, or neonatal patients (Table 22.4; see also Chapter 19).

Drug Formulations

The problems of solid dosage forms (tablets, capsules) that contain too much drug for cats or small dogs, and of injectable preparations too concentrated to permit accurate dosing, are familiar to all practitioners. Veterinarians are sometimes forced to prescribe larger-than-desired doses at less-frequent-than-ideal intervals, while hoping that safety and efficacy will not be compromised. Problems are unlikely for bactericidal and relatively nontoxic drugs, such as penicillins and cephalosporins. However, there may be difficulties with agents that are bacteriostatic (chloramphenicol, tetracyclines) or potentially toxic. Unfortunately, these problems will continue until more manufacturers can be convinced of the need to develop formulations appropriate to small animal patients.

Economic factors in practice may encourage use of cheaper generic drug products on occasions. Many of these perform similarly to the better-known brands, but the potential for differences in drug bioavailability exists. Because such differences could affect efficacy and safety, clinicians should insist that manufacturers provide adequate bioavailability data for these products before using them.

Route of Administration

The route of administration is sometimes dictated by the drug chosen. For example, if an aminoglycoside or amphotericin B is selected to treat a systemic infection, it must be given parenterally because enteral absorption is poor. More often, several routes of administration are possible and the one chosen may depend on the disease being treated, the likely duration of therapy, the temperament of the patient, and the capability of the owner.

PARENTERAL ADMINISTRATION

Injections are not routinely needed for antimicrobial therapy in dogs and cats, and some clinicians rarely use them. However, parenteral administration can be valuable to initiate treatment in severe infections where rapid systemic delivery of high drug concentrations is important. Other indications include fractious, unconscious, or vomiting patients or those with mouth pain.

The intravenous (IV) route should be used if maximum plasma drug concentrations are desired immediately after dosing, as with life-threatening infections. IV use might also be preferable in shocked or hypotensive patients, as poor peripheral perfusion may impede drug absorption from other sites.

Intramuscular (IM) or subcutaneous (SC) administration is usually safer and satisfactory in less demanding circumstances. These routes give similar bioavailability with most antimicrobial preparations, but SC administration is easier and generally causes less pain. Many formulations recommended for IM use in other species can be given to dogs and cats by SC injection, but unfamiliar preparations should be assessed in a few animals first to check for possible injection site reactions.

For IM injections, the lumbar longissimus muscle may be a better site than the thigh. The preferred location lies midway between iliac crest and last rib, and halfway between dorsal spinous processes and the lateral border of the muscle. Injection here is less likely to be intermuscular, is usually well tolerated, and avoids the risk of major nerve damage.

ORAL ADMINISTRATION

Dosage by the oral route is adequate in most infections and is generally the best method for home treatment. However, a struggle over oral medication can be counterproductive and dangerous, because of the risk of aspiration pneumonia, especially with oily medicines in cats. Some individual dogs and many cats are difficult to dose with solid dosage forms. Use of a curved hemostat can help. With a feline patient, one hand is used to grasp the scruff and an ear, the head is bent up and back on the neck until the mandible sags, then the tablet or capsule held loosely with the hemostat is pushed quickly down between tongue and palate to the pharynx, whereupon the drug is released and the instrument withdrawn. An alternative is to hold the cat's head similarly, slide a small teaspoon bearing the tablet into the oropharynx, then tilt the spoon to deposit the drug. These techniques are quick, easy, and safe when done properly.

Some owners find it easier to use liquid formulations. These may need to be reasonably palatable if a struggle is to be avoided. A plastic dropper or syringe can be used, introduced into the side of the mouth in the space behind a canine tooth, or into the pocket formed by pulling the lip commissure laterally. To minimize risks of aspiration, the head should be kept steady and almost level, not forced up or back, and the volume given each time should not exceed what the animal can swallow with ease. Nasoesophageal and orogastric intubations offer alternatives for in-hospital use.

Administration of liquids, powders, or crushed tablets mixed in food may be possible, although some patients reject medicated food. Occasionally they can be fooled into swallowing morsels of food containing a tablet or capsule, if first offered unmedicated pieces. However, the potential effect of ingesta on drug bioavailability may need to be considered.

Influence of Food on Systemic Availability of Drugs Given Orally

Interactions between food and drugs affecting drug absorption are common in human patients but are often overlooked in veterinary medicine. The most frequent outcome is reduced or delayed absorption of the drug, although sometimes absorption is increased or unaffected. The mechanisms responsible are complex and involve food-induced changes in gut physiology and direct interactions between food components and drugs. The composition of the meal, the volume of fluid ingested, and specific formulation of the drug may affect the outcome. Because of these complexities, it is not possible to give conclusive recommendations to cover all clinical situations.

It is also difficult to assess the importance of drug-food interactions, because studies comparing therapeutic efficacy under fasting and non-fasting conditions are lacking. However, it may be prudent to fast patients for 1–2 hours before and 1–2 hours after administration of agents whose absorption can be impaired substantially by food, such as most penicillins and tetracyclines. An alternative would be to increase doses given with food, but the increase required is difficult to predict. Some antimicrobial drugs can be given without regard to feeding, whereas others might be better given with food to improve absorption or reduce gastric irritation associated with dosage. Current suggestions are given in Table 22.5.

Dosing Rate and Duration of Therapy

Conventional dosage regimens for antimicrobial drugs in dogs and cats are presented in Table 22.6. These should be regarded as guidelines only. The optimum dosage regimen will vary somewhat with the case, depending on the susceptibility of the pathogen, ability of the drug to reach the infection site, and competence of the patient's defenses. Higher or more frequent dosages may be required for relatively resistant pathogens or lesions in tissues where drug penetration is poor. Smaller doses may be satisfactory in lower urinary infections, with drugs excreted adequately in the urine in active form.

It is usually apparent within 2 days or so whether treatment is having the desired effect. If the response is inadequate, the diagnosis and treatment regimen should be reevaluated. In most cases selection of a different drug is warranted, but increased dosage of the original agent could be considered if underdosing or poor tissue penetration is suspected.

Treatment duration of 4–5 days, up to 1 week, is generally adequate for the majority of acute uncomplicated bacterial infections in dogs and cats. One suggestion is to treat for a minimum of 3 days and to continue for 2 days after signs of infection have subsided. Treatment responses may be slower with chronic infections, and prolonged administration (4–6 weeks) is often needed because of existing tissue damage, impaired blood supply, and compromised local immunity. For systemic mycoses, treatment for several months is usually required.

Therapeutic Compliance

Carefully formulated therapeutic plans may be valueless if the owner does not follow the suggested dosage regimen. Problems may arise because the owner does not understand the importance of the medication or the instructions given. Furthermore, the owner's inexperience, the patient's resistance, and suboptimum formulation characteristics (eg, poor size, shape, taste, consistency) can prevent satisfactory administration and produce an angry animal and a frustrated owner. These problems are likely to be greater with cats and some less congenial small dogs.

Issues of therapeutic noncompliance have not been well studied in veterinary medicine, but Barter et al. (1996a,b) found that noncompliance was common during treatment for acute bacterial infections in dogs. Antibiotic was prescribed twice or thrice daily for 5–10 days: only 27% of 22 owners gave the prescribed number of tablets, 68% gave fewer tablets, and 5% gave more. Furthermore, only 32% of doses were given at close-to-ideal intervals (ie, 10–14 hours for twice daily, 6.5–9.5 hours for thrice daily). Reasons for these failings were not examined.

Potential difficulties with compliance should be addressed by scheduling dosing to suit the owners' routines. Linking dosage times to fixed points in the *owner's* day (eg, mealtimes, bedtime) may assist, although the *animal's* mealtimes might need changing to avoid undesirable drug-ingesta interactions. Other logical measures are to decide with the owners the dosage form they can best manage, demonstrate its use, and provide clear verbal and written instructions. Human studies have shown that increasing treatment complexity is associated with increased probability that doses will be missed. Thus, if no therapeutic difference exists between two treatment options, the one with the less complex regimen should be prescribed. Likewise, additional medications of questionable value are best avoided, because ensuing complexity could reduce therapeutic compliance with the more important drugs.

Outcome

The response to antimicrobial therapy can be most gratifying when the correct drug is used to treat an uncomplicated microbial infection in a patient that is otherwise well. By contrast, the outcome is likely to be disappointing if the wrong drug is chosen, if microbes are not responsible (or rather, viruses are), or if complicating factors have not been addressed. Additional specific and supportive measures, such as nursing, fluid therapy, and surgery, are often very important. If the response to appropriate therapy is poor or repeated relapses occur, an underlying maintaining cause should be considered, including retroviral infections in cats, other immunoparetic disorders, tumors, and foreign bodies.

Bibliography

Barter LS, et al. 1996a. Comparison of methods to assess dog owners' therapeutic compliance. Aust Vet J 74:443.

Barter LS, et al. 1996b. Owner compliance with short term antimicrobial medication in dogs. Aust Vet J 74:277.

Ettinger SJ, Feldman EC, eds. 1995. Textbook of Veterinary Internal Medicine, 4th ed. Philadelphia: WB Saunders.

Greene CE, ed. 1998. Infectious Diseases of the Dog and Cat, 2nd ed. Philadelphia: WB Saunders.

Morgan RV, ed. 1997. Handbook of Small Animal Practice, 3rd ed. Philadelphia: WB Saunders.

Nelson RW, Couto CG. 1998. Small Animal Internal Medicine, 2nd ed. St. Louis: Mosby.

Rosin E, et al. 1993a. Cefazolin antibacterial activity and concentrations in serum and the surgical wound in dogs. Am J Vet Res 54:1317.

Rosin E, et al. 1993b. Surgical wound infection and use of antibiotics. In: Slatter D, ed. Textbook of Small Animal Surgery, 2nd ed. Philadelphia: WB Saunders.

Watson ADJ, et al. 1998. Rational use of antibacterial drugs. In: NT Gorman, ed. Canine Medicine and Therapeutics, 4th ed. Oxford: Blackwell Science.

TABLE 22.2. Antimicrobial drug selection in canine infections

Site or Type of Infection	Diagnosis	Common Infecting Organisms	Comments	Suggested Drugs[a]	Alternatives
Skin and subcutis	Deep pyoderma, superficial pyoderma	Staphylococcus, secondary Escherichia, Proteus, Pseudomonas	Seek, remove underlying causes. Anti-staphylococcal drugs often succeed even if other bacteria are also present. Prolonged or intermittent dosage may be needed.	Isoxazolyl penicillin,[b] lincosamide,[c] macrolide[d]	Amoxicillin-clavulanate, chloramphenicol, sulfonamide-trimethoprim[e]
	Surface pyoderma	Staphylococcus, Streptococcus	Often secondary to skin folds or self-trauma. Local cleansing and topical antibacterials adequate.		
	Malassezia dermatitis	Malassezia pachydermatis	Identify, eliminate underlying causes. Use shampoos.	Ketaconazole	Itraconazole
	Dermatophytosis	Microsporum, Trichophyton	Topical and environmental measures needed as well. Localized lesions may not require systemic therapy.	Griseofulvin	Ketoconazole, itraconazole
	Bite wounds, traumatic and contaminated wounds	Staphylococcus, Streptococcus, Pasteurella, anaerobes	Wound irrigation debridement most important. Parenteral antimicrobial might give effective prophylaxis within 3 hours of wounding but of questionable value after 3 hours if appears	Penicillin G or V, isoxazolyl penicillin[b]	Amoxicillin-clavulanate, cephalosporin (oral, or group 1 parenteral)[f]

	Condition	Organisms	Comments		
	Anal sac inflammation, abscessation	*Escherichia, Enterococcus, Clostridium, Proteus*	uninfected. Treat empirically pending laboratory data if infected. Consider tetanus.	Amoxicillin-clavulanate	Chloramphenicol
Ear			Generally local treatment only. Systemic therapy warranted if inflammation severe, patient febrile.		
	Otitis externa	*Malassezia, Staphylococcus, Pseudomonas, Escherichia, Proteus*	Check for foreign material, hair, mites. Clean and dry canal. Initial empirical treatment often satisfactory, investigate if severe, persistent, or recurrent. Consider topical glucocorticoid or analgesic.	Topical aminoglycoside[g] or chloramphenicol, topical polymyxin[h] for Gram-negatives	Topical nystatin thiabendazole, miconazole, or clotrimazole for *Malassezia*
	Otitis media, otitis interna	As for otitis externa	Otitis externa often present. Seek contributing causes. Clean and drain; use topical antimicrobials. Avoid ototoxic drugs (topical or systemic). Microbial investigation warranted.	Amoxicillin-clavulanate	Chloramphenicol, fluoroquinolone[i]; ketoconazole or itraconazole for *Malassezia*
Eye	Superficial ocular infection	*Staphylococcus, Streptococcus, Escherichia, Proteus*	Identify and correct contributing causes (poor eyelid conformation, hairs, dust, UV light, reduced tears).	Topical neomycin-polymyxin[h]-bacitracin	Topical chloramphenicol, gentamicin

TABLE 22.2. *Continued*

Site or Type of Infection	Diagnosis	Common Infecting Organisms	Comments	Suggested Drugs[a]	Alternatives
	Penetrating eye wound	Various bacteria	Infection, uveitis possible. Sample and culture aqueous humor.	Amoxicillin-clavulanate with topical and episcleral gentamicin	Chloramphenicol (also topical) and episcleral chloramphenicol sodium succinate
Respiratory and thoracic	Bacterial rhinitis	Various resident species, usually secondary	Antibacterial drugs unlikely curative. Seek underlying cause (foreign body, allergy, fungus, tumor, virus, etc.).	Amoxicillin[j]	Sulfonamide-trimethoprim[e]
	Fungal rhinitis	*Aspergillus*, *Penicillium* rarer	Exclude nasal neoplasia. May be secondary bacterial involvement (see Chapter 17).	Topical clotrimazole	Topical enilconazole; systemic itraconazole or ketoconazole
	Infectious tracheobronchitis	*Bordetella*, viruses, *Mycoplasma*	Most recover untreated in 7–10 days, but antimicrobial therapy may hasten resolution. Secondary bacterial bronchopneumonia in some. Treat if systemically unwell.	Sulfonamide-trimethoprim[e]	Amoxicillin[j]
	Bacterial pneumonia	Single (mostly) or mixed infection involving various facultative (especially Gram-negative) bacteria and anaerobes if aspirated	Do aerobic culture and susceptibility test on material from transtracheal aspirate, bronchial wash, or lavage or from fine-needle lung aspirate; anaerobic culture if suspect aspiration.	Amoxicillin-clavulanate, sulfonamide-trimethoprim[e]	Beta-lactam,[k] with aminoglycoside[e] or fluoroquinolone[l]

548

Category	Condition	Cause	Comments	First choice	Alternative
	Pneumocystis pneumonia	*Pneumocystis carinii*	Secondary to inherited or acquired immune deficiency.	Sulfonamide-trimethoprim[e]	Pentamidine
	Pyothorax, purulent pleuritis	Various and often mixed, involving anaerobes (including *Actinomyces*) alone or in combination with aerobic-facultative bacteria (*Nocardia, Corynebacterium, Pasteurella, Staphylococcus, Streptococcus*)	Identification and susceptibility test on aerobic-facultative organisms advisable. Drainage and lavage are important.	Penicillin G,[m] amoxicillin,[j] amoxicillin-clavulanate	Lincosamide,[c] chloramphenicol. For *Nocardia*, sulfonamide[n] ± trimethoprim[e]
Alimentary and abdominal	Periodontitis, gingivitis	Resident anaerobic and facultative bacteria	Teeth cleaning, scaling, other dental treatment may be needed.	Penicillin G,[m] amoxicillin[j]	Metronidazole ± spiramycin, tetracycline,[o] clindamycin
	Malar or carnassial abscess	Resident oral flora	Extract tooth, curette alveolus, ensure drainage.	Penicillin G,[m] amoxicillin[j]	Amoxicillin-clavulanate, clindamycin
	Ulcerative gingivostomatitis	Anaerobes and other resident bacteria	Possible underlying immunodeficiency, metabolic or physical disorder. Use local treatments, possibly prolonged or intermittent systemic drugs. Consider glucocorticoid.	Penicillin G,[m] amoxicillin[j]	Metronidazole ± spiramycin, clindamycin
	Tonsillitis, pharyngitis	Resident oropharyngeal flora	Often secondary to vomiting, regurgitation cough, oral inflammation.	Amoxicillin,[j] amoxicillin-clavulanate	Sulfonamide-trimethoprim,[e] tetracycline[o]

TABLE 22.2. *Continued*

Site or Type of Infection	Diagnosis	Common Infecting Organisms	Comments	Suggested Drugs[a]	Alternatives
	Gastric helicobacteriosis	*Helicobacter*	Relation between infection and illness often unclear. Value of treatment unknown.	Metronidazole (and bismuth subsalicylate), with amoxicillin[j] or tetracycline[o]	Sulfonamide-trimethoprim[e]
	Bacterial enterocolitis	*Salmonella*	Often subclinical, sometimes significant but self-limiting. Drug indicated if systemically ill but may prolong carrier state.	Chloramphenicol	Sulfonamide-trimethoprim[e]
		Campylobacter	Possible resident or primary or secondary pathogen. Don't treat unless signs evident.	Macrolide[d]	Chloramphenicol, tetracycline[o]
		Escherichia, Clostridium, Staphylococcus, others	Normal residents, pathogenic role uncertain. Drug use questionable unless septicemia suspected.	Amoxicillin[j] amoxicillin-clavulanate	Chloramphenicol, beta-lactam[k] plus aminoglycoside[l]
	Giardiasis	*Giardia*	Infection often subclinical. Potential zoonosis.	Fenbendazole	Albendazole, metronidazole, tinidazole[p]
	Coccidiosis	*Isospora*	Infection probably irrelevant in adults or if few oocysts present. Often self-limiting.	Sulfonamide[n] ± trimethoprim[e] or pyrimethamine	Furazolidone, amprolium

Condition	Bacteria	Comments	First-choice drugs	Alternative drugs
Parvoviral enteritis	Secondary facultative and anaerobic bacteria	Fluid therapy imperative. Consider antimicrobial if severe and potential septicemia. Parenteral route best.	Amoxicillin,[j] amoxicillin-clavulanate	Beta-lactam[k] plus aminoglycoside[l]
Small intestine bacterial overgrowth	*Escherichia, Enterococcus, Staphylococcus, Clostridium*	Secondary to abnormal motility or anatomy, enteritis, maldigestion, impaired immunity. Investigation, dietary therapy required. Drug choice empirical, may need continuous or intermittent dosage.	Amoxicillin,[j] amoxicillin-clavulanate, tetracycline[o]	Metronidazole, lincosamide,[c] chloramphenicol
Colitis	Secondary infection by resident anaerobes and facultative bacteria	Bacteria irrelevant or secondary to stress, trichuriasis, immunodeficiency, viral or idiopathic disease. Dietary therapy, sulfasalazine suggested. Consider anti-anaerobe drug if unsuccessful or if acute colitis with systemic signs.	Metronidazole, chloramphenicol	Macrolide,[d] amoxicillin[j]
Cholecystitis, cholangitis	*Escherichia, Salmonella,* anaerobes	May need surgery to restore bile flow, appropriate fluid and dietary therapy.	Amoxicillin-clavulanate	Beta-lactam[k] plus either aminoglycoside[l] or fluoroquinolone[i]
Intra-abdominal sepsis (bacterial peritonitis, abscessation)	Mixed anaerobes and facultative Gram-negative bacteria	Exploration, drainage, lavage (including antimicrobial drugs) may be needed. Culture and testing essential.	Gentamicin or fluoroquinolone[i] with one of amoxicillin,[j] clindamycin, or metronidazole	Amoxicillin-clavulanate, chloramphenicol

TABLE 22.2. *Continued*

Site or Type of Infection	Diagnosis	Common Infecting Organisms	Comments	Suggested Drugs[a]	Alternatives
	Pancreatitis	Enteric bacteria		Cefotaxime, chloramphenicol	Metronidazole, lincosamide[c]
Urinary and genital	Lower urinary tract infection, cystitis	*Escherichia, Proteus, Staphylococcus, Streptococcus, Klebsiella, Pseudomonas, Enterobacter*	Usually single isolate. Seek contributing cause (calculi; tumor, urine retention, incontinence) especially if mixed infection. Culture cystocentesis sample and test susceptibility if no response or recurs (see Chapter 19).	Amoxicillin,[j] amoxicillin-clavulanate, sulfonamide-trimethoprim[e]	Tetracycline,[o] fluoroquinolone,[i] cephalexin
	Pyelonephritis	Similar to lower urinary infection, especially *Escherichia, Proteus, Staphylococcus*	Urine culture advised. Prolonged treatment, monitor response (see Chapter 19).	Amoxicillin,[j] amoxicillin-clavulanate	Fluoroquinolone,[i] sulfonamide-trimethoprim[e]
	Prostatitis	As for lower urinary infection	Often associated with urinary infection. Treat >3 weeks if acute, 6 weeks if chronic. Surgery for prostate abscess. Castration or progestin for prostatomegaly.	Sulfonamide-trimethoprim,[e] chloramphenicol	Macrolide[d] or lincosamide[c] if Gram-positive, fluoroquinolone[i] if Gram-negative
	Orchitis, epididymitis	*Escherichia, Brucella*	May be associated with urinary infection. Culture semen, urine, or needle aspirate. Consider castration.	Amoxicillin-clavulanate, sulfonamide-trimethoprim[e]	Chloramphenicol; doxycycline plus gentamicin for *Brucella*

552

Condition	Organisms	Comments	First choice	Alternative
Balanoposthitis, vaginitis	Resident bacteria, herpesvirus (prepuce) *Mycoplasma* (vagina)	Look for predisposing factors. Local cleansing and antibacterial wash sufficient.		
Metritis, pyometra	*Escherichia, Streptococcus, Staphylococcus,* other facultative anaerobes, possibly anaerobes	Ovariohysterectomy recommended. Prostaglandin plus antibiotic may be effective in *open* pyometra or metritis, but culture advisable.	Amoxicillin-clavulanate, chloramphenicol	Amoxicillin,[j] with aminoglycoside[1] or fluoroquinolone[i]
Mastitis	*Escherichia, Staphylococcus, Streptococcus*	Check milk pH (affects penetration of systemic antimicrobials). Do Gram stain or culture and test susceptibility (see Chapter 31).	Chloramphenicol (pH unimportant) if weaning possible, otherwise amoxicillin-clavulanate	If pH > 7.4: amoxicillin,[j] amoxicillin-clavulanate. If pH < 7.3: sulfonamide-trimethoprim[e] for Gram-negatives, macrolide[d] for Gram-positives
Musculoskeletal — Local bacterial myositis	*Staphylococcus, Clostridium,* other anaerobes and facultative bacteria	Flora varies with cause (trauma, bite, surgery). Drainage, culture, susceptibility test best.	Amoxicillin-clavulanate	Chloramphenicol, cephalosporin (oral, or group 1 parenteral)[f]
Osteomyelitis	Mostly *Staphylococcus,* also *Streptococcus, Escherichia, Proteus, Pseudomonas, Klebsiella,* anaerobes	Laboratory evaluation advised. Promote drainage, remove foreign material, treat long-term (see Chapter 19).	Isoxazolyl penicillin,[b] amoxicillin-clavulanate	Lincosamide,[c] isoxazolyl penicillin[b] with either aminoglycoside[1] or fluoroquinolone[i]
Discospondylitis, vertebral osteomyelitis	*Staphylococcus;* also *Streptococcus, Brucella, Escherichia, Aspergillus*	Evaluate *Brucella canis* titer; culture blood, urine, and aspirate from site to aid identification. Prolonged therapy. Curette if poor response (see Chapter 19).	Isoxazolyl penicillin,[b] amoxicillin-clavulanate	Cephalosporin (oral or group 1 parenteral).[f] For *Brucella,* doxycycline plus gentamicin

TABLE 22.2. *Continued*

Site or Type of Infection	Diagnosis	Common Infecting Organisms	Comments	Suggested Drugs[a]	Alternatives
	Septic arthritis	*Staphylococcus*, *Streptococcus*, less often anaerobes, coliforms	Possibly septicemic: culture blood, urine, joint fluid. Drain by needle or arthrotomy; use lavage (see Chapter 19).	Isoxazolyl penicillin,[b] amoxicillin-clavulanate	Cephalosporin (oral or group parenteral)[f]
Nervous system	Bacterial meningitis	*Staphylococcus*, *Pasteurella*, *Actinomyces*, *Nocardia*, sometimes anaerobes	CSF culture and susceptibility test advised (see Chapter 19).	Amoxicillin-clavulanate	Sulfonamide-trimethoprim,[e] chloramphenicol
	Cryptococcal meningo-encephalitis	*Cryptococcus neoformans*	Guarded prognosis.	Amphotericin B with flucytosine or fluconazole	Amphotericin B, fluconazole, itraconazole
	Tetanus	*Clostridium tetani*	Use nursing, antitoxin, sedation, debridement, and inject penicillin G into wound area too.	Penicillin G[m]	Tetracycline,[o] metronidazole
	Botulism	*Clostridium botulinum*	Supportive therapy mainly. Use antimicrobial only if gut colonized.	Penicillin G[m]	Metronidazole
	Hepatic encephalopathy	Normal intestinal flora	Oral antimicrobial drugs to suppress gut ammonia production; use low-protein diet, lactulose.	Amoxicillin[j]	Amoxicillin-clavulanate
Other bacterial	Actinomycosis	Various *Actinomyces* spp.	Mostly with other bacteria in infections in subcutis, thorax, abdomen, retroperitoneum. Drainage, lavage, debridement, prolonged dosage needed.	Penicillin G[m]	Chloramphenicol, erythromycin, tetracycline[o]

554

Disease	Organism	Comments	Drug of choice	Alternative drugs
Bacteremia, bacterial endocarditis	Various Gram-positive and Gram-negative facultative bacteria, or anaerobic organisms, sometimes polymicrobial	Blood culture and susceptibility test preferred. Treat parenterally for 4–10 days; then, if practicable and response satisfactory, use suitable oral therapy for 3–6 weeks.	Isoxazolyl penicillin[b] or amoxicillin[j], with aminoglycoside[l] or fluoroquinolone[i]	Cephalosporin (parenteral group 1 or 2)[f]
Brucellosis	Brucella canis	Potential zoonosis.	Doxycycline or minocycline, plus gentamicin	Other tetracycline,[o] with gentamicin or dihydrostreptomycin
Leptospirosis	Leptospira serovars canicola, copenhageni, icterohaemorrhagiae, others	Fluid and supportive therapy necessary.	Amoxicillin[j]	Penicillin G,[m] tetracycline,[o] macrolide,[d] aminoglycoside[l] (streptomycin drug of choice for kidney carrier)
Lyme borreliosis	Borrelia burgdorferi	Aspirin or other nonsteroidal anti-inflammatory for analgesia.	Doxycycline	Erythromycin, clarithromycin, amoxicillin[j]
Nocardiosis	Nocardia asteroides	Pulmonary, systemic, or solitary extrapulmonary lesions.	Sulfonamide[n] ± trimethoprim[e]	Amikacin, minocycline, erythromycin
Septicemia, neonatal	Streptococcus, Escherichia, Staphylococcus spp.		Amoxicillin-clavulanate, or parenteral sulbactam-ampicillin	Cephalosporin (oral or parenteral group 1 or 2)[f]
Tuberculosis	Mycobacterium tuberculosis, M. bovis	Prolonged therapy needed, using 2 or more of the listed drugs. Potential risk to owner.	Rifampin with isoniazid and ethambutol	Rifampin with isoniazid and pyrazinamide

TABLE 22.2. *Continued*

Site or Type of Infection	Diagnosis	Common Infecting Organisms	Comments	Suggested Drugs[a]	Alternatives
Other protozoal infections	Babesiosis	*Babesia canis*	Supportive therapy is very important, may need blood transfusion intravenous fluid with bicarbonate.	Imidocarb	Diminazene, pentamidine, phenamidine, trypan blue
		B. gibsoni	As for *B. canis*.	Diminazene	Phenamidine, pentamidine
	Cryptosporidiosis	*Cryptosporidium parvum*	Infection usually subclinical, self-limiting. Disease risk in immunocompromised animals.	Paromyocin	Azithromycin
	Hepatozoonosis	*Hepatozoon canis*	Drugs may reduce parasitemia without influencing signs. Relapses common. Use nonsteroidal anti-inflammatory for analgesia.	Imidocarb	Toltrazuril, diminazene, primaquine
	Leishmaniasis	Several *Leishmania* spp.	Resistant; infection often persists or relapses. Prognosis poor if in renal failure.	Meglumine antimonate and/or allopurinol	Sodium stibogluconate
	Neosporosis	*Neospora caninum*	Effects of tissue damage may persist even if infection eliminated.	Clindamycin	Sulfonamide[n] plus pyrimethamine?
	Toxoplasmosis	*Toxoplasma gondii*	As for neosporosis.	Clindamycin	Sulfonamide[n] plus pyrimethamine, azithromycin?, clarithromycin?

Disease	Organism	Comments	Drug of choice	Alternative
Trypanosomiasis, African	*Trypanosoma brucei, T. congolense*	Combination treatment better but relapses common.	Diminazene plus difluoromethylornithine	Diminazene
Trypanosomiasis, American	*T. cruzi*	Public health risk. Euthanasia might be preferred.	Nifurtimox	Benznidazole
Ehrlichiosis	*Ehrlichia canis, E. risticii, E. ewingii, E. phagocytophila*	Nursing, fluid therapy. Consider blood transfusion, anabolic steroid in marrow failure, glucocorticoid if thrombocytopenia or polyarthropathy.	Imidocarb	Doxycycline, minocycline, chloramphenicol
Haemobartonellosis	*Haemobartonella canis*	Transfuse blood if anemia life-threatening. Consider glucocorticoid.	Tetracycline[o]	Chloramphenicol, fluoroquinolone?[f]
Rocky Mountain spotted fever	*Rickettsia rickettsii*	Early, and supportive, therapy important. Zoonosis.	Tetracycline[o]	Chloramphenicol, fluoroquinolone[f]
Chlamydial infections	*Chlamydia psittaci*	Significance moot.	Tetracycline,[o] chloramphenicol	Macrolide,[d] fluoroquinolone[f]
Mycoplasmal infection	Various *Mycoplasma* spp.	Possible role in respiratory, urinary, and reproductive disorders; polyarthritis, colitis (see Chapter 19).	Tetracycline,[o] chloramphenicol	Macrolide,[d] fluoroquinolone[f]
Aspergillosis, disseminated	*Aspergillus terreus, A. deflectus, A. fumigatus*	Therapy may produce remission, despite persisting infection in immunocompromised patients.	Itraconazole	Amphotericin B
Blastomycosis	*Blastomyces dermatitidis*	Common sites are lung, lymph node, skin, eye, bone.	Itraconazole	Amphotericin B, plus ketoconazole

Rickettsial, chlamydial, and mycoplasmal infections (see Chapter 19)

Systemic mycoses (see Chapter 17)

TABLE 22.2. *Continued*

Site or Type of Infection	Diagnosis	Common Infecting Organisms	Comments	Suggested Drugs[a]	Alternatives
	Coccidioidomycosis	*Coccidioides immitis*	Infects lung, lymph node, bone, skin, eye, etc.	Ketoconazole	Amphotericin B ± ketoconazole; fluconazole, itraconazole
	Cryptococcosis	*Cryptococcus neoformans*	Usually involves CNS, eye, lung; often disseminated.	Amphotericin B with flucytosine and/or fluconazole	Itraconazole
	Histoplasmosis	*Histoplasma capsulatum*	Commonly disseminated; affects gut, lung, liver, spleen, associated lymph nodes.	Itraconazole ± amphotericin B	Fluconazole

[a]These selections reflect personal opinion based on review of the literature, discussion with colleagues, and clinical experience. They are intended to guide drug selection when laboratory data are lacking. Selection may change once culture and drug susceptibility test results are known. See Greene (1998) for additional information.

[b]Isoxazolyl penicillins: oxacillin, cloxacillin, dicloxacillin, flucloxacillin (see Chapter 6).

[c]Lincosamides: lincomycin, clindamycin. The latter may be preferred but is much more expensive (see Chapter 6).

[d]Macrolides: erythromycin, tylosin (see Chapter 11).

[e]Sulfonamide-trimethoprim: various sulfonamides (sulfadiazine, sulfamethoxazole, sulfadoxine, etc.) combined with trimethoprim. Ormetoprim and baquiloprim are alternatives to trimethoprim (see Chapter 14).

[f]Cephalosporins and related drugs: oral (cefachlor, cefadroxil, cephalexin, cephradine), group 1 parenteral (cefazolin, cephapirin, cephradine), group 2 parenteral (cefotaxime, ceftiofur) (see Chapter 7).

[g]Aminoglycosides, topical: neomycin, framycetin (neomycin B), kanamycin, gentamicin (see Chapter 10).

[h]Polymyxins: polymyxin B, colistin (polymyxin E) (see Chapter 9).

[i]Fluoroquinolones: ciprofloxacin, difloxacin, enrofloxacin, marbofloxacin, ofloxacin, orbifloxacin (see Chapter 15).

[j]Amoxicillin: ampicillin or hetacillin may be substituted (see Chapter 6).

[k]Beta-lactams: penicillins, cephalosporins (see Chapters 6 and 7).

[l]Aminoglycosides, system: amikacin, gentamicin, tobramycin (see Chapter 10).

[m]Penicillin G: penicillin V may be substituted for oral administration (see Chapter 6).

[n]Sulfonamides: many available, eg, sulfadimidine, sulfadiazine, sulfadimethoxine (see Chapter 14).

[o]Tetracyclines: doxycycline, minocycline, oxytetracycline, tetracycline (see Chapter 13).

[p]Tinidazole: efficacy likely but data limited.

558

TABLE 22.3. **Antimicrobial drug selection in feline infections**

Site or Type of Infection	Diagnosis	Common Infecting Organisms	Comments	Suggested Drugs[a]	Alternatives
Skin and subcutis	Superficial pustular dermatitis	*Streptococcus, Pasteurella*	Systemic drugs often unnecessary; use local cleansing, antiseptics.	Penicillin G[b]	Amoxicillin[c]
	Folliculitis, furunculosis	*Staphylococcus, Streptococcus*	Prolonged therapy may be needed for deep or recurrent lesions.	Penicillin G[b] or (for staphs) lincosamide[d]	Amoxicillin-clavulanate
	Cutaneous cryptococcosis	*Cryptococcus neoformans*	Surgical removal or debulking helpful.	Fluconazole	Itraconazole, ketoconazole plus flucytosine
	Cat fight abscess	Anaerobes, also *Rhodococcus, Pasteurella, Staphylococcus, Actinomyces*	Use hot packs and surgical drainage as necessary.	Penicillin G[b]	Amoxicillin,[c] chloramphenicol, lincosamide[d]
	Feline "leprosy"	*Mycobacterium lepraemurium?*	Surgical removal preferred (see Chapter 19).	Clofazimine[e]	Rifampin,[e] dapsone[e]
	Opportunistic mycobacterial infections	*Mycobacterium fortuitum, M. chelonae, M. smegmatis, M. phlei*	Surgical excision, debridement needed. Identification and susceptibility test advised.	Clarithromycin with rifampin or fluoroquinolone	Doxycycline (see Chapter 19)
	Variant tuberculosis syndrome	*M. tuberculosis, M. bovis variant*	Draining skin nodules, local lymphadenopathy. Rare systemic spread.	Clarithromycin with rifampin and enrofloxacin	

TABLE 22.3. *Continued*

Site or Type of Infection	Diagnosis	Common Infecting Organisms	Comments	Suggested Drugs[a]	Alternatives
Ear	Otitis	Likely secondary infection: *Malassezia, Staphylococcus, Pasteurella*	Check for *Otodectes* mites, polyps, foreign bodies. Clean and dry ear canal.	Topical aminoglycoside,[g] polymyxin,[h] or chloramphenicol	Topical nystatin, miconazole, thiabendazole, clotrimazole for *Malassezia*
Eye	Conjunctivitis	Herpesvirus or calicivirus, *Chlamydia, Mycoplasma,* secondary bacteria	*Chlamydia, Mycoplasma* may be found in conjunctival scrapings.	Topical tetracycline[i]	Topical chloramphenicol. Topical idoxuridine or trifluridine for early herpes
	Penetrating eye wound	Various bacteria	Infection, uveitis possible. Sample and culture aqueous humor.	Amoxicillin-clavulanate with topical, episcleral gentamicin	Chloramphenicol (also topical) and episcleral chloramphenicol sodium succinate
Respiratory and thoracic	Acute viral upper respiratory tract infection	Secondary bacteria: *Staphylococcus, Streptococcus, Pasteurella,* possibly *Mycoplasma*	Nursing and supportive care.	Penicillin G[b]	Amoxicillin,[c] macrolide[m]
	Chronic rhinitis-sinusitis	As above, plus anaerobes	Intermittent treatment may help control, but not cure, the condition.	Penicillin V	Amoxicillin,[c] sulfonamide-trimethoprim,[k] chloramphenicol
	Cryptococcal rhinitis-sinusitis	*Cryptococcus neoformans*	May also have pulmonary granulomas.	Fluconazole, itraconazole	Ketaconazole plus flucytosine
	Aspiration pneumonia	Mixed anaerobes and facultative bacteria	Analysis of tracheal wash fluid useful, but could treat on suspicion if aspiration occurs.	Amoxicillin,[c] amoxicillin-clavulanate	Chloramphenicol

Category	Disease	Organisms	Comments	First choice	Alternative
	Other bacterial pneumonia	*Pasteurella, Bordetella,* other facultative bacteria, anaerobes	Culture and susceptibility testing of transtracheal aspirate, bronchial wash, or lung aspirate recommended.	Amoxicillin,[c] amoxicillin-clavulanate	Sulfonamide-trimethoprim[k] chloramphenicol
	Pyothorax	Various anaerobes, (including *Actinomyces, Bacteroides*) and *Pasteurella*	Chest drainage and lavage needed. Gram-stained smears should be examined, exudate cultured.	Penicillin G,[b] amoxicillin,[c] amoxicillin-clavulanate	Lincosamide,[d] chloramphenicol
Alimentary and abdominal	Periodontitis and gingivitis	Mixed facultatives and anaerobes	Remove calculus, improve dental hygiene. If severe, consider antibiotic prior to dentistry.	Penicillin G,[b] amoxicillin[c]	Metronidazole ± spiramycin; clindamycin
	Acute ulcerative gingivostomatitis	Various resident bacteria, including anaerobes	Infection primary or secondary? Seek underlying cause. Local and supportive treatment.	Penicillin G,[b] amoxicillin[c]	Metronidazole ± spiramycin; clindamycin
	Chronic proliferative stomatitis	Bacteria secondary	Possibly viral etiology, hypersensitivity. Antimicrobials noncurative. Biopsy, treat locally, consider systemic glucocorticoid.		
	Gastric helicobacteriosis	*Helicobacter*	Relation of infection to illness often unclear. Value of treatment unclear.	Metronidazole (plus cimetidine) and amoxicillin or tetracycline[l]	

TABLE 22.3. *Continued*

Site or Type of Infection	Diagnosis	Common Infecting Organisms	Comments	Suggested Drugs[a]	Alternatives
	Bacterial enteritis	*Campylobacter*	Isolation of doubtful significance. Treatment may be unwarranted.	Erythromycin	Chloramphenicol, tetracycline[l]
		E. coli	As for *Campylobacter*.	Amoxicillin[c]	Sulfonamide-trimethoprim,[k] tetracycline[l]
		Salmonella	Mainly immunodeficient cats or kittens in poor conditions. Use drug only if systemically ill, but may prolong carrier state.	Chloramphenicol	Sulfonamide-trimethoprim[k]
	Giardiasis	*Giardia*	Inapparent carriers occur, disease rare. Potential zoonosis.	Albendazole	Fenbendazole?, metronidazole?
	Coccidiosis	*Isospora*	Coccidia may be coincidental to diarrhea. Neonates and immunosuppressed adults at risk.	Sulfonamide,[m] sulfonamide-trimethoprim[k]	Furazolidone
	Parvoviral enteritis (panleukopenia, or feline infectious enteritis)	Secondary bacteria, especially anaerobes	Treat parenterally. Fluid therapy, nursing, and supportive care essential.	Penicillin G, amoxicillin[c]	Amoxicillin-clavulanate, amoxicillin[c] plus gentamicin
	Cholecystitis, cholangiohepatitis	Coliforms, *Pasteurella*, anaerobes		Amoxicillin-clavulanate	Beta-lactam[n] plus fluoroquinolone,[f] chloramphenicol

		Organism	Comments	First choice	Second choice
Nervous system	Meningitis	*Pasteurella, Staphylococcus, Streptococcus, Cryptococcus*	Isolation and susceptibility test recommended. Guarded prognosis.	Penicillin G, amoxicillin-clavulanate Amphotericin B and flucytosine, fluconazole	Chloramphenicol, sulfonamide-trimethoprim[k] Itraconazole
Other	Hepatic encephalopathy	Normal intestinal flora	Use low-protein diet, lactulose; administer drugs orally.	Amoxicillin[c]	Metronidazole
	Bacterial lower urinary tract infections	*Escherichia, Streptococcus, Staphylococcus, Proteus*	Rare. May be secondary to idiopathic nonseptic feline urologic syndrome, calculus, tumor. Antibacterial inappropriate unless bacteriuria present.	Amoxicillin[c], amoxicillin-clavulanate	Sulfonamide-trimethoprim[k], chloramphenicol
	Bartonellosis	*Bartonella henselae,* others	Generally subclinical. Consider treatment (for 2–4 weeks) if pet maintained with immunocompromised owner, but efficacy uncertain.	Enrofloxacin	Doxycycline, rifampin
	Osteomyelitis	Mostly *Staphylococcus,* sometimes *Streptococcus* coliforms, anaerobes	Surgical intervention, susceptibility test advised.	Amoxicillin-clavulanate, isoxazolyl penicillin[o]	Cephalosporin (oral or group 1 parenteral)[p]
	Plague	*Yersinia pestis*	If enzootic areas. Human health risk. Eliminate fleas.	Aminoglycoside[q]	Doxycycline, chloramphenicol[r], fluoroquinolone[r]

TABLE 22.3. *Continued*

Site or Type of Infection	Diagnosis	Common Infecting Organisms	Comments	Suggested Drugs[a]	Alternatives
	Tuberculosis	*Mycobacterium bovis*	Rare if bovine tuberculosis controlled. Prolonged therapy. Potential risk to owner.	Clarithromycin with rifampin and/or enrofloxacin	Rifampin with isoniazid and/or ethambutol
Other protozoal infections	Babesiosis	*Babesia felis*	Hemolytic anemia; consider blood transfusion.	Primaquine	
	Cytauxzoonosis	*Cytauxzoon felis*	Often fatal despite nursing, fluids, drugs.	Imidocarb	Diminazene
	Toxoplasmosis	*Toxoplasma gondii*	Clinical disease uncommon.	Clindamycin	Sulfonamide[m] plus pyrimethamine, azithromycin?, clarithromycin?
Rickettsial, chlamydial, and mycoplasmal infections	Feline infectious anemia	*Haemobartonella*	May be secondary to immunosuppressive virus. Consider glucocorticoid with antimicrobial if primary. Transfuse blood if necessary.	Tetracycline[l]	Chloramphenicol
	Chlamydial infections	*Chlamydia psittaci*	Mainly ocular infections, possibly rhinitis pneumonia, genital infections.	Topical tetracycline[k] for conjunctivitis	Other sites: tetracycline,[i] chloramphenicol, macrolide,[j] fluoroquinolone[f]

Mycoplasmal	*Mycoplasma felis, M. gateae,* others	Possibly in conjunctivitis, pneumonia arthritis, abortion, fetal death, abscesses.	Topical: tetracycline[i] for conjunctivitis	Other sites: tetracycline,[l] chloramphenicol, macrolide,[j] fluoroquinolone[f]
Other		Various other bacterial, rickettsial, protozoal and fungal infections occur infrequently in cats. Consult Table 22.2 (canine infections) for possible treatments.		

[a]These suggestions are derived from review of the literature, discussion with colleagues, and clinical experience. Laboratory data (Gram stain of exudate or aspirate, or culture and susceptibility test) should be used to guide drug selection if available. See Greene (1998) for additional information.

[b]Penicillin G: penicillin V may be substituted for oral administration (see Chapter 6).

[c]Amoxicillin: ampicillin or hetacillin may be substituted (see Chapter 6).

[d]Lincosamides: lincomycin, clindamycin (see Chapter 11).

[e]Clofazimine, rifampin, dapsone: limited data on efficacy.

[f]Fluoroquinolones: ciprofloxacin, difloxacin, enrofloxacin, marbofloxacin, ofloxacin, orbifloxacin (see Chapter 15).

[g]Aminoglycosides, topical: neomycin, framycetin (neomycin B), kanamycin, gentamicin (see Chapter 10).

[h]Polymyxins: polymyxin B, colistin (polymyxin E) (see Chapter 9).

[i]Tetracyclines, topical: tetracycline, oxytetracycline, chlortetracycline (see Chapter 13).

[j]Macrolides: erythromycin, tylosin (see Chapter 11).

[k]Sulfonamide-trimethoprim: various sulfonamides (sulfadiazine, sulfamethoxazole, sulfadoxine, etc.) combined with trimethoprim. Ormetoprim and baquiloprim are alternatives to trimethoprim (see Chapter 14).

[l]Tetracyclines, systemic: doxycycline, minocycline, tetracycline, oxytetracycline (see Chapter 13).

[m]Sulfonamides: many available, eg, sulfadimidine, sulfadizaine, sulfadimethoxine (see Chapter 14).

[n]Beta-lactams: penicillins, cephalosporins (see Chapters 6 and 7).

[o]Isoxazolyl penicillins: cloxacillin, dicloxacillin, flucloxacillin, oxacillin (see Chapter 6).

[p]Cephalosporins, oral (eg, cefadroxil, cephalexin) and group 1 parenteral (eg, cefazolin, cephradine) (see Chapter 7).

[q]Aminoglycosides, systemic: amikacin, dihydrostreptomycin, gentamicin, kanamycin, streptomycin, tobramycin (see Chapter 10).

TABLE 22.4. Antimicrobial drugs that are potentially hazardous in renal failure, liver failure, pregnancy, or neonates

Renal Failure[a]	Liver Failure[b]	Pregnancy[a]	Neonates[a]
Aminoglycosides	Chloramphenicol	Aminoglycosides	Aminoglycosides
Amphotericin B	Clindamycin	Amphotericin B	Chloramphenicol
Chloramphenicol (cat)	Griseofulvin (cat)	Azithromycin	Fluoroquinolones
Flucytosine	Ketoconazole	Chloramphenicol	Metronidazole
Fluoroquinolones	Lincomycin	Fluconazole	Nalidixic acid
Lincomycin	Macrolides	Flucytosine	Nitrofurantoin
Nalidixic acid	Metronidazole	Fluoroquinolones	Polymyxins
Nitrofurantoin	Rifampin	Griseofulvin	Sulfonamides
Polymyxins	Sulfonamides	Ketoconazole	Rifampin
Sulfonamides	Sulfonamide-	Metronidazole	Tetracyclines
Sulfonamide-trimethoprim (cat)	trimethoprim (dog)	Nitrofurantoin	Trimethoprim
Tetracyclines (not doxycycline)	Tetracyclines	Polymyxins	
		Sulfonamides	
		Tetracyclines	
		Trimethoprim	

[a]See Chapter 19.
[b]There is little information on effects of liver failure on antimicrobial drug therapy. Some listed agents are potentially hepatotoxic; others might accumulate to toxic levels in hepatopathy. These warnings constitute relative rather than absolute contraindications.

566

TABLE 22.5. **Suggested oral administration in relation to feeding**

Better When Fasting[a]	Better with Food	Indifferent to Feeding
Azithromycin	Cefadroxil[b]	Cephalexin[b]
Cephradine	Chloramphenicol palmitate[d]	Chloramphenicol capsules, tablets[b,d]
Most erythromycin preparations[b]	Doxycycline[e]	Chloramphenicol palmitate[b]
Fluoroquinolones[c]	Griseofulvin	Clarithromycin[b]
Isoniazid	Itraconazole	Ethambutol
Lincomycin	Ketoconazole	Fluconazole
Most penicillins[b]	Metronidazole[e]	Hetacillin
Rifampin	Nitrofurantoin[e]	Spiramycin[f]
Most sulfonamides		
Most tetracyclines		

Source: Data are from human studies, except as indicated.

[a] Absorption of these drugs may be reduced or delayed by ingesta. *Fasting* means no food for 1–2 hours before and 1–2 hours after dosing.

[b] Canine data.

[c] Enrofloxacin availability is reduced by ingesta in dogs. Effects of ingesta on fluoroquinolones are considered generally mild, but milk and yogurt should be avoided.

[d] Feline data.

[e] Food may reduce gut irritation without hindering absorption significantly.

[f] Human data. Porcine data indicate better when fasting.

TABLE 22.6. Conventional dosage regimens for antimicrobial drugs in dogs and cats

Drugs	Routes	Dose (mg/kg except as indicated)	Dose Interval (h)	Comments, Cautions
Penicillins, narrow-spectrum				See Chapter 6
Cloxacillin	PO, IV, IM	12.5–25	8	PO, avoid ingesta
Dicloxacillin	PO	25	4–6	PO, avoid ingesta; non-beta-lactamase producers only
Flucloxacillin	IV, IM	25	6–8	
Methicillin	PO	15	8	PO, avoid ingesta
Oxacillin	IV, IM	25–50	6	
Penicillin G, Na or K	PO, IV, IM	15–25	8	PO, avoid ingesta
	IV, IM, SC	12.5–25 (20,000–40,000 IU/kg)	4–6	Increases plasma Na or K
Penicillin G, procaine	IM, SC	20 (20,000 IU/kg)	12–24	Once daily adequate routinely
Penicillin G, benzathine	IM	30 (40,000 IU/kg)	72–120	Highly susceptible pathogens only, very limited use
Penicillin V	PO	10 (15,300 IU/kg)	8	Avoid ingesta
Penicillins, wider-spectrum				See Chapter 6
Amoxicillin	PO	10–20	8–12	PO, ingesta have minor effect
	IV, IM, SC	7	12	
Amoxicillin-clavulanate	PO	12.5–25 (combined)	8–12	Use the higher dose for serious or systemic infections
	IM, SC	10–20 (combined)	24	
Ampicillin	PO	20–30	8	PO, avoid ingesta
	IV, IM, SC	10–20	8	
Ampicillin-sulbactam	IV, IM	20–50 (combined)	8	Alternative to injectable amoxicillin-clavulanate
Carbenicillin	IV, IM, SC	30–50	6–8	Use the lower dose for lower urinary infection, higher (to 150 mg/kg) for systemic effect
Hetacillin	PO	20–30	8	Prodrug for ampicillin
Piperacillin	IV, IM	25–50	8–12	
Ticarcillin	IV, IM, SC	20–50	6–8	See carbenicillin

Cephalosporins and relatives

				See Chapter 7 for explanation of generations and groups
Oral				
Cefaclor	PO	10–15	8	May cause vomiting, diarrhea, increased liver enzymes
Cefadroxil	PO	20–30	12	May cause vomiting, diarrhea. Ingesta increase but delay systemic availability
Cephalexin	PO	20–40	8–12	May cause vomiting, diarrhea, anorexia, salivation
Cephradine	PO	20	6–8	May cause vomiting, anorexia, diarrhea. Avoid ingesta
Group 1 parenteral				
Cefazolin	IV, IM, SC	20–30	6–8	May cause pain, phlebitis
Cephapirin	IV, IM, SC	10–30	8	May cause pain, phlebitis
Cephradine	IV, IM, SC	10–25	6–8	May cause pain, phlebitis
Group 2 parenteral				
Cefotaxime	IV, IM, SC	20–50	6–8	
Ceftiofur	SC	2–4 (dog)	12–24	Use lower dose once daily for lower urinary infection, higher dose for systemic infections
Group 3 parenteral				
Cefoperazone	IV, IM, SC	20–30	8–12	
Group 4 parenteral				
Cefoxitin	IV, IM, SC	30	6–8	A cephamycin. May cause vomiting IV, pain IM or SC
Cefotetan	IV, IM, SC	30	8–12	A cephamycin. May cause vomiting IV, pain IM or SC
Aminoglycosides				See Chapter 10. With all aminoglycosides, watch for renal, vestibular, or auditory toxicity, neuromuscular blockage, circulatory depression. Recent studies indicate administration of the total systemic dose in 1 daily
Amikacin	IV, IM, SC	15–30	24	
Dihydrostreptomycin	PO	10–20	6	
	IM, SC	20–30	24	
Gentamicin	IV, IM, SC	6.6	24	
Kanamycin	PO	10	6	
	IV, IM, SC	30	24	

TABLE 22.6. *Continued*

Drugs	Routes	Dose (mg/kg except as indicated)	Dose Interval (h)	Comments, Cautions
Neomycin	PO	10	6	bolus may reduce toxicity without compromising efficacy. Avoid in pregnancy, neonates. Potentially ototoxic in ears with ruptured eardrums. Streptomycin and dihydrostreptomycin rarely used systemically. Reserve amikacin, netilmicin, and tobramycin for bacterial infections resistant to other aminoglycosides. Consider therapeutic monitoring in geriatric and neonatal patients.
Netilmicin	IV, IM, SC	3–6	24	
Streptomycin	PO	20	6	
	IM, SC	20–30	24	
Tobramycin	IV, IM, SC	3–6	24	
Fluoroquinolones				
Ciprofloxacin	PO	5–15	12	See Chapter 15. Use lower end of dose ranges for urinary infections, higher end for soft tissue infections, osteomyelitis. *Pseudomonas*. May cause mild gastrointestinal disturbances, excitement (avoid in seizure-prone animals), nephrotoxicity (crystal deposition in tubules in alkaline urine). Avoid in pregnancy and neonatal or growing animals (cartilage lesions), and avoid or reduce dose in renal failure.
	IV	5	12	
Difloxacin	PO	5–10	24	
Enrofloxacin	PO, IV, IM, SC	2.5–10	12–24	
Marbofloxacin	PO	2	24	
Ofloxacin	PO, IV	2.5–10	12	
Orbifloxacin	PO	2.5–7.5	24	
Tetracyclines				
Chlortetracycline	PO	20	8	See Chapter 13. Oral administration preferred, painful IM. Absorption from gut generally reduced by ingesta, but doxycycline can be given with food to reduce gut
Doxycycline	PO, IV	5–10	12	
Minocycline	PO, IV	5–10	12	
Oxytetracycline	PO	20	8	
	IV, IM	10	12	

Drug	Route	Dose	Interval (h)	Comments
Tetracycline	PO IV, IM	20 10	8 12	irritation. Side effects include anorexia, vomiting, diarrhea, fever in cats, discoloration of teeth. Avoid in pregnancy, neonates, liver failure. Avoid in renal failure (except doxycycline).
Lincosamides, macrolides, and azalides				
Azithromycin	PO	5 (cat) 10 (dog)	24–48 24	See Chapter 11. IM administration may cause pain. Vomiting and diarrhea can occur with oral administration. Some erythromycin esters may be hepatotoxic; therefore avoid in liver disease. Clarithromycin is a newer macrolide. Azithromycin is an azalide. Spiramycin is often combined with metronidazole at 12.5 mg/kg.
Clarithromycin	PO	5–10	12	
Clindamycin	PO, IV, IM, SC	5–10	8–12	
Erythromycin	PO	10–20	8–12	
Lincomycin	PO IV, IM	10–20 10–20	8–12 12–24	
Spiramycin	PO	23.4	24	
Tylosin	PO IV, IM	10–20 5–10	12 12	
Sulfonamides and combinations				
Sulfadiazine	PO, IV	50–100 (double first dose in dog)	12	See Chapter 14. Generally safe but occasional adverse effects. In dogs: dry eye, dermatoses, polyarthritis, fever, blood dyscrasias, ataxia. In cats: salivation, depression, disorientation, blood cytopenias, azotemic renal failure. Potential folate deficiency. Avoid if anemic or leukopenic and in pregnancy, neonates.
Sulfadiazine-trimethoprim	PO, IV, IM, SC	30 (combined)	12–24	
Sulfadimethoxine	PO, IV, IM, SC	25 (double first dose in dog)	24	
Sulfadimethoxine-baquiloprim	PO SC	30 (combined) 30 (combined)	48 72	
Sulfadimethoxine-ormetoprim	PO	27.5 (combined, double first dose)	24	
Sulfamethoxazole-trimethoprim	PO	30 (combined)	12–24	
"Triple sulfas" (trisulfapyramidines)	PO, IV	50 (double first dose in dog)	12	

TABLE 22.6. *Continued*

Drugs	Routes	Dose (mg/kg except as indicated)	Dose Interval (h)	Comments, Cautions
Miscellaneous antibacterials				
Chloramphenicol	PO	50 (dog)	8	See Chapter 12. Few adverse effects in dogs. Oral dose safe in cats for 3 weeks, higher (60–100 mg/kg per day, divided) possible up to 1 week. Side effects: depression, inappetence, vomiting, diarrhea, reversible marrow suppression. Avoid in neonates, pregnancy, liver failure, cats with renal failure.
	IV, IM, SC	50 mg total (cat)	12	
		50 (dog)	8	
		20 (cat)	12	
Clofazimine	PO	4–8 (dog)	24	Excise or debulk lesions if possible.
		8 (cat)	24	May need prolonged therapy.
Dapsone	PO	1 (dog)	8	Reduce to 0.3–0.6 mg/kg in dogs after 2 weeks. May cause vomiting, diarrhea, anorexia, hemolysis, luekopenia, thrombocytopenia, dermatosis.
		50 mg total (cat)	12–24	
Ethambutol	PO	15 (dog)	24	Toxicity: optic neuritis, peripheral neuritis, anorexia, vomiting.
Isoniazid	PO	10–20 (dog max. 300 mg daily)		Potentially hepatotoxic, neurotoxic.
Metronidazole	PO, IV, SC	10	8	May cause anorexia, vomiting, neurological signs. Avoid in early pregnancy. Potential carcinogen. See "other antiprotozoals" for dose.
Pyrazinamide	PO	15–40	24	Hepatotoxic: gut signs, arthralgia.
Rifampin (rifampicin)	PO, IV, IM	10–20 (dog max. 600 mg daily)	2–24	Hepatotoxic; avoid in liver disease, pregnancy. Discolors tears and urine.
Tinidazole	PO	20 (dog)	12	For anaerobes. See "Other antiprotozoals" for dose.
		15 (cat)	24	
Vancomycin	IV	10–20	6–12	Infuse slowly over 30–60 minutes.

Other antiprotozoals, antirickettsials

	Route	Dose	Interval (h)	Comments
Albendazole	PO	25	12	For 2–5 days. Efficacy against feline giardiasis unknown.
Allopurinol	PO	15	12	For 26 weeks. Combine with meglumine. Maintenance treatment 20 mg/kg per day given for 1 week per month.
Amprolium	PO	100–300 mg total (dog)	24	Maximum daily dose in pups: small breeds 100 mg, large breeds 200 mg. Duration 7 days. Administer in food, water, or capsules. Toxic effects: anorexia, depression, thiamine deficiency, CNS signs.
		60–100 mg total (cat)	24	
Benznidazole	PO	5	24	For 2 months.
Clindamycin	PO, IV, IM, SC	10–20 (dog)	12	Use the higher dose in smaller dogs; duration 2–3 weeks for toxoplasmosis. See "Lincosamides, macrolides, and azalides."
		12.5–25 (cat)	12	
Difluoromethylornithine	PO	100 (dog)	8	For 6 days, with diminazene. May cause diarrhea, vomiting.
Diminazene aceturate	IM	3.5 or 7 (dog)	Once	The lower dog dose for babesiosis; higher for African trypanosomiasis; repeat in 2–4 weeks. For feline cytauxzoonosis, repeat at 72–96 hours. Pain at injection site. May cause gastrointestinal, CNS signs.
		2 (cat)	Once	
Fenbendazole	PO	50	24	For 3 days. Efficacy in feline giardiasis unknown.
Furazolidone	PO	4–10	12	For 7 days.
Imidocarb dipropionate	IM, SC	5	Once	Can repeat in 14 days. Injection painful. Causes salivation, lacrimation, diarrhea, dyspnea, depression.

TABLE 22.6. *Continued*

Drugs	Routes	Dose (mg/kg except as indicated)	Dose Interval (h)	Comments, Cautions
Meglumine antimonate	IV, SC	100 (dog)	24	For 3–4 weeks. Treat relapses similarly. Side effects: anorexia vomiting, lethargy, myalgia. Possible cardiac, renal toxicity, inflammation at injection site.
Metronidazole antibacterials	PO	15–30 (dog)	12–24	See "Miscellaneous antibacterials" for antibacterial dose, cautions.
Nifurtimox	PO	10–25 (cat)	12–24	
Paromomycin	PO	2–7 (dog)	6	Continue 3–5 months.
	PO	125–165	12	For 5 days. Repeat if needed.
Pentamidine isethionate	IM	4 (dog)	24	For 2 weeks. Pain and necrosis at injection site, hypotension, nausea, salivation, vomiting, diarrhea, anaphylaxis.
Phenamidine isethionate	SC	15 (dog)	24	For 2 days. Side effects: see pentamidine.
Primaquine	PO, IM	0.5	Once	Single dose >1 mg/kg is lethal in cats.
Pyrimethamine	PO	0.25–0.5	12	Plus sulfonamide 30 mg/kg every 12 hours, for 2 weeks. Inappetence, depression, and malaise common in cats. Give folinic acid 5 mg/day to reduce marrow suppression.
Quinacrine	PO	7 (dog) 10 (cat)	12	Treat 5 days. Transient gut upsets, anorexia, pyrexia, lethargy may occur.
Sodium stibogluconate	IV, SC	30–50 (dog)	24	For 3–4 weeks. See meglumine, which has fewer side effects.
Tinidazole	PO	44 (dog)	24	For 3 days. See "Miscellaneous antibacterials" for antibacterial dose.
Toltrazuril	PO	5	12	For 5 days.
Trypan blue	IV	10	Once	Slow infusion 1% solution.

Antifungals

Drug	Route	Dose	Interval	Comments
Amphotericin B deoxycholate	IV, SC	0.25–0.5 (dog) 0.1–0.25 (cat)	48 48	Infuse IV or inject SC in large volume. Maximum cumulative IV dose as single agent 8–12 mg/kg in dogs, 4 mg/kg in cats, higher SC (8–26 mg/kg). Nephrotoxic.
Clotrimazole	Topical	1 g in 100 ml polyethylene glycol 400	Once	Slow infusion bilaterally. See medicine texts. Repeat in 4 weeks if persists.
Enilconazole	Topical	10	12	Dilute the 10% solution 50:50 with water just before irrigating nose, sinuses. For 7–10 days.
Fluconazole	PO	5–10 (dog) 50 mg total (cat)	24 8	Liver enzymes may increase with treatment.
Flucytosine	PO	50–75 (dog) 50 (cat)	8 8	Side effects: vomiting, diarrhea, leukopenia, thrombocytopenia. Combine with amphotericin B or an azole.
Griseofulvin microsize Ultramicrosize	PO PO	25–50 5–10	12 24	May cause gut upsets; and in cats anemia, leukopenia, pruritis, ataxia, increased liver enzymes, bilirubinemia, teratogenicity.
Itraconazole	PO	5–10	12–24	May cause anorexia, increased liver enzymes and (in dogs) necrotic skin foci. Better tolerated than ketoconazole in cats.
Ketoconazole	PO	5–15 (dog) 10 (cat)	12 12–24	May cause anorexia, depression, diarrhea, vomiting, coat changes, increased liver enzymes; in dogs, reduced hormone production; in cats, fever, anemia. Avoid in pregnancy.

Source: These data are collated from many sources.
Note: For additional dosage information, see Morgan (1997) and Greene (1998). Doses and intervals are similar for dogs and cats unless otherwise indicated.

23 | Antimicrobial Drug Use in Cattle

K. G. BATEMAN

The application of antimicrobial therapy in cattle, like that in other species of domestic animals, is often based upon clinical experience and theoretical considerations rather than well-conducted clinical trials. Increasingly, however, the advent of multiperson specialist practices and the application of good record keeping and appropriate quantitative analysis mean that individual practices can conduct field trials of the treatment of common disease conditions over time. This chapter summarizes important considerations in the application of antimicrobial drugs in cattle and lists recommended treatments for individual diseases.

Principles of Antimicrobial Drug Selection and Use

Undifferentiated bovine respiratory disease (UBRD) will be used as an example of the application of the principles of selection and use of antimicrobials in the bovine because of the author's experience and the occurrence of the condition in both beef and dairy cattle, and because it is the disease that results in the greatest use of antimicrobials in cattle.

Most antimicrobials are approved for use by regulatory agencies on the basis of safety (to the animal and to the humans consuming the milk and meat) and proof that the product is an improvement over a placebo. Titration studies have been conducted to support the dosage that the manufacturer wishes to have approved. In the approval process, increasing emphasis has recently been placed on comparison with a current industry standard therapy or likely competitor in the marketplace. Unfortunately, the results are proprietary, and the veterinary practitioner sel-

576

dom has the ability to scrutinize trial design and results beyond what is provided voluntarily or under duress by the manufacturer.

Other than for a few recent clinical trials of therapy for UBRD, drugs for treatment of most bovine diseases have to be selected for use on the basis of probable organism involved, probable in vitro sensitivity pattern of the organism, and knowledge of the pharmacokinetics of the antimicrobial drug chosen. This is what some call rational therapy but what the skeptics would call a plausibility argument to justify our choice.

In the example of UBRD, *Pasteurella multocida* isolates exhibit little antimicrobial resistance and have remained susceptible to the commonly used antimicrobials. Evidence is emerging in North America that *Pasteurella haemolytica* appears to have, pretreatment, two distinct patterns of antimicrobial resistance that are serotype related and plasmid encoded. While approximately half of the serotype A1 and A2 isolates are resistant to sulfonamides, A2 isolates are generally susceptible to other commonly used antimicrobials, whereas A1 isolates demonstrate a consistent, plasmid-encoded resistance to penicillin (and therefore to ampicillin) and tetracycline. Most isolates of *P. haemolytica* that are obtained pretreatment are not antimicrobial resistant and therefore are probably A2. Once antimicrobial therapy has been applied, the isolates obtained from either the live or dead animal are almost invariably resistant to penicillin and tetracycline. There would seem to be a shift in the predominant population of *P. haemolytica* in the animal after antimicrobial exposure, and therefore posttreatment sampling will lead to erroneous conclusions.

There are well-substantiated cases in which prolonged use of an antimicrobial in a protocol has led to the selection of *P. haemolytica* with susceptibility patterns substantially different from those generally described. Recent work has shown a strong correlation between the antimicrobial susceptibility patterns of *Pasteurella* spp. obtained at illness from nasopharyngeal swabs and from bronchoalveolar lavage. Although this correlation is poor at the individual animal level, the relationship is strong enough at the group level to recommend that pretreatment nasopharyngeal swabs be obtained from a few animals where resistance to the currently employed antimicrobial is suspected as the primary cause of treatment failure.

The direct cost of most antimicrobials compared with the value of the cattle or animal involved is not usually an important issue, but relative cost of the alternative antimicrobials, likelihood of better cure rates, different withdrawal times, and lost sales (absolute for milk or delayed in the case of meat) are important factors in the choice of therapy. In many conditions in cattle, avoidance of antimicrobial therapy can be the most cost-effective choice. Salvage slaughter of residue-free cattle or even euthanasia can, under some circumstances, be an alternative to treatment, based on economical and humane grounds.

Ease of drug administration is important because clients of varying technical capabilities do most of the follow-up therapy. Unless it is extremely convenient, IV administration of antimicrobials cannot be recommended over IM or SC routes of administration in the bovine. This route of administration may, however, be indicated to avoid tissue necrosis (carcass damage) and, perhaps, injection site residues. The cost, risk of phlebitis or cellulitis, and negligible difference in clinical efficacy, where tested, do not generally favor this route.

Most antimicrobials are somewhat similar in their withdrawal times, so that this consideration may be of minimal significance, with notable exceptions. In diseases such as enzootic pneumonia of young dairy or beef calves, the animals are both so far from slaughter and of negligible salvage value that a long withdrawal time for meat is not a concern. On the other hand, a heavy feedlot steer has an appreciable salvage slaughter value. Slaughter is a viable alternative to therapy if the treatment does not have a high probability of curing the disease. Lactating dairy cows produce milk of considerable value each day, and therefore antimicrobial therapy must not be administered unless strongly indicated. The introduction of ceftiofur sodium, with no milk or meat withdrawal times, makes it worth considering at the label dose for susceptible infections in heavy feedlot cattle and lactating cows.

Treatment protocols for UBRD are based on identification of depressed and anorexic cattle that are found to be febrile (>40° C) after removal from their pen. Animals are treated for 2 days with the first-line antimicrobial. Response is evaluated on the third day, and if it is favorable, therapy is continued for an additional 1 or 2 days, for a total of 3–4 days of treatment. If a case is nonresponsive on the third day, based on a failure of the temperature to drop below 40° C, a second-line antimicrobial should be employed for 3 or 4 days. Relapses should be treated with the second-line antimicrobial or yet a third antibiotic for 3–6 days, depending on the response (temperature decline). Often, an inexpensive, relatively narrow-spectrum antimicrobial such as oxytetracycline is employed as first-line therapy, with the more expensive, broader-spectrum drugs employed as second- and occasionally third-line therapy. In light of the presence of plasmid-encoded resistance to penicillin and tetracycline, it is not advisable to use these drugs in a protocol as second-line drugs.

Long-acting oxytetracycline, tilmicosin, and florfenicol are effective antibiotics that maintain therapeutic blood levels for at least 3 days and inhibitory pulmonary tissue levels for still longer. These products have met increasing successful use in place of 3 daily injections of other conventional products. One of the most important advantages may be that their use allows the cattle to leave the hospital earlier, thus reducing their exposure to other pathogens. However, if the animal is not hospitalized, there is the risk that nonresponsive cases will not be identified and changed to second-line therapy or at least have the original therapy extended for a few days. Very experienced pen checkers may be able to evaluate response visually and avoid high case fatality; however, this aspect deserves close monitoring and assessment where single-injection therapy is employed.

The response, relapse, and case fatality rates will vary with the quality of cattle, time of year, age of calf, and feedlot management practices, including early recognition and treatment of pneumonic cattle. Generally a favorable response to therapy is considered to be a drop in the rectal temperature to below 40° C by the third day of therapy (48 hours after first treatment). Response rates (by this definition) of greater than 80% are quite acceptable. Relapse rates of greater than 20% should be cause for concern and warrant investigation of potential contributing factors. If cattle arrive at the feedlot in reasonably good condition, case fatality rates can be maintained at 3–4%.

Avoiding Selection of Antibiotic-resistant Bacteria

The selection of resistant bacteria requires exposure of the organism to antimicrobial drugs. The only sure method of preventing bacterial resistance is to avoid antimicrobial use altogether. Antimicrobial exposure should therefore be minimized. For example, many cases of subacute, clinical mastitis due to environmental organisms such as *Streptococcus uberis* or *S. dysgalactiae* will respond as well to frequent (every 4 hours) stripping as antibiotic infusion. Recently, however, there has been concern that although a clinical cure will be effected with stripping, a bacteriological cure will not. In such cases, the mastitis may become clinical in a short time or remain subclinical but cause elevation of the bulk tank somatic cell count. In the case of *Staphylococcus aureus* mastitis, the dismal bacteriological cure rate during lactation mandates stripping to be the method of choice. Such a method has the advantage of no milk withdrawal, as well as the slower emergence of resistant organisms in the herd. In the case of coliform mastitis, studies do not support the benefit of antibiotic use over frequent stripping (see Chapter 31).

For the purpose of reducing the development of resistance, we lack adequate information to make firm recommendations as to whether it is best to use different antimicrobials for specific conditions, as outlined in Table 23.1, or whether it is preferable to choose one drug suitable for a number of common conditions, use it exclusively for a time, and then use another for the next period. It is evident that all-in/all-out feedlots have less problem with antimicrobial resistance than continuous-flow feedlots or closed dairy herds that use considerable amounts of antibiotics.

Prophylactic Use of Antimicrobial Drugs

There can be no denying the clinical and subclinical biological effects that some antibiotics have under some circumstances and types of management. Before they are recommended to clients, the veterinarian should be convinced that they will have both a beneficial biological and a beneficial economic effect in the situation under consideration.

As an example, ionophore feed antibiotics such as monensin, lasalocid, and salinomycin improve feed efficiency in a cost-effective manner as well as reduce the risk of coccidiosis and acute interstitial pneumonia. On the other hand, although inclusion of chlortetracycline and/or sulfamethazine in feedlot starter rations may lower treatment rates, it may not (depending on product cost) be cost-effective.

Current interest in prophylactic use of antimicrobials for UBRD centers on the long-acting, injectable formulations of oxytetracycline and tilmicosin. They have the advantage of a quick and reliable method of administration when proper facilities are available. However, it may be difficult to anticipate that an outbreak will be severe enough to warrant mass medication and to time it accurately. Where cattle always originate from similar sources (eg, auction marts) and data available from previous groups indicate early and substantial (>30% treatment rates) outbreaks of pneumonia, injection upon arrival with long-acting oxytetracycline or tilmicosin can be cost-effective. In situations where sources and morbidity rates may not be consistent, decisions may be made on a group to group basis by deciding to medicate when a certain percentage of the cattle in a pen have been treated (eg, 10%) over a defined time period (eg, 3 days). Some suggest that mass medication be carried out whenever a pen death (untreated mortality) due to fibrinous pneumonia occurs, because lack of adequate observation of the group on the part of the manager is likely to be associated with the presence of other advanced cases in that pen.

When prophylactic antimicrobials are used, they should be directed at a specific disease condition, and an unrelated drug (to which resistance is improbable) should be used for treatment.

Residue Avoidance and Extralabel Drug Use

Veterinary drug use in food-producing species is accompanied by a duty, to the producer and the consumer, to ensure that milk and meat are free of violative residues (ie, that measurable residues are below predetermined acceptable levels; see Chapter 33). A privilege intimately associated with our obligation described above is that of prescribing drugs for purposes and at dosages different from those on the label or product insert. Extralabel drug use is practiced if the product being used is approved in that species but for a different disease, or if the product is used at a different (usually higher) dose or with an altered withdrawal time (see Chapter 34).

Off-label use generally implies that the product is not even approved for use in that species (at least in the country in question).

Each bovine practitioner and cattle producer seems to have a different comfort level with what type of antimicrobial use is morally and ethically acceptable. The time has arrived for producer and veterinary groups to adopt positions that are both realistic and responsible. The necessity for extralabel use stems from the reluctance of producers and veterinarians to stop the practice, because they feel that the competitors who continue such use will have an unfair advantage. Both groups should recognize that as long as extralabel and off-label use continues, manufacturers lose incentive to add to the list of approved uses for a product. A few large feedlot owners have ceased all extralabel antimicrobial use because they know the issue is important to consumers and they have too much to lose to risk the practice. Individual animal identification, accurate written disease treatment protocols, and treatment records are a necessity for avoiding residues in all circumstances. On-farm and in-clinic residue tests should be employed where extralabel antimicrobial use is deemed necessary.

Increasing public concerns over healthfulness and chemical residues will play an increasing role in decisions by food animal veterinarians and producers. It has never been more true, with respect to demand for our products, that perception is reality.

Injection Site Lesions

Beef quality audits in both the United States and Canada have documented unacceptably high rates of intramuscular injection site lesions (scarring) in both younger fed cattle (yearlings) and in cull cows. One recent study estimated the loss to the industry as Cdn $9.58 per head for yearlings and Cdn $6.34 for each cull cow and bull. It is imperative that subcutaneous routes of injection be used whenever possible and that intramuscular injections, when necessary, be administered in the neck. Veterinarians, producers, and equipment manufacturers all have a role in the issue.

Specific Comments on Antimicrobial Drug Use in Cattle

Listed in Table 23.2 are antimicrobials with approved uses for cattle. Table 23.1 contains recommendations for specific disease conditions commonly encountered in North America. Recommendations are made based on the following considerations: (1) the usual organism(s) involved, (2) the common resistance pattern of the organism(s), (3) some consideration of the cost of the products, and (4) the expectation that the cases are detected early enough to allow the response to be monitored and the antimicrobial changed after 48 hours if improvement is not evident. For the most part, products recommended have been restricted to those compounds with an approved (label) claim for use in the bovine. Where the dosage recommended is extralabel, it is indicated. Some antimicrobials are not approved for use in lactating dairy cows.

Enrofloxacin is approved in the United States only for use in the treatment of bovine respiratory disease. All other use in the United States is currently in violation of the regulations. However, in Europe, other fluoroquinolones, such as danofloxacin and marbofloxacin, are approved for additional purposes, including the treatment of enteric disease caused by susceptible bacteria.

It is beyond the scope of this text to discuss all product indications and cautions, but the user should always consult the product label and insert. Resources containing the label and insert information include the *Compendium of Veterinary Products* (Dechert, 1997, 1999).

Bibliography

Allen JW, et al. 1991. The microbial flora of the respiratory tract in feedlot calves: association between nasopharyngeal and bronchoalveolar lavage cultures. Can J Vet Res 55:341.

Bateman KG, et al. 1990. An evaluation of antimicrobial therapy for undifferentiated bovine respiratory disease. Can Vet J 31:689.

Dechert AA, ed. 1997. Compendium of Veterinary Products. Hensall, Ont.: North American Compendiums.

Dechert AA, ed. 1999. Compendium of Veterinary Products (USA ed.). Port Huron, MI: North American Compendiums.

Harland RJ, et al. 1991. Efficacy of parenteral antibiotics for disease prophylaxis in feedlot calves. Can Vet J 32:163.

Mechor GD, et al. 1988. Comparison of penicillin, oxytetracycline, and trimethoprimsulfadoxine in the treatment of acute undifferentiated bovine respiratory disease. Can Vet J 29:438.

Ritter L. 1991. Withholding times for procaine penicillin G in cattle. Can Vet J 32:647.

Schumann FJ, et al. 1990. Prophylactic tilmicosin medication of feedlot calves at arrival. Can Vet J 31:285.

Van Donkersgoed J, et al. 1998. Injection site surveys in Canadian yearling cattle and cull cows and bulls: fall 1997. Can Vet J 39:497

TABLE 23.1. Antimicrobial drug selection for some infections of cattle

Site	Diagnosis	Common Infecting Organisms	Comments	Suggested Drugs	Alternative Drugs
Respiratory	Enzootic calf pneumonia	Viral primaries ± *Mycoplasma* spp., *Pasteurella multocida*, *Haemophilus somnus*	Usually *P. multocida*. Occurs in both dairy and beef calves.	Oxytetracycline,[a] tilmicosin	Florfenicol, ceftiofur, trimethoprim-sulfadoxine, enrofloxacin, spectinomycin
	Pneumonic pasteurellosis	*P. haemolytica*, *P. multocida*	Ceftiofur first-line for lactating dairy cows.	Tilmicosin florfenicol	Ceftiofur, trimethoprim-sulfadoxine, enrofloxacin, spectinomycin
	Undifferentiated bovine respiratory disease (UBRD)	Virus ± *Mycoplasma* ± *P. haemolytica*, *P. multocida, H. somnus*, anaerobes	Ceftiofur first-line for lactating dairy cows.	Oxytetracycline, tilmicosin	Florfenicol, ceftiofur, trimethoprim-sulfadoxine, enrofloxacin, spectinomycin
	Chronic bacterial pneumonia	*Arcanobacterium pyogenes*, anaerobes, *H. somnus*, *Pasteurella* spp.		Penicillin G,[b] tilmicosin	Florfenicol
	Necrotic laryngitis	*Fusobacterium necrophorum*	Handle carefully due to hypoxia and give anti-inflammatories to relieve dyspnea. May require tracheostomy.	Penicillin G,[c] oxytetracycline	Ceftiofur, trimethoprim-sulfadoxine
Gastro-intestinal	Acute diffuse peritonitis	*F. necrophorum*, *A. pyogenes, E. coli*	Abomasal ulcer, uterine laceration, surgical sepsis.	Trimethoprim-sulfadoxine ± penicillin G	Sulbactam-ampicillin

TABLE 23.1. *Continued*

Site	Diagnosis	Common Infecting Organisms	Comments	Suggested Drugs	Alternative Drugs
	Acute traumatic reticulo-peritonitis	*F. necrophorum,* anaerobes, *Streptococcus* spp.	Stall rest and elevation of front end are probably as important as anti-microbial therapy. Surgery should be done in 2–3 days if it is an option and the animal is not improving.	Penicillin G, oxytetracycline	Trimethoprim-sulfadoxine
	Necrotic stomatitis/oral necro-bacillosis	*F. necrophorum*	Isolate. Feed and water with separate utensils.	Penicillin G	Oxytetracyline, ceftiofur
	Neonatal colibacillosis	Enterotoxigenic *E. coli*	Do not administer antimicrobial orally *if given at all.* Use only to treat septicemia if present. Fluids, electrolytes and bicarbonate as required are more important.	Trimethoprim-sulfadoxine, florfenicol	Sulbactam-ampicillin
	Salmonellosis	*Salmonella typhimurium, S. dublin, S. newport, S. muenster*	Only use antimicrobials for severely systemically ill patients.	Trimethoprim-sulfadoxine	Sulbactam-ampicillin
	Enterotoxemia	*Clostridium perfringens* B, C	Hyperimmune antiserum for therapy.	Penicillin	

Skin and conjunctiva	Disease	Organism	Comments	Drug of choice	Alternative
Skin and conjunctiva	Actinobacillosis	*Actinobacillus lignieresii*	Iodides may be used in conjunction with recommended antibiotics but probably affect fibrous tissue, not the bacterium.	Oxytetracycline	Trimethoprim-sulfadoxine
	Interdigital necrobacillosis	*F. necrophorum*	Mild cases in milking cows may be treated with topical copper sulfate (no need to discard milk). Preventable with copper sulfate footbath. Ceftiofur first-line for lactating dairy cows.	Penicillin G, oxytetracycline, ceftiofur	
	Stable foot rot	*Bacteroides nodosus*	Trim necrotic tissue away first. Completely preventable with copper sulfate foot bath. Parenteral antibiotics are not helpful.	Copper sulfate (topically)	
	Digital dermatitis	Undetermined	Tetracycline or lincomycin footbaths in enzootic herds (alternating with regular use of copper sulfate baths).	Oxytetracycline (topically)[d]	Lincomycin (topically)[d]
	Infectious bovine keratoconjunctivitis	*Moraxella bovis*	Ancillary therapy includes protection from sunlight. Membrana nictitans flap for advanced cases at initial visit avoids repeated handling and provides more favorable prognosis.	Long-acting oxytetracycline (parenterally)	Penicillin G topically or subconjunctivally[d] (mixed with corticosteroid unless descemetocele present)

TABLE 23.1. *Continued*

Site	Diagnosis	Common Infecting Organisms	Comments	Suggested Drugs	Alternative Drugs
	Omphalitis	E. coli, A. pyogenes, F. necrophorum, Staphylococcus spp.	Lance and flush if abscess has formed.	Trimethoprim-sulfadoxine (acute)	Penicillin G (chronic)
	Cellulitis	A. pyogenes, F. necrophorum, Staphylococcus spp.	Antibiotics recommended for prophylaxis after abdominal surgery on farm.	Penicillin G (post-cesarean section), ceftiofur (post-laparotomy when peritonitis is not a concern)	
	Ringworm	Trichophyton spp.	If extensive, examine nutrition, concurrent disease. Griseofulvin is teratogenic.	"Tincture of time"; 4% thiabendazole ointment, 2.5% iodine topically	Griseofulvin (5 mg/kg q24 hours for 7 days)[e]
	Dermatophilosis	Dermatophilus congolensis		Penicillin G	Oxytetracycline
Genital	Acute septic metritis	E. coli, A. pyogenes, Staphylococcus spp., Streptococcus spp., anaerobes, ± Clostridium spp.	Parenteral therapy is most crucial. May also infuse uterus with oxytetracycline.	Penicillin G	Trimethoprim-sulfadoxine
	Endometritis	A. pyogenes	Prostaglandin to involute uterus, then intrauterine infusion.	Cephapirin benzathine (IU)	Oxytetracycline (IU), gentamicin (IU)
	Granular vulvitis	Ureaplasma diversum	Treat only if infertility (repeat breeder).	Guarded insemination rod	Oxytetracycline (IU) 6–24 hours postbreeding
Musculo-skeletal	Traumatic tarsal/carpal cellulitis	A. pyogenes, F. necrophorum, Staphylococcus spp. anaerobes	Antimicrobial treatment ± hydrotherapy successful only in acute stage. More advanced cases need rubefacient or poultice to induce external drainage.	Penicillin G, ceftiofur	Trimethoprim-sulfadoxine, oxytetracycline

Category	Disease	Organism(s)	Comments	Treatment	Alternative
	Polyarthritis (neonatal)	E. coli, A. pyogenes	Late treatment is very unrewarding.	Florfenicol	Trimethoprim-sulfadoxine, sulbactam-ampicillin
	Polyarthritis (feedlot)	Mycoplasma bovis, H. somnus	M. bovis may be a secondary invader. Disease is positively correlated with the occurrence of UBRD.	Oxytetracycline	Florfenicol
	Blackleg	Clostridium chauvoei, (C. novyi, C. septicum)	Inject some antibiotic directly into the lesion. Prophylactic antibiotic injection and trivalent bacterin to the others in group.	Penicillin G	Oxytetracycline
	Malignant edema	C. septicum, (C. chauvoei, C. perfringens, C. novyi, C. sordellii)	Easily prevented by prophylactic antibiotics for injuries, vaginal lacerations, castration wounds. Hygiene of needles and medication is crucial.	Penicillin G	Oxytetracycline
	Actinomycosis	Actinomyces bovis	Treatment usually only halts growth of lesion.	Sodium iodide 20% IV. Repeat in 7 days.	Penicillin, isoniazid (10 mg/kg q24 hours for 28 days)
CNS	Meningitis (neonatal)	E. coli	Usually fatal.	Trimethoprim-sulfadoxine	Ceftiofur; sulbactam-ampicillin
	Listeriosis	Listeria monocytogenes	Rarely involves more than one bovine; therefore no prophylactic measures taken.	Oxytetracycline	Penicillin G

TABLE 23.1. Continued

Site	Diagnosis	Common Infecting Organisms	Comments	Suggested Drugs	Alternative Drugs
	Infectious thrombo-embolic meningo-encephalitis	H. somnus	Treatment successful if still ambulatory. Vaccination, mass medication of doubtful economic value.	Oxytetracycline	Trimethoprim-sulfadoxine, florfenicol
	Tetanus	Clostridium tetani	Vaccinate if using elastrator or bander for castration.	Penicillin G	
Urinary	Cystitis	Corynebacterium renale, Arcanobacterium pyogenes, E. coli	Treat for at least 10 days.	Penicillin G	Ceftiofur
	Pyelonephritis	C. renale	Treat for at least 10 days. Remission only temporary if infection well-established. Expect additional cases in affected herds.	Penicillin G	Ceftiofur, trimethoprim-sulfadoxine
	Leptospirosis	Leptospira hardjo, L. pomona	Treatment of entire herd with strepto-mycin to eliminate carriers is of questionable value.	Penicillin G (Chapter 19)	Oxytetracycline
Cardio-vascular	Omphalophlebitis	E. coli, Arcanobacterium pyogenes	Surgical resection if intra-abdominal mass in valuable calf (?).	Penicillin G	Trimethoprim-sulfadoxine, sulbactam-ampicillin, florfenicol
	Endocarditis	A. pyogenes, Streptococcus spp.	Antimicrobial therapy gives temporary remission only.	Penicillin G	

Myocarditis/ abscess	*H. somnus*	Usually found dead.	Oxytetracycline	Trimethoprim-sulfadoxine, florfenicol
Septicemia				
Neonatal	*E. coli, Salmonella* spp., *Streptococcus* spp.			Florfenicol, sulbactam-ampicillin
Hemophilosis	*H. somnus*	Sudden death with gross diagnosis of septicemia ± acute polyarthritis.	Trimethoprim-sulfadoxine Oxytetracycline	Trimethoprim-sulfadoxine, florfenicol
Other				
Anaplasmosis	*Anaplasma marginale*	Treatment for 3 days with oxytetracycline but sterilization with 2–4 injections of long-acting oxytetracycline q7 days.	Oxytetracycline	Imidocarb

[a]Oxytetracycline (unless otherwise noted): conventional at 6.6 mg/kg IM q24 hours or long-acting at 20 mg/kg IM q72 hours.
[b]45,000 IU/kg IM q24 hours (extralabel).
[c]Penicillin G (unless otherwise noted): 20,000 IU/kg IM q24 hours (extralabel).
[d]Extralabel route.
[e]Off-label (not approved for food animals).

TABLE 23.2.   **Suitable antimicrobials for the treatment of cattle**

Antimicrobial Drug	Dosage and Route
Individual therapy	
Cefapirin benzathine[a]	500 mg intrauterine
Ceftiofur sodium[b]	1 to 2[c] mg/kg IM q24 hours
Enrofloxacin[d]	7.5 to 12.5 mg/kg SC once
	or
	2.5 to 5 mg/kg SC q24 hours for 3 to 5 days
Florfenicol[e]	20 mg/kg IM; repeat in 48 hours
	or
	40 mg/kg SC once[f]
Gentamicin[g]	200 mg intrauterine
Long-acting oxytetracycline[h]	20 mg/kg IM or SC[i] q72 hours
Oxytetracycline	6.6 mg/kg IM q24 hours
Oxytetracycline[j]	2 to 3 gm intrauterine
Penicillin G	20,000 IU/kg[k] IM q24 hours
	or
	45,000 IU/kg[l] IM q24 hours for UBRD
Spectinomycin[m]	10 to 15 mg/kg SC q24 hours
Sulbactam-ampicillin[n,h]	2.5 ml/45 kg IM q24 hours
Tilmicosin[o,h]	10 mg/kg SC once
Trimethoprim-sulfadoxine[p]	3 ml/45 kg IM q24 hours
Mass prophylactic medication	
Long-acting oxytetracycline[h]	20 mg/kg IM or SC[i] once
Tilmicosin[o,h]	10 mg/kg SC once

[a]Metricure®, Intervet, Holland.
[b]Naxcel®, Upjohn, Kalamazoo, Michigan. (Excenel® in Canada.)
[c]2 mg/kg dose is approved in USA only.
[d]Baytril 100®, Bayer, Shawnee Mission, KS. Available only in USA.
[e]Nuflor®, Schering-Plough, Union, NJ.
[f]Single-injection SC therapy is USA claim only.
[g]Gentacin®, Schering-Plough, Union, NJ.
[h]Not approved for use in lactating dairy cows.
[i]SC claim is for only some product formulations.
[j]Kelamycin®, Vetoquinol, Joliette, Quebec.
[k]Extralabel dosage. Milk and meat withdrawal 4 and 10 days, respectively. Source: Ritter (1991).
[l]Extralabel dosage. Not for lactating cows. Meat withdrawal 20 days. Source: Ritter (1991).
[m]Adspec®, Upjohn, Kalamazoo, MI. Available only in USA.
[n]Synergistin® (60 mg/ml sulbactam, 120 mg/ml ampicillin), rogar/STB, London, Ontario. Available only in Canada.
[o]Micotil®, Elanco, Indianapolis, IN.
[p]40 mg/ml trimethoprim, 200 mg/ml sulfadoxine. Available only in Canada.

24 | Antimicrobial Drug Use in Sheep and Goats

P. I. MENZIES

General Considerations of Antimicrobial Treatment
Routes of Administration

When administering drugs to a large sheep flock, where speed of administration, minimal animal handling, and limited carcass damage are major considerations, the preferred methods of administration are subcutaneous (SC) injection, oral dosing, and incorporation into feed or water. Using a race or chute with the animals well crowded, oral drenching, or injection with an automatic gun or syringe enables rapid treatment of large numbers. SC injections are usually given behind the ear under the loose skin of the neck. Other sites available are the axilla, which is difficult to reach reliably in a race but useful for individual treatments, and the medial aspect of the thigh, which can be used if the sheep are being tipped up for another reason. Intramuscular (IM) injections should be avoided in market lambs and kids. When IM injections are necessary, they should be given in the muscle of the neck. Hind leg injections are discouraged particularly in market lambs and kids, but when large repeated volumes are required and the injections are given in the hind leg, the needle must be directed away from the femur to avoid damaging the sciatic nerve. This is particularly important in young lambs and kids. Intravenous (IV) injections are usually given in the jugular vein, which is readily accessible because it is superficial and mobile. Success of IV injection of a sheep in heavy fleece is more difficult but will be facilitated if the vein is first identified by palpation.

Considerations for treatment sites in goats are similar to those in sheep except that goats tolerate oral drenching less well. In North America, it is common for goats to be treated as individuals rather than as herds. SC injections are more frequently given in the axilla, so that

591

injection reactions are not as readily seen. Goats often exhibit more pain than sheep when given irritating drug formulations.

Both sheep and goats are frequently given udder infusions for either the treatment or the prevention of mastitis. Pretreatment samples of milk should be obtained by gently squeezing the teat rather than pulling, as this may damage the suspensory ligaments of the udder. It is important that the teat end be cleaned carefully with alcohol and that a fresh tube be used for each gland since there is great risk of the tube being contaminated from an infected gland. In sheep, the teat sphincter is sometimes difficult to penetrate with a teat infusion tube. Good restraint and careful manipulation are necessary to ensure that the tube does not become contaminated and that the teat end is not damaged.

Use of Antimicrobial Drugs in the Feed and Water

To treat or control outbreaks of disease, antimicrobial drugs such as some sulfonamides and tetracycline can be incorporated into the feed or water of sheep or goats. The most common example is a coccidiostat mixed and pelleted into lamb creep feed for the prevention of coccidiosis. Prevention or treatment of abortion in ewes or does is also sometimes treated this way. Several problems can arise from this method of treatment: (1) improper mixing (evenness or dosage), leading to toxicosis or ineffective treatment; (2) inability to ensure that all animals have consumed a therapeutic dose; (3) the danger of destruction of the rumen microflora, which leads to severe digestive disturbances such as inappetence and ketosis and which may be fatal; and (4) the danger of inactivation of an antimicrobial drug by a resistant rumen microflora. Antimicrobial drugs such as ampicillin, erythromycin, methicillin, lincomycin, oleandomycin, chloramphenicol, trimethoprim sulfa, novobiocin, and some sulfonamides (sulfathiazole, sulfamethylthiadiazole) are damaging to the rumen microflora and under some circumstances may cause fatal illness. For these reasons, antimicrobial drugs should not be administered orally (directly, in feed, or in water) to sheep and goats, with the exceptions possibly of coccidiostats and some of the sulfonamides and tetracyclines, which appear to be absorbed well from the rumen.

Monensin (a coccidiostat) has often been implicated in mixing problems in which lambs received too much of the drug, resulting in severe myopathy or death (see Chapter 16). Owners using this drug for lambs or kids must be aware of the danger in allowing other species (in particular, horses) accidental access to the medicated feed.

Antimicrobial drugs can also be added to drinking water. Problems arising from this method include the requirements for eliminating all other sources of water, difficulties with correctly calculating the capacity of the watering system, the need to ensure proper mixing of the drug, and ensuring that all animals consume enough water. This latter issue is a particular problem with sick animals or bitter-tasting medications.

Extralabel Drug Use

In North America, goats and sheep are considered minor species, with the exception that sheep are considered a major species with respect to human food safety in the United States. When licensing a new drug, few drug companies will bear the cost of the testing for efficacy and residues necessary for drug product labeling for these species. For this reason, much antimicrobial drug use in sheep and goats constitutes extralabel drug use (ELDU; see Chapters 33 and 34). ELDU is permissible, however, if the following criteria are met: a valid veterinarian-client-patient relationship (as defined by the pertinent country's veterinary medical association); reasonable evidence that the drug will not be toxic and will be therapeutically effective; unavailability of labeled therapeutic alternatives; appropriate records kept (including proper identification of animals treated); and significantly extended withdrawal times used so that no illegal residues occur. For more-detailed information regarding the regulations for ELDU in the United States, consult the Animal Medicinal Drug Use Clarification Act (AMDUCA) Guidance Brochure provided by the American Veterinary Medical Association; in Canada, consult the Food and Drug Act, as well as the provincial veterinary regulations. For information on appropriate withdrawals, the local Food Animal Residue Avoidance Databank (FARAD) should be contacted (Chapter 33). There are ongoing efforts in many countries to improve international harmonization of drug approval protocols. This is in keeping with the trend toward decreased trading restrictions, as is evidenced by trade agreements such as GATT and NAFTA.

Veterinary practitioners have limited ability to easily obtain accurate information on pharmacokinetics of new antimicrobials in sheep and goats. The data do not exist, are not published, or are not readily available to practitioners in the field. Too often the dosage, frequency of administration, length of withdrawal, and indication are extrapolated from data obtained on another species, quite possibly erroneously. This may lead to the real risk of ineffective treatment and/or residues in the meat or milk. It is in the interest of public health as well as the agricultural industry to obtain label claims for minor species and minor uses.

Some drugs, while shown to be efficacious in sheep and/or goats, are illegal for use in food-producing animals in some countries. An example is the antimicrobial class of fluoroquinolones, whose extralabel use is prohibited in food animals in the United States. However, these antibiotics are commonly used in these species in Europe. In addition, some countries have regulations against extralabel prescription of feed additives.

For example, monensin cannot be scripted into feed intended for sheep in the United Kingdom, and in the United States no drug can be scripted into feed or water for food animal species unless specifically labeled for that species, dose, and indication. For this reason, suggestions in Tables 24.1 and 24.2 should be considered in light of the specific regulations in the country where the veterinarian is practicing.

Antimicrobial Drug Selection

Antimicrobial drug selection for the treatment of common infections of sheep and goats is presented in Table 24.1 and of drug dosages in Table 24.2.

Bibliography

Apley M. 1997. AMDUCA and the food animal industry. In: Proc Am Assoc Small Rumin Pract, p49.

Bagley CV, et al. 1987. Comparisons of treatments of ovine foot rot. J Am Vet Med Assoc 191:541.

Beaulieu AJ. 1992. The IR-4 project: a national program for the approval of new animal drugs for minor species and minor uses. Accomplishments and goals for minor ruminants: FDA/CVM perspective. In: Proceedings of the IR-4/FDA Workshop for Minor Use Drugs: Focus on Small Ruminants. Bethesda, MD. Vet Hum Toxicol 35 (Suppl 2):10.

Brodie TA, et al. 1986. Some aspects of tick-borne diseases of British sheep. Vet Rec 118:415.

Bulgin MS. 1988. Losses related to the ingestion of lincomycin-medicated feed in a range sheep flock. J Am Vet Med Assoc 192:1083

Buswell JF, et al. 1989. Antibiotic persistence and tolerance in the lactating goat following intramammary therapy. Vet Rec 125:301.

Carceles CM, et al. 1995. Comparative pharmacokinetics of amoxicillin/clavulanic acid combination after intravenous administration to sheep and goats. J Vet Pharmacol Ther 18:132.

Center for Veterinary Medicine. 1995. Drug Use Guide: Sheep and Goats. CVM Memo CVMM-15. HHS Publ (FDA) 95-6019.

Cid D, et al. 1996. J Vet Pharmacol Ther 19:397.

Curry-Galvin E. 1998. Helpful tips for extralabel drug use: food animals. J Am Vet Med Assoc 9:1392.

Dargatz DA, et al. 1990. Antimicrobial therapy for rams with *Brucella ovis* infection of the urogenital tract. J Am Vet Med Assoc 196:605.

Diker KS, et al. 1994. Antimicrobial susceptibility of *Pasteurella haemolytica* and *Pasteurella multocida* isolated from pneumonic ovine lungs. Vet Rec 134:597.

Escudero E, et al. 1999. Pharmacokinetics of an ampicillin-sulbactam combination after intravenous and intramuscular administration to sheep. Can J Vet Res 63:25–30.

Espuny A, et al. 1996. Some pharmacokinetic parameters of ampicillin/sulbactam combination after intravenous and intramuscular administration to goats. Vet Q 18:136.

Grieg A, Linklater KA. 1986. Field studies on the efficacy of a long acting preparation of oxytetracycline in controlling outbreaks of enzootic abortion of sheep. Vet Rec 117:627.

Hueston WD, et al. 1989. Intramammary antibiotic treatment at the end of lactation for prophylaxis and treatment of intramammary infections in ewes. J Am Vet Med Assoc 194:1041.

König CDW. 1983. Foot rot treatment with lincomycin/spectinomycin. Proc Sheep Vet Soc 7:81.

Lashev L, et al. 1994. Species specific pharmacokinetics of rolitetracycline. J Vet Med Assoc 42:201.

McKellar QA. 1993. Therapy: chemotherapy—problems and solutions. Proc Sheep Vet Soc 17:87.

Mengozzi G, et al. 1996. Pharmacokinetics of enrofloxacin and its metabolite ciprofloxacin after intravenous and intramuscular administrations in sheep. Am J Vet Res 57:1040.

Muñoz MJ, et al. 1996. Pharmacokinetics of ciprofloxacin in sheep after single intravenous or intramuscular administration. Vet Q 18:45.

Píriz Duran S, et al. 1991. Comparative in vitro susceptibility of *Bacteroides* and *Fusobacterium* isolated from footrot in sheep to 28 antimicrobial agents. J Vet Pharmacol Ther 14:185.

Short CR. 1994. Consideration of sheep as a minor species: comparison of drug metabolism and disposition with other domestic ruminants. Vet Hum Toxicol 36:24–40.

Smith KC, et al. 1996. Other applications of the tilmicosin molecule in sheep. Proc Sheep Vet Soc 20:27.

Spence JA, et al. 1988. Development of periodontal disease in a single flock of sheep: clinical signs, morphology of subgingival plaque, and influence of antimicrobial agents. Res Vet Sci 45:324.

Taylor A. 1994. Licensed and unlicensed medicines. Proc Sheep Vet Soc 18:135.

Tice GA. 1996. The use of tilmicosin for the treatment of respiratory disease in sheep. Proc Sheep Vet Soc 20:21.

TABLE 24.1. Antimicrobial drug selection for common infections of sheep and goats

Condition	Species	Common Infecting Organism	Suggested Antimicrobial(s)	Comments
Infectious abortion				
Enzootic abortion of ewes (EAE)	Sheep and goats	*Chlamydia psittaci*	Oxytetracycline	*Prophylaxis in high-risk flocks:* tetracycline in feed for 2–3 weeks prior to breeding at a dose of 100–150 mg/head per day until lambed. *Outbreak or previous diagnosis:* long-acting tetracycline at label dosage starting 1–3 weeks before start of lambing, every 10–14 days until finished. *Outbreak:* 400–450 mg/head per day tetracycline in feed until lambing finished. Often poor efficacy because of placental damage already present. Not recommended for dairy goats because of milk withdrawal. Vaccination should also be considered.
Campylobacter abortion (Vibrionic)	Sheep	*Campylobacter fetus fetus, C. jejuni*	Penicillin G—streptomycin or tetracycline	*Prophylaxis:* injections of penicillin-streptomycin for 2–5 days or tetracycline in feed as in EAE. Antimicrobial sensitivity patterns should be established from any isolates. Vaccination in the face of an outbreak also very successful.
Listeria abortion or neurological disease	Sheep and goats	*L. monocytogenes*	Tetracycline	Injectable long-acting tetracycline to all animals at risk in the face of an outbreak.
Toxoplasma abortion	Sheep and goats	*T. gondii*	Monensin	*Monensin:* mixed in feed at a dose of 15 mg/head per day from breeding to lambing.
			Decoquinate	*Decoquinate:* mixed in feed or premix to feed at a dose of 2 mg/kg per day from breeding to lambing. Should also prevent contamination of feed by cats and kittens. Vaccine available in some countries.
Salmonella abortion	Sheep and goats	*S. typhimurium, S. abortus ovis, S. montevidio, S. dublin*	IM or SC broad-spectrum antimicrobials[a]	Often widespread by the time diagnosis is made. Antibiotics may not eliminate organism; consider culling and environmental management.
Leptospira abortion	Sheep and goats	*L. hardjo, L. pomona*	Penicillin G—streptomycin; tetracyclines	Treat all pregnant animals at risk with injections.

Condition	Species	Organism	Drug	Comments
Coxiellosis (Q fever)	Sheep and goats	*Coxiella burnetii*	Tetracycline; fluoroquinolone	Abortions are more common in goats than in sheep. Long-acting injectable (IM or SC) to all pregnant does every 10–14 days until kidded; watch withdrawal for milk in dairy goats.
Other infectious reproductive disorders				
Metritis	Sheep and goats	*Arcanobacterium pyogenes, E. coli,* mixed anaerobes	Penicillin G; broad-spectrum antimicrobials[a]	Treat for 3–4 days after clinically normal.
Lamb epididymitis	Sheep	*Haemophilus, somnus Actinobacillus seminis*	Tetracycline	*Prophylaxis:* low levels in feed in situations where rams intensively managed or injectable long-acting oxytetracycline (IM or SC). Responds poorly to treatment.
Enzootic posthitis	Sheep and goats	*Corynebacterium renale* group	Penicillin G	Remove from high-protein diet and treat locally with antibiotic ointments. May treat systemically for severe cases.
Brucella ovis ram epididymitis	Sheep	*Brucella ovis*	Long-acting oxytetracycline with dihydrostreptomycin	20 mg/kg of oxytetracycline at 3-day intervals for 5 treatments and 12.5 mg/kg of streptomycin twice daily for 7 days; decreases shedding of bacteria and improves semen quality but may not cure.
Infectious diseases of lambs and kids, systemic				
Enterotoxemia/pulpy kidney	Sheep and goats	*Clostridium perfringens* types C and D	Oral virginiamycin; penicillin G; or bacitracin	Withdraw carbohydrate source in diet. Give C and D antitoxin and a balanced electrolyte solution (BES) parenterally. Vaccinate all animals at risk.
Omphalophlebitis	Sheep and goats	*Arcanobacterium pyogenes, E. coli,* mixed anaerobes	Penicillin G; broad-spectrum antimicrobials[a]	Local drainage and treatment are important.
Watery mouth (lambs), metabolic acidosis without dehydration (kids)	Sheep and goats	Probably *E. coli* endotoxin	Oral amoxicillin; apramycin broad-spectrum antimicrobials[a]	Prevention by ensuring clean environment and good colostrum ingestion. *Watery mouth:* early prophylactic treatment with oral antibiotics. *Metabolic acidosis:* isotonic bicarbonate solutions to correct acid-base deficit followed by balanced electrolyte solution (BES).

TABLE 24.1. *Continued*

Condition	Species	Common Infecting Organism	Suggested Antimicrobial(s)	Comments
Tick-borne fever (tick pyemia)	Sheep	*Ehrlichia phagocytophila* and/or *Staphylococcus aureus*	Long-acting oxytetracycline	At 1–3 weeks of age and repeated at 5–7 weeks of age in addition to dipping with an acaracide at those times.
Erysipelothrix polyarthritis	Sheep	*E. rhusiopathiae*	Penicillin G	Treat minimum of 3 days.
Infectious diseases of lambs and kids, digestive				
Colibacillosis	Sheep and goats	Enterotoxigenic *E. coli*	Broad-spectrum antimicrobials[a]	Appropriate diagnosis is necessary; also treat with BES. Clean environment, adequate colostrum; consider vaccination. Resistance to antimicrobials is common.
Cryptosporidiosis	Sheep and goats	*Cryptosporidium* spp.	Sulfonamides	Doubtful efficacy.
Salmonella dysentery	Sheep and goats	*S. typhimurium*	Broad-spectrum antimicrobials[a]	Often poor efficacy, may not eliminate carriers.
Coccidiosis	Sheep and goats	*Eimeria* spp.	Monensin; lasalocid; decoquinate; salinomycin; amprolium; sulfonamides	Mixing should be done at a feed mill and all feeds pelleted. Some products can be mixed with salt. Dose varies with feed management. Feed from 2 weeks of age until market age. Ionophores toxic to horses and dogs. Do not allow defecation in feeders.
Infectious conditions of lamb and kids, respiratory				
Pneumonic pasteurellosis	Sheep and goats	*Pasteurella haemolytica* biotype A, *P. multocida*	Tilmicosin; oxytetracycline; ceftiofur; florfenicol; penicillin G	Long-acting oxytetracycline, tilmicosin, or florfenicol can be used as a prophylaxis and during an outbreak therapeutically. Tilmicosin should not be used in goats (therapeutic dose very close to toxic dose). Ceftiofur for daily treatment of affected animals when meat or milk withdrawal is an issue (eg, market lambs close to slaughter, lactating dairy sheep).
Pasteurella septicemia	Sheep	*P. haemolytica* biotype T	As with biotype A	This biotype shows more resistance, and because the disease is peracute, vaccination is recommended for susceptible animals.

598

Condition	Animal	Organism	Treatment	Comments
Mycoplasma pneumonia	Sheep and goats	*M. ovipneumoniae, M. arginini*	Oxytetracycline; tylosin	Often seen in conjunction with pasteurellosis (atypical pneumonia) or alone.
Mycoplasma mycoides	Goats	*M. mycoides mycoides* large-colony type	Oxytetracycline; lincomycin; tylosin	Because of the peracute form of the septicemic disease, treatment is often ineffective. If goat survives, it will probably be a carrier.
Infectious conditions of the integument				
Pinkeye (infectious keratoconjunctivitis)	Sheep and goats	*Chlamydia psittaci, Mycoplasma conjunctivae, Rickettsia conjunctivae, Neisseria ovis*	Spiramycin; oxytetracycline; tiamulin IM	Spiramycin or oxytetracycline repeated on days 1, 5 and 10; tiamulin repeated at days 1, 3, 6, 9. Oxytetracycline eye ointment. Conjunctival injection of penicillin (least effective).
Secondary infection of contagious ecthyma (orf)	Sheep and goats	*Staphylococcus aureus*	Tilmicosin	May also try local antibacterials but wear gloves, as is a zoonosis.
Dermatomycosis (lumpy wool)	Sheep	*Dermatophilus congolensis*	Long-acting oxytetracycline	Decrease humidity (ventilation) if possible; powder sheep with powdered alum to help prevent reinfection.
Caseous lymphadenitis	Sheep and goats	*Corynebacterium pseudotuberculosis*	No effective treatment	Although susceptible to penicillin, not effective because of the thick abscess wall. Recommend isolation and drainage with local disinfectants and vaccination of young stock. Cull chronically infected animals.
Infectious conditions of the foot				
Contagious foot rot	Sheep and goats	*Dichelobacter nodosus, Fusobacterium necrophorum*	Long-acting oxytetracycline; penicillin G; tinidazole; spectinomycin	10–20 % zinc sulfate with 2% weight/volume sodium lauryl sulfate or 5% formalin, as a footbath with or without foot trimming. Must remain in bath 1 hour. Repeat in 5–7 days. Can use in conjunction with systemic antimicrobials and/or vaccination. Cull chronic nonresponders.
Foot scald	Sheep and goats	*F. necrophorum*	Penicillin G; ampicillin; long-acting oxytetracycline	Zinc sulfate footbath as above.

TABLE 24.1. *Continued*

Condition	Species	Common Infecting Organism	Suggested Antimicrobial(s)	Comments
Strawberry foot rot	Sheep and goats	*D. congolensis*	As with lumpy wool	Verify that condition is not chorioptic mange.
Infectious conditions of the mammary gland				
Gangrenous mastitis	Sheep and goats	*S. aureus*, *P. haemolytica*	Tilmicosin; broad-spectrum antimicrobials[a]	Gland will be lost if animal survives, so should probably be culled.
Contagious agalactia	Sheep and goats	*Mycoplasma agalactiae*, *M. mycoides mycoides* (goats)	Tetracyclines; tylosin	Probably ineffective; animal should be culled because of the likelihood of becoming a carrier.
Subclinical and clinical mastitis	Sheep and goats	*S. aureus*, *P. haemolytica*, environmental streptococci, coagulase-negative *Staphlococcus* spp.	Tilmicosin; cloxacillin; cephapirin benzathine	Do not use tilmicosin in goats (toxic). Dry treatment to be used at the end of lactation in dairy goats or at weaning for prevention of new infections in high-risk sheep flocks. Do not split tubes.
Miscellaneous infections				
Periodontal disease	Sheep	Many species	Ineffective	Trials examining effects of tetracycline and metronidazole found no protective effect.

[a] Broad-spectrum antimicrobials include ampicillin-sulbactam, ceftiofur, fluoroquinolones, trimethoprim-sulfamethazine, or other potentiated sulfonamide combinations.

600

TABLE 24.2. **Common antimicrobial and coccidiostat drug dosages in sheep and goats**

Drug Preparation[a]	Route	Dose Rate	Units	Frequency (h)
Amoxicillin trihydrate	IM	10	mg/kg	8
Ampicillin sodium	IV, IM	10–20	mg/kg	12
Amprolium	PO, feed, water	20–50	mg/kg	24, for 5–21 days
Ceftiofur	IM	1–2.2	mg/kg	24, for 3 days
Clavulanic acid–amoxicillin	IV, IM	20	mg/kg	8
Decoquinate (0.5–1 mg/kg/day)	Complete feed	1.5 (6%)	kg/tonne[b]	In feed for period of risk
	Salt/mineral mix	22.5 (6%)	kg/tonne	Premix intake 15 g/day
Enrofloxacin (sheep)[c]	IV, IM	5	mg/kg	24
Erythromycin lactobionate	IM	3.0–5.0	mg/kg	8–12
Florfenicol	IM	20	mg/kg	48 (twice)
Lasalocid (0.5–1 mg/kg/day)	Complete feed	30	g/tonne[c]	In feed for period of risk
	Salt	500	25 kg NaCl	Loose free-choice salt
Lincomycin hydrochloride	IM	10–20	mg/kg	12–24
Monensin	In feed	11–22	g/tonne[b]	In feed for period of risk
Oxytetracycline hydrochloride	IV, IM	10	mg/kg	12–24
Oxytetracycline, long-acting	IM	20	mg/kg	48–72
Penicillin G, potassium or sodium	IV	20,000–40,000	IU/kg	6
Penicillin G, procaine	IM	20,000–45,000	IU/kg	24
Salinomycin	In feed	11–16	g/tonne[c]	In feed for period of risk
Sulbactam-ampicillin[d]	IM	10	mg/kg	12–24
Sulfonamides (sulfadimethyl-pyrimidine)	PO, drinking water	50 (loading 100)	mg/kg	24; 4 days on, 3 days off, repeat (coccidiosis)
Tilmicosin[e]	SC	10	mg/kg	Single treatment
Trimethoprim-sulfonamide	IM	24–30	mg/kg	12–24
Tylosin	IM	20	mg/kg	12

[a] Many of the drugs listed are not approved for use in sheep and goats in the United States and elsewhere, so that the use constitutes extralabel drug use. In some cases also, dose recommendations are empirical. Consult the label for details.

[b] Levels calculated based on dry-matter composition of feed. Actual dry-matter consumption by animal will vary based on feed quality and animal's age, weight, and reproductive status.

[c] Fluoroquinolones are banned from use in food-producing animals other than poultry and feeder calves (enrofloxacin only) in the United States.

[d] Sulbactam-ampicillin given once daily may have too short a half-life to be therapeutically effective in goats and sheep. Plasma levels and postantibiotic effect likely only are effective for 5–12 hours (longer level for some Gram-positive bacteria).

[e] A single SC injection of tilmicosin in goats at a rate of 30 mg/kg has resulted in acute death. This is only 3 times the recommended therapeutic dose of 10 mg/kg. For this reason, tilmicosin is not recommended for use in goats.

25 | Antimicrobial Drug Use in Swine

R. M. FRIENDSHIP

Recent changes in the swine industry have reduced its reliance on antimicrobial drugs. Some producers have depopulated herds in which endemic diseases limited performance, and they have repopulated with minimal-disease stock. New vaccines and improved management techniques have resulted in better herd health. There has been a rapid move in the North American swine industry to adopt production methods that allow all-in/all-out movement of pigs so that groups of similar-aged animals are segregated and disease transmission is thus limited (Harris, 1990; Clark et al., 1991). Disease monitoring and biosecurity have become important components of maintaining these herds of higher-health pigs.

In addition to the implementation of improved herd health measures, the swine industry has become aware of societal sensitivity to issues of food safety, including antibiotic residues in meat and fears of antibiotic-resistant bacteria developing as a result of on-farm drug use. Several countries have instituted programs to educate farmers regarding proper drug use, including the recording of all treatments and the identification of animals being medicated, to ensure that appropriate withdrawal times are observed (Lewis-Jones, 1998; Stefan, 1998). Tighter government regulations and increased testing are also being instituted.

The vast majority of antimicrobial drugs used on swine farms are incorporated into feed for the purposes of growth promotion (2–50 g/ton of feed) or for subtherapeutic use (200 g or less/ton of feed). The swine industry uses low-level feed antibiotics far more than other livestock industries (Prescott, 1997). The use of antibiotics to improve growth rate and efficiency of feed utilization is discussed in Chapter 32. The present chapter will deal primarily with antimicrobial drugs as therapeutic agents

602

and will be presented on the basis of body systems (Table 25.1). Dosages for commonly used antimicrobial drugs are presented in Table 25.2.

General Considerations of Antimicrobial Treatment

Antimicrobial drugs are generally administered to a group of pigs rather than to individuals because of the large herd size of modern swine production units. Selection of an antimicrobial agent is dependent on the drug's relative cost and legislation concerning its use. A treatment program should depend on the antibiotic sensitivity pattern of the pathogenic organism and the established MICs of the antibiotics being considered. The choice of antimicrobial drug and method of administration also depends on in-depth knowledge of the specific pig farm, including the ability of the farm workers to carry out the treatment regimen and the success or failure of different antibiotics used previously on the farm. Many health problems on modern pig farms are caused by a complex interaction of environment, management, and several disease organisms. It is important for the success of any medication program to be combined with good husbandry practices.

Route of Administration

Antimicrobials are usually delivered through a carrier (feed or water). However, parenteral injection often results in the best response, particularly in the case of acute respiratory disease or septicemia (Henry and Upson, 1992). Administration of medication to individual pigs per os is limited to nursing piglets.

Oral administration of antimicrobial drugs via the feed or water is less stressful and easier to apply to a population than parenteral treatment. Oral medication reduces injection-related side effects, including anaphylactic shock, lesions from broken needles, abscesses, and tissue damage at the injection site. Injection site damage is estimated to cost the American pork industry approximately $40 million annually as a result of trim loss at packing plants (Kolb, 1996).

Many of the most commonly used antibacterial drugs, including oxytetracycline, sulfonamides, salts of benzylpenicillin, streptomycin, trimethoprim, erythromycin, and tylosin, have been shown to cause tissue necrosis and swelling at the injection site in pigs (Rasmussen, 1978). Therefore, rather than inject medication into the valuable ham region, it is recommended that IM injections be made just behind the ear on the lateral side of the neck. This procedure will also eliminate the possibility of causing sciatic nerve damage, which has been reported as a result of improper injections into the hind leg (Van Alstine and Dietrich, 1988). SC injections can be made in the neck region under the loose skin behind the ears. In young pigs, SC injections can be given inside the flank of the abdominal wall. IV injections are usually given via the ear vein, but this technique is seldom employed in swine practice.

In-feed medication is the most common method of administering antibacterials and anthelmintics. There are, however, several disadvantages. First, this technique is wasteful in that healthy pigs receive medication, along with the diseased animals that need it. Second, sick pigs often have a suppressed appetite and therefore do not eat sufficient amounts for the drug to reach therapeutic levels in their body. In addition, many antibiotics are poorly absorbed or are destroyed by stomach acid and therefore may not achieve therapeutic levels. Commonly there is a delay in treatment while unmedicated feed is used up and the medicated feed begins to enter the feeding system. In-feed medication is most appropriate in treating enteric disease and when used as a control method over a period of several weeks.

Water medication is generally a more rapid method of treating a group of sick pigs than feed medication. There is also the advantage that sick pigs often continue to drink when they will not eat. A major disadvantage is that not all medications are water soluble. Administration of medication via water is accomplished by using either an in-line water proportioner containing a concentrated stock solution or a large tank filled with water that is at the appropriate treatment level and replaces the usual water supply. Pigs will drink approximately 8–10% of their body weight per day. As a rule of thumb, when calculating how much medication will be needed to treat a pen of pigs, one can estimate the total weight of the pigs and plan on using 5 l of medicated water/60 kg of body weight daily. Water consumption can vary depending on flow rate, wastage, ambient temperature, and dietary formulation. More precise formulas for calculating daily water intake are available (Brooks et al., 1984). Proportioners can be inaccurate (Fast and Van Ee, 1978) and may even plug, so careful attention is required to ensure that pigs receive adequate amounts of drugs.

Food Safety

Pork producers are aware of the need to produce a product in which domestic and international consumers have complete confidence. The use of antimicrobial drugs in the production of pork has created two issues of consumer concern. First, there are fears that pork produced from animals treated with antimicrobial drugs will contain harmful residues (see Chapter 33). The second major concern is the growing awareness of the emergence of antibiotic-resistant bacteria and the fear that indiscriminate use of antimicrobial agents on pig farms is contributing to this problem (see Chapter 3).

The majority of pigs receive medication at some stage in their lives. Medication of starter rations for newly weaned pigs is routine on most farms in countries that do not restrict such procedures through legislation. In a survey of swine finishing units in the Netherlands, medication had not been used in only 12.5% of finishing periods studied (Elbers et al., 1990). Similar levels of antibiotic use for finishing units has been recorded in the United States (Dewey et al., 1997) and in Canada (Dunlop et al., 1998a). In a study examining the antimicrobial resistance of fecal *E. coli* of swine on 34 farrow-to-finish herds in Canada, Dunlop et al. (1998b) concluded that there was an association between the use of medicated feeds and the prevalence of *E. coli* resistant to antimicrobials.

Antimicrobial residues, particularly sulfonamides, continue to be a problem in the swine industry. As a result of extensive testing, the prevalence of sulfamethazine residues in pork has decreased but has not been eliminated. Inadvertent contamination of feeds during preparation or storage and exposure of pigs to contaminated manure have been implicated in cases of sulfamethazine residue problems (Whipple et al., 1980). However, in most cases, antimicrobial residues in pork are caused by producers not observing appropriate withdrawal periods.

The use of medications in an off-label manner is at least partly responsible for some of the difficulties that farmers face in knowing when it is safe to ship an animal. In a U.S. study (Dewey et al., 1997), about 79% of 3,328 feeds examined contained additives being used in the labeled manner. Of the 699 feeds containing antimicrobials being used in an off-label manner, about 57% included additives at greater than the recommended concentrations or were being fed to an incorrect class of pig.

To improve the quality and safety of pork, various countries have instituted education programs for pig farmers. The use of on-farm logbooks for recording all antimicrobial drug usage has been advocated as a practical method of increasing a farmer's awareness of antibiotic use and improving adherence to withdrawal times (Elbers et al., 1990). Along with accurate and complete drug recording, there should be periodic visits by a veterinarian to review the farm's medication programs to ensure drugs are being used in a safe and efficacious manner.

Considerations in Treating Swine Respiratory Disease

The incidence and economic impact of respiratory disease have increased in countries where pig production has become intensive. The causes of respiratory disease are infectious. The emergence of viral diseases, particularly porcine reproductive and respiratory syndrome (PRRS), has created difficulty in the diagnosis and control of swine respiratory disease. Often the cause is a complex of viral and bacterial etiological agents, and the disease expression is influenced by housing and management factors.

The term *porcine respiratory disease complex* (PRDC) has been used to describe particularly severe enzootic pneumonia in the late grower-finisher stage where viral components can often be identified together with *Mycoplasma hyopneumoniae* and other bacteria (Dee, 1996).

The PRRS virus and *Mycoplasma hyopneumoniae* act synergistically to create a more severe pneumonia with a longer duration than either organism causes independently (Thacker et al., 1998). The bacterial respiratory disease agents can be categorized under the following three headings (Stevenson, 1998): (1) primary inhaled pulmonary pathogens such as *M. hyopneumoniae*, *Actinobacillus pleuropneumoniae*, and *Bordetella bronchiseptica*; (2) secondary pulmonary pathogens that require tissue or cell damage by other bacteria or viruses in order to overcome the respiratory defense, such as *Pasteurella multocida*, *Mycoplasma hyorhinis*, *Streptococcus suis*, and *Hemophilus parasuis*; and (3) blood-borne pulmonary pathogens such as *Salmonella choleraesuis*, *Arcanobacterium pyogenes*, and *Actinobacillus suis*. Eradication of primary pulmonary pathogens can be accomplished by depopulation and repopulation with specific-pathogen-free (SPF) pigs. In production systems where weaning occurs at an early age and the nursery is managed in an all-in/all-out manner on a separate site away from other age groups of swine, primary respiratory pathogens can be eliminated from the grower-finisher herd (Clark et al., 1991; Fenwick et al., 1996). Progressive atrophic rhinitis (PAR) is no longer a significant swine disease because of the widespread use of all-in/all-out management, effective vaccination, and strategic medication programs. In herds experiencing a severe outbreak of PAR, suckling piglets can be medicated by strategic injections of antibacterial drugs 4–8 times before weaning (DeJong, 1992). Potentiated sulfonamides and oxytetracycline are the antimicrobial agents of choice. Vaccination of the sow herd with a commercial bacterin containing a toxoid of the dermonecrotoxin produced by *Pasteurella multocida* should be introduced as well.

Treatment of enzootic pneumonia is generally unrewarding. In the face of a severe outbreak, the choice of medication should take into account the sensitivity of the secondary organisms as well as that of *M. hyopneumoniae*. Achieving sufficiently high drug levels in the lung tissue is difficult when using mass medication, and therefore parenteral treatment is recommended but is difficult to accomplish when dealing with a large herd. Preventative medication programs, based on pulse dosing in the feed, are becoming commonly used. Most of these programs use combinations of tetracycline with tiamulin or lincomycin (Kavanaugh, 1994; Desrosiers, 1997). Prevention of enzootic pneumonia depends on good management and environment. The incidence and severity of pneumonia is greatly increased by factors such as continuous flow of animals, large numbers of pigs in one air space, a high degree of mixing of pigs within the barn, and multiple sources, such as overcrowding, cold stress, and exposure to high levels of dust and manure gases. Mycoplasma bacterins may help reduce disease severity (Desrosiers, 1997).

Pleuropneumonia has become less of a problem in most swine rearing areas in recent years. When serious outbreaks occur, pigs can die as early as 6–12 hours postinfection. It has been shown that feed and water consumption during an outbreak can decrease by 85% (Pijpers et al., 1990). Therefore, under these circumstances, treatment must be started early, and parenteral injection is the method of choice. Many isolates of *A. pleuropneumoniae* have been shown to have developed resistance to tetracyclines and penicillin. Ceftiofur, trimethoprim-sulfadiazine, and tiamulin are appropriate alternative therapeutic agents (Daniels et al., 1998).

Considerations in Treating Swine Enteric Disease

Despite great progress in reducing enteric diseases through improved farm management practices such as all-in/all-out movement of pigs, followed by thorough washing and disinfection, there are still significant losses in the swine industry associated with diarrheal diseases. The many causes of neonatal diarrhea include *E. coli*, *Clostridium perfringens*, *Isospora suis*, *Coronavirus*, and *Rotavirus* infection.

Colibacillosis is the only one of the diseases caused by these agents that will respond to antibiotic treatment of the scouring piglet. Prompt treatment with a single injection of 5 mg gentamicin is usually sufficient to alleviate the problem. A susceptibility test on the *E. coli* could be performed if antibiotic therapy is unsuccessful. Recently, postweaning colibacillosis has become a major problem in certain regions. Treatment of diarrhea in the nursery is generally more complex than in the farrowing room because the disease is generally due to a combination of etiological agents and occurs during a period of low intestinal immunity. Apramycin and neomycin are the most widely used products for treatment of postweaning colibacillosis. Where available, colistin (polymixin E) has been shown to be a useful drug against enteropathogenic *E. coli* (Lanza, 1998). Other treatments for weanling pig scours that have been advocated include the addition of organic acids to the diet to reduce the pH and the inclusion of very high levels of zinc oxide (up to 2,500 ppm) (Melin et al., 1996).

Several bacterial enteric diseases of the young growing pig have significant economic impact on the world swine industry. Swine dysentery caused by *Serpulina hyodysenteriae* and colonic spirochetosis caused by *Serpulina pilosicoli* are diseases of the pig's large intestine that cause mucoid diarrhea. Swine dysentery is the more severe disease and is often associated with bloody diarrhea and relatively high mortality rates.

Porcine proliferative enteropathy or ileitis caused by *Lawsonia intracellularis* has been diagnosed with increasing frequency as a cause of diarrhea and slow growth. This disease is generally seen as a subclinical and chronic problem in the growing-finishing barn but can occur in an acute, hemorrhagic form that may affect young adult swine. The other enteric disease that is of growing concern is salmonellosis.

In general, production systems such as segregated early weaning and all-in/all-out management might reduce the clinical expression of all postweaning enteric diseases because barns can be cleaned and disinfected between groups and thus the bacterial challenge from the environment is reduced. However, of these diseases, only swine dysentery has been shown to be effectively eliminated by multisite production techniques and the strategic use of antibiotics to prevent the shedding of organisms from carrier animals. Swine dysentery can be eradicated from herds without depopulation by using a medication and sanitation program (Glock, 1997). Pigs acutely affected with swine dysentery must be treated by injection or via the drinking water. Initial treatment must be followed up by medication in the feed for several weeks to prevent recurrence. Resistance to dimetridazole and lincomycin is increasing, leaving carbadox and tiamulin as the most effective antimicrobial drugs to treat and eradicate swine dysentery (Molnar, 1996). Valnemulin, a pleuromutilin derivative related to tiamulin, has been shown to be highly efficacious against *S. hyodysenteriae* and *S. pilosicoli* (Wade West and Ripley, 1998). There are few controlled trials that have been conducted to evaluate the efficacy of swine dysentery drugs for the treatment of colonic spirochetosis. The antimicrobial susceptibility of *S. pilosicoli* to various drugs has been evaluated. Drugs effective in the treatment of swine dysentery have been used with general success in vivo, and 100% of isolates were found to be susceptible to carbadox and tiamulin. However, this disease appears to be associated with noninfectious factors such as feed processing, feed ingredients, and other endogenous microflora, which causes some difficulty in interpreting the results of clinical trials (Duhamel et al., 1996).

Ileitis cannot be prevented by segregated early weaning. In general, macrolides, lincosamides, pleuromutilins, tetracyclines, and carbadox appear to be effective in treating ileitis. Pigs showing clinical signs of chronic disease may not respond to treatment because the disease has progressed too far before intervention has begun. However, the acute disease does respond to prompt injections of tylosin or other effective drugs, and the inclusion of therapeutic levels of tylosin or other appropriate antimicrobials in the feed has been shown to be effective in reducing the severity of chronic ileitis (Winkelman, 1997). In general, there are two situations in which antibiotics are used in the control of ileitis. First, when replacement breeding stock are introduced, antibiotics can be used at therapeutic levels in the feed after the animals have had 2–3 weeks' exposure on the farm. Second, antibiotics (for example, 100 ppm of tylosin) in the rations of early-stage growing pigs greatly reduce the clinical impact of ileitis and improve growth performance (McOrist et al., 1997).

Salmonellosis occurs as a septicemic disease caused by *S. choleraesuis* or as an enteric problem associated with various serotypes, but particularly with *S. typhimurium*. Prompt treatment of *S. choleraesuis* will reduce mortality and bacterial shedding. Antibiotics may improve the clinical expression of enteric salmonellosis, but antimicrobial agents do not appear to reduce shedding of *S. typhimurium*. Salmonellosis is of public health concern, and the increased prevalence of antibiotic resistance strains from the use of on-farm medications is a problem. Denmark has embarked on a porcine *Salmonella* eradication program. Treatment of *S. choleraesuis* should involve parenteral treatment for the clinically ill, possibly moving these animals to an isolated pen. The remaining pigs at risk can be treated with medication in feed or water. Appropriate drugs that generally show good bacterial susceptibility in vitro include carbadox, apramycin, ceftiofur, neomycin, spectinomycin, and trimethoprim-sulfa (Winkelman, 1997).

Considerations in Treating Swine Parasitic Diseases

In modern, intensive, confinement swine operations, pigs are usually infected with only a few worm species at low levels (Roepstorff and Jorsal, 1989). Under conditions of good hygiene and management, the regular application of anthelmintics may be of little or no additional effect (Roepstorff, 1997). In herds where internal parasitism persists at an economically significant level, ascariasis is generally the most important problem. The migration of *Ascaris suum* larvae through the liver results in scarring and rejection of livers at the packing plant. In addition, larval migration in the lungs can exacerbate viral or bacterial pneumonia. The most common control method is by the regular use of anthelmintics at strategic times in the production cycle. Generally, these treatments are given via the feed to sows prior to farrowing to eliminate shedding of eggs in the farrowing room, where piglets would become exposed, and the weaned pigs are often medicated once or twice during the grower stage. Most of the modern anthelmintics available to pig farmers are effective in the control of ascarids. Ivermectin is commonly used because it is also effective against mange. If trichuriasis is present, an alternative product such as fenbendazole should be used rather than ivermectin.

External parasitism caused by mange mites and lice is no longer a significant problem in most modern swine-producing regions because of the effectiveness of modern drugs. Failure to control sarcoptic mange or lice infestation is generally due to a poor understanding of the epidemiology of organisms and apathy on the part of the herdsman (Dobson and Davies, 1992). Eradication of these parasites can be accomplished by treating the entire herd at one time with an effective drug such as ivermectin. Generally 2 treatments about 10–14 days apart are recommended to ensure that the mites or lice hatching from eggs will be killed. Where this is not feasible, treatment of the sow prior to farrowing can ensure that her piglets will not become infected.

Bibliography

Brooks PH, et al. 1984. Water intake of weaned piglets from 3–7 weeks old. Vet Rec 115:513.

Clark LK, et al. 1991. The effect of all-in/all-out management on pigs from a herd with enzootic pneumonia. Vet Med 86:946.

Daniels CS, et al. 1998. Antimicrobial susceptibility profiles of swine pathogens tested at the Iowa State University Veterinary Diagnostic Laboratory. Am Assoc Swine Pract, p59.

Dee SA. 1996. The porcine respiratory disease complex: are subpopulations important? Swine Health Prod 4:147.

DeJong MF. 1992. (Progressive) atrophic rhinitis. In: Leman AD, et al., eds. Diseases of Swine, 7th ed. Ames: Iowa State University Press, p414.

Desrosiers R. 1997. Diagnosis and control of swine respiratory diseases. Am Assoc Swine Pract, p333.

Dewey CE, et al. 1997. Associations between off-label feed additives and farm size, veterinary consultant use, and animal age. Prev Vet Med 31:133.

Dobson KJ, Davies PR. 1992. External parasites. In: Leman AD, et al., eds. Diseases of Swine, 7th ed. Ames: Iowa State University Press, p668.

Duhamel GE, et al. 1996. Prevalence of porcine spirochetosis in a multiple-site production system and antimicrobial sensitivity patterns of *Serpulina pilosicoli*. Am Assoc Vet Lab Diagn 45.

Dunlop RH, et al. 1998a. Antimicrobial use and related management practices among Ontario swine producers. Can Vet J 39:87.

Dunlop RH, et al. 1998b. Associations among antimicrobial drug treatments and antimicrobial resistance of fecal *Escherichia coli* of swine on 34 farrow-to-finish farms in Ontario, Canada. Prev Vet Med 34:2.

Elbers ARW, et al. 1990. Log-book recording on pig finishing farms in an integrated quality control (IQC) project: (1) use of drugs and vaccines. Tijdschr Diergeneeskd 115:2.

Fast H, Van Ee D. 1978. A preliminary evaluation of the accuracy of four water proportioners used to medicate hogs. Can Vet J 19:101.

Fenwick B, et al. 1996. Serological validation of the utility of early weaning in preventing sow to piglet transmission of *Actinobacillus pleuropneumoniae:* production of disease free pigs from infected breeding herds. Int Pig Vet Soc, p482.

Glock RD. 1997. Elimination and control of swine dysentery. Am Assoc Swine Pract, p379.

Harris DL. 1990. The use of Isowean 3-site production to upgrade health status. Int Pig Vet Soc, p374.

Henry SC, Upson DW. 1992. Therapeutics. In: Leman AD, et al., eds. Diseases of Swine, 7th ed. Ames: Iowa State University Press, p837.

Kavanaugh NT. 1994. The effect of pulse medication with a combination of tiamulin and oxytetracycline on the performance of fattening pigs in a herd infected with enzootic pneumonia. Ir Vet J 47:58.

Kolb JR. 1996. Vaccination and medication via drinking water. Compend Contin Educ Pract Vet 18:S75.

Lanza I. 1998. Control of infectious enteric diseases of swine. Int Pig Vet Soc, p79.

Lewis-Jones CA. 1998. Quality assurance assessment. Pig J 41:99.

McOrist S, et al. 1997. Oral administration of tylosin phosphate for treatment and prevention of proliferative enteropathy in pigs. Am J Vet Res 58:136.

Melin L, et al. 1996. The influence of zinc oxide on the intestinal microflora of piglets at weaning. Int Pig Vet Soc, p465.

Molnar L. 1996. Sensitivity of strains of *Serpulina hyodysenteriae* isolated in Hungary to chemotherapeutic drugs. Vet Rec 138:158.

Pijpers A, et al. 1990. Feed and water consumption in pigs following an *Actinobacillus pleuropneumoniae* challenge. Int Pig Vet Soc, p39.

Prescott JF. 1997. Antibiotics: miracle drugs or pig food? Can Vet J 38:763.

Rasmussen F. 1978. Tissue damage at the injection site after intramuscular injection of drugs. Vet Sci Comm 2:173.

Roepstorff A. 1997. Helminth surveillance as a prerequisite for anthelmintic treatment in intensive sow herds. Vet Parasitol 73:139.

Roepstorff A, Jorsal SE. 1989. Prevalence of helminth infections in swine in Denmark. Vet Parasitol 33:231.

Stefan GE. 1998. How the residue monitoring program will change. Proc A D Leman Conf, p197.

Stevenson GW. 1998. Bacterial pneumonia in swine. Int Pig Vet Soc, p11.

Thacker E, et al. 1998. Mycoplasma and PRRSV interactions—their possible roles in PRDC. Am Assoc Swine Pract, p351.

Van Alstine NG, Dietrich JA. 1988. Porcine sciatic nerve damage after intramuscular injection. Compend Contin Educ Pract Vet 10:1329.

Wade West G, Ripley RH. 1998. The treatment of naturally occurring swine dysentery with Encor. under field conditions. Int Pig Vet Soc, p138.

Whipple DM, et al. 1980. Tissue residue depletion and recycling of sulfamethazine in swine. J Am Vet Med Assoc 177:1348.

Winkelman N. 1997. Enteric clinical disease—"back to the basics." Am Assoc Swine Pract, p353.

TABLE 25.1. Antimicrobial drug selection in swine infection

Diagnosis	Causative Agent	Comments	Suggested Drugs	Alternatives
Enteric				
Colibacillosis	*Escherichia coli*	Test susceptibility is important because resistance is common.	Gentamicin (PO, IM), trimethoprim-sulfas (IM, PO), ceftiofur (IM), enrofloxacin (IM)[a]	Apramycin (PO), neomycin (PO)
Coccidiosis	*Isospora suis*	Piglets must be treated early, prior to clinical signs.	Toltrazuril (PO)	Amprolium (PO), decoquinate (PO), sulfonamides (PO)
Colitis	*Serpulina pilosicoli*	There is usually some response to feed changes. Controlled trials are limited.	Tiamulin (water, feed), lincomycin (water, feed), tylosin (feed), carbadox (feed)	
Intestinal parasitism	*Ascaris suum, Hyostrongylus rubidus, Esophagostomum* spp., *Trichuris suis, Strongyloides ransomi*	Confinement housing and good hygiene reduce problem.	Ivermectin (SC, feed), doramectin (IM), fenbendazole (feed), levamisole (feed, water, IM)	Pyrantel tartrate (feed), piperazine (water, feed)
Proliferative enteropathy	*Lawsonia intracellularis*	Antimicrobials need to be used very early in the disease process.	Tylosin (feed), tiamulin (feed, IM), lincomycin (feed, IM), tetracyclines (feed)	Enrofloxacin (IM),[a] carbadox (feed)
Salmonellosis	*Salmonella typhimurium*	Oral antibiotics prolong shedding and may promote resistance.		
Swine dysentery	*Serpulina hyodysenteriae*	Resistance to tylosin and lincomycin is common and increasing for dimetridazole.	Tiamulin (IM, water, feed), carbadox (feed)	Lincomycin (IM, water, feed), tylosin (IM, water, feed), dimetridazole (feed)
Clostridial enteritis	*Clostridium perfringens* (type C)	Treatment of affected piglets is non-effective after clinical signs are observed. Treat sows to reduce shedding.	Bacitracin (feed) (to sows)	

Disease	Organism	Comments	Treatment	
Respiratory				
Pasteurellosis (bronchopneumonia)	*Pasteurella multocida*	Marked resistance to sulfas, tylosin, and spectinomycin. Responds to management and environment changes.	Trimethoprim-sulfa (IM), tetracycline (IM)	Ceftiofur (IM), enrofloxacin (IM)[a]
Bordetellosis (rhinitis and bronchopneumonia)	*Bordetella bronchiseptica*		Tetracycline (IM), trimethoprim-sulfa (IM)	Enrofloxacin (IM)[a]
Pleuropneumonia	*Actinobacillus pleuropneumoniae*	Many strains resistant to tetracyclines and tylosin. Feed and water treatment is a problem because of decreased consumption.	Procaine penicillin G (IM), ceftiofur (IM), ampicillin (IM)	Tiamulin (water)
Enzootic pneumonia	*Mycoplasma hyopneumoniae*	Secondary bacteria are generally a significant problem. Tylosin and tiamulin are mycoplasmastatic.	Tetracyclines (IM), lincomycin (IM), tylosin (IM), tiamulin (IM), enrofloxacin (IM)[a]	Tiamulin (feed, water)
Lungworm	*Metastrongylus* spp.	Life cycle requires earthworm as intermediate host.	Fenbendazole (feed), ivermectin (SC), levamisole (IM, feed)	
Polysystemic				
Erysipelas	*Erysipelothrix rhusiopathiae*	Treat for several days to prevent chronic form.	Procaine penicillin G (IM), tylosin (IM)	
Glasser's disease	*Haemophilus parasuis*	Resistance is variable. Prompt treatment is essential.	Procaine penicillin G (IM), tetracyclines (IM)	Lincomycin (feed), ceftiofur (IM)
Mycoplasma polyserositis	*Mycoplasma hyorhinis*	Poor response to treatment.	Tylosin (IM), lincomycin (IM), tetracycline (IM)	Trimethoprim-sulfa (IM)
Salmonellosis	*Salmonella choleraesuis*	Need to perform sensitivity testing. Feed and water medication won't control systemic disease.	Ceftiofur (IM), enrofloxacin (IM)[a], ampicillin (IM), trimethoprim-sulfa (IM)	Apramycin (water), carbadox (feed)
Actinobacillus septicemia	*Actinobacillus suis*	Emerging disease of multi-site production nurseries.	Ampicillin (IM), trimethoprim-sulfa (IM), ceftiofur (IM), enrofloxacin (IM)[a]	

TABLE 25.1. *Continued*

Diagnosis	Causative Agent	Comments	Suggested Drugs	Alternatives
Neurological				
Streptococcal meningitis	*Streptococcus suis*	Separate sick pigs to hospital pen, provide water. Need to check antibiotic sensitivity.	Procaine penicillin G, (IM), ampicillin (IM)	Trimethoprim-sulfa (IM), ceftiofur (IM), penicillin V (water)
Edema disease	*Escherichia coli*	Ineffective if clinical signs have developed.	Apramycin (water)	Carbadox (feed)
Otitis media (middle ear infection)	*Staphylococcus, Streptococcus, Arcanobacterium pyogenes*, others	Abscessation may make treatment difficult.	Trimethoprim-sulfa (IM), ampicillin (IM)	
Tetanus	*Clostridium tetani*	Prognosis is poor. Antitoxin and relaxant could be used.	Procaine penicillin G (IM)	
Listeriosis	*Listeria monocytogenes*		Procaine penicillin G (IM), trimethoprim-sulfa (IM), tetracyclines (IM)	
Musculoskeletal				
Neonatal polyarthritis	*Streptococcus*, possibly *Staphylococcus, E. coli, A. pyogenes*	Ineffective unless treated promptly. Determine sensitivity to antibiotics.	Procaine penicillin G (IM), lincomycin (IM), tylosin (IM)	
Suppurative arthritis	*A. pyogenes*, possibly *Streptococcus, Staphylococcus*	Generally treatment is ineffective.	Procaine penicillin G (IM), lincomycin (IM), tylosin (IM)	
Mycoplasmal arthritis	*Mycoplasma hyosynoviae*	Injectable antibiotics plus corticosteroids for rapid improvement.	Lincomycin (IM), tylosin (IM), tiamulin (IM)	Tiamulin (water)
Foot rot	*Fusobacterium necrophorum*	Topical chemotherapeutic agents such as copper sulfate are helpful.	Procaine penicillin G (IM)	Tetracyclines (IM), sulfonamides (IM)

Urinary				
Cystitis	*Eubacterium suis*	Relapses are common.	Procaine penicillin G (IM), lincomycin (IM), Ivermectin (IM, feed), doramectin (IM), fenbendazole (feed)	Ceftiofur (IM), tetracycline (feed)
Parasitism	*Stephanurus dentatus*			
Reproductive				
Leptospirosis	*Leptospira* spp.	Antibiotics do not eliminate carriers.	Tetracycline (IM, feed), streptomycin (IM)	See Chapter 19.
Brucellosis	*Brucella suis*	Generally controlled by national slaughter programs. Treatment requires prolonged therapy.	Tetracyclines (IM, feed), streptomycin (IM), trimethoprim-sulfa (IM)	
Cardiovascular				
Eperythrozoonosis	*Eperythrozoon suis*	Control lice to reduce spread.	Tetracycline (IM, feed), arsenicals (feed, water)	
Skin or Subcutis				
Exudative epidermitis (greasy pig disease)	*Staphylococcus hyicus*	Treat wounds with topical disinfectants promptly. Resistance to commonly used antibiotics is a problem.	Procaine penicillin G (IM), lincomycin (IM, feed, water)	Ceftiofur (IM), enrofloxacin (IM)[a]
Lice	*Haematopinus suis*	Eradication requires 2 treatments 14–20 days apart to all pigs.	Ivermectin (SC, feed), doramectin (IM)	Phosmet (topical), malathion (topical), carbaryl (topical), lindane (topical)
Mange	*Sarcoptes scabiei*	Eradication requires 2 treatments 14–20 days apart to all pigs.	Ivermectin (SC, feed), doramectin (IM)	Phosmet (topical), malathion (topical), lindane (topical)

[a]Enrofloxacin and other fluoroquinolones cannot currently be used in swine in the United States.

TABLE 25.2. **Common antimicrobial drug dosages in pigs**

Drug	Dosing Rate (mg/kg), IM (unless specified), Interval in Hours	Feed (g/ton, US)	Water (mg/l)
Ampicillin	10–20, 12 h		
Apramycin	10–20 (oral), 12–24 h	150	100
Arsanilic acid		50–100	
Bacitracin		250	
Carbadox		50	
Ceftiofur	3–10, 24 h		
Clavulanate-amoxicillin	11–13 (oral), 24 h		
Dimetridazole		100–135	250
Enrofloxacin[a]	2.5–5, 24 h		
Erythromycin	2–20, 12–24 h		
Gentamicin	2–4, 24 h		12.5
Lincomycin	10, 24 h	100–220	33
Neomycin	10 (oral), 6 h	140	70–100
Penicillin G, procaine	20,000–45,000 IU/kg, 24 h		
Streptomycin	8–12, 8 h		
Sulfamethazine	24 (oral), 24 h	400–2,000	80–130
Tetracycline[b]	10–20, 24 h	200–800	55–110
Long-acting tetracycline	20, 48 h		
Tiamulin	10–15, 24 h	200	50
Trimethoprim-sulfamethoxazole	24–30, 12 h		
Tylosin	20–30, 12–24 h	40–100	80
Virginiamycin		100	

Note: Not all drugs listed here have been licensed for use or for use at these dosage levels by regulatory authorities. Check package inserts.

[a]Fluoroquinolones, including enrofloxacin, cannot currently be used in swine in the United States.

[b]Tetracycline, chlortetracycline, oxytetracycline.

26 | Antimicrobial Drug Use in Companion Birds

G. M. DORRESTEIN

Companion, or pet, bird medicine is a rapidly expanding field, with basic information presented in many recently published handbooks (Ritchie et al., 1994; Altman et al., 1997). It is no longer possible to write about "avian medicine," since it is now realized that at least each order has its own specific aspects (Beynon et al., 1996a,b). Major interspecies differences have become apparent as understanding of antimicrobial drug use in birds improves. The anatomy and physiology of the digestive, renal, and respiratory systems differ widely among species, and there are variations in drug distribution and the metabolism of drugs. Hand raising and treatment of newborn chicks is another new area in avian medicine (Dorrestein, 1993). As in mammals, formulation of the dosage and the presence of disease conditions may influence antimicrobial drug efficacy. In many instances, drug products are indicated that are not licensed for use in birds. Even though an antimicrobial drug may have high activity against isolated bacteria, caution should be exercised with the use of drugs that have not been evaluated clinically in the species of companion bird. Much of the material presented in this chapter is based on studies or empirical use of antibiotics in psittacines, small passerines, and pigeons, all birds that are predominantly seed eaters. With the increasing understanding and use of a number of antifungal drugs in humans, particularly some of the newer azoles (see Chapter 17), veterinarians can reconsider their approach to therapy for mycotic infections in avian patients (Orosz and Frazier, 1995). New strategies are also being developed for the treatments of avian mycobacteriosis. Recommendations for therapy of mycobacterial infections in birds include a combination of three or more drugs given concurrently for several months or longer (VanDerHeyden,

617

1997). Antiviral agents, including antiviral chemicals and interferons, are also of increased interest (Cross, 1995) (see Chapter 18).

Medicating companion birds is accomplished by the same methods of administration used in mammals but has several special considerations. In companion avian medicine, many dosage regimens have been designed largely on an empirical basis. As knowledge of antimicrobial drug disposition and metabolism in various avian species expands, it is increasingly evident that differences exist in dosage, dosing interval, and organ distribution, not only between birds and mammals but among individual avian species (Quesenberry, 1988; Carpenter et al., 1996). There is almost no drug formulation available that has been designed specifically for companion birds, even if it were possible to speak of "the companion bird" as one entity, which it is not. Optimal treatment of infectious diseases depends on diagnosis, susceptibility to the drug, potential toxicity, pharmacokinetics and pharmacodynamics of the drug, husbandry practices, and anatomical and physiological differences among the species, as well as on other considerations (see Chapter 5). The preponderance of immunosuppression in clinically ill birds, the rapid progression to life-threatening diseases, and the suspected presence of mixed infections are indications for empirical use of combination antibiotics while waiting for culture and susceptibility results (Flammer, 1994). Combination therapy with an aminoglycoside plus a beta-lactam, both bactericidal drugs that act at different target sites, can be used in the treatment of life-threatening infections caused by susceptible Gram-negative organisms (Schroeder et al., 1997).

General Considerations
Susceptibility Testing

Under optimal conditions, antimicrobial therapy is based on in vitro susceptibility testing. The MIC interpretive criteria between susceptible and resistant bacteria may be different in avian medicine from the accepted standard in human and mammalian medicine. Attainable blood levels for many drugs may be lower in birds than in mammals for the same drugs, because of short elimination half-lives and differences in bioavailability associated with various routes of administration. For example, when measuring tetracycline susceptibility, all organisms with MIC ≤ 5 µg/ml are routinely reported as susceptible. This may lead the avian clinician to consider treatment with one of the chlortetracycline or doxycycline medicated diets available commercially. However, use of these diets in treating chlamydiosis has shown that they maintain drug blood levels of only 0.5–1.5 µg/ml. It is unlikely that a microorganism with an MIC in the upper range of susceptible would be successfully treated. If it was found that the MIC was ≤1 μg/ml, use of the medicated diet would be appropriate. In avian medicine the susceptibility of the microorganism is best reported as MIC so that, when the pharmacokinetics of the drug of choice are known, an effective dosage regimen can be designed (see Chapter 5).

Route of Administration

The medication of birds may be accomplished either by individual bolus dosing or by treating an individual or flock by mixing the medication with feed or drinking water. Although the desired formulation of drugs for birds is dictated by the most practical or economical method of administration, the route of administration is often limited by the drug formulation available. Factors influencing the route of administration and dosage regimen in companion birds include flock versus individual treatment, tame or domesticated versus wild birds, large versus tiny birds, seed-eating versus meat- or fish-eating birds, so-called food specialists, anatomical and physiological differences, intestinal microflora differences, behavioral or environmental differences, availability of drug formulations, economics, and regulations. These factors not only influence the choice of the route of administration but also limit the use of the drugs available.

Drug Extrapolation

Although species are sometimes considered to be similar in their metabolism of drugs, this belief may lead either to inadequate therapy or to toxicity.

The metabolism of a drug can differ among species (sometimes even among strains of a species), since the relationship between metabolism and excretion is determined by basic metabolism and heredity. Mammals and birds differ in body temperature. The basic metabolism, however, in birds ($k = 78$) does not differ significantly from that of mammals ($k = 70$) as a class, with the exception of passerines (pigeons) ($k = 129$). Therefore, differences found in pharmacokinetics among endothermic animals are often predominantly related to differences in body weight (or rather body surface or metabolic weight, allometric scaling) and very often augmented by additional differences in metabolic pathways (see Chapter 29 for a discussion of allometric scaling). Furthermore, because of the many structural and functional differences in the digestive tract and the kidneys of birds within passerines and nonpasserines, it seems necessary to develop regimens for smaller, more uniform groups of birds (Frazier et al, 1995; Klasing, 1998).

Although chloramphenicol is no longer commonly used in avian medicine, it perfectly illustrates this point. Chloramphenicol is eliminated by biotransformation that differs among species in rate of elimination

TABLE 26.1.   Chloramphenicol half-life and plasma levels at 2 h after IM administration (dose 50 mg/kg)

Order	t½ (h)	Concentration (µg/ml)
Columbiformes (pigeons)	0.46	2.85
Psittaciformes (parrots)[a]	1.03	14.17
Anseriformes (waterfowl)	1.45	19.60
Falconiformes (birds of prey)	2.69	29.41
Galliformes (fowl)	3.46	19.21

Source: After Clark et al. (1982).
[a]Except the budgerigar.

(elimination half-life of 0.4 hours in pigeons to 5.1 hours in the cat). In general, mammalian carnivorous species conjugate drugs more slowly than herbivorous species, whereas omnivorous species are intermediate. As in mammals, notable differences in half-lives among orders of birds have been found (Table 26.1). In birds of prey, the concentration 2 hours after administration was unexpectedly high, relative to the half-life, which may indicate a lower metabolic turnover similar to that of mammalian carnivores. Individual species in an order may differ significantly. For example, the budgerigar *(Melopsittacus undulatus)* has an exceptional position among the Psittaciformes tested, since the half-life (2.1 hours) of chloramphenicol in budgerigars is twice as long as in the macaw, although the budgerigar's body weight is 20 times less. The mean calculated plasma concentration, however, at 2 hours after administration (16.6 µg/ml) in budgerigars is comparable to the mean concentration in all the Psittaciformes, indicating either a much lower bioavailability in the budgerigar or a larger volume of distribution. With regard to the pharmacokinetics of tetracyclines in psittacine species, closely related species showed differences in drug handling. For example, after oral administration of chlortetracycline via the food or IM injection of doxycycline, canary-winged parakeets *(Brotogeris versicolorus)* showed much higher blood levels than other psittacine birds studied and were higher even than blood levels of other *Brotogeris* species.

The glomerular filtration rate in some mammalian species is higher than in birds (eg, dogs, 3.96 ml/min/kg; birds, 2.98 ml/min/kg). In many avian species, especially desert species like budgerigars and zebra finches, dehydration will result in decreased glomerular filtration. This may decrease the rate of elimination of many antimicrobial drugs, and with some antibiotics (such as gentamicin and amikacin), severe renal damage due to drug accumulation may ensue.

Consequently, when adequate information is available, the therapeutic regimen should be designed specifically for each species. As a general guide, however, there is minimal variation among species in the manner by which polar compounds (eg, aminoglycosides) are eliminated by renal excretion, whereas there are wide interspecies variations and unpredictability associated with biotransformation of drugs that undergo extensive metabolism (eg, chloramphenicol, sulfonamides). Conventional dosage regimens for antimicrobial drugs in companion birds are presented in Table 26.2. Some of these are based on pharmacokinetic studies in particular species, whereas others are empirical.

Comparative Anatomy and Physiology of the Digestive System

The oral route is often used for administration of drugs to avian species. When the drug preparation is a suspension, capsule, or tablet, release from the dosage form is frequently the rate-limiting step in the overall absorption process. There are marked differences among bird species in the anatomy and physiology of the digestive system (Klasing, 1998). Therefore, variations can be expected in both the rate and the extent of drug absorption from an oral formulation. For example, in pigeons the storage function and emptying pattern of the crop result in an irregular availability of drug from tablets compared with capsules, suspensions, or solutions (Dorrestein, 1986). When chlortetracycline was given in solution, the pH of the crop was found to precipitate the antibiotic on the epithelium, with the result that elimination was delayed. In chickens the bioavailability of some macrolide antibiotics may be reduced by the *Lactobacillus* crop flora, because of inactivation. Such an effect is also to be expected in other avian species. In herbivorous and granivorous birds especially, the gizzard is a highly differentiated, powerful triturating organ. In carnivorous and piscivorous species, the relatively soft nature of the diet necessitates little mechanical disintegration, so that their gizzards are always thin walled and relatively poorly muscled. In these birds, as in mammals, gastric emptying could be the most important physiological factor controlling the rate of drug absorption after oral administration. When drugs are given in solid dosage form, release of the preparation can be slow in the case of a full, poorly differentiated stomach. In a highly differentiated stomach, in which the contents are mostly solid, the mechanical action, supported by the presence of grit, will grind the solid drug formulation and facilitate its transport to the intestines for absorption. A stable drug solution will pass quickly through the crop, esophagus, and stomach and will be available for absorption from the intestine within minutes after administration.

Most birds feeding on coarse material ingest grit, which assists in grinding food in the gizzard. The intake of grit increases divalent metal ions in the gut contents. In pigeons, absorption of both chlortetracycline and doxycycline is significantly decreased by their chelation by calcium or magnesium ions within the intestine.

Renal System in Birds

An excellent review of the avian renal system in relation to pharmacokinetic consideration of drugs excreted by renal pathways is available (Frazier et al., 1995). This review describes a number of differences, including differences in anatomy and physiology of the renal corpuscle, the reptilian- and mammalian-type tubules, the arterial and venous supplies to these different types of nephrons, the variations in the loops of Henle, the arrangement of collection ducts, and the influence of the nervous system and hormones on avian nephron function. These differences make it unlikely that the allometric equations currently used by veterinarians are appropriate for extrapolating drug dosages for birds from those described for mammals. Furthermore, significant morphological and physiologic differences exist in the kidneys of different avian species. To date, pharmacokinetic studies have been conducted in only a few species of birds. More studies are needed before broad-based assumptions about drug regimens can be made that adequately address the diversity of birds encountered by veterinarians.

Respiratory System in Birds

The difference between birds and mammals in their response to nebulization is the result of the unique anatomy and physiology of the avian respiratory system. Anatomical differences in lung structure and the lack of physical activity in the sick bird will, even under optimal technical conditions, reduce drug access to only 20% of the lung tissue in many species; thus a negligible amount may reach the air sacs. At rest there is no air exchange in most of the respiratory tract. Nevertheless, therapeutic levels have been reported in the lungs and air sacs after nebulization in several species. Because the avian lung differs from that of mammals in that the air capillaries are not dead-end saccules, nebulization therapy could be an effective treatment. The air capillaries of birds range between 0.5 and 2 mm, and the parabronchi vary in size from 3 to 10 μm in diameter. To establish local drug levels in the lungs and air sacs, particles or drops should be 1–3 μm. In chickens, aerosolized particles between 3–7 μm are generally deposited on a mucosal surface of the nasal cavity and trachea. The systemic availability of the drugs administered by nebulization is low, so that its primary use is to humidify air and to treat local respiratory tract disease. To maintain local drug concentrations in the therapeutic range for an adequate time is a problem. Therefore, in treating bacterial infections of the respiratory epithelium, bactericidal may be superior to bacteriostatic antibiotics. The usefulness of nebulization for treating mycotic infections requires further evaluation. Local therapeutic levels of drugs in the respiratory tract, (eg, amphotericin B) can be attained by intratracheal application.

Methods of Drug Administration

Routes of administration of medications in birds include medicated water, medicated food, oral, injectable (IM, IV, subcutaneous, intraosseous, intratracheal), topical, nebulization, and sinus and nasal flushes. Selection of routes of administration is based on severity of infection, number of birds to be treated, ability of the owner to administer the medication, and formulation available. Parenteral administration of medications is suggested for critically ill birds. A flock of birds are often treated with medicated food or water, but therapeutic drug concentrations are seldom achieved in companion and aviary birds on water treatment alone. Availability and absorption after oral administration are influenced by the crop (including its microflora, pH), gizzard function and morphology, the presence of grit, form and function of the intestines, and the presence of a functional cecum and its microflora.

Flock versus Individual Treatment

Companion birds and zoo birds are kept in flocks, breeding colonies, or large numbers of breeding couples confined to separate flight pens (eg, backyard poultry, pigeons, canaries and other finches, budgerigars, parakeets and many parrot species). On the other hand, many companion birds are housed individually or in pairs in households (eg, canary, budgerigar, parrot, myna bird). The approach to medication will depend on the situation. Techniques differ when dealing with the individual tame companion bird or wild bird, a large flock of recently imported birds, a breeding flock, or a baby bird that is being hand-fed. Since many drugs are rapidly eliminated in birds, the maintenance of therapeutic levels requires frequent dosage, which necessitates excessive handling of the birds. Individual handling and physical restraint are stressful and must be minimized. The value of frequent administration of drugs must be weighed against the stress caused by handling.

Individual Oral Dosage Forms of Drugs

Direct oral administration is difficult in psittacines because it is difficult to get them to open their mouths, and some birds refuse to swallow medications, but this administration method is commonly practiced in pigeons, waterfowl, and gallinaceous birds. Do not use oral medication in critically ill birds, because they may aspirate medication.

TABLETS

In human medicine, solid dosage forms such as compressed tablets are the most commonly used means for administering medication. Such dosage forms are less popular for birds because the administration can be both time-consuming and uncertain. In birds there are additional problems in that the body weight may be low (15–500 g), and the tablets available may contain too much drug. Administering part of a tablet will make the dosage uncertain. The problem of tablet strength is partly compensated for by the higher metabolism of the bird, which requires a higher dosage per kilogram body weight. The difficulty can be overcome by grinding the tablet, making a suspension, and feeding it by crop cannula. Many birds have a crop that forms a storage organ. The unpredictable emptying time of the crop, the lack of a large volume of fluid, and the relatively high pH make the crop different from the mammalian stomach. Administration of amoxicillin or ampicillin tablets to pigeons resulted in a very irregular absorption pattern, which did not allow prediction of a reasonable dosage regimen (Dorrestein, 1986). The same effect was seen after administration of prolonged-release tablets of ronidazole. Administration in an empty crop improved the uniformity of the pharmacokinetics. Coated tablets are of no use in birds with a muscular gizzard, which will destroy the coating and give HCl and pepsin full access to the drug.

There are tablets marketed for pigeons; these are antiparasitic drugs (carnidazole, clazuril, levamisole, and praziquantel). Those drugs need to be dosed only once to be effective, and the onset of activity after administration is not critical. Most of these tablets do not need to be administered in an empty crop and will not disintegrate before reaching the gizzard, resulting in a bolus delivery. In antimicrobial therapy the use of tablets is satisfactory only when the drug has a bactericidal action and when peak concentrations are more important than a constant blood concentration.

In some cases tablets are useful because they constitute a uniform dosage system. In these cases the tablet formulation is used to medicate the drinking water. These tablets should be made of a hydrophilic matrix that will provide quick and complete release in vitro in a few seconds in distilled water. Dissolution could be a problem unless effervescent tablets are used (eg, potassium bicarbonate and winestone acid).

CAPSULES

Capsules are good alternative dosage forms to tablets. The capsule is a tasteless, easily digested, unit dose container. In pigeons, capsules readily release drug into the crop and show high bioavailability. They are preferably administered into an empty crop. Capsules are especially useful for the treatment of individual birds. In psittacines this dosage form will be difficult to deliver because of the beak anatomy.

In avian medicine the capsule may be used as a container for drugs to be applied to the food or in the drinking water. It gives an exact measure for medication of a small volume of water. In individual companion birds (eg, parrots), the addition of drugs to a favorite food increases the chance of acceptance. Oral suspensions, ground tablets, or the contents of capsules may be applied to fruits, peanut butter sandwiches, fresh corn, cooked sweet potatoes, monkey biscuits, or any other relished items.

SOLUTIONS AND SUSPENSIONS

Aqueous solutions are the simplest and probably the most economical veterinary dosage forms for oral use but are seldom used on a large scale for direct administration to birds. The disadvantage of all liquid dosage forms is that the administration may result in regurgitation or inhalation, and either some of the dose may be lost or aspiration pneumonia may occur. These preparations can be mixed with food and administered by gavage, especially in hand-fed baby birds or sick birds requiring fluids and nutrients. Hand-fed babies are easily medicated in their food. Most medications that are used in self-feeding birds can be used in hand-feeding babies. However, hand-feeders and recently weaned young birds of nest dwellers, in many cases, consume twice the volume of food consumed by adult birds, so that most medications added to the mash should be halved. To medicate nestlings and fledglings, the drug should be given in soft food. This will be fed to them by their parents. Also in this case the amount fed to these fledglings will be twice as much per kg of body weight as would be fed to adult birds.

Oral suspensions developed for pediatric use are particularly useful in avian medicine. Most are very palatable, and the concentrations are appropriate for small birds. In larger birds or in cases where a more concentrated solution is required, the drug may be given in capsules. In most cases, aqueous fluids and suspensions are used to medicate drinking water or food with small amounts of drug. Sometimes it is necessary to adjust the pH of a solution to keep the drug dissolved in sufficient concentration. High concentrations of chlortetracycline can be maintained in solution only at a low pH. Because the pH in the crop of pigeons is close to the isoelectric point for tetracyclines, the drug will precipitate on the crop wall when administered as an oral solution.

Parenteral Dosage Forms

Parenteral administration is the most exact and effective method for administering antimicrobial drugs to companion birds. This route is used mainly in individual birds that are difficult to handle for oral medication (like many psittacines), critically ill birds, or in birds that are unconscious. An exception is the treatment against chlamydiosis with doxycycline or long-acting oxytetracycline, because an injection will provide adequate blood levels for almost 1 week. In general the parenteral drug preparations used in birds are the same as those used in humans and domestic animals.

INTRAMUSCULAR INJECTION

IM injection, especially in many psittacines, is often easier than oral administration. The parenteral preparations are most commonly administered IM in the pectoral or leg muscles. The venous plexus, which lies between the superficial and deep pectoral muscle, should not be punctured. A disadvantage is the relatively large volume that may have to be injected. Therefore, individual birds should be carefully weighed and appropriate dilutions and syringes should be used to enable accurate dosing. General guidelines for acceptable injection volumes in psittacines and small passerines are as follows: macaw and cockatoo, 1 ml; Amazon or African gray parrot, 0.8 ml; cockatiel and small conures, 0.2 ml; and budgerigars, canary, and finch, 0.1 ml. Repeated injections in the same side of the breast or the use of irritating drugs IM may result in muscle necrosis or atrophy. Of 50 different drug preparations injected in budgerigars, most caused severe muscle damage. Eight out of 13 preparations tested in hens caused necrosis, the greatest tissue damage occurring after injections of tetracyclines and sulfonamides. Use of oxytetracycline containing polyvinylpyrrolidone as a vehicle produced lesions that were far less severe and more quickly repaired than those produced by oxytetracycline in propylene glycol. Different vehicles for doxycycline caused varying degrees of damage and also resulted in large differences in drug bioavailability. The IM injection of irritating formulations increases the muscle enzyme activity in serum.

In pigeons and parrots the greatest advantage of parenteral administration seems to be the slow release of drug from some formulations. A practical example is the IM administration of doxycycline for the treatment of chlamydiosis. Blood concentrations exceeding 1 µg/ml are maintained for 5–6 days when large doses (75–100 mg/kg) are injected into the pectoral muscles. Dosage regimens requiring only 8–10 injections over a 45-day period have proven efficacious in a variety of psittacine species. This regimen is practical for treating either individuals or small groups of birds. A problem is the large volume to be injected, up to 5 ml/kg, which is comparable to 2.5 l in a 500-kg cow. The use of long-acting injectable oxytetracycline, 50–100 mg/kg subcutaneously every 2–3 days, would safely maintain plasma concentrations of >1µg/ml. This can be used as an alternative to medicated feed or oral dosing for the treatment of chlamydiosis in psittacine birds.

Drugs administered in the posterior pectoral muscle or legs may pass through the renal portal system prior to entering the general circulation.

Sympathetic stimulation tends to open the valves in the renal portal system, resulting in a direct flow of the blood from the caudal part of the bird to the caudal vena cava.

SUBCUTANEOUS INJECTIONS

Subcutaneous injections in the neck region, between the wings, or the groin are often a preferable alternative when relatively large volumes are injected. But because of minimal amounts of dermis and the low elasticity of the skin, part of the fluid may flow out. Irritating drugs may cause skin necrosis and ulceration.

INTRAVENOUS AND INTRAOSSEUS INJECTIONS

Intravenous injections should be reserved for emergencies and single-dose drug administration. Because of the fragility of avian veins and the uncooperative nature of most birds, continuous IV administration is difficult in the avian patient, unless the bird is anesthetized. The vein of choice in the passerines and psittacines is the right jugular vein. In pigeons the brachial vein is more easy accessible. Hematomas are common. Veins may also be needed for blood withdrawal for diagnostic tests. Intraosseous administration allows stable access to the intravascular space if repeated IV-equivalent drug administration is required.

OTHER INJECTION SITES

Intratracheal injection is a route for delivery of therapeutics to the lungs and airways of birds (Jenkins, 1997). Volumes up to 2 ml/kg of water-soluble medication may be administered safely. A small-diameter metal feeding needle is used to administer the drug. The bird is restrained in a towel, and the beak is held open using a speculum or gauze loops. The medication is injected into the trachea with some force. The bird is then released and allowed to cough and clear its throat.

Nasal flush is often important in the successful treatment of infraorbital sinus infections. Antibiotics or antifungals can be used in lower dose than recommended for nebulization (Table 26.3). The bird is restrained, and the head is held lower than the body. The syringe is pressed against the nostril, the fluid is flushed into the sinuses, and the fluid exits the opposite nostril and through the choana and mouth. Use isotonic solutions and minimal pressure. The amounts of fluids for nasal flushing are 1–3 ml for a budgerigar up to 10–15 ml for a large macaw or cockatoo (Jenkins, 1997; Rupley, 1997).

Sinus flush is used to deliver medication directly into the infraorbital sinus for treatment of sinusitis. The bird is restrained with the head secure. The needle is inserted midway between the commissure of the beak and the medial canthus of the eye. The needle is directed under the zygomatic arch at a 45-degree angle to the side of the head. The sinus is more easily entered if the mouth is held open. Once the sinus has been entered, sterile water and an antibiotic or antifungal solution may be used for treatment of sinusitis. The same concentration can be used as recommended for nasal flush (Table 26.3). Inject only nonirritating solutions (Rupley, 1997).

Medication of Feed or Water

The major method of administering drugs to poultry and many other birds is via feed and drinking water. This method is largely based on convenience and the difficulties associated with individual administration to large numbers of birds. For most drugs, however, for reasons discussed below, water medication in psittacines, passerines, pigeons, and most other birds is unreliable and should not be used.

FEED MEDICATION

In companion bird medicine the addition of antimicrobial drugs to food stuffs is a reliable way of medicating birds, as long as the birds are still eating normally. The total intake of drug with the food during the day should be equal to the desired daily dose calculated on an individual base. Crushed tablets, oral suspensions, and powders can be mixed with moist foods. However, the interactions between a drug and food cannot be entirely predicted, and dosage forms need to be evaluated. The only proof of bioavailability is pharmacokinetic study. Most companion birds are seed-eating (dehusking their seeds) or grain-eating birds; neither type of food is suitable for mixing drugs homogeneously.

For the treatment of chlamydiosis in psittacines, considerable experience has been accumulated with chlortetracycline (0.5–1.0%) medicated food such as mashes, pellets, and impregnated seeds. In larger psittacines, a chlortetracycline mix consisting of rice, hen scratch, brown sugar, and water can be used. This must serve as the sole source of food for 45 days. To reduce interference with chlortetracycline absorption, the calcium content of these diets is reduced to 0.7%. Pelleted feeds are an excellent means for delivering chlortetracycline while providing a balanced diet. Unfortunately, some species are very reluctant to accept pellets. Because of the negative influence of divalent metal ions on the bioavailability of tetracyclines, grit-mineral administration has to be stopped during treatment. During egg production and breeding, this can result in soft-shelled eggs and rickets in the chicks. Extensive use of pelleted feeds in quarantine stations has shown a varying degree of acceptance among common species. Amazon parrots, Pionus parrots, African parrots, and most conures and cockatoos usually accept pellets readily. Many other birds will not easily accept pellets (when available) or a medicated soft food. To solve this problem, a mash (soft food mixed with seed) provided daily appears to be satisfactory.

Use of doxycycline and enrofloxacin in a food mix or added to water showed that a nonhomogeneous mixture (mash, adhesion to seeds) resulted in unpredictable blood levels in budgerigars. Only impregnated, dehulled seeds gave reproducible and reliable results. Other drugs could be applied in this manner.

A practical method of adding drugs to a grain mixture is by coating a moist food, which is then added to the mixture. This method is often used for pigeons and backyard poultry. These birds do not dehusk their grain but swallow it completely. In pigeons, buttermilk is used for preparing the premix. Freshly cooked, whole kernel corn is inexpensive and well accepted by large and medium-sized psittacine species. Canned or fresh corn can be used. Rice may also be readily accepted. Yogurt as a base for administering drugs is often readily accepted by psittacines. Budgerigars, cockatiels, and Australian parakeets may be more reluctant to accept these foods. Toucans may be easily medicated by the injection of drugs into grapes. The acceptance of medicated food might be improved by adding drugs that have a higher bioavailability (eg, minocycline 500 mg/kg of food or doxycycline 200 mg/kg of food). In contrast to the situation with tablets, the storage of medicated food in the crop of many birds is an advantage. From this reservoir there is a continuous delivery of drug. Pharmacologically, food medication can simulate a slow-release system, which provides decreased fluctuations in drug concentrations in tissues.

WATER MEDICATION

In companion avian medicine the addition of antimicrobial agents to the drinking water is often the only practical means of drug administration. This is the least stressful method for medicating birds, especially with drugs that are palatable. Theoretically the bird will frequently self-dose during the day. However, studies in parrots, pigeons, and chickens showed that therapeutic blood levels for many drugs were not attained via the drinking water, because of factors such as nonacceptance, poor solubility, and day length. One problem associated with water medication in birds is the night period in which they do not drink. In addition, wide variations exist among avian species in water intake pattern. As a guide, the volume of water consumed by the bird needs to contain the calculated daily dose in mg/kg. Often the daily dose is not ingested either because the drug is poorly soluble or the patient will not drink the medicated water. In the latter case this may result in dehydration. Many drugs are stable for only a short time in water, which necessitates frequent changes.

Although therapeutic blood concentrations may not be achieved with many antibiotics, levels in the intestine may be sufficient to control enteric infections. The use of medicated water can be valuable for reducing the spread of disease, which might have arisen through contaminated water.

Medicated water may be rejected because of color or taste. Xerophilic birds, which are adapted to dry and hot climates (ie, budgerigars, Zebra finches, Australian parakeets), may not consume any water containing dissolved medications. In breeding flocks the male bird may consume large volumes of water in order to feed the female in the nest, resulting in toxic drug levels in the male.

Other Administration Routes
TOPICAL MEDICATION
Topical medications include skin application, eyedrops, and ointments. External applications should be used carefully and sparingly because they will stick the feathers together. When ingested through preening behavior, many topical formulations are toxic.

NEBULIZATION
Nebulization can be an important adjunct to the management of respiratory disease (Jenkins, 1997). A particle size less than 3 μm is required to have local effect in the lungs and air sacs. Several inexpensive nebulization units are available (Acorn II Nebulizer, Marquest Medical) that produce suspended particles in the size range of 0.5–6 μm. Many commercial humidifiers and vaporizers do not produce particles this small. If there is considerable airway congestion or lack of flow, this form of treatment may not reach the tissues needing it the most.

Most IV formulations and some antifungal medications can be mixed with saline for nebulization. Initiate nebulization with a broad-spectrum antibiotic before culture and susceptibility results (Table 26.3), and alter selection of antibiotic based on susceptibility testing. Nebulize for 10–30 minutes, 2–4 times daily, in conjunction with systemic therapy (Rupley, 1997).

Treatment of Chlamydiosis
Either tetracyclines or enrofloxacin may be used for the treatment of chlamydiosis (psittacosis) in companion birds (Table 26.4). The duration of treatment with tetracyclines is 30 days for small psittacines and 45 days for large psittacines. Enrofloxacin should be administered for 21 days to all species. Although effective treatment of chlamydiosis has been documented, practical experience indicates that total eradication of chlamydia is often difficult, probably because of inadequate drug levels for too short a time.

Bibliography

Altman RB, et al, eds. 1997. Avian Medicine and Surgery. Philadelphia: WB Saunders.

Beynon PH, et al. 1996a. BSAVA Manual of Psittacine Birds. Cheltenham, UK: Br Small Anim Vet Assoc.

Beynon PH, et al. 1996b. BSAVA Manual of Raptors, Pigeons, and Waterfowl. Cheltenham, UK: Br Small Anim Vet Assoc.

Bougerol C. 1990. Antibiotherapie chez les oiseaux. Rec Med Vet 166:361.

Bush M, et al. 1981. Pharmacokinetics of cephalothin and cephalexin in selected avian species. Am J Vet Res 42:1014.

Carpenter JW, et al. 1996. Exotic Animal Formulary. Manhattan, KS: Greystone.

Clark CH, et al. 1982. Plasma concentrations of chloramphenicol in birds. Am J Vet Res 43:1249.

Cross G. 1995. Antiviral Therapy. Semin Avian Exot Pet Med 4:96.

Devriese LA, Dutta GN. 1984. Effects of erythromycin-inactivating Lactobacillus crop flora on the blood levels of erythromycin given orally to chicks. J Vet Pharmacol Ther 7:49.

Dorrestein GM. 1986. Studies on pharmacokinetics of some antibacterial agents in homing pigeons (Columba livia). Thesis, Utrecht University.

Dorrestein GM. 1993. Avian Pediatric Pharmacology. Semin Avian Exot Pet Med 2:110.

Dorrestein GM, Verburg E. 1988. Pharmacokinetics of Baytril. in homing pigeons after different administration routes. Proc 6th Conf Avian Dis Munich.

Dorrestein GM, et al. 1998. Comparative study of Synulox and Augmentin after intravenous, intramuscular, and oral administration in collared doves (Streptopelia decaocto). Proc 11th Symp Avian Dis Munich.

Flammer K, 1994. Antimicrobial therapy. In: Ritchie BW, et al., eds. Avian Medicine: Principles and Application. Boca Raton, FL: Wingers, p434.

Frazier DL, et al. 1995. Pharmacokinetic considerations of the renal system in birds: Part I, Anatomic and physiologic principles of allometric scaling. Part II, Review of drugs excreted by renal pathways. J Avian Med Surg 9:92 and 104.

Gylstorff J, Grimm F. 1987. Vogelkrankheiten. Stuttgart: Verlag Eugen Ulmer.

Jakoby JR, Gylstorff I. 1983. Comparative research on the medicated treatment of psittacosis. Berl Munich Tieraerztl Wochenschr 96:261.

Jenkins RJ, 1997. Hospital techniques and supportive care. In: Altman RB, et al., eds. Avian Medicine and Surgery. Philadelphia: WB Saunders, p232.

Klasing KC. 1998. Anatomy and physiology of the digestive system. In: Lasing KC, ed. Comparative Avian Nutrition. Wallingford, UK: CAB International, p9.

Orosz SE, Frazier DL. 1995. Antifungal agents: a review of their pharmacology and therapeutic indications. J Avian Med Surg 9:8.

Orosz SE, et al. 1996. Pharmacokinetic properties of itraconazole in blue-fronted Amazon parrots (Amazona aestiva aestiva). J Avian Med Surg 10:168.

Quesenberry KE. 1988. Avian antimicrobial therapeutics. In: Jacobson ER, Kollias GV, eds. Exotic Animals. New York: Churchill Livingstone.

Ritchie BW, et al., eds. 1994. Avian Medicine: Principles and Application. Boca Raton, FL: Wingers.

Rupley AE. 1997. Manual of Avian Practice. Philadelphia: WB Saunders.

Schroeder EC, et al. 1997. Pharmacokinetics of ticarcillin and amikacin in blue-fronted Amazon parrots (Amazona aestiva aestiva). J Avian Med Surg 11:260.

Tully NT. 1997. Formulary. In: Altman RB, et al., eds. Avian Medicine and Surgery. Philadelphia: WB Saunders, p671.

VanDerHeyden N. 1997. New strategies in the treatment of avian mycobacteriosis. Semin Avian Exot Pet Med 6:25.

TABLE 26.2. Conventional dosage regimens for antimicrobial drugs in pet birds (parrots and pigeons)

Drugs	Routes	Dose (mg/kg)	Interval (h)	Study/species[a]	Reference	Remarks
Beta-lactams						
Cloxacillin	IM	100–200	24	Emp/birds	1	*Staphylococcus* spp.
Ampicillin-Na	IM	150	12–24	Kin/pigeon	5	Only Gram-positives
Ampicillin-trihydrate	PO	25	12–24	Kin/pigeon	5	Only Gram-positives
	PO	120–175	12–24	Kin/pigeon/parrot	5	Gram-negatives
Amoxicillin-Na	IM	50	12–24	Kin/pigeon	5	Only Gram-positives
		250	12–24	Kin/pigeon	5	Gram-negatives
Amoxicillin-trihydrate	PO	20	12–24	Kin/pigeon	5	Only Gram-positives
	PO	100	12–24	Kin/pigeon	5	Gram-negatives
	PO	150–175	12–24	Emp/psitt	12	
Amoxicillin, long-acting	IM	100	48	Kin/pigeon	5	Only Gram-positives
Amoxycillin–clavulanic acid	IM	50/10	8–12	Kin/pigeon/psitt	7	Gram-positives
	PO	100/25	8–12	Kin/pigeon/psitt	7	Gram-positives
	IM	100/20	8–12	Kin/pigeon/psitt	7	Gram-negatives
	PO	200/50	8–12	Kin/pigeon/psitt	7	Gram-negatives
	PO	50/10–100/20	12	Kin/pigeon/psitt	7	Intestinal infections
Carbenicillin	IM	100–200	8–12	Emp/psitt	12	Synergistic aminoglycosides (as are all beta-lactams)
	IV	100–200	8–12	Emp/psitt	12	
	IT	100	24	Emp/psitt	12	*Pseudomonas* infections
Ticarcillin	IM, IV	150–200	6–8	Kin/psitt	11	Synergistic aminoglycosides
Cefotaxime	IM, IV	75–100	6–8	Emp/birds	12	
Cefoxitin	IM, IV	50–75	6–8	Emp/birds	12	
Ceftriaxone	IM, IV	75–100	4–6	Emp/birds	12	
Ceftazidine	IM, IV	75–100	6–8	Emp/birds	12	
Ceftiofur	IM	50–100	6	Emp/birds	12	
Cephalexin monohydrate	PO	50–100	8	Emp/birds	12	
Cephalothin	IM, IV	100	2–6	Kin/cranes, emus	3	
Cephradine	PO	35–50	2–6	Kin/birds	2	
		35–50	6	Emp/birds	12	

Drug	Route	Dose	Interval (h)			Comments
Piperacillin	IM, IV	200	6–8	Emp/birds	12	Synergistic with aminoglycosides
		75–100	4–6	Emp/psitt	12	
Polymyxins						
Polymyxin B	PO	50,000 IU/kg	12	Emp/birds	4	Enteric infections
Aminoglycosides						
Neomycin	PO	10	24	Emp/birds	4	
Streptomycin	PO	50–100	24	Emp/chicken	8	
	PO	100–200	24	Emp/pigeon	4	
	IM	10–30	8–12	Emp/birds	12	
Kanamycin	IM	10–20	12	Emp/birds	4	
Gentamicin	IM	2.5–10	6–12	Kin/birds	12	Nephrotoxicity
	PO	40	8–24	Emp/psitt	12	Intestinal tract infection
Amikacin	IM, IV	15–20	8–12	Kin/psitt	11	Nephrotoxicity
		20–40	12–24	Emp/psitt	12	
Tobramycin	IM, IV	2.5–5	12	Emp/birds	12	
Spectinomycin	IM, SC	25	8	Emp/pigeon	4	
	PO	30	24	Emp/birds	8	
	PO	150–250	24	Emp/chicken	12	Flock treatment enteritis
Lincosamides, Macrolides, and Pleuromutilins						
Lincomycin	PO	75–100	12–24	Emp/birds	12	Overdose caused death
	PO	50	24	Emp/birds	4	
Lincomycin/spectinomycin	PO	100	24	Emp/pigeon	12	
Clindamycin	IM	10–20	24	Emp/birds	12	
Erythromycin	PO	50–100	12	Emp/psitt	12	
Spiramycin	IM	25	24	Emp/pigeon	4	
	PO	250	24	Emp/birds	8	
Tylosin	IM	10–40	6–8	Kin/birds	12	
	PO	50	24	Emp/birds	4	
Tiamulin	PO	25–50	24	Emp/birds	8	
Oleandomycin	IM	25	24	Emp/pigeon	4	
	PO	50	24	Emp/pigeon	4	

TABLE 26.2. Continued

Drugs	Routes	Dose (mg/kg)	Interval (h)	Study/species[a]	Reference	Remarks
Chloramphenicol						
Chloramphenicol succinate	IM	100	6	Kin/pigeon	4	
		50	8–12	Kin/parrot	4	
		50–80	12–24	Kin/other	4	
Chloramphenicol palmitate	PO	50–100	6–12	Emp/psitt	12	
Tetracyclines						
Chlortetracycline	PO	40–50	8	Kin/pigeon	5	Grit
	PO		12	Kin/pigeon	5	No grit
	Diet	0.25–1.0%	45 days	Kin/psitt	12	
Oxytetracycline	IM, SC	15–50	12–24	Emp/birds	12	Tissue damage
Oxytetracycline, long-acting	IM, SC	50–100	48–72	Kin/psitt	12	
Tetracycline	PO	50	8	Emp/psitt	12	
Doxycycline	PO	25	12	Kin/pigeon	5	Grit
		7.5	12	Kin/pigeon	5	No grit
Doxycycline (vibramycin-IV)	IM, SC	75–100	5–7 days	Kin/pigeon	5	
				Kin/psitt	9	
Sulfonamides and Potentiators						
Trimethoprim	PO	15–20	8	Kin/pigeon	5	
Trimethoprim + sulfatroxazole	PO	10/50	12	Kin/pigeon	5	
Trimethoprim + sulfamethoxazole	PO	10/50	24	Kin/pigeon	5	
Fluoroquinolines						
Flumequine	IM, PO	30	8–12	Kin/pigeon	5	Vomiting
Ciprofloxacin	PO, IM	15–20	12	Emp/birds	12	
Enrofloxacin	IM, SC	5–10	24	Kin/pigeon	6	
	PO	10–20	12–24	Kin/pigeon/psitt	6	
	Food	250–1,000	24	Kin/psitt	12	
Miscellaneous Antimicrobial Drugs						
Furazolidone	PO	15–20	24	Emp/pigeon	4	
Furaltadone	PO	15–20	24	Emp/pigeon	4	

Antifungal Drugs

Drug	Route	Dose (mg/kg)	Interval (h)	Basis	Ref	Comments
Amphotericin B	IV	1.5	8–12	Emp/birds	14	5–7 days
	IT	1	8–12	Emp/birds	14	5–7 days
Nystatin	PO	100,000–300,000 IU/kg	8–12	Emp/psitt	14	7–10 days
Miconazole	IM, IV	10–20	8–24	Emp/birds	12	*Candida* or *Cryptococcus* infection
Ketoconazole	PO	20–30	12	Kin/birds	12, 14	14–30 days? liver damage?
Itraconazole	PO	5–10	12–24	Kin/psitt/birds	12, 13	14 days, in orange juice
Fluconazole	PO	2–5	24	Emp/birds	12, 14	7–10 days
5-Fluorocytosine	PO/gavage	30–50 (120)	6–12	Emp/psitt	12, 14	With amphotericin B, 14–28 days
Chlorhexidine	PO	5–10	24	Emp/birds	12	Toxic for finches
Enilconazole	Aerosol	—	—	—	12	Only disinfection equipment
Caprylic acid	PO	250	24	Emp/birds	12	
Tuberculostatics, in combination of 3 or more drugs					15	Initial therapy should include rifabutin, ethambutol, and ether azithromycin or clarithromycin
Isoniazid	PO	5–15	12	Emp/birds	12, 15	GI and CNS disorder
Rifampin	PO	10–20 (45)	12–24	Emp/birds	12, 15	
Rifabutin	PO	15–45	24	Emp/psitt	15	
Ethambutol	PO	15–30 (85)	12–24	Emp/birds	12, 15	For combination treatment
Streptomycin	PO	20–40	24	Emp/psitt	15	
Amikacin	IM	15–30	12–24	Emp/psitt	15	
Ciprofloxacin/enrofloxacin	PO	15–30	12–24	Emp/psitt	15	
Clofazamine	PO	6–12	24	Emp/psitt	15	
Clarithromycin	PO	85	24	Suggested	15	
Azithromycin	PO	45	24	Suggested	15	

Antiviral Drugs

Drug	Route	Dose (mg/kg)	Interval (h)	Basis	Ref	Comments
Acyclovir	PO, IM, IV	25–80	8	Emp/psitt	10	Up to 400 mg/kg food

References: 1, Bougerol (1990); 2, Bush et al. (1981); 3, Clark et al. (1982); 4, Devriese and Dutta (1984); 5, Dorrestein (1986); 6, Dorrestein and Verburg (1988); 7, Dorrestein et al. (1998); 8, Gylstorff and Grimm, (1987); 9, Jakoby and Gylstorff (1983); 10, Cross (1995); 11, Schroeder et al. (1997); 12, Tully (1997); 13, Orosz et al. (1996); 14, Orosz and Frazier (1995); 15, VanDerHeyden (1997).
[a]Emp, means empirical dose recommendations; Kin/studies (eg. Kin/psitt) means dose recommendations based on pharmacokinetic studies in psittacines.

TABLE 26.3. **Some medications commonly nebulized**

Medication[a]	Dosage[b]	Administration[c]
Amikacin sulfate[d]	50	15 min BID
Amphotericin B[e]	10	15 min BID
Carbenicillin[e]	200	15 min BID
Cefotaxime[e]	100	10-30 min BID-QID
Erythromycin[e]	100	15 min BID
Gentamicin[e]	50	15 min BID
Piperacillin[e]	100	10-30 min BID-QID
Tylosin	100	10-60 min BID

Sources: Adapted from Jenkins (1997) and Rupley (1997).
[a]For nasal flush and sinus flush use dosage in 250 ml.
[b]Dosage in mg in 10 ml saline.
[c]Administration time and frequency.
[d]Discontinue use if polyuria develops.
[e]Injectable.

TABLE 26.4. **Suggested drugs for the treatment of chlamydiosis (psittacosis) in pet birds**

Drug	Dose	Administration
Tetracyclines[a]		
Doxycycline injection (vibramycin-IV, Pfizer)	75–100 mg	SC, IM every 5–7 days
Oxytetracycline, long-acting	50–100 mg	SC every 2–3 days
Enrofloxacin	10–20 mg	PO, IM, SC
Medicated food		
Doxycycline hyclate	200–400 ppm	
Chlortetracycline HCl		
Budgerigars	500 ppm	
Other psittacines	1,000–2,000 ppm	
Enrofloxacin	100–200 ppm	
Medicated drinking water (pigeons only)		
Enrofloxacin	100–200 ppm	

[a]Tetracyclines in small psittacines for 30 days, in large psittacines for 45 days. Enrofloxacin in all birds 21 days.

27 | Antimicrobial Drug Use in Poultry

A. C. TANNER

Recent legislative changes have affected the availability of antimicrobials approved for use in poultry. Approval of fluoroquinolones for therapeutic use in the United States is encouraging, although this has been accompanied by considerable debate as to the risk versus its benefit. In Europe, the nutritional use of a number of antimicrobials has been prohibited over concerns that food-animal use could lead to widespread cross-resistance, which in turn may adversely affect the use of some human antimicrobials. Although the scientific and legal validity of this action is the subject of fierce debate, it is clear that an inability to use antimicrobials to influence the growth parameters of commercial poultry will significantly affect the economics of the industry and thus the cost to the consumer.

With antimicrobial use in commercial birds under scrutiny, it is important to remember that even the best treatment programs can never replace good management. The positive effects of effective biosecurity, sound flock management practices, and scrupulous hygiene on bird health cannot be understated. In this chapter, the role of antimicrobial therapy in the control of disease is discussed, together with the prophylactic use of antimicrobials to prevent secondary bacterial infections, often the cause of greatest economic loss. Also considered are the use of antimicrobials to influence growth and practical considerations associated with flock medication, including dose calculations and the use of automated water medication systems.

The modern broiler has been selected for growth rate, feed efficiency, and fleshing rather than for robustness and resistance to disease. The present hybrids can be especially susceptible to disease toward the end of the growing period, when investment in the bird is at its greatest. Disease outbreaks often lead to extensive carcass condemnations at processing, resulting in significant economic losses to the grower. It is in light of all these important factors that the critical role of medication in the poultry industry must be considered.

Antibacterial drugs and anticoccidials account for the largest proportion of antimicrobial use in poultry. Of the top 10 causes of chicken morbidity, most are infectious diseases that can be controlled by antimicrobial drugs (colibacillosis, airsacculitis, *Staphylococcus* spp. infections, omphalitis, coccidiosis, and *Mycoplasma gallisepticum* infection). Despite this fact, in a recent survey of broiler carcasses condemned for disease, 43% showed lesions consistent with colisepticemia.

General Considerations of Antimicrobial Use in Poultry

Antimicrobial drugs are used within the poultry industry in three principal ways: therapeutic, prophylactic, and nutritional. Although many outbreaks of clinical disease are self-limiting, therapeutic programs are designed to minimize economic losses due to the disease. Prophylactic use of antimicrobials occurs before signs of disease become evident, in an attempt to avert clinical disease. The commercially raised bird is exposed to infectious agents for most of its life yet may exhibit clinical signs of disease only when subjected to some additional stress. The most important causes of additional stress are vaccination (particularly with live viral vaccines), extremes of ambient temperature (especially overheating), excessive ammonia (>25 ppm) from poor ventilation and fecal degradation in wet litter, transport, contamination of feed with mycotoxins, change in diet, or additional medications such as anthelmintic administration. With experience, a poultry veterinarian can accurately predict when an infectious disease outbreak might occur in response to these factors and can initiate prophylactic medication. Incorporating low concentrations of some antimicrobials into the feed can increase growth rate, feed efficiency, or both (see Chapter 32). In these cases, there is an economic benefit to the farmer, provided that the cost of medication does not exceed the gain in productivity. The use of subtherapeutic levels of antimicrobials is not without disadvantage. Consumers perceive these additives to be unhealthy, and nutritional use of additives may increase the frequency with which bacterial resistance is selected (see Chapter 3). Nevertheless, the practice is widespread, and a considerable number of antimicrobials are currently approved for nutritional use in poultry.

Selection of Appropriate Antimicrobials

The most important consideration in the choice of a poultry antimicrobial is the cost-to-benefit ratio. Since the cost of medication never outweighs the economic benefit, the first decision facing the poultry veterinarian is whether or not to initiate any treatment at all. It may make more economic sense to limit the effect of a disease outbreak by advancing the processing date, even though the birds may not yet have reached their target market weight. Another important consideration is drug withdrawal time. Use of medication may mean that, with broilers, the grow-out period would have to be extended to comply with mandatory withdrawal times or, in laying flocks, there may be reduced hatchability or compulsory destruction of eggs during the withdrawal period. Such considerations may preclude treatment of illness. In the equation of medication cost versus economic benefit, the cost of medication can be precisely calculated. Estimation of the economic benefit is, however, much more difficult and often relies on empirical guidelines specific to individual poultry producers.

Once the decision to treat has been made, the antimicrobial susceptibility of the target pathogen must be considered. In part because of bacterial resistance, older and less expensive drugs are generally less effective in controlling disease. These drugs can sometimes be used effectively by increasing the dose (often to 3–4 times the recommended level) or extending the duration of treatment. Both of these strategies can affect the drug withdrawal time.

Route of Administration

The two routes of administration available are parenteral injection or oral administration. Although individual injection, correctly performed, delivers a precise dose, this method is labor-intensive and results in considerable stress in the birds. Injection is best conducted at the hatchery where automated injection systems are available, with valuable birds such as breeders or turkeys or where labor costs are less of a consideration. The oral route is by far the most practical, and antimicrobials can be administered either through the feed or in the water.

Feed medication is particularly effective for the long-term prophylactic administration of antimicrobials. For therapeutic purposes, incorporation of antimicrobials into feed is less effective because of the time necessary to manufacture a suitable medicated feed and because inappetence and the inability to compete for food are common in sick birds. Environmental factors such as high ambient temperatures may also reduce feed intake.

Water medication is most effective for the treatment of outbreaks of microbial disease but equally well can be used for short-term prophylaxis. The main advantages of medicating the drinking water are rapid response, with medication reaching the birds within a relatively short time, and convenience of administration. A few disadvantages exist.

Water consumption can vary considerably, and allowances must be made in the incorporation rate of the drug to avoid misdosing. Palatability problems may arise because any drug "flavor" will be more noticeable in water than in feed. A number of useful antimicrobials have limited solubility and can only be suspended in water, leading to potential problems of sedimentation and water line blockage. Finally, there are a number of common impurities in drinking water that will affect drug activity. Despite these considerations, water medication is the favored mode of antimicrobial administration in disease outbreaks, especially for large production units.

Drug Interactions
CONCURRENT USE OF ANTIMICROBIALS
A number of adverse interactions between antimicrobial drugs have been reported (Table 5.1). For example, the concurrent oral administration of neomycin with penicillin can reduce absorption of the latter, and spectinomycin will antagonize tetracycline absorption. Drug interactions can be avoided by observing the recommendations contained in manufacturers' data sheets.

ENVIRONMENTAL INTERACTIONS
Photodegradation of some antimicrobials will occur in direct sunlight. To minimize this, medication tanks should have close-fitting light-proof lids, proportioner stock solutions should not be exposed to direct sunlight, and house water systems should be constructed of opaque, light-proof plastics. High ambient temperatures cause excessive water consumption, leading to overdosing by consumption of medicated water in significantly less time than the recommended medication period. Conversely, lower ambient temperature can lead to underdosing. Reduced feed consumption can lead to underdosing of in-feed medication. At its maximum approved level, the anticoccidial nicarbazin increases the risk of heat stress mortality in broiler chicks exposed to high humidity or to ambient temperatures approaching 38° C. Nicarbazin at a reduced dose level, in combination with narasin, may be more appropriate where heat stress is a concern.

CHEMICAL INTERACTIONS
When chicken houses are supplied with city water, chlorine is present to lower the level of microbiological contaminants and maintain water quality. In addition, bleach solution is frequently added to the house water system by the poultry grower to minimize the growth of algae in pipes and water troughs. Chlorine inactivation of some antimicrobials— for example, the fluoroquinolones—has been reported. Excessive levels of

iron, calcium, and magnesium ions will reduce the absorption of tetracyclines. High levels of these cations can be found in some drug premixes, such as nystatin, and concurrent use is a potential source of tetracycline malabsorption. Conversely, long-term feeding of low calcium or magnesium diets to facilitate medication with tetracyclines may result in nutritional disorders. Concurrent administration of citric acid (in a 1:1 ratio) can enhance tetracycline absorption from medicated water. Copper sulphate has been reported to impair the action of nitarsone.

MISCELLANEOUS INTERACTIONS
Inactivation of some antimicrobials will occur when they are in contact with metal containers. One example is chlortetracycline; its manufacturers recommend making up fresh medication every 12 hours where galvanized water troughs are used, as opposed to every 24 hours with plastic watering systems. Antimicrobial drug stock solutions should not be made up in, or administered from, galvanized containers. Similarly, apramycin and gentamicin in solution are rapidly inactivated when mixed or stored in rusty containers. Few water filters can remove colloidal particles, a common contaminant of well water that may adsorb some antimicrobials and limit their bioavailability. Algal growth, which will interfere with medication and obstruct watering systems, should be controlled by regular cleaning and the use of light-proof plastic pipes and tanks. Binding agents that are used in pelleted feed, for example bentonite, can cause malabsorption of antimicrobials such as bacitracin.

Probiotics

In the normal healthy bird the natural intestinal flora provides a stable, effective barrier against colonization of the intestine by pathogenic microorganisms. However, when the chick first hatches, this flora is absent, and later stress or antimicrobial drug use can disrupt or alter its composition, allowing colonization by pathogens, in particular *Salmonella* spp. A number of feed supplements, called probiotics, which comprise mixtures of normal gut bacteria, are available to aid in returning the poultry intestinal flora to its normal composition and to prevent pathogen colonization. Although often efficacious experimentally, this principle of competitive exclusion has not been well accepted for commercial use. This may change in the United States with the recent approval of a spray-administered probiotic and the increasing interest in using antimicrobial therapy in combination with competitive exclusion.

Drug Withdrawal Time

A critical factor in the medication of all food animals is the statutory drug withdrawal time, the period during which an antimicrobial must not be administered prior to slaughter of the animal for consumption. This is an integral part of the regulatory approval process and is designed to ensure that no significant drug residue is present in the bird at slaughter. The stated drug withdrawal times are appropriate only when the drug is used as directed by the manufacturer and may be significantly extended by extralabel use. Where antimicrobials are approved for administration only to young chicks or poults, a withdrawal time may not be specified. This is because such birds are considered too small for consumption, not because these drugs have a zero withdrawal time.

Current Practices in Antimicrobial Drug Use in Poultry
Drugs Affecting Growth
A number of antimicrobial drugs are approved for nutritional use in poultry to improve pigmentation, growth rate, feed efficiency, or egg production. The level of incorporation is below that generally considered to be therapeutic, but in most cases little information is available on the mode of action (see Chapter 32). Table 27.1 lists drugs approved for nutritional use in poultry. Occasionally, concurrent use with other antimicrobials, such as some anticoccidials, can negate the growth-promoting effects. Under these circumstances the nutritional claim is for improved pigmentation (of skin, leg scale, eye ring, or comb).

TABLE 27.1. **Antimicrobials approved for nutritional use in poultry**

Antimicrobial	Use Level[a]	Withdrawal Time (days)
Arsanilic acid or sodium arsanilate	0.01%	5
Avilamycin	5–10 g/tonne	0
Avoparcin	7.5–15.0 g/tonne	0[b]
Bacitracin (methyl disalicylate or zinc)	4–50 g/ton	0
Bambermycins	1–20 g/tonne	0
Chlortetracycline	10–100 g/ton	0
Lincomycin	2–4 g/ton (chickens)	0
Oxytetracycline	5–50 g/ton	0[c]
Penicillin (procaine)	2.4–50 g/ton	0
Roxarsone	0.0025–0.005%	5
Spiramycin	5–20 g/tonne	0
Tylosin	4–50 g/ton (chickens)	0[b]
Virginiamycin	5–15 g/ton (chickens)	0[b]
	10–20 g/ton (turkeys)	0[b]

Note: Approved inclusion rates may vary. Therefore the manufacturer's data sheet should be consulted for dose, withdrawal time, approved cross-clearances and conditions of use.
[a]1 ton (U.S.) is equivalent to 1.016 tonnes (metric).
[b]Use recently prohibited in EU member states.
[c]In low-calcium feeds (0.18–0.55% dietary calcium) withdraw 3 days prior to slaughter.

Anticoccidial Drugs

Coccidiosis is a disease of production, markedly encouraged by the conditions prevalent in the modern broiler house. More often than not, morbidity caused by *Eimeria* spp. results in loss of production rather than mortality. Coccidiosis is an ongoing problem, requiring constant attention and, especially in the case of broilers, continuous in-feed medication with anticoccidials. The strategy of medication for layers is different because most anticoccidial therapy must cease by the time the bird comes in to lay, to avoid the potential deposition of drug residues in the egg. With these birds, the objective is to prevent clinical coccidiosis while still encouraging the development of active immunity during the first 14–20 weeks of life. There is increasing use of coccidial vaccines to stimulate bird immunity.

The ideal anticoccidial drug, developed for continuous in-feed medication, should have no adverse effects on either growth rate or feed efficiency, should be active against all economically important species of coccidia, and should require no withdrawal time, with no possibility of drug residues at processing. Coccidiosis is generally well controlled using currently available ionophore drugs, but the susceptibility of *Eimeria* species varies considerably, with *E. maxima*, *E. acervulina*, and *E. tenella* considered the most difficult species to control. Resistance, or at least reduced susceptibility in the target population, can also arise.

It is necessary for anticoccidial drugs to be compatible with a wide range of compounds that may be administered to the bird concurrently during the production cycle. Details of approved drug combinations (cross-clearances) can be found in individual manufacturers' data sheets.

Clinical coccidiosis outbreaks commonly occur when the anticoccidial drug is omitted from feed during antibacterial therapy, typically around 3–4 weeks of age. Combinations of antibacterials with anticoccidials help prevent this type of outbreak. In addition, potentiated sulfonamides (eg, sulfadimethoxine and ormetoprim in a 5:3 ratio), which have both anticoccidial and antibacterial efficacy, can be useful. Combinations of anticoccidial drugs can be synergistic. Narasin and nicarbazin, for example, possess greater activity in combination than either drug does alone. Finally, when narasin or certain ionophore anticoccidials are used concurrently with tiamulin, both activity and toxicity are synergized. This is the only significant toxic interaction of anticoccidials with other medication, although in some instances combining an anticoccidial with a performance enhancer may result in reduced performance enhancement during the period the combination is fed. It should be noted that some anticoccidials can depress bird growth when fed in the absence of significant coccidial challenge.

The intensive use of most drugs is accompanied by the development of tolerance or a reduction in the susceptibility of the target population. A number of strategies have been developed to prolong the useful life of anticoccidials, while still controlling coccidiosis. The most popular anticoccidial use programs include *continuous programs,* in which the drug is given continuously in both starter and grower feed, with unmedicated finisher feed given for 5–7 days prior to processing; *shuttle programs,* in which one drug is given in the starter feed, followed by a different drug in the grower feed, again with an appropriate unmedicated feed withdrawal period; and *rotation programs,* in which either a continuous or a shuttle program is used, but the anticoccidials are changed seasonally or annually. Shuttle programs take advantage of the different anticoccidial properties of the drugs, matching spectrum of activity, potency, and drug cost against risk of infection, while lessening the potential for resistance development. It is generally accepted that rotational programs provide increased drug efficacy at the time of change by letting coccidia regain sensitivity during the off time of each drug.

Antimicrobials currently approved for use against coccidiosis in poultry are summarized in Table 27.2. Regulatory approvals, dose regimens, and cross-clearance with other drugs vary by country, and the manufacturers' data sheets should be consulted prior to drug use.

Antimicrobial Drug Use for Other Infections

The extensive use of prophylactic anticoccidials has reduced the economic impact of coccidiosis, so that respiratory pathogens, in particular *Escherichia coli,* remain the major reason for clinical outbreaks of disease in intensively reared poultry. Infection by *E. coli* commonly progresses to airsacculitis and septicemia and results in significant economic loss at processing. In addition, resistance to currently available antibacterials is more frequently encountered in *E. coli* than in any of the other bacterial pathogens of poultry.

Because of their viral nature, no cost-effective chemotherapeutic control methods exist for many poultry pathogens, so that their control relies on alternative methods. Examples of these include vaccination of growing birds against Marek's disease, infectious bronchitis, or Newcastle disease; vaccination of breeder stock against avian encephalomyelitis or duck viral hepatitis; biosecurity, with vaccination only where disease is prevalent, for control of laryngotracheitis; depopulation of affected houses to prevent spread of avian tuberculosis or coronaviral enteritis; improved husbandry and ventilation in cases of *Aspergillus* sp. infection; or control of the insect vector to prevent avian malaria.

ANTIMICROBIAL DRUG USE PRIOR TO HATCH

Fumigation is widely used to prevent entry of contaminating microorganisms into the egg. However, in turkeys or where mycoplasmal infection is endemic, antimicrobial drugs are employed extensively for treating eggs to minimize the transmission of pathogenic microorganisms from dam to hatching poults. Egg dipping is most commonly used, although egg injection techniques have been developed. During egg dipping, a pressure differential is established between the inside and the outside of the egg to allow penetration of the antimicrobial. Initially, temperature was used to establish this differential. More recently, vacuum techniques have become available. The aim of both methods is to get approximately 0.2 ml of antimicrobial solution into the egg. Both gentamicin and enrofloxacin, at 500 ppm, are approved for this purpose. Injection of antimicrobials, such as lincomycin-spectinomycin, into the airspace of eggs has also shown promising results for the control of vertically transmitted infections such as *Mycoplasma gallisepticum* in chickens. With turkeys, experimental egg injection of gentamicin, enrofloxacin, tylosin, and josamycin have all been successful in reducing vertical transmission of mycoplasmas.

ANTIMICROBIAL DRUG USE IN NEWLY HATCHED CHICKS

A number of antimicrobials (eg, doxycycline, gentamicin, sarafloxacin, spectinomycin) have been approved for use in the young chick to control early mortality. These drugs can be administered in the water or injected SC into the newly hatched chick, often concurrently with vaccination against Marek's disease. Antimicrobial drug use at this time is particularly cost-effective because the small size of a newly hatched chick requires the administration of less drug to attain clinically useful levels.

ANTIMICROBIAL DRUG USE FOLLOWING VACCINATION

Although administration of antimicrobial drugs does not halt the progression of viral disease in poultry, the drugs can be of use in preventing secondary bacterial infections. In particular, the use of live, attenuated viral vaccines, such as Newcastle disease and infectious bronchitis, can increase the susceptibility of birds to bacterial infection, and prophylactic administration of antimicrobial drugs postvaccination can be especially effective in preventing secondary infection by *E. coli*.

Antimicrobial Drugs of Choice

Table 27.3 summarizes the indications for use of antimicrobial drugs currently approved for the treatment of poultry in North America. Where no medication period is specified, the antimicrobial should be used throughout the period of risk or until clinical signs are no longer apparent. Recommended drug dosage is shown in Table 27.4.

ANTIMICROBIAL DRUGS CURRENTLY UNDER DEVELOPMENT

Many of the antimicrobials listed in Table 27.3 are no longer efficacious at the manufacturers' recommended dose and duration. This has led to extensive extralabel use of them as the only option for controlling disease outbreaks. There is a clear need to license newer antimicrobial drugs for which resistance is not a problem and which are efficacious against difficult-to-control infections. Approval is being sought for a number of antimicrobial drugs with important potential for food animal use. Some of these antimicrobials have already been approved for use in poultry in Europe and/or South America, where the drug approval process proceeds more quickly than in North America. A summary of relevant compounds is shown in Table 27.5. Where available, appropriate references detailing poultry use studies have been cited in the Bibliography.

Principles of Water Medication

Understanding the principles of water medication is essential for treatment to be successful. It is arguable that the most accurate dose recommendation for a soluble product is that specified on a weight-for-weight basis, for example, mg/kg. However, it is common to see recommendations based on parts per million (ppm) or even birds per packet of drug. While tables of average water consumption are available from most chick breeders, many factors can affect day-to-day water consumption of poultry. The most significant factor is ambient temperature, with higher temperatures increasing water consumption. Consequently, to ensure correct administration of drugs via the water supply, consumption should be monitored using an in-line water meter. This device is easily fitted and provides an inexpensive and reliable method for measuring water intake. Water intake, however, should always be recorded for a complete 24-hour period, because consumption rates vary throughout the day and night.

When medication is supplied through a gravity water system, the requisite amount of drug is dissolved in a bulk tank adjacent to or above the poultry house, which ideally holds sufficient water to supply bird needs over a 24-hour period. To medicate birds, the bulk tank is filled, the drug is added at the dose rate recommended, and the medicated water is supplied to the house. However, very thorough mixing is required to ensure a homogeneous mix of drug in the large volume of water, and bulk tanks are often too small to hold the volume of water consumed in 24 hours by older birds, necessitating a multiple-dosing schedule. Consequently, it is often preferable to use a proportioner system.

A proportioner device is a liquid dispenser that introduces a medicated solution into the house water supply in a fixed ratio of medicated stock solution to water consumed and is powered by the flow of water into the poultry house rather than by electricity. With proportioner systems, the dose rate can be quickly and easily adjusted, and the birds are not left without water if there is a higher consumption rate than expected. Mechanical failure can occur if these devices are not adequately maintained, and some models can be less reliable at low flow rates, such as those encountered with young chicks. Calculation of the correct dose rate is less easy than with a gravity system, with which the appropriate amount of drug can be mixed directly into the bulk tank. By contrast, a proportioner system requires a concentrated stock solution to be formulated that, when introduced into the water system at the ratio chosen, medicates the drinking water at the recommended rate. The dosing ratio can be adjusted on most proportioners but is generally set at 1:128, equivalent to 1 ounce of stock solution per 1 U.S. gallon of drinking water. Using the previous day's consumption of house water as a guide, one can easily calculate the volume of stock solution required to medicate the birds over a 24-hour period. An example of a typical dose calculation for a proportioner system would be to measure the volume of water consumed in the 24 hours prior to medication, say, 512 U.S. gallons; calculate amount of drug required to meet manufacturer's recommendations based on average bird weight or age and number of birds in the house; set proportioner ratio to 1:128 (1 ounce/U.S. gallon); calculate volume of stock solution that will medicate 512 U.S. gallons (512/128, or 4 U.S. gallons); dissolve the 24-hour dose of medication in 4 U.S. gallons of water to give the correct concentration of stock solution. This will provide the manufacturer's recommended dose of medication in 512 gallons of drinking water, the amount estimated to last the birds for 24 hours. Each day's medication should be based upon the previous day's water consumption. This allows for changes in bird water consumption attributable to growth or compensatory feeding as morbidity decreases in response to treatment.

Other factors can affect the success of water medication in controlling disease. Drinkers must be well maintained, since leaking drinkers will cause an overestimation of water consumption, will waste medication, and will lead to underdosing. Water troughs must be clean because feed or algal deposits can lead to drug inactivation, again resulting in underdosing. The effect of impurities in the house water, which can limit drug availability, have been discussed earlier in this chapter.

Bibliography

Afifi NA, El-Sooud KA. 1997. Tissue concentrations and pharmacokinetics of florfenicol in broiler chickens. Br Poult Sci 38:425.

Alls AA, et al. 1963. The mechanics of treating hatching eggs for disease prevention. Avian Dis 7:89.

Calnek BW, et al. 1997. Diseases of Poultry, 10th Ed. Ames: Iowa State Univ Press.

Jordan FTW, Horrocks BK. 1996. The minimum inhibitory concentration of tilmicosin and tylosin for *Mycoplasma gallisepticum* and *Mycoplasma synoviae* and a comparison of their efficacy in the control of *Mycoplasma gallisepticum* in broiler chicks. Avian Dis 40:326.

Küther K. 1987. Coccidiosis in broiler production and experience with lerbek. Zootech Int (Oct).

McCapes RH, et al. 1977. Antibiotic egg injection to eliminate disease. Avian Dis 21:57.

McGinnis CH, et al. 1978. The effect of nosiheptide, a new antibiotic, on body weight gain and feed efficiency in broiler chickens. Poult Sci 57:1641.

Muirhead S. 1998. Feed Additive Compendium. Minnetonka, MN: Miller, p36.

Pardue SL, Luginbuhl GH. 1998. Improvement of poult performance following *Bordetella avium* challenge by administration of a novel oxy-halogen formulation. Avian Dis 42:145.

Reynolds DJ, et al. 1997. Evaluation of combined antibiotic and competitive exclusion treatment in broiler flocks infected with *Salmonella enterica* serovar Enteritidis. Avian Pathol 26:83.

Sakaguchi Y, et al. 1988. Esafloxacin, a new quinolone derivative: its in vitro antibacterial activity against chicken pathogens. Proc 17th World Poult Congr Jap, p1265.

Sumano H, et al. 1998. Antibacterial activity, pharmacokinetics, and therapeutic efficacy in poultry of a new cephalosporin-fluoroquinolone (CQ) molecule. J Appl Anim Res 13:169.

Tanner AC, et al. 1991. A comparison of danofloxacin and tylosin in the treatment of induced *Mycoplasma gallisepticum* infection. Proc 40th West Poult Dis Conf Mex, p268.

Yamamoto K, et al. 1988. Myplabin (miporamicin), a new macrolide antibiotic. Proc 18th World Poult Congr Jap, p1256.

Yogaratnam V. 1995. Analysis of the causes of high rates of carcass rejection at a poultry processing plant. Vet Rec 137:215.

TABLE 27.2. Antimicrobials approved for treatment and control of coccidiosis in poultry

Antimicrobial	Use Level[a]	Withdrawal Time (days)	Use/Comments
Amprolium	0.004–0.025%	0	Prevention in and/or treatment of broilers, replacement chickens, layers, turkeys, and pheasants. Dose level determined by severity of exposure, and degree of immunity desired.
Clopidol	0.0125–0.025%	0–5	Prevention. Withdrawal time varies with dose and use of bird.
Decoquinate	0.003%	0	Prevention in broilers.
Diclazuril	1 g/tonne	5	Prevention in broilers.
Halofuginone	1.36–2.72 g/ton	4–7	Prevention in broilers, replacement layers and breeders, and turkeys. Withdrawal time longest for turkeys.
Lasalocid	68–113 g/ton	0	Prevention in broilers, turkeys, and partridges.
Maduramicin	4.54–5.45 g/ton	5	Prevention in broilers. Higher dose may adversely affect growth rate in the absence of clinical coccidiosis.
Monensin	54–110 g/ton	0	Prevention in broilers, replacement chickens, turkeys, and bobwhite quail. Dose level determined by severity of exposure. May lead to reduced weight gains in the absence of clinical coccidiosis.
Narasin	54–72 g/ton	0–5	Prevention in broilers. Toxic to turkeys.
Narasin + Nicarbazin	54–90 g/ton	5	Prevention in broilers. Combination is synergistic in the ratio of 1:1. Toxic to turkeys.
Nicarbazin	0.012–0.02%	4–9	Prevention of infection by *Eimeria acervulina, E. brunetti, E. maxima, E. necatrix,* and *E. tenella.*

TABLE 27.2. *Continued*

Antimicrobial	Use Level[a]	Withdrawal Time (days)	Use/Comments
Robenidine	0.0033%	5	Prevention in broilers and turkeys.
Salinomycin	40–60 g/ton	0–5	Prevention in broilers, replacement chickens, and quail.
Semduramicin		0	Prevention in broilers.
Sulfamethazine (soluble)	58–124 mg/lb per day	10	Treatment of clinical coccidiosis in chickens and turkeys.
Sulfadimethoxine (soluble)	0.025–0.05%	5	Treatment of clinical coccidiosis in broilers and turkeys.
Sulfadimethoxine + ormetoprim	0.0125% 0.0075%	5	Prevention in broilers and replacement chickens. Prevention in turkeys at half this level. Combination is synergistic in the ratio of 5:3.
Sulfaquinoxaline (soluble)	0.025–0.04%	10	Control of clinical coccidiosis in chickens and turkeys.
Sulfaquinoxaline (500 mg/g) + trimethoprim (165mg/g)	30 mg/kg	7–9	Treatment of clinical coccidiosis in chickens and turkeys.
Tetracyclines (oxy-, chlor-)	200 g/ton	3	Prevention and control of *Eimeria necatrix* and *E. tenella*. Not normally considered a drug of choice.
Toltrazuril	7 mg/kg	21	Treatment of clinical coccidiosis in broiler breeders and layer replacements.
Zoalene	0.004–0.0187%	0	Prevention and control in broilers, replacement chickens, and turkeys. Dose level determined by severity of exposure and degree of immunity required.

Note: Approved use level, type of bird, and withdrawal time may vary. Therefore the manufacturer's data sheet should be consulted for confirmation of withdrawal period, approved cross-clearances with other medicated feed additives, and conditions of use.

[a] 1 ton (U.S.) is equivalent to 1.016 tonnes (metric).

TABLE 27.3. **Antimicrobial drug selection for infections of poultry**

Site	Diagnosis	Causative Organism	Suggested Drugs	Alternative Drugs	Comments
Upper respiratory tract, lung, air sac	Chronic respiratory disease (CRD)	*Mycoplasma gallisepticum*	Erythromycin, fluoro-quinolones,[a] lincomycin-spectinomycin, tetracycline,[b] tylosin	Furazolidone,[c] spectinomycin, spiramycin	All drugs PO except oxytetracycline (PO, SC) and spectinomycin (SC); enrofloxacin approved for egg dipping
	Mycoplasma respiratory disease, airsacculitis	*M. synoviae, M. meleagridis*	As *M. gallisepticum*		
	Infectious coryza	*Haemophilus paragallinarium*	Erythromycin, sulfonamides,[d] tetracycline	Ormetoprim-sulfadimethoxine	All drugs PO except tetracycline (intranasal)
	Complicated chronic respiratory disease (CCRD), colibacillosis	*E. coli* with/without *M. gallisepticum*	Fluoroquinolones,[a] gentamicin, lincomycin-spectinomycin, tetracycline,[b] ceftiofur	Erythromycin, ormetoprim-sulfadimethoxine, spectinomycin	All drugs PO except gentamicin, ceftiofur, and spectinomycin (SC)
	Respiratory disease	*Ornithobacterium rhinotracheale*	Ceftiofur,[c] tetracyclines[c]	Spectinomycin,[c] erythromycin[c]	All drugs PO except ceftiofur and spectinomycin (SC)
Soft tissue, septicemia	Erysipelas	*Erysipelothrix rhusiopathiae*	Penicillin G	Penicillin-streptomycin	PO except pencillin-streptomycin (IM)
	Fowl cholera	*Pasteurella multocida*	Tetracycline[b]	Novobiocin, ormetoprim-sulfadimethoxine, spectinomycin, sulfonamides[d]	All drugs PO except oxytetracycline (IM) and spectinomycin (SC)
	Fowl typhoid	*Salmonella gallinarium*	Fluoroquinolones,[a] furazolidone,[c] gentamicin	Apramycin,[c] spectinomycin, sulfonamides[d]	All drugs PO except gentamicin and spectinomycin (SC)
	Infectious serositis	*Riemerella anatipestifer*	Novobiocin, ormetoprim-sulfadimethoxine, sulfonamides[d]		All drugs PO

651

TABLE 27.3. *Continued*

Site	Diagnosis	Causative Organism	Suggested Drugs	Alternative Drugs	Comments
	Infectious synovitis	*M. synoviae*	As *M. gallisepticum*		
	Arizonosis, paracolon	*Salmonella arizona*	As fowl typhoid		
	Paratyphoid	*Salmonella*	As fowl typhoid		
	Pseudomonas infection	*P. aeruginosa*	Gentamicin		Administer at 1 day of age (SC)
	Pullorum disease	*Salmonella pullorum*	As fowl typhoid		
	Staphylococcal septicemia, breast blisters	*Staphylococcus aureus*	Erythromycin, novobiocin, pencillin G	Tetracycline[b]	PO
	Staphylococcal synovitis	*Staphylococcus* spp.	As *S. aureus*		
	Vibrionic hepatitis	*Campylobacter* spp.	Furazolidone,[c] erythromycin	Oxytetracycline, neomycin	All drugs PO
Intestinal tract	Crop mycosis	*Candida albicans*	Nystatin		PO
	Hexamitiasis	*Hexamita meleagridis*	Furazolidone,[c] tetracycline[b]		All drugs PO
	Histomoniasis	*Histomonas meleagridis*	Dimetridazole,[c] furazolidone[c]	Nifursol, nitarsone, ronidazole[c]	All drugs PO
	Leucocytozoonosis	*Leucocytozoon smithi*	Clopidol		PO
	Necrotic enteritis	*Clostridium perfringens*	Bacitracin, lincomycin	Virginiamycin	All drugs PO
	Nonspecific enteritis	Poorly defined	Bacitracin, neomycin, nitrofurazone,[c] penicillin	Furazolidone,[c] streptomycin, tetracycline[b]	All drugs PO
	Ulcerative enteritis, quail disease	*Clostridium colinum*	Furazolidone[c]	Bacitracin	All drugs PO

Note: Regulatory approval is necessary for antimicrobial administration to food animals. The manufacturer's data sheet should be consulted for information on dose, duration, and withdrawal times. Not all the drugs shown here have been approved for these purposes in commercial poultry.

[a] Includes danofloxacin, enrofloxacin, and sarafloxacin. Not all are approved for food animal use; extralabel use of fluoroquinolones is illegal in the United States.

[b] Includes chlortetracycline, doxycycline, oxytetracycline, and tetracycline.

[c] Not approved for food animal use in some countries, including the United States.

[d] Includes sulfadimethoxine, sulfamethazine, sulfaquinoxaline, and sulfathiazole.

TABLE 27.4. Recommended dosage of antimicrobial drugs for prophylactic and therapeutic use in poultry

Drug	Prophylactic		Therapeutic		
	g/ton (U.S.)	mg/l	g/ton (U.S.)	mg/l	Other
Amoxicillin	—	—	—	—	15–20 mg/kg[c]
Apramycin	—	—	—	—	0.25–0.5 g/l[c]
Bacitracin	50–100	—	100–200	—	—
Ceftiofur	—	—	—	—	0.08–0.2 mg/chick[a]
Chlortetracycline	50–200	—	100–500	106–264.5	—
Clopidol	113–227	—	—	—	—
Dimetridazole	98–197	—	453	—	—
Doxycycline	—	—	—	50	—
Enrofloxacin	—	—	—	—	10 mg/kg[c]
Erythromycin	92.5–185	—	92.5–185	115.6–250	—
Furazolidone	50–100	—	100–200	—	—
Gentamicin	—	—	—	—	0.2–1.0 mg/chick[a]
Lincomycin	2	—	2	17	—
Lincomycin + spectinomycin	—	—	—	530–833	5 mg/lb
Neomycin	—	35–80	35–226	—	50–65 mg/lb
Nifursol	50	—	—	—	—
Nitarsone	170	—	—	—	—
Nitrofurazone	—	—	50	—	—
Novobiocin	—	—	200–350	—	7–14 mg/lb
Nystatin	50	—	50–100	—	—
Ormetoprim + sulfadimethoxine	34.05 + 56.75 to 68.1 + 113.5	—	136.2 + 227 to 272.4 + 454	—	—
Oxytetracycline	50–200	—	100–500	26.5–105.8	6.25–200 mg/bird
Oxytetracycline + neomycin	—	—	100–200 + 35–40	—	—

653

TABLE 27.4. *Continued*

Drug	Prophylactic		Therapeutic		
	g/ton (U.S.)	mg/l	g/ton (U.S.)	mg/l	Other
Penicillin	50–100	—	100	—	1,500,000 IU/gal
Penicillin + streptomycin	—	—	—	—	20,000 IU + 25 mg/lb
Romidazole	54.4	—	—	—	—
Sarafloxacin	—	—	—	—	0.1 mg/chick[a]
					20–40 ppm
Spectinomycin	—	132	—	264–530	2.5–10 mg/chick[a]
Spiramycin	—	—	—	400	—
Streptomycin	—	—	—	66–100	25 mg/lb
Sulfachlorpyridazine + trimethoprim	—	—	—	—	24 mg total activity/kg[c]
Sulfadiazine + trimethoprim	—	—	—	—	15 mg total activity/kg[c]
					300 g total activity/tonne (in feed)
Sulfadimethoxine	—	—	—	250–500	—
Sulfamethazine	—	—	—	1000	—
Sulfaquinoxaline + trimethoprim	—	—	—	—	110–273 mg/kg
Sulfaquinoxaline	—	—	—	397	30 mg total activity/kg[c]
Sulfathiazole	—	—	—	1000	—
Tetracycline	—	100–200	—	200–400	25–50 mg/bird[b]
Tylosin	—	—	800–1000	530	15–25 mg/bird[b]
Virginiamycin	5–20	—	—	—	—

Note: Although these dosages are those recommended for use by the manufacturer, the approved dose, duration, and withdrawal period should always be confirmed prior to drug use in poultry for human consumption.

[a]Subcutaneous.
[b]Intranasal.
[c]Oral.

TABLE 27.5. **Some antimicrobials under development with potential utility in poultry**

Generic Name (Compound Class)	Indications (Proposed Dose Level)
Acetyl isovaleryl (macrolide)	Antimycoplasmal
Apramycin (aminocyclitol)	Antibacterial (500 mg/l)
CQ (cephalosporin/fluoroquinolone)	Antibacterial (3 mg/kg)
Danofloxacin (fluoroquinolone)	Antibacterial/antimycoplasmal (5mg/kg)
Esafloxacin (fluoroquinolone)	Antibacterial/antimycoplasmal (2.5–20 mg/kg)
Florfenicol (chloramphenicol derivative)	Antibacterial
LL-E19020	Nutritional (0.01–50 mg/kg)
Meticlopindol/methylbenzoquate (pyridinol/4-hydroxyquinolone)	Anticoccidial, synergistic combination 20%:1.67% (108 ppm total activity)
Miporamicin (macrolide)	Antibacterial (100 ppm)
Neoviridogrisein	Nutritional
Norfloxacin (fluoroquinolone)	Antibacterial
Nosiheptide (peptide)	Nutritional (5–10 g/ton feed)
Oxyhalogens	Antibacterial (0.008–0.016%)
Tilmicosin (macrolide)	Antimycoplasmal (100–300 mg/l)

28 Antimicrobial Drug Use in Rodents, Rabbits, and Ferrets

P. BURGMANN

Antimicrobial therapy in rodents and rabbits entails greater risk than in most other species because inappropriate therapy can result in death of the patient due to enterotoxemia. In a laboratory animal setting, unnecessary prophylactic use of antimicrobials can also interfere with experimental studies or result in antimicrobial resistance and in the emergence of infections that were previously subclinical. Due to the inherent risk, practitioners must resist the urge to administer antimicrobials indiscriminately and must carefully consider the following questions before any therapy is instituted. For a more thorough discussion of the following, see Rosenthal (1998).

First, what are the nutritional status and husbandry situation of the patient? Although laboratory settings are well controlled, rodents kept as pets are often fed stale pellets and are exposed to high levels of ammonia in inadequately cleaned cages. Guinea pigs are often presented with low-grade hypovitaminosis C, even if not showing clear signs of scurvy. Dietary indiscretions resulting in carbohydrate overload are common in overindulged pet rabbits. Instituting antimicrobial therapy in pet practice without correcting such deficits is tantamount to malpractice.

Second, what is the nature of the infection? Is it acute or chronic, and what is the most likely pathogen? Whenever possible, culture and sensitivity results are essential, as many of these species cannot tolerate a second course of antibiotics because of the risk of dysbiosis. Which organ

The author gratefully acknowledges Dr. Dean Percy's contributions to the earlier version of this chapter in the second edition of this book.

system is involved, and can the chosen antibiotic reach the site of infection? Abscesses in these animals tend to be walled off and caseous and must be lanced or excised for therapy to be effective. Establishing these basic parameters allows the practitioner to form a reasonable prognosis and a clear rationale for the therapeutic approach and length of treatment required.

Finally, which drug is the safest, at what dose, and which route of administration is most efficacious? Given the small and delicate nature of the species involved, restraint is often difficult, and parenteral therapy can have its own limitations.

The following sections will address most of these issues in greater detail. With the passage of time, certain diseases lessen in importance in laboratory animal medicine and others emerge, while the diseases encountered in pet practice are often different altogether. The tables presented do not represent a complete list of recognized bacterial diseases in rabbits, rodents, and ferrets but rather are summarized lists of those diseases most likely to be encountered in private practice or a laboratory animal setting at the present time. Drugs recommended for specific conditions are also given.

Antimicrobial Toxicity

It is now fairly common knowledge that the incidence of antimicrobial toxicity in rabbits and rodents is relatively high when compared with that of other species. Antimicrobial therapy can lead to suppression of normal bacterial flora, resulting in subsequent dysbiosis, enteritis, and finally enterotoxemia and death, most commonly caused by iota toxin production by *Clostridium spiroforme*. Mice, rats, ferrets, and possibly gerbils are relatively resistant to dysbiosis, but hamsters, guinea pigs, chinchillas, and rabbits are susceptible. The susceptibility of hedgehogs to dysbiosis is not yet known but will likely become clearer as these pets increase in popularity and more references become available in the literature.

Antibiotics most likely to induce dysbiosis include amoxicillin, ampicillin, penicillin, clindamycin, and lincomycin, whereas cephalosporins and erythromycin are considered intermediate. Tetracyclines may cause dysbiosis in guinea pigs but appear to be less likely to do so in other species. Antibiotics least likely to induce dysbiosis include the aminoglycosides, chloramphenicol, fluoroquinolones, metronidazole, and the sulfonamides.

Other adverse side effects of antimicrobial therapy have also been observed. Streptomycin and dihydrostreptomycin toxicity has occurred in mice, hamsters, gerbils, and guinea pigs. Deaths often occur within minutes after treatment and are likely caused by direct effects on the cardiovascular system (Wightman et al., 1980; Carpenter et al., 1996). Deaths attributed to the toxic effects of procaine have occurred in mice, guinea pigs, and rabbits following treatment with procaine penicillin G (Morris, 1995). The nephrotoxic potential of aminoglycosides can be decreased by ensuring that fluids are administered concurrently, particularly if the animal is older or even mildly dehydrated. Involution of lymphoid tissue and an impaired immune response were observed in rabbits on prolonged oral tetracycline treatment (Stetsenko et al., 1981). In addition, prolonged or inappropriate antimicrobial therapy may result in the development of antibiotic-resistant strains of bacteria.

When prescribing antimicrobial treatment for rabbits raised for meat production, it is essential that the veterinarian be aware and inform the client of regulations concerning those drugs approved for use and their recommended withdrawal times for this species.

Drug Dosages

In recent years a number of formularies that include small mammals have been published, gathering together sources that have long been scattered throughout the scientific literature. Yet, as each author hastens to add, it is important to remember that many of the dosages presented are empirical and not based on pharmacokinetic or controlled efficacy trials. Assembling dosages from such a nebulous array of sources results in some myths becoming self-perpetuating. For example, for years tetracycline in the drinking water was advocated for use in rabbits, until pharmacokinetic study revealed that administration by this route is an ineffective method of achieving therapeutic blood concentrations (Percy and Black, 1988). Similarly, intramuscular penicillin at 40,000 IU/kg has long been advocated for use against *Treponema* in rabbits, yet trials have indicated that this drug may cause mortality at this dose (Harkness and Wagner, 1995).

In order to compensate for this deficiency, various allometric equations have been proposed as a means of extrapolating dosages among species (Morris, 1995). However, allometry assumes that there are no interspecies differences in metabolism, which is not always the case, particularly when treating smaller mammals. Still, at present, although no equation has achieved universal acceptance, allometry is considered an acceptable method for drug calculations when dosages are not available.

The tables provided give dosages and drug choices that are currently considered reasonably safe and efficacious (Tables 28.1–28.12). However, further drug dosage research is needed, and it remains the practitioner's responsibility to apply new data as they become available and to be aware that very few of the drugs listed are licensed for use in rabbits and rodents and that the choice of drug is at the discretion of the practitioner and is considered extralabel use.

Routes of Administration

Various routes of administration are used in rabbits and rodents, and each has its advantages and disadvantages.

Medicating the drinking water is advantageous in that no stress of capture or restraint is involved and large numbers of animals can be treated easily. However, this method of drug administration has many disadvantages. Exact dosage is impossible, since factors that influence drug dosage, such as water intake, body weight, disease status, dehydration, obesity, age, and sex, vary among individuals. Animals fed dry rations consume more water than those receiving fluid from other sources such as fresh fruits or vegetables. Interspecies differences must also be considered. For example, guinea pigs consume relatively large amounts of water, whereas gerbils consume very little. In rabbits, food intake is closely linked with water consumption. If the water is unpalatable, food consumption decreases. To be suitable for administration in the drinking water, an antibiotic should be soluble and stable in water, palatable, and well absorbed from the gastrointestinal tract. Table 28.1 gives average daily food and water intakes of various species. Recommended dosages for administration in food or drinking water is given in Table 28.3.

Direct oral dosing is much preferred to medication of the drinking water, since the amount administered can be accurately determined based on the needs of the individual. Provided that the animal consumes the entire offering, the drug can be hidden in a small piece of fruit, cooked sweet potatoes, or corn or applied to a half-inch square of toast and covered with peanut butter. In this case no restraint is involved, and stress is minimized. Once again, palatability is essential to prevent drug refusal. If

TABLE 28.1. **Daily food and water intake per 100 g of body weight**

Species	Food (dry weight, g)	Water (ml)
Mouse	15	15
Hamster	10–12	8–10
Gerbil	5–8	4–7
Rat	10	10–12
Guinea pig	6	10–12
Hedgehog	—[a]	—[a]
Chinchilla	4 pellets; ad lib hay	—[b]
Rabbit	5 pellets; ad lib hay	10
Ferret	4–55	6–10

[a]Currently undetermined, hedgehog diets in captivity are still experimental. For several diet suggestions, see Johnson-Delaney (1996).
[b] Data unavailable.

the drug is administered PO directly, proper restraint techniques are essential to minimize regurgitation, exhalation, or aspiration. For all small rodents and ferrets, a firm scruff grip will pull back the lips sufficiently to allow oral dosing. Guinea pigs, chinchillas, and rabbits can be easily dosed if an assistant can restrain the animal while the drug is administered. Another alternative is to wrap the rabbit, chinchilla, or guinea pig in a towel and administer the medication via a syringe placed just behind the incisors. If the drug is given slowly, the licking response can be evoked, and the oral medication can be administered by one person. Hedgehogs (*Atelerix albiventris*) provide their own challenges in that, when threatened, they will curl tightly into a ball, making medication administration difficult. In this species, medicating the food or water or SC injection is often the most useful approach.

Parenteral administration is indicated for drugs that are inactivated or poorly absorbed from the gastrointestinal tract or where rapid onset of pharmacological action is required. Because very small volumes are required, a 0.5-ml tuberculin syringe with a 27-gauge needle is ideal in the smaller species. Even then, most commercially available substances are too concentrated and require dilution before use. Wherever possible, use the same diluent already present in the drug solution.

SC administration is best if applicable, because tissue damage to the small muscle mass available in most species limits the use of IM injection. Tetracyclines, tylosin, and sulfonamides are, however, particularly irritating to tissues, especially when dissolved in a propylene glycol base, and may cause localized tissue necrosis and sloughing when given subcutaneously. SC injections can be given in the loose skin of the scruff or under the skin of the underbelly, where the skin is thinner and more easily penetrated by the 27-gauge needle. When IM injection is required, use the lumbar muscles or the muscles of the quadriceps or gluteals in all species. Remember that the sciatic nerve runs immediately caudal to the femur and should be avoided, or lameness may result.

IV injections are difficult to administer and best avoided. When required, mice, gerbils, and rats can be injected into the lateral tail vein; hamsters can be injected into the femoral vein; and the saphenous, cephalic, or jugular vein are accessible in the guinea pig, chinchilla, rabbit, and ferret. Interosseus administration may provide a better alternative in the smaller species, particularly if an indwelling catheter is already in place there for fluid administration. The catheter can be placed in the proximal head of the femur, which is the most accessible long bone for this purpose.

Topical drug preparations have a limited application in rabbits and rodents. Eyedrops and ointments are useful in all species, but topical creams and ointments are generally ineffective in the smaller rodents because of their fastidious grooming habits. Creams and ointments can, however, be used in rabbits, ferrets, and guinea pigs, provided they are applied to an area not easily accessible for grooming. Rodents are relatively susceptible to the toxic side effects of drops, creams, or ointments containing steroids, and they should be used with caution in these species. Nebulization of antibiotics for respiratory tract infections is helpful in all species and is a useful adjunct to oral or parenteral therapy.

Bibliography

Bishop Y, ed. 1996. The Veterinary Formulary, 3rd ed. London: Pharmaceutical Press.

Carpenter JW, et al. 1996. Exotic Animal Formulary, 1st ed. Manhattan, KS: Greystone.

Collins BR. 1995. Antimicrobial drug use in rabbits, rodents, and other small mammals. In: Antimicrobial Therapy in Caged Birds and Exotic Pets, An International Symposium. Trenton, NJ: Veterinary Learning Systems.

Foltz CJ, et al. 1996. Evaluation of various oral antimicrobial formulations for the eradication of *Helicobacter hepaticus*. Lab Anim Sci 46:173.

Harkness JE, Wagner JE. 1995. The Biology and Medicine of Rabbits and Rodents, 4th ed. Philadelphia: Williams and Wilkins.

Hawk CT, Leary SL. 1995. Formulary for Laboratory Animals. Ames: Iowa State Univ Press.

Hillyer EV, Quesenberry KE, eds. 1997. Ferrets, Rabbits, and Rodents Clinical Medicine and Surgery. Philadelphia: WB Saunders.

Hoefer HL. 1994. Hedgehogs. In: Exotic Pet Medicine II. Philadelphia: WB Saunders. Vet Clin North Am Small Anim Pract 24(1):113.

Hrapkiewicz K, et al. 1998. Clinical Laboratory Animal Medicine, 2nd ed. Ames: Iowa State Univ Press.

Johnson-Delaney CA. 1996. Exotic Companion Medicine Handbook for Veterinarians. Lake Worth, FL: Wingers.

Laber-Laird K, et al. 1996. Handbook of Rodent and Rabbit Medicine. Oxford: Elsevier Science.

Lipman NS, et al. 1992. Utilization of cholestyramine resin as a preventive treatment for antibiotic (clindamycin) induced enterotoxaemia in the rabbit. Lab Anim 26:1.

Matsushita S, Suzuki E. 1995. Prevention and treatment of cilia-associated respiratory bacillus in mice by use of antibiotics. Lab Anim Sci 45:503.

McKay SG, et al. 1996. Use of tilmicosin for treatment of pasteurellosis in rabbits. Am J Vet Res 57:1180.

Morris TH. 1995. Antibiotic therapeutics in laboratory animals. Lab Anim 29:16.

Percy DH, Black WD. 1988. Pharmacokinetics of tetracycline in the domestic rabbit following intravenous or oral administration. Can J Vet Res 52:5.

Richardson VCG. 1997. Diseases of Small Domestic Rodents. Oxford: Blackwell Science.

Rosenthal KL. 1998. Bacterial infections and antibiotic therapy in small mammals. Compend Contin Educ Pract Vet 20 (Suppl 3A):13.

Smith AJ. 1992. Husbandry and medicine of African hedgehogs *(Atelerix albiventris)*. J Small Exot Anim Med 2:21.

Stetsenko ON, et al. 1981. Tetracycline effect on immune and hematopoietic systems of intact rabbits. Antibiotic 26:856.

Wightman SR, et al. 1980. Dihydrostreptomycin toxicity in the Mongolian gerbil, *Meriones unguiculatus*. Lab Anim Sci 40:71.

TABLE 28.2A. **Recommended dosages of antimicrobial drugs in laboratory animals**

Drug	Mice	Hamsters	Gerbils	Rats	Guinea Pigs
Amikacin[a]	10 mg/kg SID, SC, IM	10 mg/kg SID, SC, IM	10 mg/kg SID, SC, IM	10 mg/kg SID, SC, IM	10 mg/kg SID, SC, IM
Ampicillin[b]	20–100 mg/kg BID, PO, SC	Do not use	20–100 mg/kg BID, PO, SC	20–100 mg/kg BID, PO, SC	Do not use
Chloramphenicol palmitate	50–200 mg/kg TID, PO	50–200 mg/kg TID, PO	50–200 mg/kg TID, PO	50–200 mg/kg TID, PO	50 mg/kg BID, PO
Chloramphenicol succinate	30–50 mg/kg BID, SC, IM	30–50 mg/kg BID, SC, IM	30–50 mg/kg BID, SC, IM	30–50 mg/kg BID, SC, IM	30–50 mg/kg BID, SC, IM
Chlortetracycline[c]	25 mg/kg BID, SC, IM	20 mg/kg BID, SC, IM	—[d]	6–10 mg/kg BID, SC, IM	—[c,d]
Ciprofloxacin[e]	15–20 mg/kg SID, PO	15–20 mg/kg SID, PO	15–20 mg/kg SID, PO	15–20 mg/kg SID, PO	15–20 mg/kg SID, PO
Doxycycline[c]	2.5–5 mg/kg BID, PO	2.5–5 mg/kg BID, PO	2.5–5 mg/kg BID, PO	2.5–5 mg/kg BID, PO	2.5–5 mg/kg BID, PO[c]
Enrofloxacin[e]	5–10 mg/kg SID, PO, SC, IM	5–10 mg/kg SID, PO, SC, IM	5–10 mg/kg SID, PO, SC, IM	5–10 mg/kg SID, PO, SC, IM	5–10 mg/kg SID, PO, SC, IM
Gentamicin[a]	5 mg/kg SID, SC, IM	5 mg/kg SID, SC, IM	5 mg/kg SID, SC, IM	5 mg/kg SID, SC, IM	5 mg/kg SID, SC, IM
Metronidazole	20–60 mg/kg BID, PO	20–60 mg/kg BID, PO	20–60 mg/kg BID, PO	20–60 mg/kg BID, PO	20–40 mg/kg BID, PO
Neomycin	50 mg/kg SID, PO	100 mg/kg SID, PO	100 mg/kg SID, PO	50 mg/kg SID, PO	30 mg/kg SID, PO
Oxytetracycline[c]	10–20 mg/kg TID, PO	16 mg/kg SID, SC	10 mg/kg BID, TID, PO	10–20 mg/kg TID, PO	—[c,d]
Tetracycline[c]	10–20 mg/kg BID, TID, PO	10–20 mg/kg BID, TID, PO	10–20 mg/kg BID, TID, PO	10–20 mg/kg BID, TID, PO	10–20 mg/kg BID, PO[c]
Trimethoprim sulfadiazine[f]	30 mg/kg SID, SC, IM	30 mg/kg SID, SC, IM	30 mg/kg SID, SC, IM	30 mg/kg SID, SC, IM	30 mg/kg SID, SC, IM
Trimethoprim sulfamethoxazole	30 mg/kg BID, PO	15–30mg/kg BID, PO	30mg/kg BID, PO	30mg/kg BID, PO	30 mg/kg BID, PO
Tylosin[f,g]	10 mg/kg SID, PO, SC, IM	10 mg/kg SID, PO, SC, IM[g]	10 mg/kg SID, PO, SC, IM	10 mg/kg SID, PO, SC, IM	10 mg/kg SID, PO, SC, IM[g]

[a]Nephrotoxic; best given with fluids.
[b]Prolonged treatment with penicillin or its derivatives may result in changes in microbial flora and diarrhea.
[c]May induce dysbiosis, particularly in guinea pigs.
[d]Data on safety, efficacy, and dosage not currently available.
[e]May cause arthropathies in growing animals.
[f]May cause tissue necrosis when given subcutaneously.
[g]Toxicity has been reported in hamsters and guinea pigs.

TABLE 28.2B. Recommended dosages of antimicrobial drugs in laboratory animals

Drug	Hedgehogs	Chinchillas	Ferrets	Rabbits
Amikacin[a]	—[d]	10 mg/kg SID, SC, IM	10 mg/kg SID, SC, IM	10 mg/kg SID, SC, IM
Ampicillin[b]	10 mg/kg BID, SC, IM	Do not use	5–10 mg/kg BID, PO	Do not use
Chloramphenicol palmitate	50 mg/kg BID, PO	50 mg/kg BID, PO	50 mg/kg BID, PO	50 mg/kg BID, PO
Chloramphenicol succinate	30–50 mg/kg BID, SC, IM	30–50 mg/kg BID, SC, IM	30–50 mg/kg BID, SC, IM	30–50 mg/kg BID, SC, IM
Chlortetracycline[c]	—[d]	50 mg/kg BID, PO	—[d]	50 mg/kg BID, PO
Ciprofloxacin[e]	15–20 mg/kg SID, PO	15–20 mg/kg SID, PO	15–20 mg/kg SID, PO	15–20 mg/kg SID, PO
Doxycycline[c]	—[d]	2.5–5 mg/kg BID, PO	2.5–5 mg/kg BID, PO	2.5–5 mg/kg BID, PO
Enrofloxacin[e]	5–10 mg/kg SID, PO, SC, IM	5–10 mg/kg SID, PO, SC, IM	10 mg/kg SID, PO, SC, IM	10 mg/kg SID, PO, SC, IM
Gentamicin[a]	—[d]	5 mg/kg SID, SC, IM	5 mg/kg SID, SC, IM	4 mg/kg SID, SC, IM
Metronidazole	25 mg/kg BID, PO	20–40 mg/kg BID, PO	20 mg/kg BID, PO	20–40 mg/kg BID, PO
Neomycin	—[d]	15 mg/kg SID, PO	30 mg/kg SID, PO	30 mg/kg SID, PO
Oxytetracycline[c]	50 mg/kg SID,PO	50 mg/kg BID, PO	20 mg/kg TID, PO	50 mg/kg BID, PO
Tetracycline[c]	10–20 mg/kg BID, PO	50 mg/kg BID, PO	25 mg/kg BID, TID, PO	50 mg/kg, BID, PO
Tilmicosin	—[d]	—[d]	—[d]	25 mg/kg SID, SC
Trimethoprim sulfadiazine[f]	30 mg/kg SID, SC, IM	30 mg/kg SID, SC, IM	30 mg/kg SID, SC, IM	30 mg/kg SID, SC, IM
Trimethoprim sulfamethoxazole	30 mg/kg BID, PO	30 mg/kg BID, PO	30 mg/kg BID, PO	30 mg/kg BID, PO
Tylosin[f,g]	10 mg/kg SID, PO, SC, IM	10 mg/kg SID, PO, SC, IM	10 mg/kg SID, PO, SC, IM	10 mg/kg SID, PO, SC, IM

[a]Nephrotoxic; best given with fluids.
[b]Prolonged treatment with penicillin or its derivatives may result in changes in microbial flora and diarrhea.
[c]May induce dysbiosis, particularly in guinea pigs.
[d]Data on safety, efficacy, and dosage not currently available.
[e]May cause arthropathies in growing animals.
[f]May cause tissue necrosis when given subcutaneously.
[g]Toxicity has been reported in hamsters and guinea pigs.

TABLE 28.3. Recommended dosages of antimicrobials administered in drinking water or in food

Drug	Mice	Hamsters	Gerbils	Rats	Guinea Pigs	Chinchillas	Rabbits
Chloramphenicol	0.5 mg/ml[a]	—[b]	0.83 mg/ml	—[b]	1 mg/ml	—[b]	1.3 mg/ml
Dimetridazole	1 mg/ml	0.5 mg/ml	0.5 mg/ml	1 mg/ml	—[b]	0.8 mg/ml	0.2 mg/ml
Enrofloxacin[c]	0.05–0.2 mg/ml	0.05–0.2 mg/ml	0.05–0.2 mg/ml	0.05–0.2 mg/ml	0.05–0.2 mg/ml	0.05–0.2 mg/ml	0.05–0.2 mg/ml
Neomycin	2.6 mg/ml	0.44 mg/ml	2.6 mg/ml	2.6 mg/ml	—[b]	—[b]	0.2–0.8 mg/ml
Oxytetracycline[d]	0.4 mg/ml	0.25–1 mg/ml	0.8 mg/ml	0.4 mg/ml	1 mg/ml[d]	1 mg/ml	1 mg/ml
Sulfamerazine	1 mg/ml or 0.25 mg/g diet	1 mg/ml	1 mg/ml	1 mg/ml or 0.25 mg/g diet	1 mg/ml	1 mg/ml	1 mg/ml
Sulfamethazine	1 mg/ml	1 mg/ml	1 mg/ml	1 mg/ml	1–5 mg/ml	1–5 mg/ml	1–5 mg/ml or 5–10 mg/g diet
Sulfaquinoxaline	1 mg/ml	1 mg/ml	1 mg/ml	1 mg/ml or 0.5 mg/g diet	1 mg/ml	1 mg/ml	1 mg/ml or 0.6 mg/g diet
Tetracycline[d]	2–5 mg/ml	0.4 mg/ml	2–5 mg/ml	2–5 mg/ml or 1–5 mg/g diet	0.7 mg/ml[d]	0.3–2 mg/ml	1 mg/ml
Tylosin[e]	0.5 mg/ml	0.5 mg/ml[e]	0.5 mg/ml	0.5 mg/ml	0.5 mg/ml[e]	—[b]	—[b]

[a]Per ml of drinking water.
[b]Data on safety, efficacy, or dosage are not available.
[c]May cause arthropathies in growing animals.
[d]May induce dysbiosis, particularly in guinea pigs.
[e]Toxicity has been reported in hamsters and guinea pigs.

TABLE 28.4. Antimicrobial treatment in mice

Site	Clinical Signs/Diagnosis	Common Infecting Organisms	Comment	Suggested Drugs
Skin and subcutis	Scabbing over shoulders and back, dermatitis, abscesses	*Staphylococcus aureus, Streptococcus* spp., mite infestation	Secondary to primary wounds caused by fighting or self-trauma due to acariasis	Ampicillin; chloramphenicol; tetracyclines
Respiratory	Rhinitis, dyspnea, otitis media, upper respiratory tract disease, pneumonia	*Mycoplasma pulmonis*	Often concurrent with Sendai virus or CAR bacillus; decrease intracage ammonia levels	Tylosin; fluoroquinolone; tetracyclines
	Dacryoadenitis, sneezing, dyspnea, pneumonia	*Pasteurella pneumotropica*	Often concurrent with Sendai virus or CAR bacillus; decrease intracage ammonia levels	Chloramphenicol; fluoroquinolones; tylosin; aminoglycosides[a]
	Pneumonia	Cilia-associated respiratory (CAR) bacillus	Primary, or opportunist in association with respiratory pathogens	Sulfamerazine; ampicillin; sulfonamides[b]
Gastrointestinal	Stunted growth, diarrhea, rectal prolapse, death; transmissible murine colonic hyperplasia	*Citrobacter freundii*	Genotype, age, and diet influence course and severity of disease	Tetracyclines; neomycin; metronidazole
	Liver disease, death; chronic active hepatitis	*Helicobacter hepaticus*[c]		
	Anorexia, dehydration, diarrhea, death; Tyzzer's disease	*Clostridium piliforme*	Concurrent fluid therapy essential	Tetracyclines

665

TABLE 28.4. Continued

Site	Clinical Signs/Diagnosis	Common Infecting Organisms	Comment	Suggested Drugs
Urogenital	Oophoritis, salpingitis, metritis, infertility, abortions	M. pulmonis, P. pneumotropica, Klebsiella oxytoca		Tylosin; fluoroquinolones; tetracyclines
	Urethral gland obstruction, preputial gland abscesses	P. pneumotropica, S. aureus		Chloramphenicol; fluoroquinolones; aminoglycosides[a]
CNS	Head tilt, torticollis, circling	M. pulmonis, Streptococcus spp.		Chloramphenicol; tylosin; fluoroquinolones
	Eye abscesses, conjunctivitis, panophthalmitis	P. pneumotropica		Tetracyclines; aminoglycosides[a]
General	Septicemia, death; mice that survive acute infection may have chronic arthritis, limb deformity, limb amputation; streptobacillosis	Streptobacillus moniliformis	Zoonotic potential	Ampicillin; tetracycline

[a]Refers to systemic use of amikacin or gentamicin.
[b]Includes trimethoprim-sulfonamide combinations.
[c]Treatment of choice: amoxicillin 1.5–3 mg/30 g per day; metronidazole 0.69 mg/30 g per day; bismuth subsalicylate 0.185 mg/30 g per day combined PO.

TABLE 28.5. Antimicrobial treatment in hamsters

Site	Clinical Signs/Diagnosis	Common Infecting Organisms	Comment	Suggested Drugs
Skin and subcutis	Cheek pouch abscesses, abscesses	*Staphylococcus aureus, Streptococcus* spp.*, Pasteurella pneumotropica, Actinomyces* spp.	Drain and flush; complete excision of abscess beneficial	Chloramphenicol; tetracyclines; fluoroquinolones
	Swollen lymph nodes, lymphadenitis	*Staphylococcus aureus, Streptococcus* spp.		Chloramphenicol; tetracyclines; fluoroquinolones
Respiratory	Sneezing, dyspnea, upper respiratory tract disease, and/or pneumonia	*P. pneumotropica, Streptococcus pneumoniae, Streptococcus* spp.	Secondary to poor nutrition, husbandry	Chloramphenicol; fluoroquinolones; tetracyclines
		Cilia-associated respiratory (CAR) bacillus	Opportunist in association with respiratory pathogens	Sulfamerazine; ampicillin; sulfonamides
Gastrointestinal	Diarrhea, stained perineum, lethargy, anorexia, rectal prolapse; proliferative ileitis	*Lawsonia intracellularis*	Especially in 3-to-10-week-olds; difficult to treat successfully; concurrent fluid therapy essential	Tetracyclines; fluoroquinolones
	Enteritis	*E. coli, Clostridium* spp.	Concurrent fluid therapy essential	Fluoroquinolones; metronidazole; tetracyclines
	Anorexia, dehydration, diarrhea, death; Tyzzer's disease	*Clostridium piliforme*	Concurrent fluid therapy essential	Tetracyclines
	Catarrhal enteritis in weanlings	*Giardia muris*		Metronidazole
CNS	Squinting, rubbing eye, corneal ulceration	*Pasteurella* spp., *Streptococcus* spp.	Topical treatment	Chloramphenicol; tetracyclines

TABLE 28.6. Antimicrobial treatment in gerbils

Site	Clinical Signs/Diagnosis	Common Infecting Organisms	Comment	Suggested Drugs
Skin and subcutis	Red, crusty nares, staining on forepaws; nasal dermatitis	*Staphylococcus aureus, Staphyloccocus* spp.*, Streptococcus* spp.	Secondary to irritation due to Harderian gland secretions	Chloramphenicol; sulfonamides;[a] fluoroquinolones
	Midventral marking gland infection, dermatitis	*S. aureus, Streptococcus* spp.		Chloramphenicol; sulfonamides;[a] fluoroquinolones
Gastrointestinal	Lethargy, anorexia, diarrhea, sudden death; Tyzzer's disease	*Clostridium piliforme*	Highly susceptible	Tetracyclines
	Diarrhea, death; salmonellosis	*Salmonella enteritidis, S. typhimurium,* *E. coli*	Concurrent fluid therapy essential	Chloramphenicol; fluoroquinolones
	Enteritis, diarrhea, dehydration			Chloramphenicol; fluoroquinolones

[a]Includes trimethoprim-sulfonamide combinations.

668

TABLE 28.7. Antimicrobial treatment in rats

Site	Clinical Signs/Diagnosis	Common Infecting Organisms	Comment	Suggested Drugs
Skin and subcutis	Abrasions/ulcerations over shoulders and back; dermatitis	*Staphylococcus aureus*	Secondary to primary wounds caused by self-trauma	Ampicillin; chloramphenicol; tetracyclines
	Abscesses, furunculosis, mastitis	*Pasteurella pneumotropica, Klebsiella pneumoniae*	Secondary opportunist; drain and flush abscesses	Chloramphenicol; fluoroquinolones; aminoglycosides[a]
	Mastitis	*P. pneumotropica*	Hot compresses, drainage	Chloramphenicol; fluoroquinolones; aminoglycosides[a]
Respiratory	Sneezing, dyspnea, vestibular disease, depression, chromodacryorrhea; upper respiratory tract disease and/or pneumonia	*Mycoplasma pulmonis*	Common; improve nutrition, husbandry; decrease intracage ammonia levels	Combination enrofloxacin 10 mg/kg and doxycyline 5 mg/kg beneficial; tylosin
	Serosanguinous to mucopurulent nasal discharge, rhinitis, conjunctivitis, otitis media	*Streptococcus pneumoniae, Corynebacterium kutcheri, P. pneumotropica*	Synergistic interaction between organisms and also Sendai virus, coronavirus	Combination enrofloxacin 10 mg/kg and doxycyline 5 mg/kg beneficial; tylosin
		Cilia-associated respiratory (CAR) bacillus		Sulfamerazine; ampicillin
Gastrointestinal	Diarrhea, dehydration, anorexia, death; Tyzzer's disease	*Clostridium piliforme*		Tetracyclines
Urogenital	Infertility, oophoritis, salpingitis, metritis, pyometra	*M. pulmonis*		Tylosin; fluoroquinolones; tetracyclines
	Preputial gland abscesses	*Staphylococcus aureus, P. pneumotropica*		Chloramphenicol; fluoroquinolones
CNS	Head tilt, circling, torticollis, otitis interna	*M. pulmonis ±* secondary bacterial invaders		Fluoroquinolones; chloramphenicol; Tylosin
General	Bacteremia, septicemia, multiorgan abscessation and infarction	*Streptoccocus pneumoniae*		Ampicillin

[a]Refers to systemic use of amikacin or gentamicin.

669

TABLE 28.8.   Antimicrobial treatment in guinea pigs

Site	Clinical Signs/Diagnosis	Common Infecting Organisms	Comment	Suggested Drugs
Skin and subcutis	Enlarged lymph nodes, cervical lymphadenitis	*Streptococcus zooepidemicus*	May cause septicemia; complete surgical excision of infected lymph nodes beneficial	Chloramphenicol; fluoroquinolones
	Wet chin, "slobbers"	Oral microflora (eg, *Staphylococcus aureus*)	Secondary to malocclusion	Chloramphenicol; sulfonamides[a]
	Mastitis	*Klebsiella, Staphylococcus* spp., *Streptococcus* spp., *Pasteurella* spp., *E. coli, Proteus* spp.	Hot compresses, milk out infected glands	Amikacin; fluoroquinolones; sulfonamides
	Swollen, ulcerated foot; ulcerative pododermatitis; osteomyelitis	*S. aureus, Actinomyces* spp.	Secondary to trauma	Chloramphenicol; fluoroquinolones
Respiratory	Rhinitis, tracheitis, otitis media, upper respiratory tract disease, and/or pneumonia	*Bordetella bronchiseptica*	Commonly carried by dogs and rabbits; some success with *Bordetella* bacterins	Amikacin; fluoroquinolones; chloramphenicol
		Streptococcus pneumoniae, S. zooepidemicus, Klebsiella pneumoniae		Amikacin; fluoroquinolones; chloramphenicol
Gastrointestinal	Anorexia, diarrhea, enteritis, death	*Clostridium* spp., *Salmonella typhimurium, S. enteriditis, E. coli, Yersinia pseudotuberculosis, Pseudomonas aeruginosa, Listeria monocytogenes*	Concurrent fluid therapy essential; amikacin best for *P. aeruginosa*	Chloramphenicol; aminoglycosides[b]

	Anorexia, ascites, diarrhea, death; Tyzzer's disease	*Clostridium piliforme*	Recent weanlings, predisposed by crowding, poor sanitation	Tetracyclines
	Diarrhea, coccidiosis	*Eimeria caviae*	Most common in juveniles	Sulfonamides
	Failure to gain, weight loss, diarrhea, death; cryptosporidiosis	*Cryptosporidium wrairi*	In humans, newer macrolides such as roxithromycin and azithromycin have shown some efficacy	
Urogenital	Endometritis, abortions, stillbirths	*B. bronchiseptica, Streptococcus* spp.		Chloramphenicol; aminoglycosides[b]
	Cystitis	*Streptococcus pyogenes, Staphylococcus* spp., fecal coliforms	Urinary calculi often present	Sulfonamides;[a] fluoroquinolones
Eye	Ocular discharge, conjunctivitis	*Chlamydia psittaci, B. bronchiseptica, S. pneumoniae*	Topical treatment; rule out concurrent hypo-vitaminosis C	Tetracyclines
General	Anorexia, soft stools, dyspnea, splenitis, hepatitis, lymphadenitis, septicemia, death	*Salmonella typhimurium, S. enteriditis*	Concurrent fluid therapy essential	Chloramphenicol; fluoroquinolones

[a]Includes trimethoprim-sulfonamide combinations.
[b]Refers to systemic use of amikacin or gentamicin.

TABLE 28.9. Antimicrobial treatment in hedgehogs (*Atelerix albiventris*)

Site	Clinical Signs/Diagnosis	Common Infecting Organisms	Comment	Suggested Drugs
Skin and subcutis	Dermatitis, abscesses	*Staphylococcus aureus*, *Streptococcus* spp., various external parasites	Secondary to acariasis or bite wounds; concurrent antiparasitic therapy should be considered	Ampicillin; chloramphenicol
	Granulomatous subcutaneous lesions, lymphadenitis	*Mycobacterium* spp.	Zoonotic potential	Treatment unknown
Respiratory	Anorexia, catarrhal rhinitis; upper respiratory tract disease and/or pneumonia	*Bordetella bronchiseptica*, *Pasteurella multocida*, *Corynebacterium* spp.	Cytomegalovirus, verminous pneumonia may also be involved	Fluoroquinolones; sulfonamides;[a] tetracyclines
Gastrointestinal	Gingivitis, periodontitis	Multiple etiologies	Improve diet; extractions may be beneficial	Metronidazole
	Anorexia, diarrhea, weight loss, enteritis; salmonellosis	*Salmonella tilene*	Concurrent fluid therapy essential; zoonotic potential	Chloramphenicol; fluoroquinolones
	Diarrhea; coccidiosis	Organism not specified		Sulfonamides
	Diarrhea; giardiasis	*Giardia* spp.		Metronidazole
Urogenital	Leptospirosis	*Leptospira* spp.	Zoonotic potential	Ampicillin; tetracyclines
General	Septicemia, death; tularemia	*Francisella tularensis*		Aminoglycosides[b]
	Chronic wasting, submandibular lymphadenopathy, acute, fatal septicemia	*Yersinia pseudotuberculosis*	Zoonotic potential	Aminoglycosides;[b] fluoroquinolones; tetracyclines
	Q fever	*Coxiella burnetii*	Zoonotic potential	Tetracyclines; fluoroquinolones

[a]Includes trimethoprim-sulfonamide combinations.
[b]Refers to systemic use of amikacin or gentamicin.

TABLE 28.10. Antimicrobial treatment in chinchillas

Site	Clinical Signs/Diagnosis	Common Infecting Organisms	Comment	Suggested Drugs
Skin and subcutis	Abscesses	Staphylococcus aureus, spp., Streptococcus spp., Pseudomonas spp.	Secondary to primary wounds; complete surgical excision beneficial	Chloramphenicol; tetracyclines; fluoroquinolones
Respiratory	Anorexia, upper respiratory tract disease and/or pneumonia	Pasteurella multocida, Bordetella spp., Streptococcus pneumoniae, Pseudomonas aeruginosa	Amikacin best for P. aeruginosa	Amikacin; fluoroquinolones; tetracyclines
Gastrointestinal	Diarrhea, enteritis, sudden death	Yersinia enterocolitica, Clostridium perfringens, E. coli, Proteus spp., Salmonella typhimurium, S. enteriditis, Pseudomonas aeruginosa, Listeria monocytogenes, Corynebacterium spp.	Concurrent fluid therapy essential; sulfonamides[a] best for L. monocytogenes	Aminoglycosides;[b] fluoroquinolones; sulfonamides
	Diarrhea; giardiasis	Giardia spp.		Metronidazole
Urogenital	Depression, abortions Metritis, fever, purulent vulvar discharge	L. monocytogenes E. coli, Pseudomonas spp., Staphylococcus spp., Streptococcus spp.	Highly susceptible	Sulfonamides; tetracyclines Aminoglycosides;[b] fluoroquinolones
CNS	Depression, ataxia, convulsions, sudden death	L. monocytogenes	Highly susceptible	Sulfonamides;[a] tetracyclines
General	Septicemia, death	Streptococcus spp., Enterococcus spp., Pasteurella multocida, Klebsiella pneumoniae, Actinomyces spp., Fusobacterium necrophorum		Chloramphenicol; fluoroquinolones

[a]Includes trimethoprim-sulfonamide combinations.
[b]Refers to systemic use of amikacin or gentamicin.

673

TABLE 28.11. Antimicrobial treatment in rabbits

Site	Clinical Signs/Diagnosis	Common Infecting Organisms	Comment	Suggested Drugs
Skin and subcutis	Dermatitis, abscesses	*Pasteurella multocida, Staphylococcus aureus*	Can be located anywhere on the body; complete surgical excision of abscess beneficial	Chloramphenicol; tetracyclines; fluoroquinolones
	Wet chin, dewlap; "slobbers"	*Pseudomonas aeruginosa*	May turn fur green	Amikacin
	Ulceration of face, metacarpals, plantar metatarsals; necrobacillosis	*Fusobacterium necrophorum*	Occurs under unsanitary conditions	Metronidazole; chloramphenicol; tetracyclines
	Mastitis	*S. aureus, Pasteurella* spp., *Pseudomonas* spp.	Hot compresses and milk out affected glands often	Amikacin; fluoroquinolones; chloramphenicol; tetracyclines
Respiratory	Nasal discharge, conjunctivitis, upper respiratory tract disease and/or pneumonia	*Pasteurella multocida*	Common	Fluoroquinolones; tetracyclines; tilmicosin?; aminoglycosides[a]
		Bordetella bronchiseptica, S. aureus, Pseudomonas aeruginosa	Usually secondary to *Pasteurella*	Amikacin; fluoroquinolones; tetracyclines
Gastrointestinal[c]	Constipation to mucoid diarrhea, bloat, anorexia, borborygmus; mucoid enteropathy	Probably multiple etiologies	Major cause of morbidity and mortality in 7-to-14-week-olds	Metronidazole; chloramphenicol
	Diarrhea, death; Tyzzer's disease	*Clostridium piliforme*		Tetracyclines
	Diarrhea, death; colibacillosis	*E. coli*	Especially neonates 1–14 days old and weanlings	Sulfonamides; fluoroquinolones, amikacin

Category	Clinical signs	Organism	Comments	Treatment
	Diarrhea, enterotoxemia, death	*C. spiroforme*	Weanlings especially susceptible	Metronidazole; chloramphenicol
	Diarrhea, death	*Salmonella* spp., *Pseudomonas* spp.	Concurrent fluid therapy essential	Chloramphenicol; fluoroquinolones
	Diarrhea, coccidiosis	*Eimeria* spp.	Hepatic or intestinal; improve sanitation	Sulfonamides
		Lawsonia intracellularis		Tetracyclines; tylosin; metronidazole
Urogenital	Reddening, edema of external genitalia, to dry, scaly, slightly raised areas; venereal spirochetosis	*Treponema cuniculi*		Tetracyclines; chloramphenicol
	Abortion	*Listeria monocytogenes, Pasteurella multocida*		Sulfonamides;[b] chloramphenicol tetracyclines
	Cystitis	*E. coli, Pseudomonas* spp.		Sulfonamides;[b] fluoroquinolones
	Orchitis, metritis	*Pasteurella multocida, Staphylococcus aureus*		Chloramphenicol; tetracycline; gentamicin
CNS	Clear to white discharge from one or both eyes; conjunctivitis	*P. multocida, S. aureus*	Treat topically; flush tear ducts	Chloramphenicol; tetracyclines; aminoglycosides
	Head tilt, nystagmus, torticollis	*P. multocida*	Usually due to otitis media	Chloramphenicol; fluoroquinolones
General	Lethargy, anorexia, pyrexia, septicemia	*P. multocida, L. monocytogenes*		Fluoroquinolones; aminoglycosides; tetracyclines; chloramphenicol

[a]Refers to systemic use of amikacin or gentamicin.
[b]Includes trimethoprim-sulfonamide combinations.
[c]Where applicable, supportive therapy should include IV or IO fluids, cisapride or metoclopramide, high-fiber diet, metronidazole 20 mg/kg BID; cholestyramine at 2 g per 20 ml water BID by gavage may bind bacterial toxins.

TABLE 28.12. Antimicrobial treatment in ferrets

Site	Clinical Signs/Diagnosis	Common Infecting Organisms	Comment	Suggested Drugs
Skin and subcutis	Dermatitis, abscesses	Staphylococcus spp., Streptococcus spp., Corynebacterium spp., Pasteurella spp., Actinomyces spp., E. coli	Secondary to bite wounds; debride and flush	Ampicillin; chloramphenicol; fluoroquinolones
	Cervical masses with sinus tracts containing thick yellow-green pus; actinomycoses	Actinomyces spp.	Debride and flush	Ampicillin; tetracyclines
	Skin black, dam ill, dehydrated; acute gangrenous mastitis	Staphylococcus spp., coliforms	Immediate surgical excision of infected gland; contagious between dams	Ampicillin; fluoroquinolones
	Glands firm, scarred, not painful or discolored; chronic mastitis	Staphylococcus intermedius	Contagious between dams; appears insiduously when kits 3 weeks old	Treatment generally ineffective
Respiratory	Dyspnea, cyanosis, upper respiratory tract disease and/or pneumonia	Streptococcus zooepidemicus, S. pneumoniae, E. coli, Klebsiella pneumoniae, Pseudomonas aeruginosa, Bordetella bronchiseptica, Listeria monocytogenes	Secondary to influenza virus, respiratory syncytial virus, canine distemper virus	Ampicillin; tetracyclines; fluoroquinolones
		Pneumocystis carinii		Sulfonamides
		S. pneumoniae, S. zooepidemicus, K. pneumoniae		Amikacin; fluoroquinolones; chloramphenicol

System	Clinical signs	Etiology	Comments	Treatment
Gastrointestinal	Dental tartar, gingivitis, periodontal disease	Multiple etiologies	Improve diet; dentistry	Metronidazole
	Diarrhea, wasting, black tarry stool, anemia, gastritis, gastric, duodenal ulceration; H. mustelae gastritis	Helicobacter mustelae	Rule out foreign body, lymphoma, Aleutian disease, coronavirus	See footnote[a]
	Diarrhea, wasting, tenesmus, prolapsed rectum; proliferative bowel disease	Lawsonia intracellularis		Chloramphenicol; tylosin
	Acute gastric distension, dyspnea, cyanosis, sudden death; gastric bloat	Thought to be due to Clostridium perfringens overgrowth	Treat as for bloat in canine patients	Metronidazole
	Fever, bloody diarrhea, lethargy; salmonellosis	Salmonella neuport, S. typhimurium, S. choleraesuis	Zoonotic potential	Chloramphenicol; fluoroquinolones
	Weight loss, diarrhea, vomiting, granulomatous inflammation; mycobacteriosis	Mycobacterium spp.	Zoonotic potential	See Chapter 19
	Diarrhea, coccidiosis	Eimeria spp.		Sulfonamides
	Diarrhea; giardiasis	Giardia spp.		Metronidazole
Urogenital	Straining, hematuria; cystitis	Staphylococcus spp., Proteus spp.	Urolithiasis often present	Fluoroquinolones; ampicillin; sulfonamides

[a]Treatment of choice amoxicillin 10 mg/kg BID PO, metronidazole 20 mg/kg BID PO, and bismuth subsalicylate 17 mg/kg BID PO combined.

29 | Antimicrobial Drug Use in Reptiles

E. R. JACOBSON

Infectious diseases are an important cause of illness and mortality in captive reptiles (Jacobson, 1980; Austwick and Keymer, 1981; Clark and Lunger, 1981; Cooper, 1981). Although a wide variety of bacteria have been incriminated as either primary or secondary pathogens, infections caused by Gram-negative bacteria are most common. *Aeromonas hydrophila, Klebsiella oxytoca, Morganella morganii, Providencia rettgeri, Pseudomonas aeruginosa,* and *Salmonella arizonae* are prominent among the microorganisms isolated from healthy and ill captive reptiles. These bacteria become invasive when conditions decrease the resistance of the host, select for pathogenic organisms (Cooper, 1981), and/or follow primary viral infection, such as ophidian paramyxovirus pneumonia (Jacobson, 1992). Some species of reptiles seem particularly prone to infection with specific bacteria. The American alligator, *Alligator mississippiensis,* for example, is susceptible to *Aeromonas hydrophila* infections. A new *Neisseria* species, *N. iguanae,* has been isolated from the oral cavity and bite wounds of the green iguana, *Iguana iguana* (Barrett et al., 1994). A chronic upper respiratory disease has been described in the desert tortoise *(Gopherus agassizii)* and other tortoises (Jacobson et al., 1991) and a new mycoplasma, *Mycoplasma agassizii,* has been identified as the causative agent of this disease (Brown et al., 1995). A new mycoplasma also has been identified as the cause of arthritis and pneumonia in Nile crocodiles *(Crocodylus niloticus)* and the American alligator (Mohan et al., 1995; Clippinger et al., 1996). While infections with chlamydia have been reported in reptiles (Jacobson et al., 1989; Jacobson and Telford, 1990; Homer et al., 1994), whether the scarcity of reports is because they have been missed or whether infections with chlamydia are uncommon in reptiles is unknown.

678

Mycotic infections are commonly seen in all major groups of captive reptiles, with the integumentary and respiratory systems most often involved (Austwick and Keymer, 1981; Migaki et al., 1984). While *Microsporum* and *Trichophyton*, which cause dermatomycotic infections in mammals, appear rarely to affect reptiles, other mycotic infections such as fusariosis, geotrichosis, phycomycosis, and chromomycosis are common. Predisposing factors such as suboptimal cage temperature and foul environmental conditions are generally involved.

Antimicrobial therapy is an important component in medical management of reptiles that are affected with bacterial or mycotic disease. Selecting the appropriate antimicrobial agent is more difficult than for mammals because of the diversity of the behavioral, anatomic, and physiological features of the variety of species within the class Reptilia. Since limited pharmacokinetic studies of only some antimicrobial agents have been performed in only a small number of reptilian species, dosage is either extrapolated from one species or is empirical.

Antimicrobial Drug Selection

When selecting an antimicrobial drug to treat an infectious disease in a reptile, identification of the causative microorganism is of primary importance. If a lesion is present, a biopsy specimen should be obtained for cytologic and histologic examination in addition to collecting a swab specimen for culture. This approach is required to interpret the significance of the microorganism cultured (Tables 29.1–29.3). In reptiles suspected of being septic, blood culture should be performed. Techniques for collecting specimens from reptiles have been described elsewhere (Jacobson, 1992).

Following isolation and identification of the causative bacteria, the MICs of potentially effective antimicrobial agents should be determined. Selection of the most appropriate antimicrobial agent will depend upon the results of quantitative susceptibility tests together with the following considerations: site of infection and type of lesion; pharmacodynamic properties and pharmacokinetic characteristics of antimicrobial agents in the species of reptile affected; and the clinical condition, size, temperament, and immune status of the ill reptile. The clinician should select an antimicrobial drug that will attain therapeutic concentrations at the site of infection. The dosage form and route of administration will be largely governed by the species of reptile.

Certain biological features of reptiles influence response to treatment. The development of granulomatous inflammation is common in reptiles affected with bacterial diseases (Montali, 1988). This limits penetration of most antimicrobial agents to the site of infection. In cases where mature granulomas are located subcutaneously, the lesion should be removed surgically to facilitate access of the antimicrobial drug to the affected tissue. Another unique feature of some reptiles is the spectacle (Millichamp et al., 1983), which embryologically represents a fusion of the upper and lower eyelids that become transparent. It is located over the cornea in all snakes with eyes and in some lizards. Infections of the subspectacular space are common in snakes, and topically applied antimicrobial agents do not appear to penetrate this barrier. In treating reptiles with subspectacular infections, a wedge should be excised from the spectacle and then the appropriate antimicrobial drug applied directly onto the globe and within the space.

Pharmacokinetic characteristics of antimicrobial drugs in reptiles have been reported for exceedingly few of the 6,400 species of reptiles. This is not surprising in view of the relatively few researchers interested in pharmacokinetics of antimicrobials in reptiles and the lack of funds for such studies. The small number of pharmacokinetic studies that have been performed indicate that the half-life of antimicrobial drugs eliminated by excretion (unchanged) is considerably longer in reptiles than in mammalian species. In a study of chloramphenicol elimination, which takes place mainly by hepatic metabolism, the apparent half-life of chloramphenicol in bull snakes was 5.2 hours, whereas it is 1–3 hours in mammalian species, with the exception of cats (Bush et al., 1978). Since reptiles constitute a highly diverse collection of species, the validity of interspecies extrapolation of pharmacokinetic data is highly questionable. Enrofloxacin (5 mg/kg, IM) persisted in blood of box turtles for a prolonged period (Aucoin, pers. comm., 1991), whereas IM injection of the drug (10 mg/kg) provided therapeutic blood concentrations for only 24 hours in Hermann's tortoise (Sporle et al., 1991). Intraspecies differences in dosage may also exist, depending on age and size. For example, a hatchling Burmese python, *Python molurus,* weighing 125 g would probably require a higher dose of antibiotic per kg body weight than an adult python weighing over 100 kg. Metabolic scaling, based on daily minimum energy expenditure rather than live body weight (see below), has been suggested as a method for estimating antimicrobial dosage regimens (Sedgewick et al., 1984), but problems are encountered when this approach is used (Jacobson, 1996).

When selecting an antimicrobial drug, one should consider the immune status of the ill reptile. Since many ill reptiles, especially those with chronic infections, appear to be immunocompromised, bactericidal antibiotics are generally preferred (Jacobson, 1987). Furthermore, since the immune system of reptiles is affected by temperature, it is imperative to maintain the ill reptile under optimum environmental conditions. Ambient temperature has been shown to affect the disposition kinetics of amikacin. Gopher snakes *(Pituophis melanoleucus catenifer)* were given amikacin (5 mg/kg, IM) and housed at ambient temperatures of 25° C and 37° C. When they were housed at 37° C, the apparent volume of distribution was larger and body clearance of amikacin was higher, while the apparent half-life of the drug did not change significantly (Mader et al., 1985). The mean residence time of amikacin was significantly shorter in gopher tortoises, *Gopherus polyphemus*, acclimated at 30° C (22.7 ± 0.5 hours) than at 20° C (41.8 ± 3.2 hours), and body clearance of the drug in the tortoises acclimated at 30° C was approximately twice that in the tortoises at 20° C (Caligiuri et al., 1990). In addition, oxygen consumption was approximately twice as great in the tortoises at the higher acclimation temperature. Snakes affected with respiratory disease have recovered without antimicrobial therapy by maintaining them at an elevated environmental temperature (Ross, 1984), in the technique of thermotherapy. In another study in ball pythons *(Python regius)*, snakes were either acclimated at 25° C or 37° C and serum concentrations of amikacin were determined following intracardiac and IM administration (3.5 mg/kg) (Johnson et al., 1997). No significant pharmacokinetic differences were found among the snakes housed at these temperatures. Thus these findings are not consistent with the few other studies showing temperature effects on blood concentrations of antimicrobial drugs in reptiles.

Size and temperament of a reptile influence antimicrobial drug selection and the method of administration. Most species of reptiles weigh less than 100 g, and many lizards are under 30 g as adults. The clinician may be limited to those antibiotics that can easily be diluted to a concentration that can be precisely and safely injected. At the other end of the spectrum are those reptiles that are quite large in size and dangerous to approach. In such cases the clinician may have to choose a drug that can be administered in a relatively small volume via an injection dart. In dangerous reptiles, such as venomous snakes, a drug administered every few days rather than daily would be preferred. Some reptiles are extremely timid and nervous and may not be suitable for injection. In such cases the antibiotic will have to be administered orally, preferentially in food if the animal is still feeding. Thus, the route of administration will also influence the choice of antibiotics to be administered.

The microorganisms that commonly infect various locations and the drugs recommended for treating these infections are listed in Tables 29.1–29.3.

Methods of Administration

In most cases, antimicrobials will be given by injection, either SC or IM. The author generally administers oral antimicrobials only in those cases where there is primary infection of the gastrointestinal tract, in those species that do not tolerate injections and have to be medicated in their feed, and for those disease conditions requiring a drug that is available only in an oral form. In farming operations of reptiles such as with crocodilians and sea turtles, when large numbers of reptiles are ill and have to be treated, it may not be practical to administer drugs by injection. In such cases, oral medication is generally the preferred route of administration.

Several problems exist with oral medication of reptiles. First, very few pharmacokinetic studies have been performed on drugs administered orally to reptiles. Thus, for the vast majority of antimicrobials, the dose selected will not be based on science. The gastrointestinal transit time varies greatly between the various groups and species of reptiles, being the slowest in the large herbivorous reptiles. Even in some carnivorous reptiles the transit time may be quite prolonged. Thus, in these animals it may be difficult to achieve optimum therapeutic concentrations of antimicrobials in blood following administration of oral medicaments.

Although many oral medicaments can be administered in the food of ill reptiles that are feeding, orally medicating reptiles that are not feeding may not be simple. Venomous snakes and large crocodilians are dangerous to handle and manipulate for administration of oral drugs. It may be impossible to extricate the head beyond the shell margins and to force open the mouths of many species of turtles and tortoises. The keratinized epidermal hard parts over the mandibles and dentary bones are easily traumatized, and extreme care must be taken in trying to force open the mouth. It is particularly difficult to administer oral drugs to the giant tortoises. These reptiles will have to be anesthetized and a pharyngostomy tube inserted for oral medication (Norton et al., 1989).

As a generalization, snakes are the easiest group of reptiles to medicate orally. The mouths of most snakes are simple to open, and because the glottis is in an extremely cranial position, it is easily avoided. A lubricated French catheter or nasogastric tube can be passed down the esophagus of the snake with minimal resistance. Catheters that are very rigid should be avoided. It is important to have the snake relatively straight when passing the catheter. Since the cranial esophagus is extremely thin in most species, the end of the catheter should be round and smooth. The stomach of most snakes is from one-third to halfway down the distance from the head to cloaca, but it is not necessary to pass a catheter as far as this organ. In most situations passing the catheter halfway between the stomach and oral cavity is satisfactory.

Most of the antibiotics commonly used in reptile medicine are administered IM or SC. The problem with IV administration of antibiotics is that, except in tortoises, peripheral vessels cannot be visualized (Jacobson et al., 1992). Although blood can be collected from a number of sites in different species of reptiles (Olson et al., 1975; Samour et al., 1984), most of this sampling is "blind" and may not be suitable for repetitive infusions. With SC and IM drug administrations, the author tends to avoid administering drugs that require large volumes per kilogram of body weight, especially if the drug is irritating to surrounding tissues. For instance, the author has had several snakes develop necrotizing skin lesions following injection of more than 1 ml of enrofloxacin at a single site.

Since most species of reptiles have a renal portal system, with blood from the caudal half of the body going to the kidneys before reaching systemic circulation, it has been recommended that SC and IM injections be given in the cranial half of the body. However, there are few studies that have looked at this potential problem scientifically. In a study in red-eared sliders, *Trachemys scripta elegans,* blood from the caudal region of the body did not necessarily flow through the kidney via the renal portal system (Holz et al., 1997a). Blood draining the caudal portion of the body in the red-eared slider perfuses the liver in addition to, or instead of, the kidneys. Thus hepatic metabolism also must be considered. When red-eared sliders received either gentamicin (10 mg/kg) or carbenicillin (200 mg/kg) in a forelimb or hindlimb, no significant differences were found in any of the pharmacokinetic determinants in turtles treated with gentamicin, whereas those that received carbenicillin in a hindlimb had significantly lower blood levels for the first 12 hours postinjection than those that received it in a forelimb (Holz et al., 1997b). However, since blood levels for both injection sites were still well above the MIC for organisms generally treated with carbenicillin, this difference was not considered clinically significant. Still, the renal portal system varies in development between various groups of reptiles and further work is needed before broad generalizations can be made. This is particularly important when injecting drugs that are potentially nephrotoxic and those that are eliminated primarily through the renal system.

Snakes are the easiest reptiles to inject because of the large dorsal muscle masses associated with the ribs and vertebrae. In lizards, the muscle masses associated with the forelimbs are not very substantial, and small volumes of drug will be needed in these animals. Tortoises, especially the large tortoises, have extremely thick epidermal hard parts on the cranial aspect of their forelimbs, so that injections are generally made through the thinner skin on the caudal (posterior) aspect of the forelimbs.

Metabolic Scaling

Metabolic scaling has become popular in attempting to determine the most appropriate dosage of an antibiotic in a species or size range of animal for which no pharmacokinetic studies have been conducted. Since pharmacokinetic studies have been performed in only a handful of the 6,400 species of extant reptiles, most dosages of antibiotics (and other drugs) are given based upon extrapolation from one species to another. In using metabolic scaling, dosages of drugs administered are based upon metabolic size rather than mass. In expressing metabolic rate (P_{met}, or minimum energy costs) as a function of body mass (M_b) in kilograms, for most mammals the following allometric equation best describes this relationship (Kleiber, 1961):

$$P_{met} = 70M_b^{0.75}$$

A similar allometric equation [MEC = $10(kg)^{0.75}$] has been suggested for use in reptiles (Sedgwick et al., 1984; Pokras et al., 1992). In a recent review of the subject, no single equation was considered appropriate for all reptiles because the mass constant varies from 1 to 5 for snakes and from 6 to 10 for lizards; no values for chelonians or crocodilians are available (Jacobson, 1996). In regard to reptiles, the major problem with this approach is a general lack of metabolic data for most reptiles. Additionally, there appears to be significant variability in these data among those groups where scientific studies have been performed. For instance, Bartholomew and Tucker (1964) in analyzing metabolic data on lizards ranging in size from 2 g to 4.4 kg, calculated the allometric equation to be $P_{met} = 6.84M_b^{0.62}$. This is different from findings by Bennet and Dawson (1976) for 24 species of lizards, ranging from 0.01 to 7 kg, for which the equation $P_{met} = 7.81M_b^{0.83}$ was determined. Furthermore, when one looks at studies with snakes, still different equations can be calculated (Galvao et al., 1965). In determining resting metabolic rate of 34 species from genera of boas and pythons, the mass exponents of different species showed considerable variation (Chappell and Ellis, 1987). The problem with metabolic scaling is that reptiles represent a heterogenous group of vertebrates, and thus no single equation relating metabolic rate to body mass can be developed for calculating antibiotic dosages. Differences in body temperature, season, reproductive status, nutritional, and overall physiology are just of few of the variables that may ultimately influence metabolic rates and thus make single equation application invalid. Although on the surface this appears to be better than extrapolation, developing a single equation for all reptiles may not be valid. Metabolic scaling will be most useful when calculating doses in a species for which a specific equation has been determined.

Dosage Regimens

Suggested dosage regimens for antimicrobial drugs in the various species of reptiles are presented in Table 29.4.

Bibliography

Austwick PKC, Keymer IF. 1981. Fungi and actinomycetes. In: Cooper JE, Jackson OF, eds. Diseases of the Reptilia, vol 1. London: Academic Press.

Barrett SJ, et al. 1994. A new species of *Neisseria* from iguanid lizards, *Neisseria iguanae* sp. nov. Lett Appl Microbiol 18:200.

Bartholomew GA, Tucker VA. 1964. Size, body temperature, thermal conductance, oxygen consumption, and heart rate in Australian varanid lizards. Physiol Zool 37:341.

Bennet AF, Dawson WR. 1976. Metabolism. In: Gans C, Dawson WR, eds. Biology of the Reptilia, Physiology A, vol. 5. New York: Academic Press, p127.

Brown MB, et al. 1995. *Mycoplasma agassizii* causes upper respiratory tract disease in the desert tortoise. Infect Immun 62:4580.

Bush M, et al. 1976a. Biological half-life of gentamicin in gopher snakes. Am J Vet Res 39:171.

Bush M, et al. 1976b. Preliminary study of antibiotics in snakes. Am Assoc Zoo Vet Annu Proc, p50.

Bush M, et al. 1977. Preliminary study of gentamicin in turtles. Annu Proc Am Assoc Zoo, p71.

Bush M, et al. 1978. Biological half-life of gentamicin in gopher snakes. Am J Vet Res 39:171.

Caligiuri RL, et al. 1990. The effects of ambient temperature on amikacin pharmacokinetics in gopher tortoises. J Vet Pharmacol Ther 13:287.

Chappell MA, Ellis TM. 1987. Resting metabolic rates in boid snakes: allometric relationships and temperature effects. J Comp Physiol B 157:227.

Clark CH, et al. 1985. Plasma concentrations of chloramphenicol in snakes. Am J Vet Res 46:2654.

Clark HF, Lunger PD. 1981. Viruses. In: Cooper JE, Jackson OF, eds. Diseases of the Reptilia, vol. 1. London: Academic Press.

Clippinger TL, et al. 1996. Mycoplasma epizootic in a herd of bull alligators *(Alligator mississipiensis)*. Annu Proc Am Assoc Zoo Vet, p230.

Cooper JE. 1981. Bacteria. In: Cooper JE, Jackson OF, eds. Diseases of the Reptilia, vol. 1. London: Academic Press.

Galvao PE, et al. 1965. Heat production of tropical snakes in relation to body weight and body surface. Am J Physiol 209:501.

Gamble KC, et al. 1997. Itraconazole plasma and tissue concentrations in the spiny lizard *(Sceloporus sp.)* following once daily dosing. J Zoo Wildl Med 28:89.

Helmick KE, et al. 1997. Preliminary kinetics of single-dose intravenously administered enrofloxacin and oxytetracycline in the American alligator *(Alligator mississipiensis)*. Proc Am Assoc Zoo Vet, p27.

Hilf M, et al. 1991. Pharmacokinetics of piperacillin in blood pythons *(Python curtus)* and in vitro evaluation of efficacy against aerobic Gram-negative bacteria. J Zoo Wildl Med 22:199.

Holz P, et al. 1997a. The anatomy and perfusion of the renal portal system in the red-eared slider *(Trachemys scripta elegans)*. J Zoo Wildl Med 28:378.

Holz P, et al. 1997b. The effect of the renal portal system on pharmacokinetic parameters in the red-eared slider *(Trachemys scripta elegans)*. J Zoo Wildl Med 28:386.

Homer BL, et al. 1994. Chlamydiosis in green sea turtles. Vet Pathol 31:1.

Hungerford C, et al. 1997. Pharmacokinetics of enrofloxacin after oral and intramuscular administration in savanna monitors *(Varanus exanthematicus)*. Annu Proc Am Assoc Zoo Vet, p89.

Jacobson ER. 1980. Infectious diseases of reptiles. In: Kirk RW, ed. Current Therapy, vol 7. Philadelphia: WB Saunders.

Jacobson ER. 1987. Reptiles. In: Harkness J, ed. Veterinary Clinics of North America. Philadelphia: WB Saunders.

Jacobson ER. 1992. Laboratory investigations. In: Lawton MPC, Cooper JE, eds. Manual of Reptiles. Br Small Anim Vet Assoc 50.

Jacobson ER. 1996. Metabolic scaling of antibiotics in reptiles: basis and limitations. Zoo Biol 15:329.

Jacobson ER, Telford SR. 1990. Chlamydia and poxvirus infection of monocytes in a flap-necked chameleon. J Wildl Dis 26:572.

Jacobson ER, et al. 1988. Serum concentration and disposition kinetics of gentamicin and amikacin in juvenile American alligators. J Zoo Anim Med 19:188.

Jacobson ER, et al. 1989. Chlamydial infection in puff adders, *Bitis arietans*. J Zoo Wildl Med 20:364.

Jacobson ER, et al. 1991. Chronic upper respiratory tract disease of free-ranging desert tortoises *(Xerobates agassizii)*. J Wildl Dis 27:296.

Jacobson ER, et al. 1992. Techniques for sampling and handling blood for hematologic and plasma biochemical determinations in the desert tortoise *(Xerobates agassizii)*. Copeia, p237.

Jenkins JR. 1991. Medical management of reptiles. Compend Contin Educ Pract Vet 13:980.

Johnson JH, et al. 1997. Amikacin pharmacokinetics and the effects of ambient temperature on the dosage regimen in ball pythons (*Python regius*). J Zoo Wildl Med 28:80.

Kleiber, M. 1961. The Fire of Life: An Introduction to Animal Energetics. New York: John Wiley.

Klingerberg RJ. 1996. Therapeutics. In: Mader ER, ed. Reptile Medicine and Surgery. Philadelphia: WB Saunders, p299.

Klingenberg RJ, Backner B. 1991. The use of ciprofloxacin, new antibiotic, in snakes. Proc 15th Int Symp Captive Propag Husb Reptiles Amphibians, p127.

Kolmstetter CM, et al. 1997. Metronidazole pharmacokinetics in yellow ratsnakes (*Elaphe obsoleta quadrivitatta*). Annu Proc Am Assoc Zoo Vet, p26.

Lawrence K. 1984. Preliminary study on the use of ceftazidime, a broad spectrum cephalosporin antibiotic, in snakes. Res Vet Sci 36:16.

Lawrence K, et al. 1984. A preliminary study on the use of carbenicillin in snakes. J Vet Pharmacol Ther 7:119.

Lawrence K, et al. 1986. Use of carbenicillin in 2 species of tortoise (*Testudo graeca* and *T. hermanni*). Res Vet Sci 40:413.

Mader DR, et al. 1985. Effects of ambient temperature on the half-life and dosage regimen of amikacin in the gopher snake. J Am Vet Med Assoc 187:1134.

Maxwell LK, Jacobson ER. 1997. Preliminary single-dose pharmacokinetics of enrofloxacin after oral and intramuscular administration in green iguanas (*Iguana iguana*). Annu Proc Am Assoc Zoo Vet, p25.

Migaki G, et al. 1984. Fungal diseases of reptiles. In: Hoff GL, et al., eds. Diseases of Amphibians and Reptiles. New York: Plenum.

Millichamp N, et al. 1983. Diseases of the eye and ocular adnexae in reptiles. J Am Vet Med Assoc 183:1205.

Mohan K, et al. 1995. Mycoplasma-associated polyarthritis in farmed crocodiles (*Crocodylus niloticus*) in Zimbabwe. Onderstepoort J Vet Res 62:45.

Montali R. 1988. Comparative pathology of inflammation in the higher vertebrates (reptiles, birds, and mammals). J Comp Pathol 99:1.

Norton TM, et al. 1989. Medical management of a Galapagos tortoise (*Geochelone elephantopus*) with hypothyroidism. J Zoo Wildl Med 20:212.

Olson GA, et al. 1975. Techniques for blood collection and intravascular infusions of reptiles. Lab Anim Sci 25:783.

Page CD, et al. 1991. Multiple dose pharmacokinetics of ketoconazole administered to gopher tortoises (*Gopherus polyphemus*). J Zoo Wildl Med 22:191.

Plowman CA, et al. 1987. Septicemia and chronic abscesses in iguanas (*Cyclura cornuta and Iguana iguana*) associated with a *Neisseria* species. J Zoo Anim Med 18:86.

Pokras MA, et al. 1992. Therapeutics. In: Beynon PH, et al., eds. Manual of Reptiles. Kerkshire, UK: Br Small Anim Vet Assoc, p194.

Prezant RM, et al. 1994. Plasma concentrations and disposition kinetics of enrofloxacin in gopher tortoises (*Gopherus polyphemus*). J Zoo Wild Med 25:82.

Raphael B, et al. 1985. Plasma concentrations of gentamicin in turtles. J Zoo Anim Med 16:138.

Raphael BL, et al. 1994. Pharmacokinetics of enrofloxacin after a single intramuscular injection in Indian star tortoises. J Zoo Wildl Med 25:88.

Ross RA. 1984. The Bacterial Diseases of Reptiles. Stanford, CA: Institute for Herpetological Research.

Samour HJ, et al. 1984. Blood sampling techniques in reptiles. Vet Rec 114:472.

Sedgewick CJ, et al. 1984. Scaling antimicrobial drug dosage regimens to minimum energy cost rather than body weight. Annu Proc Am Assoc Zoo Vet, p15.

Sporle H, et al. 1991. Blood levels of some anti-infectives in the Hermann's tortoise (*Testudo hermanni*). In: 4th Int Colloq Pathol Med Reptiles Amphibians, p120.

Young LA, et al. 1997. Disposition of enrofloxacin and its metabolite ciprofloxacin after IM injection in juvenile Burmese pythons (*Python molurus bivittatus*). J Zoo Wildl Med 28:71.

TABLE 29.1. Antimicrobial drug selection in chelonian infections

Site or Type	Diagnosis	Common Infecting Organisms	Suggested Drugs
Skin and subcutis	Epidermitis/dermatitis	*Citrobacter freundii, Serratia, Proteus morganii, Providencia rettgeri, Pseudomonas aeruginosa, Mycobacterium chelonae*	Amikacin, enrofloxacin
		Mucor	No known treatment
			Immersions in malachite green solution
	Subcutaneous abscesses	*Pasteurella testudinis, Escherichia coli, Providencia*	Amikacin
		Bacteroides, Fusobacterium	Metronidazole
Oral cavity	Stomatitis	*Aeromonas hydrophila, Pseudomonas aeruginosa, Vibrio* spp.	Amikacin, ceftazidime, enrofloxacin
Respiratory tract	Pneumonia	*P. aeruginosa, Morganella morganii, Serratia marcescens, Acinetobacter calcoaceticus*	Amikacin, ceftazidime, enrofloxacin
		Bacteroides, Fusobacterium	Metronidazole
		Aspergillus, Geotrichum candidum, Beauvaria, Penicillium lilacinum, Paecilomyces fumosoroseus	Ketoconazole
	Rhinitis	*Pasteurella testudinis, Mycoplasma*	Enrofloxacin, tylosin
Gastrointestinal tract	Enteritis	*Pseudomonas aeruginosa, Salmonella* spp., *Aeromonas hydrophila, Flavobacterium meningosepticum*	Trimethoprim/sulfadiazine, ciprofloxacin
	Liver Abscesses	*Bacteroides, Clostridium, Fusobacterium*	Metronidazole
	Septicemia	*Salmonella* spp., *A. hydrophila, P. aeruginosa, Flavobacterium meningosepticum*	Amikacin/ceftazidime, enrofloxacin
Skeletal	Osteomyelitis	*Pseudomonas, Klebsiella*	Amikacin/ceftazidime
Eye and adnexa	Conjunctivitis	*Mycoplasma*	Enrofloxacin
Ear	Otitis interna	*Pseudomonas, Escherichia coli, Proteus, Pasteurella testudinis*	Amikacin, enrofloxacin
		Bacteroides, Fusobacterium	Metronidazole

TABLE 29.2. Antimicrobial drug selection in crocodilian infections

Site or Type	Diagnosis	Common Infecting Organisms	Suggested Drugs
Oral cavity	Stomatitis	*Aeromonas hydrophila*	Tetracycline, amikacin
Skin	Epidermitis/dermatitis	Unidentified filamentous organism resembling *Dermatophilus*	No known effective antimicrobial
Respiratory tract	Pneumonia	*Morganella morganii, Klebsiella oxytoca, Pseudomonas aeruginosa, Serratia marcescens*	Amikacin/ceftazidime
		A. hydrophila, Citrobacter freundii, M. morganii, Providencia rettgeri, E. coli, Salmonella arizona	Amikacin/ceftazidime, enrofloxacin
		Beauvaria	Ketoconazole
Yolk infection	Omphalitis	*A. hydrophila*	Tetracycline, amikacin
Liver	Hepatitis	*S. arizona, E. coli, A. hydrophila*	Amikacin/ceftazidime, enrofloxacin
Eye	Uveitis	*A. hydrophila*	Amikacin/ceftazidime, tetracycline
Cardiovascular	Septicemia	*S. arizona, A. hydrophila*	Amikacin/ceftazidime, enrofloxacin

TABLE 29.3. Antimicrobial drug selection for infections in lizards and snakes

Site or Type	Diagnosis	Common Infecting Organisms	Suggested Drugs
Oral cavity	Stomatitis	*Pseudomonas aeruginosa, Aeromonas hydrophila*	Amikacin/ceftazidime, enrofloxacin
Skin and subcutis	Abscesses	*Proteus, E. coli, Providencia, Pseudomonas, Salmonella, Serratia, Clostridium*	Amikacin/ceftazidime, enrofloxacin
		Fusobacterium, Bacteroides	Metronidazole
	Bacterial dermatitis	*Citrobacter, Klebsiella, Pseudomonas, Neisseria*	Amikacin/ceftazidime, enrofloxacin
	Mycotic dermatitis	*Geotrichum, Fusarium, Chrysosporium*	Ketoconazole, itraconazole
Respiratory tract	Pneumonia	*Pseudomonas aeruginosa, P. maltophilia, Salmonella arizona, Providencia rettgeri, A. hydrophila, Morganella morganii*	Amikacin/ceftazidime, piperacillin, enrofloxacin
Gastrointestinal tract	Enteritis	*S. arizona, P. aeruginosa, A. hydrophila, E. coli*	Trimethoprim/sulfadiazine, ciprofloxacin
	Hepatitis	*P. aeruginosa, P. maltophilia, M. morganii, S. arizona, P. rettgeri*	Amikacin/ceftazidime, enrofloxacin
		Clostridium	Metronidazole
Skeletal	Osteomyelitis	*Proteus, E. coli, Pseudomonas*	Amikacin/ceftazidime, enrofloxacin
Eye	Subspectacle infections	*Pseudomonas* spp., *Providencia rettgeri, Proteus* spp.	Topical gentamicin
	Uveitis	*Pseudomonas* spp., *Klebsiella pneumoniae*	Amikacin
	Conjunctivitis	*Pseudomonas* spp.	Amikacin, enrofloxacin
Cardiovascular	Septicemia	*A. hydrophila, P. aeruginosa, S. arizona*	Amikacin/ceftazidime, enrofloxacin

TABLE 29.4. Conventional dosage regimens for antimicrobial drugs in reptiles

Drugs	Species	Route of Administration	Dose	Dose Interval	References
Amikacin	Alligator	IM	2.25 mg/kg	96 h	Jacobson et al. (1988)
	Tortoise	IM	5 mg/kg	48 h	Caligiuri et al. (1990)
	Snakes	IM	5 mg/kg; 2.5 mg/kg	1st dose; thereafter 72 h	Mader et al. (1985); Johnson et al. (1997)
Ampicillin	Tortoise	IM	50 mg/kg	12 h	Sporle et al. (1991)
Carbenicillin	Snakes	IM	400 mg/kg	24 h	Lawrence et al. (1984)
	Tortoise	IM	400 mg/kg	48 h	Lawrence et al. (1986)
Cefoperazone	Tegu	IM	125 mg/kg	24 h	Klingenberg (1996)
	False water cobra	IM	100 mg/kg	96 h	
Ceftazidime	Snakes	IM, IV	20 mg/kg	72 h	Lawrence (1984)
	Loggerhead sea turtle				
Chloramphenicol	Snakes	SQ	50 mg/kg	12–72 h, depending on species	Bush et al. (1976a)
Ciprofloxacin	Snake	Oral	2.5 mg/kg	48–72 h	Klingenberg and Backner (1991)
Doxycycline	Tortoise	IM	50 mg/kg; 25 mg/kg	1st dose; 72 h	Sporle et al. (1991)
Enrofloxacin	Box turtle	IM	5 mg/kg	96–120 h	Aucoin, pers. comm, 1991
	Hermann's tortoise	IM	10 mg/kg	24 h	Sporle et al. (1991)
	Gopher tortoise	IM	5 mg/kg	24–48 h	Prezant et al. (1994)
	Star tortoise	IM	5 mg/kg	12–24 h	Raphael et al. (1994)
	American alligator	IV	5 mg/kg	36 h	Helmick et al. (1997)
	Green iguana	IM	5 mg/kg	24 h	Maxwell and Jacobson (1997)
	Savanna monitor	IM	10 mg/kg	5 days	Hungerford et al. (1997)
	Burmese python	IM	10 mg/kg	48 h	Young et al. (1997)

Gentamicin	Alligator	IM	1.75 mg/kg	72–96 h	Jacobson et al. (1988)
	Aquatic turtles	IM	6–10 mg/kg	48–120 h	Bush et al. (1977)
					Raphael et al. (1985)
Itraconazole	Snakes	IM	2.5 mg/kg	72 h	Bush et al. (1978)
Ketoconazole	Spiny lizard	PO	23.5 mg/kg	Daily	Gamble et al. (1997)
Metronidazole	Tortoise	Oral	15–30 mg/kg	24 h	Page et al. (1991)
	Yellow rat snake	PO	20 mg/kg	48 h	Kolmstetter et al. (1997)
Nystatin	All species	Oral	100,000 IU/kg	24 h	Jacobson (1980)
Oxytetracycline	American alligator	IV	10 mg/kg	96 h	Helmick et al. (1997)
Piperacillin	Snakes	IM	100 mg/kg	24 h	Hilf et al. (1991)
Trimethoprim/ sulfadiazine	All species	IM	30 mg/kg	1st 2 doses 24 h apart, then every 48 h	Jacobson (1987)
Tylosin	All species	IM	5 mg/kg	24 h	Jenkins (1991)

30 | Antimicrobial Drug Use in Aquaculture

D. J. ALDERMAN

Aquaculture is the most rapidly growing and, in many parts of the world, the only growing area of animal husbandry. In 1994 one fish in five consumed by the human population came from aquaculture; in 1996 it was one in four (Subashinghe et al., 1999). Although this current overview inevitably concentrates on the more mature intensive aquaculture industries of the developed world, the greatest aquaculture production is in Asia and involves extensive culture systems. Intensive aquaculture is largely based on carnivorous fish species fed with artificial diets and with control over the complete host life cycle. In contrast, extensive aquaculture depends largely on natural feed and on wild-caught feed. This means that the range of disease problems encountered by the different types of aquaculture systems differs fundamentally. Together with a lack of formal controls, or inadequate enforcement of controls, on the use of medicines in many countries with extensive aquaculture, this means that the use of and needs for veterinary medicinal products in the two types of aquaculture differ markedly.

Both intensive and extensive aquaculture systems continue to expand with the introduction of new culture species and of new culture methods. In view of these continuing developments, it is tautological to state that this chapter is written at a time of considerable and continuing change in all aspects of the use of veterinary medicines in aquaculture. Among these changes are the development of some new aquacultural therapeutics with a steadily evolving regulatory environment, inevitably imposing restrictions and greater costs on the industry, and, more promisingly, the development and introduction of effective vaccines, particularly in the intensive salmonid husbandry sector. Drugs new to aquaculture

692

have become available mainly as a result of the development of data to allow the expansion of claims for existing products from other areas of veterinary medicines. This is likely to continue to be the case for the foreseeable future in Europe and North America.

In 1991, the Office International des Epizooties organized an international conference entitled "Chemotherapy in Aquaculture: From Theory to Reality." In their introductory overview, Michel and Alderman (1992) considered that, in attempting to control infectious disease where controls on transfer of infectious disease pathogens failed, vaccination was the next most valuable approach to control. In the early 1990s, however, vaccines were available only for a limited range of bacterial pathogens, namely *Aeromonas salmonicida, Yersinia ruckeri,* and *Vibrio anguillarum,* and the use of antimicrobials in particular was seen to be essential for control of infectious disease. Toward the end of the 1990s, more-effective vaccines were available against a wider range of bacterial pathogens. Vaccines for prevention of virus diseases are beginning to appear commercially (eg, infectious pancreatic necrosis, or IPN), and others are in an advanced state of development. Nonetheless, several important bacterial pathogens of salmonids remain without effective vaccines *(Flavobacterium psychrophilum, Piscirickettsia salmonis, Renibacterium salmoninarum).* Although considerable research effort has been devoted to development of vaccines to control both topical and systemic protozoan parasites, these are some years from becoming available for practical disease control, and vaccines for fungal and crustacean fish pathogens are even further away. Those protozoan and metazoan pathogens that cannot be cultured in the laboratory environment present considerable problems to the vaccine producer. To control such pathogens, the aquaculture industry may be the first animal husbandry area for which biotechnology product vaccines are developed.

Before the era of effective vaccines, as intensive salmonid aquaculture developed, many bacterial diseases were or became widespread (eg, furunculosis, enteric redmouth disease), and many of the possible husbandry improvements (eg, reduced stocking densities) were regarded as conflicting with the demands of increased production. Given these limitations, the introduction of chemotherapeutic drugs into aquaculture started early (Alderman, 1988), and chemotherapy rapidly became considered as the most effective and flexible weapon against infectious disease. However, it was also realized early that chemotherapy was a palliative rather than a final solution to problems of disease and that its use in the aquatic environment was associated with considerable practical problems. Some, such as development of resistance to antimicrobials by fish pathogens in the aquatic environment, became a real and practical problem within a few years. Others, such as the potential hazards that intensive use of drugs could represent for the environment itself and for human health have become the subject of attention only relatively recently (Alderman and Hastings, 1998).

Disease Groups

Fish diseases are caused by a wide range of infectious organisms, including viruses, bacteria, fungi, and protozoan and metazoan parasites. Viral diseases are widespread and have a major adverse effect on the production of shrimp and oysters, as well as of carp and salmonids. Because viral diseases are not readily susceptible to control by chemotherapy, despite their considerable significance as pathogens, viruses will not be considered further here.

Bacterial diseases are of equal or greater practical importance in aquaculture, many acting as secondary opportunistic invaders that can take opportunity of any cause of weakness in fish to overcome the natural host defenses. Opportunistic bacteria are widespread in the aquatic environment and are a threat every time handling or other husbandry operations are undertaken. However, their harmful effects rarely persist and generally cease with the removal of the original predisposition. Many other bacteria are true pathogens, and all fish culture systems suffer outbreaks of primary bacterial infections, as do invertebrate hatchery systems that are particularly susceptible. The main groups of bacteria involved in fish mortalities are listed in Table 30.1, illustrated by species of major economic significance for the aquaculture industry. In fish, Gram-negative bacteria usually produce septicemic infections characterized by hemorrhagic and/or necrotic lesions, outbreaks of which, if intervention is commenced early, are usually responsive to antimicrobial agents. Chronic infections, which progress more slowly and may result in granulomatous internal lesions, are more commonly associated with Gram-positive bacteria (eg, *Mycobacterium*). Such chronic conditions are more difficult to treat successfully. In vertically ova-transmitted infections (eg, renibacteriosis, piscirickettsiosis) and where infection may be intracellular, it is difficult to ensure that effective drug concentrations are achieved within the affected cells or tissues, and only partially effective treatments at best exist.

In general, the majority of important bacterial pathogens of fish are Gram-negative. Of the Gram-positives, *Renibacterium salmoninarum* (salmonid bacterial kidney disease, BKD) and *Streptococcus* spp. are associated with significant disease problems in farmed fish. The latter is a problem particularly in Japan in rainbow trout and in yellowtail, and as for BKD, best success in therapy has been associated with the application of erythromycin. Other Gram-positives such as *Mycobacterium* spp. and (rarely) *Nocardia* spp. are associated with chronic infections. *Mycobacterium marinum* is associated with granulomatous lesions ("fish tuberculosis") and zoonotic infections ("aquarist's finger"). Attempts at therapy of such infections in fish are rarely reported.

Mycoses are significant in all aquaculture species. Oomycetes produce superficial infections in freshwater fish, particularly under stressful conditions or where superficial wounds and abrasions occur. Such infections are susceptible to chemotherapy, although for food fish species the traditional use of malachite green is no longer acceptable, because of persistent tissue residues of a suspect carcinogen.

Protozoans are responsible for often opportunistic infections ranging from topical to systemic. Like some fungal infections, topical infections are controllable by chemotherapy, although the range of available effective treatments is limited now that malachite green can no longer be countenanced for use with food species. Systemic protozoan infections, largely associated with Myxosporida and Microsporida such as *Kudoa* and PKX (causative organism for proliferative kidney disease, PKD) in fish and *Bonamia* in oysters, are responsible for the most serious losses. Such pathogens are more refractory to treatment, and their practical significance is thus enhanced by the lack of effective chemotherapy. Their life cycles are often poorly understood, so that parasites such as *Myxosoma cerebralis* (the agent of salmonid whirling disease) have only relatively recently been recognized as being one stage in a life cycle of a parasite that includes tubificid worms as alternate hosts.

Many metazoan parasites of fish have been described, some having a multiple host life cycle that cannot easily be completed in intensive farm conditions. Some cause problems in extensive and cage culture; external parasites can proliferate in all environments where convenient fish species favor their development, and they present a constant threat in all kinds of facilities. Parasitic crustaceans find suitable conditions for their development in marine cage farm conditions when naturally infected waters exist nearby. Under such conditions, sea lice cause extensive damage and mortality in farmed salmonids. The use of effective treatments of fish ectoparasites is limited by many environmental and drug residue factors.

Regulatory Constraints on Use of Antimicrobials in Aquaculture

No matter how effective an antimicrobial agent or parasiticide has been shown to be, such products are of no value if their use is either prohibited or not permitted by national or regional regulation. Prohibition and lack of permission are not identical. In Europe and North America, regulatory controls requiring that veterinary medicines are safe and effective before being approved for use have been developing over the last 30 years. Previously, requirements allowed regulators a considerable degree of discretion as to the details required from applicants for approval. In almost every case these regulations were formulated initially with human medicines and subsequently with "conventional" veterinary medicines (ie, medicines for farm mammals) in mind. The more-specific regulatory needs for assessment of aquaculture products have had to be fitted into the existing framework, presenting considerable problems for both regulators and manufacturers.

Regulatory frameworks vary from detailed to lax, but strict regulations may not be rigorously enforced. Thus the regulations of countries such as Norway and Japan need to be considered in terms of the range of approved products in their markets. Japan has some 29 antimicrobials authorized for use in various fish species (Okamoto, 1992). In Norway the Norwegian Medical Control Authority has maintained a centralized record of the amount of drugs prescribed for many years, whereas members of the European Union are only now introducing such requirements. Norway has 6 products currently approved for use in salmon farming, while European Union member states average 4 approved antimicrobials. Even fewer products are authorized specifically for food fish use in the United States and Canada (only ormetoprim-sulfadimethoxine and oxytetracycline in the United States). These differences reflect a stricter approach to preapproval scrutiny requirements, the earlier introduction of such requirements, the size and national importance of the industry, and hence the likely return to pharmaceutical companies from gaining regulatory approval.

In Europe, the critical initial regulatory requirement is for a maximum residue limit (MRL) to be established, the U.S. equivalent of tolerance. In both cases these are the levels of residue of a veterinary medicine that may be present in animal tissues without presenting any hazard to consumers. The European approval system places greater emphasis on residue levels than does the United States. In contrast, safety to the host for European approvals in general requires demonstration that (at least) a double dose, double exposure time presents no hazard (confusingly called [host] tolerance), whereas the effects of higher doses (3×, 5×, and 10×) are required by the United States. Safety critical studies must be carried out to good laboratory practice standards, with concomitant costs.

Application of strict regulatory requirements has inevitably resulted in few antimicrobials being approved for use in aquaculture. Both North American and European regulations now permit the use of therapeutics approved for use in other species, both animal and human in the United States termed off-label or extralabel use under the Animal Medicinal Drug Clarification Act of 1994 (see Chapter 34). In Europe the "veterinary cascade" system was established by Directive 90/676/EEC to establish the prescribing cascade (Alderman 1999). This limits veterinarians treating food-producing animals to prescribing veterinary medicines containing only substances authorized for use in food-producing species (or authorized for use in humans, since it is the safety of consumers that is relevant).

Thus, where there is no suitable product to treat fish, a suitable product approved in other food-animal species may be prescribed in Europe and in the United States. In Europe, the use of this prescription route requires the imposition of a standard withdrawal period of 500 degree-days by the prescribing veterinarian. North American and European regulations are specifically aimed at food species, with the object of protecting the consumer.

Lack of antimicrobial drugs approved for aquaculture inevitably means an increasing reliance on off-label use. Measures designed to improve consumer safety by ensuring that only approved veterinary medicines are used have produced so few approved drugs that off-label use has become common. Recognition of this problem has markedly shifted the approach of regulatory authorities in the United States and in Europe. The Center for Veterinary Medicine of the U.S. Food and Drug Administration (FDA), in response to the provisions of the Animal Drug Availability Act of 1996, has published a report (U.S. FDA, 1998) containing proposals to increase the legal availability of animal drugs for minor uses and minor species (MUMS). The U.S. Code of Federal Regulations in effect defines fish as a minor species (21 CFR 514.1[d]). The FDA's conclusion from this report is that no effective change can be made without amendment of federal statutes to allow better access for minor uses, because the present "scientifically best" standards have resulted in virtually no drugs for such use being available. In much the same vein, the European Medicines Evaluation Agency (EMEA) published two notes for guidance (Committee for Veterinary Medicinal Products, 1997, 1998). In Europe the Salmonidae are regarded as major food species, and the EMEA proposes that MRLs established for Salmonidae may be extended to other fish species. Indeed it also proposed an extrapolation, whereby an MRL established for a substance in muscle in a major mammalian species might be applied to Salmonidae and thus to other fin fish. It will, however, be some time before these proposals and other moves on international harmonization for aquaculture drugs and biologics make available additional veterinary medicines for aquaculture (Schnick et al., 1997).

Pharmacokinetic Considerations

The performance of pharmacokinetic studies in fish presents unique problems but has some major advantages over studies carried out in mammals. The principal advantage is that fish as individual animals are inexpensive, and therefore it is economical both to include many individuals in a study and to study behavior of veterinary residues in edible tissues rather than in serum. Special difficulties, apart from the cost of special experimental facilities needed, relate to the problems of applying drugs to fish under experimental conditions. If experimental medication is not supplied orally in feed, then oral bolus and IV routes may be used, but only after anesthetizing the fish. Normally if fish are to be anesthetized, they should be starved for 24 hours before and after anesthesia, resulting in abnormal gut conditions for the medication. In any case, anesthesia may alter the behavior of the fish and have a difficult-to-quantify effect on uptake, distribution, and/or metabolism. A number of studies report collection of serum from cannulated fish. This has the advantage of allowing the kinetics of a drug to be studied in a single animal, but the effects of cannulation on a fish, which is a relatively small animal, must be regarded as having an unquantifiable effect on behavior and metabolism. The low cost of an individual fish means that reasonable numbers of fish may be used in any pharmacokinetic study. European guidelines require 10 fish for analysis at each time because of known fish-to-fish variations. Thus not only may fish-to-fish variation be accounted for by increased numbers, but drug residue levels in specific tissues may also be studied, together with classical serum concentration–based pharmacokinetic modeling. Since the reason for carrying out pharmacokinetic studies on fish is usually to establish withholding periods, the ability to do so on specific edible tissues is a major advantage. The metabolic rates of fish are determined by environmental temperatures, specifically water temperatures. This means that tissue levels achieved in medication, persistence of veterinary drug residues, and thus time needed to deplete below MRL in edible tissues is heavily influenced by water temperatures (see Table 4.7). In climates in which water temperatures do not change rapidly, this may not represent a significant problem, but in temperate climates where seasonal changes result in (sometimes rapid) changes in water temperatures, the effects on residue depletion may be significant. In Europe, a degree-day definition of withholding period is used to reduce the chance of inadvertent breach of residue requirements. Data must be supplied on uptake and depletion at two temperatures relevant to the intended use of the drug to support the proposed withholding period, and if such data indicate that temperature does not play any significant effect on the pharmacokinetic performance, then a fixed withholding period may be allowed. A degree-day–based withholding period is generally appropriate for most drugs commonly approved for aquaculture use, provided that the fish are exposed only to temperatures within their normal physiological range. For drugs used off-label where no data is available to determine withholding periods, a standard minimum withholding time of 500 degree-days is advised.

Selection of Antimicrobial Drugs

Ideally, the use of an antimicrobial agent should result from reliable diagnosis of the disease and pathogen involved, followed by determination of the most effective drug. The latter would involve a laboratory determination of the antibiotic sensitivity of the specific pathogen, taking into account factors such as the pharmacokinetic and pharmacodynamic properties of the drug. This is another "best scientific practice," which in the real world of fish production is never practical during an active fish mortality, where speed, efficacy, and cost of treatment are paramount. At best, some of these factors can be considered after treatment has commenced to confirm that the decision already made, based on experience of the farm and stocks concerned, was correct.

To demonstrate the impracticality of the "best scientific practice" approach, consider the question of determining antibiotic sensitivity once the putative pathogen has been isolated in pure culture, at best 48 hours after sampling. No agreed methodology for testing antibiotic sensitivity of fish pathogenic bacteria exists, let alone an agreed method for interpreting these results. Given these limitations, one laboratory's resistant isolate may be another's susceptible isolate, so that the value of such interpretations in arriving at clinical decisions on selection of therapeutic regimes must currently be regarded skeptically, and such "best scientific practice" must be seen as impractical. In November 1998 a European Commission workshop addressed this problem, and draft methodologies were agreed on for recommendation to the aquaculture community. These were recommendations for methods, and the further step of agreeing on methods of interpretation of the results derived from these methods has still to be taken. Even when agreed-upon methods and interpretations are in place, the time between the commencement of disease outbreaks, determination of the susceptibility of the pathogen, and the delivery of medicated feed militate against observance of the scientifically ideal approach.

Routes of Application: Problems and Constraints

No matter whether antimicrobials are authorized for use in food species, are used off-label, or are used with ornamental and pet fish, their use in aquaculture is limited by major practical constraints. Almost all treatments can be administered by parenteral injection, as is usual in other areas of veterinary practice. However, with fish this is costly in time and labor, requiring that fish be caught and anesthetized, with associated stress. This is impractical except for fish of high individual value, such as brood stock and ornamental fish and would be disastrous to stocks undergoing epizootic mortality. Most fish treatments are carried out on farms producing table fish and on animals of low inherent individual worth and already subject to farm and disease stresses. Under such conditions, not only must the route of application be economical and practical to apply, but the cost of the drug itself will often be of overriding importance.

If the parenteral route is excluded, then the practical routes in aquaculture species are bath and oral. Bath treatments are easy to carry out with products of high solubility by immersing fish in concentrated solutions or by adding the drugs directly to the fish's environment. For antimicrobials, bath treatments are restricted to use in recirculating units or in tanks of limited size, as much for reasons of cost as of potential environmental impact. Recirculating systems normally depend on biofilters to remove wastes from the recirculated water, and such biofilters depend on bacteria. Therefore the use of antimicrobial agents in recirculating systems is normally impossible because of the inevitable deleterious effects on the essential bacterial flora of the biofilter system. Since the ways in which drugs are absorbed by fish are only partly understood for only a few drugs, it is difficult to determine dose to ensure appropriate tissue concentrations of active product with the bath method. The difficulty is increased with antimicrobials such as the tetracyclines, which are complexed by divalent cations with major reductions in bioavailability. When a bath treatment is carried out in the form of a flush treatment (ie, in flowing, not static, water), the dose determination becomes even more difficult. Bath treatments have therefore found their most widespread application in the treatment of topical infections of fry or fingerling stages and of older fish suffering skin and gill infections and topical parasitic infections. In farmed fish outside the hatchery, bath treatments are mainly used to control parasites such as sea lice (*Lepeophtheirus* spp.), using insecticides such as dichlorvos and azimethiphos or hydrogen peroxide. The large volumes of insecticide-treated water employed present marked handling and environmental difficulties for organophosphate and other insecticides, while hydrogen peroxide presents shipping and transport problems because the explosive hazards of the bulk material mean that it cannot be shipped on passenger-carrying ferries.

Therefore, in all but these limited cases, the only practical way to ensure good uptake of controlled and effective amounts of an antimicrobial drug in fish is by the oral route, particularly for antibacterials. The oral route permits controlled dosing of large numbers of fish under intensive culture conditions with minimal loss of the product into the environment, so that even high-cost compounds can be employed in cases of emergency. Inevitably, there are limitations to the oral route of administration. Thus absorption from the gut must be adequate to achieve therapeutic levels in target organs. Some compounds can render medicated feed unpalatable, and palatability can vary from species to species. Additionally, the method of medication of fish feed can vary. In some cases, feed manufacturers produce medicated feed in which the drug is incorporated into the feed itself. The principal problems for the manufacturer in doing this are the small batch size and the contamination of the feed manufacturing plant. Feed manufacturers may thus be reluctant to incorporate medication into the feed itself. The alternative method is to "surface-dress" medication onto feed, normally using an agent such as fish oil as both a carrier and an adhesive agent to attach the medication to the feed. Production of medicated feeds at feed manufacturing plants has the advantage that proper control of incorporation rates is possible even with very active products, but against this is the need for rapid availability at the farm, often impractical with remote sites. With the "top-dress" approach to feed medication, whether manufactured in a feed plant or on a farm, there are further potential complications. To aid proper distribution of the medicine onto the feed, the product is usually formulated as a medicated premix. The premix will consist of the active ingredient itself, together with appropriate bulking agents. Selection of an inappropriate bulking agent can severely affect bioavailability, particularly for premixes used in the aquatic environment. Where on-farm mixing of medicated feeds is practiced, dust hazards for the user of the premix will be more difficult to control than in a feed plant environment. On-farm mixing of medicated feed has, in the past, involved mixing by shaking the drug or premix with feed in a dustbin, an approach certain to lead to inadequate distribution of the active ingredient. However, with even relatively simple equipment and with properly designed protocols, on-farm mixing of medicated feeds can produce an effective product.

A range of carrier and adhesive agents, from sodium alginate to water, has been described for medication of fish feed. In such studies the effect of such agents rarely seems to have been the subject of as much thought as that given to the drugs under trial. Not only may the drug itself present palatability problems, but the carrier, whether possessing adhesive properties or not, will also have implications for palatability and drug availability. Even the use of fish oil, a normal constituent of fish feed, used in this way results in a change of taste of the feed, with a greater concentration of oil on the surface. One of the few studies of this type found that cheaper vegetable oil was as effective as a carrier and adhesive agent as fish oil and that both alginate and water were poor, especially in terms of leaching properties. Label recommendations from suppliers of antimicrobials and premixes for use in aquaculture do not always give adequate guidance for preparation of medicated feeds. For example, should the premix be suspended in the adhesive agent and then poured into the feed in an operating mixer, or should the dry premix be added to the dry feed in the mixer drum and then mixed before addition of the adhesive agent and further mixing? In fish stocks where clinical disease is developing, it is inevitable that there will be a loss of appetite. Since medicated feed is likely to be supplied only to such fish, any change in taste of the feed will be likely to further increase the chances of poor acceptance of the feed.

This problem cannot easily be solved. Under laboratory conditions for studies of drug uptake, it is perfectly practical to reduce the palatability effects by acclimating the fish to the carrier agent by feeding coated ordinary feed in advance of the medication study. This is not a practical option for use on the farm. Any reduced acceptance of feed makes leaching properties of medicated feed more important by increasing drug loss if the fish are slow to feed. Poor and uneven attachment of the drug increases loss to the water between the time the feed is offered and its consumption. Uneven coating and uneven particle size increase the probability that fish will receive uneven and/or inadequate medication.

These factors combine to make dose control markedly more difficult in fish than in homeothermic species. The range of water types from hard (high levels of divalent cations) to soft (presence of humic acids) to seawater (divalent cations again) means that some compounds may be bound or inactivated by organic matter and inorganic ions (eg, oxytetracycline). The efficacy and toxicity of certain products changes according to the water quality, so much so that in complex environmental systems farmers may be unable to predict the full effects of a treatment. Feeding habits of fish also introduce degrees of uncertainty in the dosage of medicinal compounds. Many species exhibit hierarchical behavior, which results in competition for food and thus exacerbates uneven distribution of the drug within stock. To attempt to compensate for all of these complex interactions, it has often become practice to supply higher doses than those recommended for mammals, even though such practice has the disadvantage of increasing the potential impact of drug use on the environment and the risks of persistent residues. Equally there is a tendency for therapeutic regimes to be extended, with a 10-day medication period being most common. The reasons for this appears to be the view that fish feeding habits are such that an extended period is necessary to ensure that as many fish as possible receive sufficient drug. Perhaps equally as common is the view that, since 10 days is the most frequent recommended period for medication for control of bacterial disease in fish, this period can be proposed in order to minimize the amount of data required and avoid the cost of conducting full-dose titration studies.

An antimicrobial that is costly to develop will be expensive to use. Given the low individual value of most farmed fish, the economic return from the use of an expensive antimicrobial to control a disease outbreak may be insufficient to justify its use. When a pathogen is resistant to available cheaper antimicrobials, farm managers may decide that it is more efficient to kill out a fish stock and start again, rather than to use a more expensive drug.

The fact that it is rarely possible to determine the probable efficacy of any proposed therapy before it is carried out is one of the most difficult aspects of chemotherapy in aquaculture. Even if knowledge from previous outbreaks or from rapid identification of the causative organism can sometimes provide pointers to drug selection, there still remains a significant risk of failure, and the requirement to change the drug when the laboratory result is known cannot be eliminated. Such a procedure does not conform to good practice for antibiotic therapy, but it is unrealistic to expect a fish farmer to remain inactive when fish are dying. Practical and economic factors mean that fish treatments cannot in practice easily adhere to the same approaches as those that should prevail in terrestrial veterinary medicine.

With the very limited range of approved drugs for aquaculture use, the problems outlined above apply with even greater force to products used off-label. Here the prescribing veterinarian may have some experience with the product concerned but will have limited ability to control the effects of palatability, and the particle size of available product or premix may well be inappropriate for use in the aquatic environment. In most regulatory jurisdictions, off-label use is permitted only for products designed for administration by the same route of administration. Thus only products approved for oral administration should be used off-label for oral administration to fish.

Drug Classes Used in Aquaculture

Attempts to control ectoparasites in fish culture date back to when formalin was used in 1909 to control *Costia* infections. Other topical "disinfectants," including copper and malachite green, were used in the 1920s and 1930s, and quaternary ammonium compounds in the 1940s. Trials with antimicrobial agents against systemic bacterial infections in aquaculture commenced as early as the drugs became available, particularly in the United States, where sulfamerazine was introduced in 1948. As new drugs were introduced into human and veterinary medicine, suitable representatives were soon investigated for application to fish. Although aquaculture continues to expand and although many drugs appear under test in the scientific literature, the range of veterinary medicines that are legitimately available to fish farmers is limited and has been reduced in recent years, as discussed earlier. The few major drug groups to consider remain generally as outlined in Alderman and Michel (1992). The major antimicrobial groups are listed in Table 30.2. The numerous "topical disinfectants" and miscellaneous antiparasitics that have been proposed may be found in detail in Hoffman and Meyer (1974) and Stoskopf (1992).

Topical Disinfectants

The topical disinfectants are a disparate group, including salt, formalin, malachite green, copper sulphate, quaternary ammonium compounds, and others. Of various degrees of efficacy, these are partly interchangeable products employed to eliminate topical parasites such as opportunistic bacteria, protozoans, and fungi. The most useful, malachite green, presents major tissue residue problems and is a suspected mutagen and carcinogen. Of these compounds, formalin is widely used and is approved for use in the United States.

Sea Lice Treatments

Originally the organophosphates dichlorvos and azimethiphos were used to control sea lice parasites in sea cages, but they are no longer used extensively. Hydrogen peroxide is now the most common treatment (together with improved husbandry), although host toxicity increases with water temperature. Ivermectin is an effective oral agent for sea lice control but is used off-label, resulting in persistent tissue residues that require a withholding period of 3 months, during which time reinfection may readily occur. Newer sea lice control agents are under development (and some are available in some markets) and, like ivermectin, are effective by the oral route.

Antimicrobial Drugs

The antimicrobial drugs include the following: sulfonamides, tetracyclines, beta-lactams, quinolones, macrolides, nitrofurans, sulfonamides, chloramphenicol and related drugs, and aminoglycosides. Sulfonamides, including potentiated sulfonamides, have been widely used in the last 15 years in many countries. Of the tetracyclines, the most widely used is tetracycline, although doxycycline and chlortetracycline have been used. Although oxytetracycline is the most widely approved antibiotic for use in aquaculture in the world, complexing of tetracyclines with divalent cations means that bioavailability is poor in freshwater and very poor in seawater. If aquaculture was a completely new industry and a de novo research program was set up to select the most appropriate antimicrobials for development for that new industry, the tetracyclines would appear to be the most inappropriate choice for inclusion in that program. Amoxicillin is the major beta-lactam antibiotic in use. Rapid selection for resistance can occur for example, with *Flavobacterium psychrophilum*, but beta-lactams may present fewer environmental problems than other antibiotics, since they are rapidly broken down in the environment and do not persist in the way that tetracyclines and quinolones may do. First introduced into aquaculture in Japan, the older quinolones oxolinic acid and flumequine have achieved wide usage in Europe, and the fluoroquinolone sarafloxacin is now approved in much of Europe. No quinolone has been approved for aquaculture in the United States, where off-label use of these compounds is prohibited. Erythromycin, a macrolide, is the only drug with reported effect against renibacteriosis (bacterial kidney disease, or BKD). Its ability to prevent vertical transmission is still in dispute. Nitrofurans such as nitrofurazolidone and nifurpirinol were once widely used, but their use is now generally prohibited because of their carcinogenic potential. Chloramphenicol was once used widely, but its use is now discouraged or prohibited in most countries, because of its toxicity for people. Florfenicol and thiamphenicol do not present the same toxicity problems, and the former is now approved for use in some countries (eg, Norway). Aminoglycosides such as kanamycin, neomycin, and streptomycin appear quite frequently in reports of antibiotic susceptibility tests on bacterial pathogens isolated from fish. Although there is currently a streptomycin-penicillin combination approved for use in Norway, the aminoglycosides have found little general acceptance for general aquaculture use, partly because uptake by the oral route is poor. Gentamicin, kanamycin, and neomycin are reported as effective against bacterial infections of elasmobranchs (sharks) under aquarium conditions (Stoskopf et al., 1986).

Antimicrobial Resistance and Environmental Constraints

Major concerns about the use of antimicrobial agents in aquaculture relate, first, to the potential for selection for antibiotic resistance and the possibility that this might directly or indirectly present a health hazard to humans, and, second, to the potential for adverse environmental effects rising from their use. Problems of antibiotic residues in edible tissues also potentially exist but have been addressed by setting residue limits and ensuring that suitable withholding periods are used. Off-label use continues to present a problem, particularly if fixed withholding periods are used, since some off-label uses might result in detectable residues being present at slaughter. Even if such residues are within tolerance (MRL) for the tissues of other food-producing animals, since there is no tolerance set for fish meat, the residues, if detected, are illegal.

Selection for antibiotic resistance occurs in fish pathogens, particularly with continuing long-term use over a number of years. The proportion of isolates showing resistance to each antimicrobial has fluctuated considerably in different years (Tsoumas et al., 1989). In the 1990s in Europe there was a general decrease in numbers of resistant fish pathogens isolated, corresponding to the decreasing number of cases of furunculosis and therefore of isolates tested, since increasingly effective vaccines have displaced therapeutic use of antibiotics in the European salmon industry (Alderman and Hastings, 1998). Fish pathogens in which plasmid-mediated resistance to antimicrobials have been identified include *Aeromonas salmonicida, A. hydrophila, Edwardsiella tarda, Pasteurella piscicida, Pseudomonas fluorescens,* and *Vibrio anguillarum* (Aoki, 1988) and

Yersinia ruckeri (DeGrandis and Stevenson, 1985). Transferable R plasmids have been found in *A. salmonicida* that encode resistance to chloramphenicol, sulfonamide, and streptomycin (in Japan) and to combinations of sulfonamide, streptomycin, spectinomycin, trimethoprim, and/or tetracycline (in Ireland) (Aoki, 1997). Even wider multiple resistance is commonly encountered in isolates of *Aeromonas* spp. from ornamental fish. Although plasmid-mediated resistance to quinolones has not been reported in fish pathogens, laboratory studies have shown how chromosomally mediated resistance to oxolinic acid can readily be selected in the presence of the antibacterial (Tsoumas et al., 1989). Such studies deliberately set out to exert maximum selection pressure for antibiotic resistance in the absence of any competing microorganisms. These problems of resistance and its significance for human health are extensively discussed in Alderman (1999) and Alderman and Hastings (1998). Fish are poikilotherms, and almost all of their pathogens are adapted to grow at the normal temperature range of their hosts. Most therefore do not survive at mammalian body temperatures, so that the possibility, particularly in temperate climates, that antibiotic resistance in fish pathogens might represent a human health hazard may be judged to be slight (Alderman and Hastings, 1998). In warmer climates, particularly where control of antibiotic use is poorly enforced, the risks may be greater. In most developed countries, although there is regulation of the use of antibiotics in food-animal species, there is a much wider use of antibiotics off-label for companion animal species, and fish are no exception. Ornamental fish may have very high individual value, and desire to find an effective therapy can lead to use of a wide range of antibiotics. Imported ornamental fish may already be carrying multiply-resistant bacterial strains on import, rendering subsequent attempts at therapy useless. Unrestricted use of drugs also occurs in many shrimp farms in tropical regions. Infection by *Vibrio* spp. can severely limit the production of shrimp larvae, resulting in the routine use of oxytetracycline and selection of resistant *Vibrio* spp.

The potential for adverse environmental impact from the use of antibiotics in aquaculture exists. With in-feed antimicrobials, despite all attempts to ensure efficient use, a proportion of the medicated feed will not be consumed and will fall to the bottom of the pond or cage. Additionally some of the antibacterial agent will leach from the treated feed pellets, and a further proportion will be excreted (metabolized or unmetabolized) by the fish. In sites with fast water movements, there will be greater dispersal of solid and particulate material than in sites with poor flows. Waste feed pellets will also be eaten by fish and invertebrates in the vicinity of the farm. Residues of oxolinic acid have been found in wild fish, crabs, and mussels in the vicinity of a farm up to 13 days posttreatment. Samuelsen et al. (1992) and Coyne et al. (1994) reported transient residues of oxytetracycline in mussels growing directly under a marine cage. In marine salmon farms in Norway and Finland, the use of oxytetracycline coincided with an increased frequency of resistant microflora and fish pathogens in the sediments beneath the cages (Bjorklund et al., 1991; Samuelsen et al., 1992). However, a study on the use of oxytetracycline in two marine salmon farms in Ireland found no significant rise or else only a transitory rise in the frequency of resistance in under-cage sediments (Kerry et al., 1994). Alderman and Hastings (1998) and Alderman (1999) review these and other reports in detail. While excessive use of antimicrobials may be expected to produce adverse effects, the potential for adverse environmental impact by the reasonable use of antibiotics in aquaculture remains to be determined, despite considerable research.

Tissue Antimicrobial Drug Residues

It is normal in approving veterinary medicines to impose a withholding period, between last drug treatment and slaughter for human consumption, expressed in terms of days. This is appropriate for use with mammals in which metabolic rates and therefore drug residue elimination rates are not environmentally determined, but not for fish, since environmental temperatures play a critical role in their metabolic rates. Early aquaculture drug approvals were based on fixed withholding periods, but pharmacokinetic studies have shown that drug residues were more persistent in colder water, with a demonstration of a near 10% reduction for each degree centigrade for oxytetracycline. Fixed temperature-linked withholding periods may be suitable for relatively constant temperature waters, but rapidly fluctuating water temperatures are found on many freshwater fish farms in temperate climates. In Europe the degree-day withholding period is now generally used. This approach enables a single withholding period to be set that can be applied to any farm at any time of year, with the expectation that it accurately reflects the varying residue excretion rates being imposed by variable water temperatures. A degree-day withholding period is defined as the water temperature on each day cumulated over time; thus water temperatures (in degrees centigrade) of 11, 12, 11, 13, 12, 10, 9, 9, 8, 8, and 7 over 10 successive days corresponds to 110 degree-days. The concept is very familiar to fish farmers, who have long used it as a means of defining parameters such as the length of time for fish eggs to hatch after fertilization. For off-label use, where no residue depletion data exist, a minimum of 500 degree-days is imposed, which should be extended if the prescribing veterinarian has any reason to believe that a longer period should be used.

Bibliography

Alderman DJ. 1988. Fisheries chemotherapy: a review. In: Muir JF, Roberts RJ, eds. Recent Advances in Aquaculture 3. London: Croom Helm.

Alderman DJ. 1999. Requirements for the approval of veterinary therapeutics or growth enhancers in fish production. In Beconi-Barker M, et al., eds. Xenobiotic Metabolism in Fish. London: Plenum. (In press.)

Alderman DJ, Hastings TS. 1998. Antibiotic use in aquaculture: development of antibiotic resistance.potential for consumer health risks. Int J Food Sci Tech 33:139.

Alderman DJ, Michel C. 1992. Chemotherapy in aquaculture today. In: Michel C, Alderman DJ, eds. Chemotherapy in Aquaculture Today. Paris: Office Intern Epizooties.

Aoki T. 1988. Drug-resistant plasmids from fish pathogens. Microbiol Sci 5:219.

Aoki T. 1997. Resistance plasmids and the risk of transfer. In:E-M Bernoth, ed. Furunculosis: Multidisciplinary Fish Disease Research. London: Academic Press.

Bjorklund HV, et al. 1991. Residues of oxolinic acid and oxytetracycline in fish and sediments from fish farms. Aquaculture 97:85.

Committee for Veterinary Medicinal Products. 1997. Note for guidance on the establishment of maximum residue limits for minor species, EMEA/CVMP/153a/97-FINAL. London: European Medicines Evaluation Agency, Veterinary Medicines Evaluation Unit.

Committee for Veterinary Medicinal Products. 1998. Note for guidance on the establishment of maximum residue limits for Salmonidae and other fin fish, EMEA/CVMP/153b/97-FINAL. London: European Medicines Evaluation Agency, Veterinary Medicines Evaluation Unit.

Coyne R, et al. 1994. Concentration and persistence of oxytetracycline in sediments under a marine salmon farm. Aquaculture 123:31.

DeGrandis SA, Stevenson, RMW. 1985. Antimicrobial susceptibility patterns and R plasmid.mediated resistance in the fish pathogen *Yersinia ruckeri*. Antimicrob Agents Chemother 27:938.

Hoffman GL, Meyer FP. 1974. Parasites of freshwater fishes: a review of their control and treatment. Neptune City, NJ: TFH Publications.

Kerry J, et al. 1994. Frequency and distribution of resistance to oxytetracycline in micro-organisms isolated from marine fish farm sediments following therapeutic use of oxytetracycline. Aquaculture 123:43.

Michel C, Alderman DJ. 1992.Chemotherapy in Aquaculture: From Theory to Reality. Paris: Office Intern Epizooties.

Okamoto A. 1992. Restrictions on the use of drugs in aquaculture in Japan. In: Michel C, Alderman DJ, eds. Chemotherapy in Aquaculture Today. Paris: Office Intern Epizooties.

Samuelsen OB, et al. 1992. Residues of oxolinic acid in wild fauna following medication in fish farms. Dis Aquat Org 12:111.

Schnick RA, et al. 1997. Worldwide aquaculture drug and vaccine registration progress. Bull Eur Assoc Fish Pathol 17:251.

Stoskopf MK. 1992. Fish Medicine. Philadelphia: WB Saunders.

Stoskopf MK, et al. 1986. Therapeutic aminoglycoside antibiotic levels in brown sharks *(Carcharhinus plumbeus)*. J Fish Dis 9:301.

Subashinghe R, et al. 1999. Health management strategies: towards sustainable aquaculture. Proc 2nd Int Conf Sustainable Aquaculture, Norway. Rotterdam: Balkema.

Tsoumas A, et al. 1989. *Aeromonas salmonicida:*development of resistance to 4-quinolone antimicrobials. J Fish Dis 12:493.

U.S. Food and Drug Administration. 1998. Proposals to increase the legal availability of animal drugs for minor species and minor uses. Report of ADAA Minor Use/Minor Species Working Group. Docket No. 97N-0217, Federal Register 63 FR 58056 10/29/98.

TABLE 30.1. Principal bacterial pathogens of fish

Pathogen	Host	Disease	Environment
Enterobacteriaceae (Gram-negative)			
Edwardsiella tarda	Channel catfish, eel, carp, goldfish, and tilapia	Red pest disease	Southern USA, SE Asia, warm freshwater
E. ictaluri	Channel catfish	Enteric septicemia	USA, Thailand, warm freshwater
Yersinia ruckeri	Salmonids	Enteric redmouth	N America, Europe, freshwater
Vibrionaceae (Gram-negative)			
Vibrio anguillarum	All fish	Vibriosis	Ubiquitous, marine
V. salmonicida	Atlantic salmon	Hitra, cold-water vibriosis	Northern Europe, marine
V. viscosus	Atlantic salmon	Winter ulcer disease	Northern Europe, marine
Vibrio spp.	Mollusks and crustaceans	Larval infections	Ubiquitous, marine
Aeromonas salmonicida	Salmonids	Furunculosis	Ubiquitous
A. hydrophila	All fish	Septicemia	Freshwater
Pasteurellaceae (Gram-negative)			
Pasteurella piscida	Yellowtail, sea bass, sea bream	Pseudotuberculosis	Marine, Japan, Mediterranean
Pseudomonadaceae (Gram-negative)			
Pseudomonas anguilliseptica	Eel	Red spot disease	Japan
Flavobacteriaceae (Gram-negative)			
Flexibacter columnaris	All fish	Columnaris disease	Freshwater
Flavobacterium psychrophilum	Salmonids	Cold-water disease Rainbow trout fry syndrome (RTFS)	Freshwater N America Freshwater, Europe, Chile
Mycobacteriaceae (Gram-positive, acid-fast)			
Mycobacterium spp.	All fish	Tuberculosis	Marine, aquaria
Nocardiaceae (Gram-positive)			
Nocardia kampachi	Yellowtail	Nocardiosis	Japan, marine
Nocardia spp.	Crustaceans	Nocardiosis	Ubiquitous
Coryneforms (Gram-positive)			
Renibacterium salmoninarum	Salmonids	Bacterial kidney disease	Freshwater, N America, Europe
Cocci (Gram-positive)			
Streptococcus spp.	All marine fish	Septicemia	Marine
Aerococcus viridans	Lobster	Gaffkemia	Marine
Rickettsia-like organisms (RLOs)			
Piscirickettsia salmonis	Salmonids	Piscirickettsiosis	Chile, Europe, Canada

TABLE 30.2. **Major antimicrobial drugs used in aquaculture**

Product	Route	Dose (mg/kg fish per day)	Indication
Antibiotics			
Beta-lactams			
Ampicillin			
Amoxycillin			
	Oral	50–80 mg/kg 10 days	Gram-negative bacteria
Benzylpenicillin (with streptomycin)			
Aminoglycosides			
Neomycin	Oral	50–80 mg/kg 10 days	Gram-negative bacteria
Kanamycin	Bath	20 mg/l	
Tetracyclines			
Tetracycline	Oral	50–80 mg/kg 10 days	Gram-negative bacteria
Oxytetracycline			
Doxycycline	Bath	20 mg/l	
Macrolides			
	Oral	50 mg/kg 10 days	Bacterial kidney disease
Erythromycin	Bath (eggs)	2 mg/l 1 h	
Chloramphenicol group			
	Oral	50–80 mg/kg 10 days	Gram-negative bacteria
Florfenicol	Bath	20 mg/l 1 h	
	Oral	50–80 mg/kg 10 days	Gram-negative bacteria
Thiamphenicol	Bath	20 mg/l 1 h	
Synthetic Antibacterial Agents			
Sulfonamides			
Sulfamethazine			
Sulfadimethoxine	Oral	200 mg/kg 10 days	Gram-negative bacteria
Sulfaguanidine			
Potentiated sulfonamides			
Trimethoprim + sulfadiazine (1:5)		50 mg/kg 10 days	Gram-negative bacteria
	Oral		
Ormetoprim + sulfadimethoxine		50 mg/kg 5 days	
Quinolones			
Oxolinic acid	Oral	10–30 mg/kg 10 days	Gram-negative bacteria
Flumequine			
Sarafloxacin	Oral	10 mg/kg 5 days	Gram-negative bacteria

Note: Only oxytetracycline and ormetoprim-sulfadiazine are approved for use with food fish in the United States.

31 | Antimicrobial Drug Use in Bovine Mastitis

R. J. ERSKINE

Effective and economical mastitis control programs rely on prevention rather than treatment. Herds practicing mastitis prevention produce higher-quality milk at less cost than herds that do not. Nonetheless, therapeutic intervention is an important part of a control program for bovine mastitis. This chapter will describe the strategies of antimicrobial therapy for bovine mastitis, with a practical emphasis.

The concept of administering intramammary infusions of antiseptic solutions as a treatment for mastitis caused by infectious agents has been present for at least a century. Widespread availability and use of antimicrobials in animal agriculture in the 1950s cultivated the development of a wide variety of commercial products for intramammary infusion in the 1960s and 1970s. Initial successes suggested 75% efficacy (cures) in both lactating and dry-cow formulations. However, there has been growing realization that in many cases therapeutic attainments fall short of expectations. Chronic intramammary infections (IMI) with extensive fibrotic change caused by pathogens such as *Staphylococcus aureus* pose difficult therapeutic problems, and it is unlikely that typical labeled-dose regimens, which may provide effective antibacterial concentrations above MIC for 24–48 hours, will eliminate the pathogen from affected mammary glands. Additionally, the major developmental thrust for antimicrobials as a treatment for mastitis has been directed against Gram-positive organisms, particularly staphylococci and streptococci. However, in many herds the emergence of pathogens with greater resistance to antimicrobial therapy, such as Gram-negative rods and *Mycoplasma bovis,* has been a substantial cause of loss.

Nonetheless, mastitis remains the most frequent reason for antimicrobial use on dairy farms and thus contributes to a substantial portion of total drug and veterinary costs incurred by the dairy industry. Although these costs are minimal, relative to the economic losses attributable to lost production resulting from inflammation, application of management practices that decrease the prevalence of contagious pathogens, such as *Streptococcus agalactiae* and *Staphylococcus aureus*, has shifted the focus of mastitis control and economic losses to IMI caused by environmental pathogens that are associated with more frequent episodes of clinical mastitis. The cost of clinical mastitis is greater than U.S. $100/case and $40 to $50 per cow in a herd per year. Discarded milk following treatment may account for as much as 70% of lost marketable milk, and in herds that do not have a judicious treatment program, losses from discarded milk alone can exceed $100 per cow per year. Thus, there is increased awareness among producers of treatment-related costs, and the economic cost of extensive antimicrobial therapy for mastitis.

Michigan Department of Agriculture records, collected from Michigan dairies that had at least one occurrence of inhibitory residues in marketed milk in 1995-1997, revealed that antimicrobial therapy of mastitis accounts for 90% of the occurrences. Furthermore, both the consuming public and the regulatory sector have increased their awareness of the possible health hazards posed by antimicrobials and other drugs in milk used for human consumption (see Chapter 33). Whether these concerns are real or perceived, frequency of milk testing and regulatory control of drug use on dairy farms are increasing and are likely to increase in complexity. Thus, because of accountability to dairy producers and the consuming public, we must address two key issues other than efficacy. Therapy must be economically viable and must not increase risk of drug residues in marketed milk.

Considerations before Treatment
Assessing Efficacy

Therapy of infectious disease should assist host defenses in eliminating invading pathogens and/or reduce pathophysiological consequences of infection without degrading host defenses. Logically, emphasis in research and clinical application of antimicrobial drugs for mastitis treatment has focused on the elimination of infectious agents. However, therapeutic success for some IMIs may be better measured by evaluating reduction of clinical symptoms, rather than total elimination of the pathogen from the gland. Ultimately, the best outcome of mastitis therapy is a positive effect on the amount of marketed milk received from the treated cow, along with long-term survival of the cow as a milk producer in the herd.

Determination of IMI status and definition of cures are dependent on bacteriologic culture of milk samples and on the sensitivity and specificity of this technology to assess the outcome correctly. The conventional definition of an IMI is either the presence of the same microorganism in 2 of 3 consecutive cultures (different sampling dates) or the presence of the pathogen in both samples of duplicate samples (collected at the same time). If these guidelines are followed, the chance of determining an IMI based on false positive isolations from contamination is relatively low. One isolation from a single sample of the contagious pathogens *Streptococcus agalactiae* and *Staphylococcus aureus* is probably indicative of an IMI, because of the high prevalence of these organisms as intramammary pathogens and the low rate of environmental contamination of milk samples with these pathogens. Mammary gland quarters that have an IMI caused by a particular pathogen before treatment but do not have an IMI caused by the same pathogen after treatment would be defined as cured. Conversely, quarters that remain bacteriologically positive after treatment are not cured. Although this is a rather simple premise of efficacy, a survey of mastitis therapy trials can result in numerous, and perhaps misleading, definitions of bacteriologic cures. The number of times a quarter is sampled before and after therapy, the volume of milk sample inoculated, the sample used to inoculate the culture medium, the time when sampling occurs, and elapsed time between collection of consecutive samples are dissimilar among many reports. In both research and in clinical practice, the definition of cures is often insufficiently conservative. Misleading belief in bacteriologic cures that are really false-negative culture results can readily develop if care is not taken in data analysis, particularly when assessing therapeutic outcomes for IMI caused by such invasive pathogens as *S. aureus* and *Streptococcus uberis* and by Gram-negative rods such as *Pseudomonas* and *Klebsiella*. Bacteria exposed to antimicrobials may be inhibited in growth and can remain so for some time after the termination of therapy. Intracellular survival, abscess formation, and L forms, an antimicrobial-induced variant of *Staphylococcus aureus* and some other Gram-positive bacteria that lacks a cell wall, can reduce the probability of successful isolation of bacteria following routine aerobic culture of milk samples. A 30-day refractory period of decreased probability to isolate bacteria in milk has been demonstrated for *S. aureus* IMI, and *Pseudomonas aeruginosa* can be isolated from affected quarters subsequent to a case of clinical mastitis more than 12 months after initial therapy, despite repeated negative cultures. Additionally, many chronic IMIs result in intermittent shedding of bacteria in milk so that one, or even two samples, collected after treatment may be inadequate to ensure the absence of bacteria in the affected quarter. The conclusion is that bacteriologic cures should be reviewed critically before success of therapy can be affirmed.

The other potential goal of therapy is to attain clinical cures, with or without bacteriologic cures. This may be desirable to allow an affected cow's milk to be sold or to ameliorate a potential severe or life-threatening IMI. Clinical cures attained by antimicrobial therapy can be more obvious than bacteriologic cures, but assessment can be tainted by subjective outcomes. Clinical mastitis is defined as abnormal milk, with or without quarter enlargement and systemic signs. Return to normal appearance is accepted as a clinical cure; however, relapses (ie, clinical mastitis cases that become apparent again before milk withholding periods following therapy are complete) and recurrences should be noted as part of the therapeutic evaluation. Particularly for systemic (acute) clinical mastitis cases, clinical chemistries and/or objective measures such as heart rate and rectal temperature can be measured. Best indicators for efficacy are dry matter intake, milk production, the amount of produced milk actually marketed, and culling/death rates after treatment.

Pharmacokinetic Considerations
Intramammary administration by infusion through the teat canal offers a direct method of obtaining relatively high concentrations of drug in the affected quarter of the gland. For this reason, this method of administration continues to be the most frequently employed and can be particularly successful with Gram-positive cocci that are susceptible to beta-lactam drugs as a means to reduce the signs of clinical mastitis and, in some instances, to eliminate IMI. Additionally, intramammary infusions can help eliminate existing IMI or prevent new IMI caused by Gram-positive cocci during the dry period. Nonetheless, there are drawbacks to this route of administration. Most of the products labeled for use in dairy cattle have been directed for use against Gram-positive cocci and thus have little or no activity against Gram-negative pathogens. Various extra-label products have been employed clinically and in research to broaden the potential spectrum of activities over that available in commercial products. With such products, it is difficult to ascertain correct milk and meat withdrawal periods following extralabel drug use. Intramammary infusion with preparations not prepared under sterile conditions can result in superinfection caused by environmental pathogens. Often the secondary IMI caused by such pathogens as *Pseudomonas aeruginosa*, *Candida* spp., and *Nocardia* spp. result in worse clinical implications than if no intramammary infusion was administered at all. Additionally, it is difficult to ascertain correct milk and meat withdrawal periods following extralabel drug use. Fibrin casts and microabscess formation typical of more chronic IMI interfere with distribution of infused drugs to the site of infection in the terminal alveoli, thus not allowing effective concentrations

at the site of IMI. Finally, the relatively short duration of dosing typical of intramammary therapy limits the period of effective concentration in the gland needed to eliminate more chronic or invasive IMI. For these reasons, the systemic administration of antimicrobials has received attention as an adjunct or alternative therapy to intramammary therapy.

As a basis for practical pharmacokinetics of mastitis therapy, Ziv (1980) suggested that the ideal antibiotic for parenteral mastitis therapy would (1) have low MIC against the majority of udder pathogens, (2) have high bioavailability from IM injection sites, (3) be weakly basic or otherwise non-ionized in serum, (4) be sufficiently lipid soluble, (5) have a low degree of protein binding, (6) have a long $t_{1/2}$ in the body, (7) retain activity in inflammatory secretions, and (8) have clearance from body organs and tissues similar to the clearance of the drug from the blood—ie, not result in drug accumulation in specific organs. Systemically administered sulfonamides, penicillins, aminoglycosides, and early-generation cephalosporins do not readily penetrate the mammary gland. Macrolides, trimethoprim, tetracyclines, and fluoroquinolones distribute well to the mammary gland; however, only the fluoroquinolones have broad-spectrum activity against many Gram-negative pathogens. This class of drugs is undergoing intense scrutiny for use in food-producing animals, because of bacterial resistance concerns for humans, and is therefore banned by the Food and Drug Administration for any dairy-bred bovine in the United States.

Systemic use of antimicrobials has been moderately successful for improving cure rates as compared with intramammary infusions for chronic *S. aureus* IMI in dry cows and lactating cows (Owens et al., 1988; Soback et al., 1990; Sol et al., 1990). Antimicrobials such as fluoroquinolones and tetracyclines would be good pharmacokinetic candidates because of their large volume of distribution (lipophilic) and relatively long half-life. Because of a high degree of resistance to antimicrobials in commercial intramammary products, systemic antimicrobial therapy with alternative antimicrobial drugs has been attempted for the treatment of acute mastitis caused by Gram-negative bacteria. In general, poorer results are attained than with Gram-positive pathogens, although drug selection for some of the studies did not follow sound pharmacologic principles. For example, ceftiofur (IV) has high protein binding and therefore low bioavailability, erythromycin (IM) has poor efficacy against coliforms, and gentamicin is not lipid soluble and therefore does not diffuse into tissues. Treatment of experimental *E. coli* infections with cefquinome, a third-generation cephalosporin that has good tissue distribution and low MIC for Gram-negative bacteria, was determined to be beneficial in reducing deleterious clinical outcomes of experimentally induced infections (Shpigel et al., 1997). Thus, from a pharmacologic perspective, mastitis treatment should utilize bacterial culture and apply sound pharmacokinetic and pharmacodynamic principles if systemic therapy is indicated as an adjunct for intramammary dosing. Most parenteral dosing involves extralabel drug use. This frequently increases the risk of antimicrobial residues in milk and meat of treated cows, as well as the need to withhold products from market for longer periods of time.

The Cow's Point of View

Cows that have concurrent metabolic disease or inadequate nutrition or are subjugated to stress, including calving, are more likely to be affected by infectious agents. Although neutrophil efficiency for phagocytosis and killing in the mammary gland is poorer than in other tissues, it is the most critical defense mechanism of the mammary gland, once the teat end barrier is breached by an invading pathogen. In vitro, neutrophil phagocytosis and killing are positively correlated with beneficial clinical outcomes of experimental IMI, and thus preventive measures such as core-antigen vaccines and antioxidant supplementation of dietary rations, which improve antibacterial function of neutrophils, reduce the incidence and severity of clinical mastitis. Conversely, increased incidence and severity of clinical mastitis cases in cows in the periparturient period are believed in part to be caused by impeded ability for neutrophil migration into the gland. Additionally, the understanding of mammary resistance to infection has increased, so that the neutrophil is now recognized to be part of a larger, complex symphony of immune effectors that includes macrophages, lymphocytes, immune modulators such as cytokines, inflammatory mediators, and acute phase reactants. Potential differences among cows in immune response, coupled with the realization of the diverse nature of pathogens that invade the bovine mammary gland, result in highly variable responses to even the best of preventive programs. Based on the premises that antibiotics do not eliminate an infection without a functional immune system, and that ability to manipulate immune function is limited at the time of treatment, mastitis therapy should be initiated on an assessment, even on a crude scale, of immune competence of the treated cow. Some crude predictions of therapeutic failure include intramammary infections in older cows, infections of long duration, consistent shedding of pathogens over time, and multiple infected quarters. Genetic markers in dairy cattle may in the future allow identification of potentially immune-impaired breeding lines, as well as target therapeutic efforts and expectations of treated animals.

Antimicrobial Therapy of the Lactating Cow
Treatment of Acute Clinical Mastitis—Coliforms

Acute, or systemic, mastitis is most often caused by coliform (lactose-fermenting Enterobacteriaceae) and other Gram-negative organisms.

However, numerous other pathogens, including *Mycoplasma bovis,* Gram-positive cocci, Gram-negative rods, and mycotic organisms can result in severe mastitis. Cases can be life threatening to the cow and are often accompanied by marked production loss. If the cow survives, affected cows often perform poorly and may undergo premature culling. From a cowside appraisal, treatment of these cases is a forced decision—ie, treatment is indicated, if only to relieve the cow of systemic signs. Supportive care is usually indicated and, in the case of coliform mastitis, may be the most beneficial component of the therapeutic regimen. The obvious basis for antimicrobial therapy is knowledge of the causative pathogen. However, this is not attainable for some hours after initial case recognition, and thus the practical problem remains of basing treatment on best clinical guess. In addition, most antimicrobial therapeutic regimens currently used as a treatment of coliform mastitis in the United States are not labeled for use in dairy cows. As a result, in the United States, the veterinarian or herd manager often formulates therapeutic management of coliform cases using extralabel drugs.

Experimental challenge models have clarified much of the pathophysiology of mastitis resulting from infection with Gram-negative organisms. Following infection, bacterial numbers in milk increase rapidly. Depending on the size of the challenge, peak bacterial concentrations in milk often occur within a few hours. Typically, a subsequent rapid decline in bacterial concentration follows neutrophil migration into the gland. Though often severe, experimental coliform infections usually clear spontaneously and rarely are more than 10 days in duration. The resulting inflammation and leukocytosis in the affected quarter may persist for weeks, or the quarter may become agalactic, despite inability to isolate bacteria on culture.

Much of the inflammatory and systemic changes observed during the course of acute coliform mastitis result from the release of lipopolysaccharide (LPS) endotoxin from the bacteria. Although there is considerable release of LPS during the rapid proliferation of the Gram-negative bacteria, the majority of release occurs following bacterial phagocytosis and killing by neutrophils. The release of LPS results in subsequent activation of the cyclooxygenase and lipoxygenase pathways, releasing prostaglandins, leukotrienes, and thromboxanes, compounds that are potent mediators of local inflammatory and systemic circulatory events. LPS induces the release of macrophage-derived cytokines, initiating a wide range of systemic responses to inflammation, including fever, leukocytosis, protein synthesis and release by hepatocytes, and serum iron sequestration, collectively termed the acute phase response. Consequently, in order to reduce the severity of acute coliform mastitis, either bacterial growth must be inhibited to reduce exposure of the quarter and the cow to LPS, or the effects of the LPS release must be neutralized. From a practical standpoint, therapy of acute coliform infections cannot begin until clinical signs appear. Clinical recognition of coliform mastitis usually occurs after peak bacterial numbers have been attained. Thus, by the time therapy is initiated, maximal release of LPS has likely occurred. This raises concerns regarding the advantages of antimicrobial therapy in alleviating the effects of acute coliform mastitis. Thus, the primary therapeutic concern is the treatment of endotoxin-induced shock with fluids, together with other supportive care. The reader is referred to other sources for in-depth reviews of these concepts (Anderson, 1989; Erskine et al., 1993).

Antimicrobial therapy may be of secondary importance relative to supportive treatment of endotoxic shock, but it remains a practical part of a therapeutic regimen for acute mastitis. Although useful for determining the pathogenesis of coliform IMI, experimental challenge models cannot be considered as universally applicable for all cases. Occasionally, coliform infections result in chronic mastitis. Septicemia can occur, although it is believed to be an infrequent result of infection. In addition, numerous other pathogens cause acute clinical mastitis, which can be difficult to distinguish from cases caused by coliforms at initial presentation. Chronic IMI caused by pathogens such as *S. aureus* can become acute or even gangrenous at times of neutropenic dysfunction, such as parturition. Severe overwhelming IMIs that lead to sepsis have been recorded for pathogens such as *Pseudomonas aeruginosa* and *Bacillus cereus*. The need for antimicrobial therapy in cows with grossly abnormal milk but with improved appetite, attitude, and milk production should be evaluated critically. Unnecessary extension of therapy in these instances results in increased discarded milk expense for the dairy producer and risk of antimicrobials in marketed milk.

Selection of a potentially efficacious antimicrobial agent for the therapy of acute coliform mastitis is primarily dependent on in vitro culture and sensitivity. A review of antimicrobial susceptibility data for Gram-negative pathogens is presented in Table 31.1. Antimicrobials such as aminoglycosides and cephalosporins are often selected for use, because a higher proportion of isolates display sensitivity or lower MIC to drugs of this class than to available penicillins or macrolides. Selection of aminoglycosides, however, appears to be erroneous, for reasons discussed above and confirmed by experimental data. Gentamicin IM was not more efficacious in preventing agalactia or death resulting from acute clinical mastitis, or in improving other clinical outcomes, when compared with administration of erythromycin IM or no systemic antimicrobials (Jones and Ward, 1990). In addition, cows experimentally challenged with *E. coli* and dosed with 500 mg of intramammary gentamicin as frequently as

TABLE 31.1. Antimicrobial susceptibility (%) of Gram-negative pathogens

Pathogen	Gram-negative	Coliform	Coliform	Gram-negative	Coliform	Coliform	Coliform	E. coli
Number of Isolates	214[a]	1,695[b]	172[c]	46[d]	53[e]	70[f]	ND[g]	27[h]
	%							MIC90 (µg/ml)
Amoxicillin	ND	ND	ND	ND	ND	ND	59	>200
Ampicillin	ND	48	44	61	ND	73	20	200
Cephalothin	53	65	79	83	87	79	ND	128
Erythromycin	ND	ND	ND	ND	0	ND	ND	ND
Gentamicin	96	ND	91	98	100	96	ND	2
Neomycin	48	87	63	48	55	83	68	ND
Norfloxacin	ND	ND	ND	ND	ND	ND	ND	<0.25
Novobiocin	ND	ND	ND	ND	0	ND	ND	ND
Penicillin	0	4	ND	0	0	1	ND	ND
Spectinomycin	ND	ND	ND	ND	ND	ND	45	128
Streptomycin	69	60	34	30	42	59	55	ND
Sulfadiazine-trimethoprim	ND	ND	ND	72	ND	ND	82	128
Tetracycline	30	66	24	43	60[i]	61	68	>200

Note: Data expressed as percentage of isolates susceptible from disk assay, except for *E. coli* (Muckle et al., 1986). ND, not done.
[a]McDonald et al. (1977).
[b]Davidson (1980).
[c]Larson et al. (1981).
[d]Anderson et al. (1982).
[e]Schultze (1983).
[f]Anderson (1989).
[g]Mackie et al. (1988); 4-year study.
[h]Muckle et al. (1986).
[i]Oxytetracycline.

every 12 hours did not have lower peak bacterial concentrations in milk, duration of infection, convalescent somatic cell or serum albumin concentrations in milk, or rectal temperatures than those of untreated challenged cows (Erskine et al., 1992). Additionally, gentamicin readily diffused through the milk:blood barrier, as indicated by detectable concentrations in serum throughout the treatment period and the first 12 hours after the last dose. Consequently, urine gentamicin concentrations were detectable 14 days after the last infusion, and concentrations of 1 µg of gentamicin/g in renal tissue were detected in cows 6 months after the trial. The American Veterinary Medical Association has approved a voluntary ban on the extralabel use of aminoglycosides in cattle.

Ceftiofur sodium, a third-generation cephalosporin, has been reported to have excellent activity against Gram-negative pathogens, with a suggested MIC for *E. coli* of 0.25–1.0 µg/ml. However, mammary tissue and milk concentrations of ceftiofur following systemic treatment remain below these concentrations (Owens et al., 1990; Erskine et al., 1993). This is probably a consequence of low bioavailability because of a high degree of protein binding, as previously discussed. Three doses of parenteral sulfadiazine-trimethoprim have also failed to achieve clinical improvement in experimental *E. coli* infections (Pyorala et al., 1994). However, three doses IM of cefquinome, a third-generation cephalosporin with good tissue distribution, was found to improve clinical outcome of experimentally infected cows when compared with use of cloxacillin or ampicillin (Shpigel et al., 1997). This is one of the few studies that demonstrated efficacy for parenteral use of antimicrobials in cows with experimental coliform mastitis, but it also demonstrates the importance of selecting antimicrobials with low MIC for targeted organisms in addition to beneficial pharmacokinetic properties.

Treatment of Acute Clinical Mastitis—Noncoliforms

Therapy for causative pathogens of acute mastitis other than coliforms has not been well studied. In general, results can be expected to be poor for Gram-negative and Gram-positive rods, mycotic or algal organisms, and for *Mycoplasma bovis*. Some benefit may be gained in reducing the clinical severity, and perhaps in outright bacteriologic cure, of IMI caused by Gram-positive cocci. For these pathogens, parenteral administration of antimicrobials that exhibit relatively good activity against these organisms and distribute well to the gland, such as oxytetracycline, fluoroquinolones, and macrolides, may be the best choices for therapy.

PSEUDOMONAS SPECIES

Aminoglycoside susceptibility is often reported, and outside the United States, chloramphenicol, polymixin B or C, and furazolidone have been reported to have success. However, these conclusions are based on clinical observations and not on controlled studies, and the reality is that antimicrobial therapy is not likely to achieve bacteriologic cures or affect clinical outcome. *Pseudomonas* IMI can become dormant, and virtually undetectable from bacteriologic culture of milk, only to recur as severe mastitis months after therapy. In other words, false-negative cultures from affected cows following a case of severe mastitis are common. Additionally, fatal septic involvement of these IMIs has been reported. Thus, treatment should be focused on supportive care and on antimicrobial use to prevent sepsis. Effective control, by reducing the exposure of udders to the reservoir of infection, is critical when approaching mastitis outbreaks caused by this organism.

SERRATIA SPECIES

Serratia spp. are not readily invasive, and for IMI to occur, large numbers of bacteria must be placed on or near the gland. About half of the infections are reported to be clinical, although subclinical herd outbreaks are possible, and new IMI can occur during the dry period. The clinical nature of IMI caused by these organisms may depend on the initial exposure, and chronic infections that last much longer than typical Gram-negative infections may occur. Spontaneous recovery has been reported. Thus, as with *Pseudomonas* spp., treatment for the purpose of bacteriologic cure is not likely to be beneficial.

ARCANOBACTERIUM PYOGENES

Arcanobacterium (Actinomyces) pyogenes is one of several organisms involved in the etiology of European "summer mastitis." It is frequently associated with teat injury and clinical mastitis observed in dry cows. Cases are predominantly malodorous and clinical; however, because the clinical signs are not specific, diagnosis and therapy should be based on milk culture and antimicrobial susceptibility. Long-acting antibiotic treatment has been reported to be successful at dry off, and tylosin has been reported to be effective in Denmark (Katholm, 1988). However, because of decreased production and low rate of cure, culling is frequent. For more typical cases of clinical mastitis in lactating cows, treatment of this pathogen should be attempted with intramammary infusions of beta-lactams. Because of the intense propensity of this organism to form purulent abscesses, it is recommended to include systemic administration of procaine penicillin G or oxytetracycline. More-chronic IMIs are not likely to be cured bacteriologically, and therapy of recurring cases should be approached judiciously, as bacteriologic cures become unlikely and high concentrations of the pathogen are often shed, raising concern over the potential reservoir of infection that affected cows become for herdmates.

NOCARDIA SPECIES, YEASTS, AND FUNGI

Infection with *Nocardia* spp. and *Candida* spp. are characterized by sudden onset of udder swelling and lack of positive clinical response to conventional antimicrobial therapy. Some cases, particularly caused by *Candida*, are subclinical. Clinical cases are often associated with extended antimicrobial treatment and contaminated udder infusions or devices. Because the clinical signs are similar to bacterial infections, diagnosis should be based on milk culture. Treatment should include discontinuation of antimicrobial therapy and culling of chronically infected cows. Clinically recovered cows may shed organisms for up to 8 months. Clotrimazole, ketoconazole, miconazole, nystatin, and sulfamethoxypyridazine have all been used, with reported clinical success, in the treatment of *Candida*. However, these studies were based on clinical impressions, and none of these drugs is approved for use in food-producing animals in the United States.

OTHER PATHOGENS

Prototheca zopfii, a colorless alga, is a common inhabitant of the dairy environment, being associated with wet areas contaminated with manure. Chronic subclinical and clinical infections occur, and successful treatments have not been reported. Infected cows should be isolated and removed from the herd. Mycoplasmal infections occur primarily during milking, and carrier cows are the major reservoir of infection. Routine microbiological identification procedures will not detect the presence of these organisms in milk, as special media and growth conditions are required. Successful treatment methods have not been discovered for *Mycoplasma* mastitis, and because of the potential contagious nature of infection, infected cows should be segregated or culled from noninfected cows in the herd.

Occasionally, premature agalactia in chronically infected quarters, particularly quarters infected with pathogens refractile to therapy, is promoted as an alternative to culling the cow. This may have some benefit in genetically superior animals within a herd or in cows that are to be maintained until calving. The goal is to eliminate the infection by causing fibrosis of the affected quarter, thus reducing the risk of further pathogenic change or systemic effects on the cow, as well as reduced risk of infection for other cows. Infusion of 60 ml of 2.0% chlorhexidine-diacetate (Nolvasan, solution—Fort Dodge) into affected quarters is administered twice at 24-hour intervals. The quarter should be stripped out before the second infusion. Care should be taken that milk from noninfected quarters is not sent to market before prior testing for inhibitors in milk. This regimen is not recommended for a majority of chronically infected animals and should be used judiciously by practitioners.

Treatment of Mild Clinical Mastitis

Of bacteriologic cultures of milk samples collected from cows with clinical mastitis, 30–35% will not yield any microorganism. Unlike treatment of severe clinical mastitis cases, treatment of mild cases (abnormal milk with or without local inflammation of the affected quarter, no systemic signs) is a more voluntary therapeutic decision. Many mild mastitis cases are coliform IMIs that are resolved before treatment is necessary. Additionally, numerous mild clinical mastitis cases are temporary setbacks in the balance between pathogen and host defenses that occur in more chronic IMIs. A high proportion of clinical cases, particularly those caused by Gram-positive cocci, observed in cows during the first 60 days after calving are manifestations of infections that started during the dry period. Additionally, chronic IMIs often display recurring episodes of clinical mastitis at regular intervals, and a small proportion of cows often account for a disproportionate number of cases. This poses the major question about treatment of mild clinical cases. Does antimicrobial therapy enhance cure rate over that attained by no treatment (spontaneous cure)? Therapeutic and spontaneous cure rates for clinical mastitis cases caused by coliforms and staphylococci are very similar. However, by contrast, it may be advantageous to treat streptococcal IMIs if they are not chronic. Information on therapeutic efficacy of mild clinical mastitis cases is not extensive. In one study, clinical symptoms were resolved in 74% of clinical cases caused by *Streptococcus uberis* and 84% of cases caused by *S. dysgalactiae* after a single intramammary infusion of cefoperazone (Wilson et al., 1986). Bacteriologic cure was achieved in only 60–65% of the cases. A comparison of cure rate in treated and untreated cows was not reported. In a study of three Californian dairies, bacteriologic cure assessed at 4 and 20 days after treatment with amoxicillin, cephapirin, or oxytocin (no antimicrobial) did not differ for mild clinical mastitis cases caused by any pathogen, although antimicrobial treatment resulted in better clinical cure rates for cases caused by pathogens other than streptococci and coliforms (Guterbock et al., 1993). Thus, renewed interest in a "no antibiotic" approach to mild clinical mastitis cases promotes a convenient regimen to avoid costs of discarded milk and residue risks that are inherent in antimicrobial therapy. However, an economic analysis of the California data determined that although milk production and survival in the herd did not differ between antimicrobial- and non-antimicrobial-treated cows, the rates of both relapses and recurring cases were higher in non-antimicrobial-treated cows, especially among streptococcal cases. A case report from a Colorado dairy also reported a marked increase in the incidence of clinical mastitis, in the prevalence of IMI, and in the subsequent increase in herd somatic cell count associated with streptococcal IMI following adoption of a no-antibiotic approach to clinical mastitis (Cattell, 1996). Administration of supportive care, IV oxytet-racycline, and intramammary cephapirin to cows with varying degrees of clinical mastitis severity resulted in a higher frequency of normal udder appearance at 10 days (clinical cure) and bacteriologic cure in 14 days for streptococcal IMIs and clinical cure for coliform IMI than in cows administered supportive care only (Morin et al., 1998).

The conclusion is that common sense and individual herd history should determine the course of therapeutic planning for mild clinical mastitis cases in dairy herds. For initial occurrences of clinical episodes for any affected quarter, especially those caused by streptococci, labeled use of commercial intramammary infusions is the best approach. However, if infected quarters recur with regularity, and in the absence of systemic signs, repeated treatment of what now has become chronic IMI is not warranted. Any moderate increase in cure rates gained by extensive parenteral therapy for chronic IMI in lactating cows will not overcome the expense of discarded milk and other related treatment costs.

Treatment of Subclinical Intramammary Infections

As with mild clinical mastitis cases, subclinical mastitis does not present an urgent potential loss of gland function or life to the cow. No significant economic losses will occur as a result of prolonging initiation of therapy until bacterial culture can be completed. Antimicrobial susceptibilities of isolated pathogens often reveal potentially beneficial therapy with beta-lactam and macrolide drugs (Tables 31.2 and 31.3).

TABLE 31.2. **Antimicrobial susceptibility (%) of *Staphylococcus aureus***

Number of Isolates	214[a,e]	—[b,e]	28[f]	106[g]
	%			MIC$_{90}$ (µg/ml)
Ampicillin	47	33	ND	ND
Cephalothin	100[c]	100[c]	100	1
Erythromycin	94	98	96	0.5
Gentamicin	ND	ND	100	ND
Neomycin	89	94	86	1
Novobiocin	97	98	93	0.25
Penicillin	0	30	4	ND
Streptomycin	ND	ND	39	4
Tetracycline	88	88	93	0.5[d]

Note: Data expressed as percentage of isolates susceptible from disk assay, except Craven et al. (1986). ND, not done.
[a]Clinical isolates.
[b]Subclinical isolates.
[c]Cephaloridine.
[d]Oxytetracycline.
[e]Mackie et al. (1988).
[f]Schultze (1983).
[g]Craven et al. (1986).

TABLE 31.3. **Antimicrobial susceptibility (%) of streptococci**

Number of Isolates	7[a]	41[a]	5[b]	257[a]	68[b]	52[b]	96[c]
Pathogen	Streptococcus agalactiae	S. dysgalactiae	S. dysgalactiae	S. uberis	S. uberis	Enterococci	Gram-positive cocci
Ampicillin	ND	ND	ND	ND	ND	ND	59
Cephalothin	100[d]	100[d]	80	100[d]	96	63	96
Cloxacillin	ND	ND	60	95	81	10	ND
Erythromycin	100	100	100	97	72	48	ND
Gentamicin	ND	63	100	11	72	67	82
Neomycin	ND	ND	80	ND	29	44	89
Novobiocin	ND	ND	80	ND	88	48	ND
Penicillin	100	100	100	100	93	60	49
Streptomycin	ND	ND	10	ND	10	35	39
Tetracycline	100	27	100	98	66	48	63

Note: Data expressed as percentage of isolates susceptible from disk assay. ND, not done.
[a]McDonald et al. (1976).
[b]Schultze (1983).
[c]Anderson et al. (1982).
[d]Cephoxazole.

However, many subclinical IMIs selected as potential therapy candidates are chronic, and particularly in the case of *Staphylococcus aureus*, prediction of therapeutic outcome by in vitro testing is poor in chronically infected quarters when compared with predictions regarding newly acquired IMIs (Owens et al., 1997). Thus, drug distribution following intramammary administration may not be efficacious, because of extensive fibrosis and microabscess formation in the gland. In addition, it is critical to assess the cow's immune status from a perspective of duration of infection, number of quarters infected, and other variables, as previously discussed.

Therapy is administered on the premise that treatment costs will be outweighed by compensatory production gains following elimination of infection. In the case of contagious pathogens, elimination of an IMI may also result in a decrease of the reservoir of infection for previously noninfected cows. Most often, the predominant pathogens causing subclinical mastitis are streptococci and staphylococci. In particular, the contagious pathogens *Streptococcus agalactiae* and *Staphylococcus aureus* offer a study in opposites with respect to therapeutic strategies.

Prevalence of *S. agalactiae* IMI can be rapidly reduced by "blitz" treatment. With this method an entire herd, or more economically, all the infected cows in a herd, are treated with antimicrobials. The most efficacious and cost-effective regimen is to employ intramammary beta-lactam therapy using approved commercial intramammary products, although use of erythromycin has been successful. All four quarters of infected cows should be treated to ensure elimination of the pathogen from the cow and prevent possible within-cow cross-infection of a noninfected quarter by an infected quarter. Cure rates can often be from 70% to 90%. Much of this success relies on the high degree of antimicrobial susceptibility of *S. agalactiae*, as well as its being essentially an obligate udder pathogen. It is necessary to monitor treated herds by somatic cell count and bacteriology to further identify and treat cows that were not initially identified as being infected. Usually, 30-day monitoring intervals after each treatment will be successful. A small percentage of cows will not respond to therapy and are best segregated or culled. Additionally, failure to use postmilking teat dipping and total dry-cow treatment to prevent new IMIs while eliminating existing IMIs by blitz treatment will ultimately result in considerable expense and frustration on the part of the producer, as well as possible reinfection of the herd. Parenteral therapy is not likely to offer any benefit over intramammary therapy, and in one study, 90% cure rates were achieved with intramammary penicillin-novobiocin therapy as opposed to 9% with IM ceftiofur, an elegant demonstration as to the importance of using pharmacokinetic considerations for parenteral drug selection (Erskine et al., 1996).

Other common streptococci causing IMI are *S. dysgalactiae, S. bovis,* and *S. uberis.* As with *S. agalactiae,* most of these streptococci are very susceptible in vitro to penicillin. Despite this apparent susceptibility, these streptococcal infections are not as easily cured as those caused by *S. agalactiae.* Controlled clinical data on the therapy of streptococcal infections is not extensive. Intramammary administration of beta-lactams or, if parenteral treatment is desired, procaine penicillin G administered at 22,000 IU/kg of body weight twice daily is considered a good drug regimen. However, efficacy and cost-effectiveness of this therapeutic regimen are at present difficult to assess. Furthermore, penicillins are poorly distributed to the mammary gland following parenteral administration. In strains with in vitro susceptibility to a combination of penicillin and novobiocin, intramammary therapy has obtained cure rates of 90% for subclinical IMIs caused by *S. agalactiae, S. uberis,* and *S. dysgalactiae* and 77% for other streptococci (Owens et al., 1997). Thus, in vitro susceptibility correlates well with clinical outcome for IMIs caused by streptococci.

Staphylococcus aureus IMIs often result in deep-seated abscesses. Therapy is difficult, especially since resistance to antimicrobial drugs (particularly beta-lactams) is more common than in streptococci, and *S. aureus* may survive within phagocytic cells following phagocytosis, where antimicrobial concentrations are reduced. Additionally, *S. aureus* has numerous extracellular substances that impart an ability to survive in the presence of a hostile host immune system. Consequently, elimination of infections by antimicrobial treatment is often not successful.

Experimentally induced *S. aureus* IMIs have cure rates of 25–55% of infected quarters when evaluated for 21–60 days after infection. However, natural infections are usually of longer duration before detection and subsequent therapy and thus are more refractory to therapy. The use of intramammary cefaperazone for the treatment of naturally occurring clinical *S. aureus* mastitis resulted in bacteriologic cures for only 39% of the cases, as measured 14 days after treatment (Wilson et al., 1986). However, as with experimental infections, these results may be optimistic, because assessment of bacteriologic cures depends on the time period during which the infection is monitored after treatment; relapses of 28 days after treatment have been reported. Treatment of IMIs caused by *S. aureus* identified as susceptible to penicillin-novobiocin resulted in cures of 70% in quarters with IMI of 14 days duration and 35% in chronically infected quarters (Owens et al., 1997). This not only reaffirms the difficulty in attaining successful therapy but also suggests a poor correlation between in vitro culture and susceptibility and therapeutic outcome in chronic IMIs caused by this organism. Consequently, novel combinations of drugs, including parenteral treatment regimens, may be needed to eliminate a higher proportion of infections. In experimental infections in lactating cows, the combined use of IM procaine penicillin G and intramammary amoxicillin achieved a better cure rate (18 of 35 infected quarters) than intramammary amoxicillin alone did (10 of 40 infected quarters (Owens et al., 1988). Parenteral administration as an adjunct to intramammary therapy has been further supported by an additional study that determined that administration of 11 mg/kg of oxytetracycline in addition to intramammary antimicrobials improved cure rates for lactating cows with *S. aureus* IMI over cure rates in cows that received intramammary infusions only (Sol et al., 1990). Additionally, therapy that is administered for longer periods than those typical for labeled intramammary regimens (4 days rather than 2 days) maintains drug concentrations above MIC of *S. aureus* in the gland for longer times and results in better efficacy (Ziv and Storper, 1985).

These studies suggest that therapy of chronic subclinical IMI may be more successful when it includes parenteral as well as intramammary therapy and is preferentially administered for periods long enough to ensure drug levels above MIC, to allow effective killing of the pathogen. However, cure rates attained may not be much better than those attained from spontaneous cure. Additionally, definitions of cure must be made critically, and affected quarters monitored bacteriologically for at least 30 days to encompass the refractory period when IMI are present but bacteria may not be isolated.

Antimicrobial Therapy of Dry Cows

The dry (nonlactating) period of the lactation cycle is a critical time for dairy animals. The major proportion of calf growth occurs during this time, and metabolically this is the most critical time for the cow to prepare for the next lactation. The mammary gland also undergoes marked biochemical, cellular, and immunological changes. Involution of the mammary parenchyma begins 1–2 days after the end of lactation and continues for 10–14 days. During this time, the gland is particularly vulnerable to new IMI, and in conjunction with the periparturient period, these are the times of greatest risk for new IMI in the lactation cycle of the cow. However, the involuted mammary gland offers the most hostile immune environment for bacterial pathogens of the lactation cycle. The most important defense, as with lactating cows, remains the teat canal. This barrier is enhanced by the formation of a keratin plug. Additionally, populations of macrophages and lymphocytes, and concentrations of complement and immunoglobulins, that can help orchestrate more efficient phagocytosis all increase. Lactoferrin, a potent iron-chelating protein, also markedly increases in dry-cow secretions, thus helping to inhibit growth of Gram-negative bacteria, particularly *E. coli*. As dry periods are usually 45–60 days in length, doses or formulations that allow extended drug presence in the gland are of minimal concern with regard to milk residues and discarded milk costs. Consequently, the dry period is an ideal time to attain synergy between antimicrobial therapy and immune function to eliminate pathogens from the gland and not incur the extensive costs typical of lactating-cow therapy. Intramammary administration of antimicrobials at the end of lactation has been a standard of dairy mastitis management for 30 years. In addition to the important role that dry-cow therapy has in eliminating existing IMI, one of the most critical roles of dry-cow therapy is the prevention of new IMI. However, most commercial dry-cow products have little or no activity against Gram-negative pathogens. These products will not be effective when administered at the start of the dry period for new IMI caused by this class of microbes, which begins in association with the periparturient period. Although cure rates for all pathogens (those IMIs that existed prior to the dry period but were not detected following calving) have been reported in initial studies as averaging 75%, efficacy of conventional dry-cow treatments in eliminating more chronic IMI such as those caused by *Staphylococcus aureus* may be lower. More-recent reports have cited success and failure of intramammary infusions at dry-off for curing IMI during the dry period. Undoubtedly, success may vary from herd to herd and from cow to cow. The importance of repeat sampling to detect the true prevalence of subclinical IMI was discussed earlier. Many studies do not use consistent sampling methods to identify infected quarters before or after the dry period. Thus, it is possible that the discrepancies among studies may be accounted for in the differences of experimental methods used to determine IMI.

As with lactational therapy, the use of systemic administration as an adjunct to intramammary administration has stimulated interest in potential alternative therapeutic regimens. SC norfloxacin nicotinate administered at the start of the dry period achieved a better cure rate and a lower new infection rate over the dry period for *S. aureus* infections than the rates in untreated cows and cows administered intramammary cephapirin benzathine preparations (Soback et al., 1990). However, in a Michigan study, cows administered IM oxytetracycline and intramammary cephapirin did not have better cure rates for quarters infected with *S. aureus* than cows treated with cephapirin only (Kaneene and Miller, 1992), although this study was performed in a herd with a prevalence of *S. aureus* in 50% of the cows, and the IMIs were chronic and of long duration. This may have had an important bearing on the success of therapy. Additionally, we should not limit our evaluation of dry-cow therapy on the success of eliminating IMI caused by *S. aureus* only. For many other Gram-positive cocci, therapeutic efficacy can be 80–90%.

Attempts to enhance immune function and clearance with immune modulators, either solely or synergistically with antimicrobials, are also an area of potential future importance for mastitis therapy. Recombinant cytokines are becoming available. Cytokines that have demonstrated promise for use in the prevention and/or treatment of bovine mastitis are interleukin-1 (IL-1), interleukin-2 (IL-2), interferons, and colony-stimulating factor. Intramammary IL-1β and IL-2 increase mammary gland polymorphonuclear leukocyte diapedesis, and IL-2 activates inducible superoxide production. However, field trials using intramammary IL-2 as an adjunct therapy with intramammary cephapirin determined little or no benefit of IL-2 in curing or preventing IMI in the dry period. IL-2 has been associated with abortions in treated cattle 3–5 days after infusion. Future research may elucidate potential uses of immune modulation, but because the bioagents in this class are potent and have complex actions, care will be necessary to attain the desired antimicrobial effect without other side effects.

Thus, the important considerations for dry-cow treatment are as follows: (1) Commercial dry cow treatment is generally effective against Gram-positive cocci in preventing, as well as eliminating IMI; (2) because of enhanced immune function and decreased discarded milk costs, dry cows should be preferentially treated rather than lactating cows for subclinical and chronic IMI; (3) most commercial intramammary products have little efficacy against Gram-negative pathogens; and (4) treatment of more-chronic IMIs should include systemic drug regimens, preferably antimicrobials that distribute well in mammary tissue, such as tetracyclines, macrolides, and fluoroquinolones, where these are allowed for such a purpose.

Antimicrobial Therapy of Heifers

By convention, heifers were considered to be essentially free of IMI before calving and, except for the rare case, needed little therapeutic attention until after lactation, when the risk of infection increased. Many IMIs in calving heifers are caused by staphylococcal species other than *S. aureus,* which have a high rate of spontaneous cure. However, it is apparent that under some herd conditions, a substantial portion of heifers at calving are infected, and additionally some of the IMIs can be caused by pathogens such as *S. aureus.* There is a geographical element of risk to this problem, and fly-bite dermatitis of the teat end, which compromises this important physical barrier to infection, may play a role in the pathogenesis. The potentially most significant problems have been reported in relation to IMIs caused by staphylococci, which are known to colonize skin and readily increase in numbers in the presence of lesions. Clinical investigations

TABLE 31.4. **Framework for designing therapeutic protocols for mastitis**

	Severe Clinical Mastitis (systemic involvement)	Mild Clinical Mastitis, Initial Case	Mild Clinical Mastitis, Recurrence	Subclinical Mastitis
Supportive fluids, anti-inflammatory drugs, electrolytes, nutritional supplements	Indicated as primary therapy, especially if cow is in shock	Not indicated	Not indicated	Not indicated
Intramammary antimicrobials	Labeled use of commercial products suggested	Labeled use of commercial products suggested	Judicious use if economically viable and not a chronic IMI	Lactating cows: indicated for *Streptococcus agalactiae,* generally not recommended for other pathogens. Dry cows: recommended for all cows
Parenteral antimicrobials	Broad-spectrum in activity, and milk and meat withholding times strictly followed	Not indicated	Generally not indicated; judicious use if economically viable and not a chronic IMI	For chronic IMI caused by Gram-positive cocci, as an adjunct therapy to intramammary infusion at dry-off; treatment of lactating cows with subclinical IMI is not recommended

have indicated intramammary infusions of lactating-cow preparations of beta-lactams 7 days before expected calving dates as a means to reduce the rate of IMI at calving. However, as with cows, strict teat end antisepsis should be followed before infusion to prevent any contamination; labor to handle animals for treatment can be extensive; and the risk of antimicrobial residues in milk following calving is greater than in untreated heifers. This is not a recommended management program for many dairies. However, if herd records indicate that an undesirable proportion of first-lactation animals are infected at calving, particularly with staphylococci, then this regimen may be suitable to reduce losses.

Therapeutic Protocols

A framework for therapeutic protocols is shown in Table 31.4.

Bibliography

Anderson KL. 1989. Therapy for acute coliform mastitis. Compend Contin Educ Pract Vet 11:1125.

Anderson KL, et al. 1982. Diagnosis and treatment of acute mastitis in a large dairy herd. J Am Vet Med Assoc 181:690.

Cattell MB. 1996. An outbreak of *Streptococcus uberis* as a consequence of adopting a protocol of no antibiotic therapy for clinical mastitis. Proc 35th Annu Meet Natl Mastitis Counc, p123.

Craven N, et al. 1986. Antimicrobial drug susceptibility of *Staphylococcus aureus* isolated from bovine mastitis. Vet Rec 118:290.

Davidson JN. 1980. Antibiotic resistance patterns of bovine mastitis pathogens. Proc 19th Annu Meet Natl Mastitis Counc, p181.

Erskine RJ, Eberhart RJ. 1990. Herd benefit-to-cost ratio and effects of a bovine mastitis control program that includes blitz treatment of *Streptococcus agalactiae*. J Am Vet Med Assoc 196:1230.

Erskine RJ, et al. 1992. Intramammary gentamicin as a therapy for experimental *Escherichia coli* mastitis. J Am Vet Med Assoc 53:375.

Erskine RJ, et al. 1993. Advances in the therapy of mastitis. Vet Clin North Am 9:499.

Erskine RJ, et al. 1995. Ceftiofur distribution in serum and milk from clinically normal cows and cows with experimental *Escherichia coli*–induced mastitis. Am J Vet Res 56:481.

Erskine RJ, et al. 1996. Intramuscular administration of ceftiofur sodium versus intramammary infusion of penicillin/novobiocin for treatment of *Streptococcus agalactiae* mastitis in dairy cows. J Am Vet Med Assoc 208:258.

Erskine RJ, et al. 1998. Recombinant bovine interleukin-2 and dry-cow therapy: efficacy to cure and prevent intramammary infections, safety, and effect on gestation. J Dairy Sci 81:107.

Guterbock WM, et al. 1993. Efficacy of intramammary antibiotic therapy for treatment of clinical mastitis caused by environmental pathogens. J Dairy Sci 76:3437.

Jones GF, Ward GE. 1990. Evaluation of systemic administration of gentamicin for treatment of coliform mastitis in cows. J Am Vet Med Assoc 197:731.

Kaneene JB, Miller RA. 1992. Description and evaluation of the influence of veterinary presence on the use of antibiotics and sulfonamides in dairy herds. JAVMA 201:68.

Katholm J. 1988. Pyogenes mastitis—improved therapy. Dan Veterinaertidskr 71:257.

Kirk JH. 1991a. Diagnosis and treatment of difficult mastitis cases, part 1. *Agri-Practice* 12:5.

Kirk JH. 1991b. Diagnosis and treatment of difficult mastitis cases, part 2. *Agri-Practice* 12:15.

Larson VL, et al. 1981. Therapy of acute toxic mastitis. Proc 20th Annu Meet Natl Mastitis Counc, p168.

Mackie DP, et al. 1988. Antibiotic sensitivity of bovine staphylococcal and coliform isolates over four years. Vet Rec 123:515.

McDonald JS, et al. 1977. Antibiotic sensitivity of aerobic Gram-negative rods isolated from bovine udder infections. Am J Vet Res 38:1503.

McDonald TJ, et al. 1976. Antibiograms of streptococci isolated from bovine mammary infections. Am J Vet Res 37:1185.

Morin D, et al. 1998. Comparison of antibiotic administration in conjunction with supportive measures versus supportive measures alone for treatment of dairy cows with clinical mastitis. J Am Vet Med Assoc 213:676.

Muckle CA, et al. 1986. Susceptibility of *Escherichia coli* from bovine mastitis to new antimicrobial drugs. Can J Vet Res 50:543.

Newbould FHS. 1974. Antibiotic treatment of experimental *Staphylococcus aureus* infections of the bovine mammary gland. Can J Comp Med 38:411.

Oliver S, et al. 1992. Influence of prepartum antibiotic therapy on intramammary infections in primigravid heifers during early lactation. J Dairy Sci 75:406.

Owens WE, et al. 1988. Antibiotic treatment of mastitis: comparison of intramammary and intramammary plus intramuscular therapies. J Dairy Sci 71:3143.

Owens WE, et al. 1990. Determination of milk and mammary tissue concentrations of ceftiofur after intramammary and intramuscular therapy. J Dairy Sci 73:3449.

Owens WE, et al. 1997. Comparison of success of antibiotic therapy during lactation and results of antimicrobial susceptibility tests for bovine mastitis. J Dairy Sci 80:313.

Pyorala S, et al. 1994. Efficacy of two therapy regimens for treatment of experimentally induced *Escherichia coli* mastitis in cows. J Dairy Sci 77:453.

Schultze WD. 1983. Effects of a selective regimen of dry cow therapy on intramammary infection and on antibiotic sensitivity of surviving pathogens. J Dairy Sci 66:892.

Sears PM, et al. 1987. Isolation of L-form variants after antibiotic treatment in *Staphylococcus aureus* bovine mastitis. J Am Vet Med Assoc 191:681.

Sears PM, et al. 1990. Shedding patterns of *Staphylococcus aureus* from bovine intramammary infections. J Dairy Sci 73:2785.

Shpigel NY, et al. 1997. Efficacy of cefquinome for treatment of cows with mastitis experimentally induced using *Escherichia coli*. J Dairy Sci 80:323.

Soback S, et al. 1989. Pharmacokinetics of ceftiofur administered intravenously and intramuscularly to lactating cows. Isr J Vet Med 45:118.

Soback S, et al. 1990. Systemic dry cow therapy in control of subclinical *Staphylococcus aureus* infections. Proc Int Symp Bovine Mastitis, p134.

Sol J, et al. 1990. Factors affecting the result of dry cow treatment. Proc Int Symp Bovine Mastitis, p118.

Weaver LD, et al. 1986. Treatment of *Streptococcus agalactiae* mastitis in dairy cows: comparative efficacies of two antibiotic preparations and factors associated with successful treatment. J Am Vet Med Assoc 189:666.

Wilson CD, et al. 1986. Field trials with cefaperazone in the treatment of bovine clinical mastitis. Vet Rec 118:17.

Wilson DJ, et al. 1990. *Serratia marcescens* mastitis in a dairy herd. J Am Vet Med Assoc 196:1102.

Yamagata M, et al. 1987. The economic benefit of treating subclinical *Streptococcus agalactiae* mastitis in lactating cows. J Am Vet Med Assoc 191:1556.

Ziv G. 1980. Practical pharmacokinetic aspects of mastitis therapy–2: practical and therapeutic applications. Agri-Practice (March):469.

Ziv G. 1992. Treatment of acute mastitis. Vet Clin North Am 8:1.

Ziv G, Storper M. 1985. Intramuscular treatment of subclinical staphylococcal mastitis in lactating cows with penicillin G, methicillin, and their esters. J Vet Pharmacol Ther 8:276.

Ziv G, et al. 1990. Incidence of new *S. aureus* infections during the dry period in antibiotic-treated and non-treated infected and non-infected cows. Proc Int Symp Bovine Mastitis, p123a.

32 | Growth Promotion and Feed Antibiotics

T. J. SHRYOCK

Antibiotics have been administered as medicated feedstuffs to healthy livestock and poultry to promote feed efficiency and improve the rate of weight gain for more than 50 years (Gustafson and Bowen, 1997). Antibiotics used in this manner have been termed growth promoters, production enhancers, digestive enhancers, or feed additives. Since the concentration of antibiotic in the feed is lower than what is used for therapeutic purposes, the term *subtherapeutic* is often used to describe this application. *Subtherapeutic* does not necessarily equate to *sub-MIC* concentrations (ie, concentrations below the MIC derived from in vitro susceptibility testing) against intestinal microflora. Generally, growth promoters are incorporated into the feed ration at a feed mill and then provided to the animal. Currently, growth promotion uses are approved in cattle, swine, and poultry (and several minor species), but none are approved for aquaculture. Most countries allow growth promoters to be used in their animal production industries to maximize productivity in highly competitive commercial environments. Although the focus of this chapter is growth promotion, it must be recognized that disease prevention can also occur. It is difficult to separate the two effects when evaluating animal performance data, because many of the improvements related to weight gain and feed efficiency are intimately associated with preventing subclinical disease in an otherwise apparently healthy animal.

The use of antibiotics to improve animal productivity has been highly regulated over the years because of potential human health concerns. Consequently, a variety of safety studies on residues, toxicology, worker safety, and food safety are required. Strict policies on residue avoidance are enforced to assure a safe product. In spite of these

735

safeguards, controversy has continued for several decades on the magnitude of selection of antibiotic-resistant bacteria in food animals and its implications to human medicine.

Regulatory Review Criteria

To assure the safety and efficacy of antibiotics used as growth promoters, government regulatory authorities have developed and refined stringent requirements, and the manufacturer must provide satisfactory data to receive a product registration. Target species studies include safety (biological, toxicological, macroscopic, and histological); microbiological (antibacterial spectrum, cross-resistance to therapeutic antibiotics, resistance selection, effects on digestive tract microflora, effects on shedding and colonization of pathogens, and field studies to monitor for antibiotic resistance); and metabolism and residues. Studies on excreted residues or on environmental toxicology are necessary. The final area of data is toxicological (environmental, acute and chronic toxicity, mutagenicity, carcinogenicity, reproductive toxicity, and metabolite toxicity). Based on these types of studies, withdrawal periods are established so that any residues will be safely below agreed-upon limits. Specific information on the approval criteria and regulatory process for antibiotics used as feed additives in the United States and those in the European Union have been separately described (Lawrence, 1998; National Research Council, 1999), although other countries have similar regulatory agencies and requirements. An interesting contrast between the two regulatory systems is the recognition in the United States that the same concentration used for growth promotion may also have disease prevention claims, whereas in the European Union there can be none. This may become problematic when data on control of disease at growth promotion levels are available (Tsinas et al., 1998).

Antibiotics approved as feed additives for growth promotion in the United States are listed in Table 32.1 and those in the European Union are in Table 32.2. Following the recommendations of the Swann Committee in 1969, most growth promoters in Europe are either nontherapeutic antibiotics, ionophores, or synthetic compounds—hence the exclusion of tetracyclines and penicillins. In 1996, avoparcin was suspended from the list of European Union–approved products, pending a reevaluation of the potential medical impact associated with the selection of glycopeptide-resistant enterococci during its use. Following this precedent, in late 1998, the European Agriculture Council and Commission voted to invoke the "precautionary principle" for tylosin, bacitracin, spiramycin, and virginiamycin, thereby prohibiting them from feed additive use (ie, nontherapeutic use), effective July 1999.

TABLE 32.1. Antibacterial feed additives approved for growth promotion in cattle, swine, and poultry in the United States

Drug	Antibiotic Class	Cattle	Swine	Poultry
Arsenicals	Arsenical		+	+
Bacitracin	Polypeptide	+	+	+
Bambermycins	Glycophospholipid	+	+	+
Carbadox	Quinoxaline		+	
Tetracyclines	Tetracycline	+	+	+
Chlortetracycline, sulfamethazine, penicillin			+(<75 lb)	
Lasalocid	Ionophore	+		
Lincomycin	Lincosamide		+(>75 lb)	+
Monensin	Ionophore	+		
Penicillin	Beta-lactam		+	+
Tiamulin	Pleuromutilin		+	
Tylosin	Macrolide	+	+	
Virginiamycin	Streptogramin	+	+	+

Source: Feed Additive Compendium (1999).

TABLE 32.2. Antibacterial feed additives approved for growth promotion in cattle, swine, and poultry in the European Union

Drug	Antibiotic Class	Cattle	Swine	Poultry
Avoparcin[a]	Glycopeptide	+	+	+
Bacitracin[b]	Polypeptide	+ (calves)	+	+
Flavophospholipid	Glycophospholipid	+	+	+
Monensin	Ionophore	+		
Salinomycin	Ionophore		+	
Spiramycin[b]	Macrolide	+ (calves)	+	+
Tylosin[b]	Macrolide		+	
Virginiamycin[b]	Streptogramin	+ (calves)	+	+
Avilamycin	Orthosomycin		+	+
Carbadox[a]	Quinoxaline		+(<4 months)	
Olaquindox[a]	Quinoxaline		+(<4 months)	

Source: Corpet (1996); Commission on Antimicrobial Feed Additives (1997); Lawrence (1998).
[a]Suspended or withdrawn.
[b]Authorization withdrawn under EU Council Directive 70/524/EEC; effective July 1999.

Mechanism of Action

In healthy animals the role of the normal digestive tract bacterial flora has been studied, but not completely elucidated, by comparing germ-free animals to animals raised conventionally and by comparing the response of each group to antibiotic administration (Coates, 1980; Ratcliffe, 1991). Conventional animals are mildly impaired in growth performance and efficiency of feed conversion when compared with gnotobiotic, or "germ-free," animals, possibly because the presence of weakly pathogenic bacteria in the intestines of conventional animals is deleterious. When a low concentration of an antibiotic was administered, only the growth response of the conventionally grown animals matched that of the germ-free group; the antibiotic had no effect on the germ-free group. Because antibiotics in the digestive tract of animals are likely to inhibit the growth and/or metabolism of susceptible populations of bacterial flora, and most of the antibiotics used for growth promotion have a Gram-positive spectrum of activity, Gram-positive bacteria such as clostridia, enterococci, bacilli, and others seem likely candidates. In essence, the administration of an antibiotic serves to allow a conventionally raised animal to grow like an optimally growing germ-free animal.

Additional studies on the physiological, nutritional, metabolic, microbiological, and immunological effects associated with the use of antibiotic feed additives demonstrate the complexity of their mode of action (Hays, 1969; Visek, 1978; Commission on Antimicrobial Feed Additives, 1997). Table 32.3 describes the reported effects, which can be summarized as follows: (1) inhibit growth or metabolism of harmful gut bacteria; (2) decrease elaboration of toxic substances, including bacterial toxins; (3) reduce bacterial destruction of essential nutrients; (4) increase synthesis of vitamins and other growth factors; (5) improve efficiency of nutrient absorption by modifying the gut wall; (6) reduce intestinal mucosal epithelial cell turnover; and (7) reduce intestinal motility. Recent work has shown that antibiotics administered to immune system–stimulated animals allowed them to grow at rates similar to those of min-

TABLE 32.3.   **Some physiological, nutritional, and metabolic effects ascribed to antibiotic feed additives**

Physiological Effects[a]		Nutritional Effects		Metabolic Effects	
Gut food	–	Energy retention	+	Ammonia production	–
Gut wall	–	Gut energy loss	–	Toxic amine production	–
Gut wall length	–	Nitrogen retention	+	Alpha-toxin production	–
Gut wall weight	–	Limiting amino acid supply	+	Fatty acid oxidation	–
Gut absorptive capacity	+	Vitamin absorption	+	Fecal fat excretion	–
Fecal moisture	–	Vitamin synthesis	–	Liver protein synthesis	+
Mucosal cell turnover	–	Trace element absorption	+	Gut alkaline phosphatase	+
Stress	–	Fatty acid absorption	+	Gut urease	–
Feed intake	±	Glucose absorption	+		
		Calcium absorption	+		
		Plasma nutrients	+		

Source: Commission on Antimicrobial Feed Additives (1997).
[a]+, increase; –, decrease.

imally stressed, nonmedicated animals. The effect of the antibiotics in this phenomenon may be to modulate intestinal bacteria whose components stimulate cytokines, such as tumor necrosis factor (which exerts a catabolic or negative growth effect), and thereby allow the animal to grow efficiently.

Usage Practices and Benefits

Over the course of the last half of the twentieth century, numerous changes in the production of food animals have taken place, most notably the consolidation of production toward large, company-operated farms that raise the vast majority of livestock and poultry indoors in groups (the notable exception remains feedlot beef cattle). Improvements in animal genetics, herd/flock management, medicines, feedstuffs, and hygiene have allowed increased production of meat and other foods of animal origin to meet the demand in a safe, cost-efficient manner. The use of antibiotics to facilitate growth promotion has evolved during this period, so that today a wide variety of application strategies abound regarding product choice, age of animal medicated, duration of medication, and use of professional consultation (Dewey et al., 1997). The incorporation rate of most antibiotics is on the order of 5–125 ppm (or g/ton), which equates to only a few mg/kg on a daily intake basis.

The percentage improvement in performance of pigs fed antibiotics has been summarized in Table 32.4. The efficacy of growth promotion use has been constant over the two periods compared and for the two categories of pigs reported. The growth response is greater in the starter than in the grower-finisher, an observation consistent with actual use practices (Dewey et al., 1997). Recent information suggests that growth promoters reduced the variation in size of slaughter animals and thereby improved the ability to process the carcass and improved the quality of the meat product.

The economic benefits of using antibiotics in production animals have been described from various perspectives in the United States and

TABLE 32.4. Percentage improvement in performance of pigs fed antimicrobials for specific years

| Years | Periods[a] | Improvement (%) | |
		Daily Gain	Feed/Gain
1950–1977	Starter	16.1	6.9
	Grower-finisher	4.0	2.1
1978–1985	Starter	15.0	6.5
	Grower-finisher	3.6	2.4

Source: Zimmerman (1986).

[a]Starter period from about 8 to 26 kg and grower-finishers period from 27 to 92 kg body weight.

Europe, including the consequences of their discontinued use (USDA, 1978; Council of Agricultural Scientists, 1981; MacKinnon, 1986; Zimmerman, 1986; Commission on Antimicrobial Feed Additives, 1997; Lawrence, 1998; National Research Council, 1999). Although the return per animal (in terms of gain accrued from the use of growth promotion) is small, the cumulative effect on an industry that produces millions of animals (and billions of chickens) each year is economically significant. For an individual producer, the profit margin attributed to the use of a growth promoter has sometimes made the difference between profit and loss. Finally, in order to maintain animal production in the absence of growth promoters, an increase in animals was projected that would increase the need for the environmental resources.

The ecological benefits of using antibiotics in production animals accrue from the more efficient production of animals by reducing days to market, quantity of feed required, nitrogen and phosphorous excretion, manure, and water consumption (Lawrence, 1998). A reduced need for feed means less land (and associated herbicides, etc.) required for crop production.

Manufacturing Issues

Feed additives are manufactured under strict guidelines as premix products (Feed Additive Compendium, 1999). The final medicated feedstuff is manufactured at the feed mill to conform to tight inclusion range specifications for potency, then bagged or delivered in bulk to the farm, where it is used before the expiration date. Assays for potency and cross-contamination are routinely performed. Although rare, it is possible that the clean-out between batches of different medicated feedstuffs results in the inadvertent administration of a feed additive to a species for which it was not intended, resulting in an adverse consequence.

Worker safety issues are considered in the manufacture of medicated feedstuffs. Dust particles are controlled by minimizing inhalation through personal respirators and containment processes. Newer methods of medicating feedstuffs use a liquid premix sprayed onto the feed to minimize cross-contamination and inhalation of premix dust particles. Some workers may be allergic to the antibiotics (eg, penicillin) and should avoid the handling of such products.

Public Health and Environmental Concerns
Antibiotic Residues in Meats

During the regulatory review process, withdrawal times are established for meat and other edible tissues to allow the animal to eliminate the antibiotic naturally. Acceptable limits for residue are set as part of this process. When an edible tissue is assayed and found to exceed this limit, a violative residue is reported, the product is condemned, and the producer is penalized. In order to avoid this situation, producers, industry associations, and companies have developed quality assurance programs to document the use of antibiotics and to observe the proper withdrawal times. Consequently, the rate of violative residues is extremely low for antibiotics in general (0.12% in 1997; National Research Council, 1999) in spite of the high numbers of animals processed (see Chapter 33).

Salmonella Reservoir

Concern has been raised that an enhanced excretion of enteric pathogens, particularly salmonella, is attributable to the use of antibiotics in feed (which are presumed to disrupt normal protective flora that competitively exclude the pathogens) (Solomons, 1978; Corpet, 1996). To address this issue, manufacturers provide data to regulatory authorities that demonstrate that feed additives do not increase the prevalence, quantity, or duration of salmonella in medicated animals compared to nonmedicated controls and, furthermore, that antibiotic susceptibility is not significantly altered in the salmonella (Solomons, 1978; Lawrence, 1998). A review of research studies on antibiotic effects and salmonella suggests that discrepancies in outcomes may be due to the various study designs employed (Commission, 1997). There are fewer studies on enteric bacteria other than salmonella.

Antibiotic-resistant Food-Borne Bacteria

The public health implications of antibiotic-resistant food-borne bacteria, attributable to growth promotion use in animals, have been studied by numerous committees for more than three decades (CAS, 1981; Institute of Medicine, 1989; Gustafson et al., 1997; Lawrence, 1998; National Research Council, 1999). Although antibiotic-resistant bacteria have been detected in medicated animals and humans, definitive proof that these bacteria have caused treatment failures in humans is lacking. Microorganisms of concern include not only salmonella but also, more recently, campylobacter and enterococci (see Chapter 3). Since enterococci have developed resistance to many "last-resort" antibiotics used in human medicine (eg, vancomycin), newer analogs are being developed from the classes currently used as growth promotion antibiotics (eg, streptogramins, orthosomycin). These issues are discussed in more detail in Chapter 3.

Environmental Concerns

Since medicated feedstuffs are consumed and then excreted via the urine and feces of animals, the potential exists for biologically active antibiotic or metabolites, as well as antibiotic-resistant bacteria, to enter the environment via the waste stream from production facilities (Commission, 1997). Manufacturers of feed additives supply environmental fate studies to regulatory agencies that describe the soil half-life of the antibiotic and related metabolites, as well as data on soil-associated organisms, fish, wildlife, and plants.

Current Status and Future Developments
Monitoring Programs

Within the past several years, because of concerns related to antibiotic resistance (particularly in enterococci), antibiotic susceptibility testing of isolates from various sources is under way in a number of countries in order to develop a baseline of data to monitor resistance. These programs are sponsored by feed additive manufacturer associations, by government agencies, and by other groups in both the United States and Europe.

New Antibiotic Growth Promoters

Several antibiotics have been described as potential new growth promoters. Ardacin (a glycopeptide) and efrotomycin have been described but not marketed (Corpet, 1996). Alexomycin, a novel class, has been identified as a possible new product candidate with no medical use constraints.

Bibliography

Coates ME. 1980. The gut microflora and growth. In: Lawrence TLJ, ed. Growth in Animals. Boston: Butterworths.

Commission on Antimicrobial Feed Additives. 1997. Antimicrobial feed additives. Swed Gov Off Rep 132. Stockholm, Sweden.

Corpet DE. 1996. Microbiological hazards for humans of antimicrobial growth promoter use in animal production. Rev Med Vet 147:851.

Council of Agricultural Scientists. 1981. Antibiotics in animal feeds. Counc Ag Sci Tech Rep 88. Ames, IA.

Dewey CE, et al. 1997. Associations between off-label feed additives and farm size, veterinary consultant use, and animal age. Prev Vet Med 31:133.

Feed Additive Compendium. 1999. Minnetonka, MN: Miller.

Gustafson RH, Bowen RE. 1997. Antibiotic use in animal agriculture. J Appl Microbiol 83:531.

Hays VW. 1969. Biological basis for the use of antibiotics in livestock production. In: The use of drugs in animal feeds. Washington, DC: National Academy of Sciences.

Institute of Medicine. 1989. Human health risks with the subtherapeutic use of penicillin or tetracyclines in animal feed. Washington, DC: National Academy Press.

Lawrence K. 1998. Growth promoters in swine. Proc 15th Int Pig Vet Soc Congr, p337.

MacKinnon JD. 1986. The role of growth promoters in pig production. Pig Vet Soc 17:69.

National Research Council, Committee on Drug Use in Food Animals. 1999. The use of drugs in food animals: benefits and risks. Washington, DC: National Academy Press.

Ratcliffe B. 1991. The role of the microflora in digestion. In: In Vitro Digestion for Pigs and Poultry. Fuller, MF, ed. Wallingford, UK: Commonwealth Agricultural Bureau.

Solomons IA. 1978. Antibiotics in animal feeds—human and animal safety issues. J Anim Sci 46:1360.

Tsinas AC, et al. 1998. Control of proliferative enteropathy in growing/fattening pigs using growth promoters. J Vet Med 45B:115.

U.S. Department of Agriculture. 1978. Economic effects of a prohibition on the use of selected animal drugs. USDA Ag Econ Rep 414. Washington, DC.

Visek WJ. 1978. The mode of growth promotion by antibiotics. J Anim Sci 46:1447.

Zimmerman DR. 1986. Role of subtherapeutic levels of antimicrobials in pig production. J Anim Sci 62 (Suppl 3):6.

33 | Antimicrobial Drug Residues in Food-producing Animals

S. F. SUNDLOF, A. H. FERNANDEZ, and J. C. PAIGE

Adulteration of the food supply by foreign chemicals is an important and costly problem to the livestock industry. Consumer health-related concerns has led to public demand for national governments to establish regulatory programs that ensure that unsafe residues do not contaminate the food supply. The failure of governments to adequately address public concerns over drug residues in animal-derived foods has affected international markets for meat and poultry resulting in embargoes and other nontariff trade barriers.

Causes and Incidence of Residue Violations in the United States

Chemicals that persist as residues in food animals can be classified as drugs, pesticides, environmental contaminants, and naturally occurring toxicants. Of these, drugs are the most frequently detected chemicals, the overwhelming majority of which are antimicrobials.

Unlike environmental contaminants and naturally occurring toxicants, drugs are intentionally administered to food-producing animals. When administered in accordance with the approved labeling, the prevalence of violative drug residues in animal products will be less than 1% of such products. Residue violation rates greater than 1%, therefore, generally indicate that the drug has been used in some manner that was inconsistent with the labeling. The fact that antimicrobial drugs account for most of the residue violations detected by U.S. Department of Agriculture monitoring implies that extralabel use is more common for these drugs than for other therapeutic agents. During the period between 1960 and

744

1972, the prevalence of violative antimicrobial drug residues in swine, lambs, calves, and fat cattle slaughtered in the United States was 30%, 21%, 18%, and 7%, respectively (Huber, 1971). Prior to 1962, approximately 13% of all milk produced in the United States contained residues of antimicrobial drugs (Huber, 1971). Since 1962 the prevalence of antibiotic residues in milk declined to well below 1%. This figure may be misleading, however, because the required method used to test milk for antimicrobial drugs was very sensitive to the beta-lactam antibiotics but not sensitive to other classes of antimicrobial drugs. Studies using more-sensitive detection methods indicate that the prevalence of oxytetracycline and sulfamethazine residues in milk may be as high as 40% and 70%, respectively (Brady and Katz, 1988; Collins-Thompson et al., 1988; Grassie, 1988).

The U.S. Department of Agriculture's Food Safety and Inspection Service (FSIS) is responsible for the monitoring and surveillance of red meat and poultry for residues of drugs and other chemicals. The FSIS National Residue Program consists of a system based on hazard analysis and critical control point (HACCP), which is consistent with the principles of risk analysis. Under the monitoring program, a statistically based selection of random samples from healthy-appearing animals is collected at slaughter, and these samples are analyzed for specific chemical compounds. The number of samples chosen for a given compound in a particular animal species is designed to assure detection of a national problem that affects a specified percentage of the animal population of interest. Generally, the number of samples will provide 95% probability of detecting at least one violation when 1% of the animal population sampled contains residues at violative concentrations. Each year, FSIS analyzes approximately 40,000 samples from all market classes of food-producing animals (cattle, swine, chickens, and turkeys).

Unlike the monitoring program in which healthy-appearing animals are sampled on a random basis, the surveillance program (enforcement testing) focuses on obtaining samples from animals suspected to contain violative drug residues in their tissues. Examples of these suspect animals include culled dairy cows, bob veal calves (calves <3 weeks of age and weighing <68 kg), any animal with visible evidence of an injection site, any animal showing evidence of an infectious disease, or animals of a given production class for which a high incidence of residue violations has been detected through the monitoring program. Carcasses from suspect animals sampled under the surveillance program are usually retained at the abattoirs until the results of the residue testing are available. Approximately 350,000 samples are analyzed each year under the surveillance program (Patel et al., 1997). In-plant tests used during enforcement testing provide a rapid screening method to detect the presence of residues. Such tests include the Sulfa-On-Site (SOS), Calf Antibiotic and Sulfonamide Test

(CAST), Swab Test on Premises (STOP), and the Fast Antimicrobial Screen Test (FAST).

The most frequently occurring antimicrobial drugs causing residues in 1993–1997 include penicillin, oxytetracycline, and gentamicin. Penicillin residues accounted for 26–35% of all the violative residues reported in 1993–1997. Most of the violative penicillin residues occurred in culled dairy cows, cow-beef, and bob veal. Streptomycin residues accounted for 15% of all violative residues in 1993, but the prevalence has since declined to about 7%. The prevalence of oxytetracycline residues has remained relatively constant, accounting for 11–17% of all violative residues. Although sulfamethazine has remained the most frequently reported residue over time, in 1996 and 1997 there were more violative residues of sulfadimethoxine than sulfamethazine. The prevalence of gentamicin residues appears to be increasing over time accounting for 13% of all violative residues in 1997, whereas neomycin residues remained relatively constant, accounting for 5% of all violative residues (Table 33.1). The bovine species accounted for 91% (1,179 of 1,292) of the reported violations, with culled dairy cows contributing to 60% of the violations, bob veal 16%, cows-beef 9%, and other subclasses of bovine 6% (Table 33.2).

Several factors contribute to the drug residue problem, but most violations result from use of the drug in some manner that is inconsistent with the labeling. Analysis of the probable causes for violative residues in the United States reveal that failure to observe withdrawal times, drugs administered in error, treatment of animals with greater than labeled

TABLE 33.1. **Antimicrobial residue violations in the United States in 1997 reported by slaughter class under the USDA/FSIS Surveillance Program**

Animal Class	Number of Residues	%
Cows, dairy	769	60
Bob, veal	204	16
Cows, beef	120	9
Steers	39	3
Barrow/guilt/market hogs	39	3
Horses	25	1.9
Heifers	20	1.5
Bulls/stags/boars	14	1.1
Formula-fed veal	13	1.0
Sows	8	0.6
Goats	8	0.6
Non-formula-fed veal	7	0.5
Heavy cows	7	0.5
Young chickens	7	0.5
Rabbits	6	0.46
Young turkeys	2	0.15
Lambs/yearlings	2	0.15
Other (geese 1, buffalo 1)	2	0.15
Total	1,292	100

TABLE 33.2. Antimicrobial residue violations in the United States from 1993 to 1997 reported under the USDA/FSIS Surveillance Program

Antimicrobial	1993		1994		1995		1996		1997		Total 1993–1997	
Penicillin	856	(31)	629	(28)	563	(26)	520	(29)	449	(35)	3,017	(29)
Oxytetracycline	409	(15)	304	(13)	376	(17)	255	(14)	139	(11)	1,483	(14)
Sulfamethazine	394	(14)	293	(13)	180	(8)	119	(7)	104	(8)	1,090	(11)
Other	146	(5)	371	(16)	208	(10)	183	(10)	84	(7)	992	(10)
Streptomycin	416	(15)	177	(8)	99	(5)	123	(7)	117	(9)	932	(9)
Tetracycline	166	(6)	154	(7)	188	(9)	201	(11)	66	(5)	775	(8)
Gentamicin	150	(5)	108	(5)	122	(6)	168	(9)	171	(13)	719	(7)
Neomycin	143	(5)	120	(5)	264	(12)	89	(5)	47	(4)	663	(6)
Sulfadimethoxine	101	(4)	101	(4)	161	(7)	136	(8)	115	(9)	614	(6)
Total	2,781	(100)	2,257	(99)	2,161	(100)	1,794	(100)	1,292	(101)	10,285	(100)

Note: Numbers in parentheses are percent of total violative antimicrobial residues.

doses, failure to use the appropriate route of administration, and improper maintenance of medication records are identifiable risk factors (Paige et al., 1999). Adherence to withdrawal times may be considered burdensome, inconvenient, and expensive in that nonmedicated feed must be provided during the withdrawal period, and this requires the changing of feed programs and containers for the short time at the end of the feeding period (Huber, 1971). Improper maintenance of treatment records or the failure to identify treated animals adequately can lead to abbreviated withdrawal periods. When drugs are administered to animals at dosages greater than those specified in the labeling, or when drugs are used in species for which they are not approved, withdrawal periods must be estimated. These estimated withdrawal periods may be inadequate in duration to prevent violative drug residues from persisting in the carcass, milk, or eggs. Attempting to salvage, for slaughter purposes, terminally ill animals that have recently been treated with antimicrobial drugs is a common cause of violative drug residues, especially in culled dairy cows. Educational intervention during follow-up investigations by regulatory authorities can prevent similar events from recurring in the future.

Effect of Food-borne Drug Residues on Human Health
Regulation of Veterinary Drugs

Before any drug can be approved in the United States for use in a food-producing animal, an extensive toxicologic evaluation of the drug and its metabolites must be undertaken to ensure that any residues persisting in animal-derived foods do not pose a health threat to the consumer. A battery of four toxicologic tests is required to satisfy human food-safety requirements for any new animal drug intended for use in a food-producing animal species:

1. Metabolism studies for identification of residues for toxicological testing. Metabolite identification in the target species, metabolite identification in a laboratory animal species.
2. Toxicological testing in laboratory animals. Genetic toxicity tests, acute toxicity tests, subchronic (90-day) toxicity tests, a 2-to-3-generation reproduction study with a teratology component in rats. Lifetime carcinogenicity studies in two rodent species *only* if genetic toxicity tests indicated that the drug or metabolites are potentially carcinogenic (the decision by FDA to require lifetime carcinogenicity studies is based on a decision tree process referred to as *threshold assessment*), other specific toxicity tests as needed.
3. Residue depletion studies in the target species.

4. Regulatory analytical methodology for identification and quantitation of marker residues in animal tissues, milk, or eggs. Determinative method for quantitation of marker residues, confirmatory method for structural identification when the determinative method is not sufficiently specific.

For an in-depth discussion of the drug approval requirements in the United States, consult the reference Sponsored Compounds in Food-Producing Animals (1985) and Chapter 34.

Based on the results of the toxicity tests, regulatory agencies establish an acceptable daily intake (ADI). The ADI represents a level of daily intake of a chemical that, during an entire lifetime, appears to be without appreciable risk to the health of the consumer. The maximum residue limit (MRL) is the maximum concentration of a marker residue in edible tissues, milk, or eggs that is legally permitted or recognized as acceptable. The MRL is calculated such that daily intake of food with residues at the MRL will result in a total daily consumption of residues in quantities at or below the ADI. In establishing MRLs, consumption estimates for the various foods are taken into account so that foods consumed infrequently or in small amounts are allowed greater MRL values than those foods likely to be consumed daily or that represent a major component of the diet. ADIs are based on the total residue of a chemical present in food (parent compound and all metabolites), whereas MRLs are based on a single, measurable marker residue, which may be the parent compound or any of its metabolites. In the United States and some other countries, the term *tolerance* is used in place of the term *MRL*.

In addition to the standard battery of toxicology testing, antimicrobial drugs may require additional evaluation to ensure the safety of the public. Residues of antimicrobial animal drug raise special human safety concerns with regard to allergenicity and effects on the human intestinal microflora. Allergic reactions are manifested in many ways, from life-threatening anaphylactic reactions to lesser reactions such as rashes. Although animal drug residues do not cause primary sensitization of individuals, because exposures are too low and for short duration, violative residues of animal drugs in food have caused allergic reactions in sensitive individuals. Violative residues of penicillin are the most frequently cited cause of allergic reactions in persons consuming residues. Many other animal drugs, including tetracyclines, sulfonamides, and aminoglycosides, can cause allergic reactions in sensitive individuals.

The indigenous bacteria that populate the gastrointestinal tract of humans provide a barrier to infectious agents, metabolize toxins and carcinogens, produce vitamins, and aid in food digestion. Therapeutic concentrations of some antimicrobials perturb the gastrointestinal ecosystem, causing adverse health effects. Abnormal or soft stools or diarrhea are considered adverse biological effects in the human food safety evaluation. Although soft stools and diarrhea following administration of antimicrobials are generally considered to be indirect biological effects rather than a true toxic effect of the drug, these effects are the result of perturbations of the intestinal microflora and therefore are considered adverse effects of the drug. Further, there exists the potential that overgrowth of pathogenic microorganisms could cause colitis or septic conditions, especially in immunocompromised individuals; colonization resistance sustained by indigenous anaerobes within the intestine could be compromised, resulting in increased susceptibility to invasion by pathogenic organisms; metabolic activity of the flora could be altered, resulting in altered metabolism of different compounds; and populations of antimicrobial-resistant strains of enteric pathogens may emerge, resulting from selective pressure by antimicrobials.

Therefore, the following studies may be required to establish an ADI based on microbiologic rather than toxicologic endpoints: (1) changes in the colonization resistance properties of the microflora; (2) changes in the metabolic activity of the intestinal microflora; (3) changes in antimicrobial resistance patterns of the microflora; and (4) changes in the number and composition of the microorganisms that constitute the intestinal microflora. To date, there have been few studies to determine the lowest dose of antibiotic required to perturb the normal human flora. Nevertheless, MRLs are being established by national authorities and international bodies based on microbiologic ADIs.

The Codex Alimentarius Commission on Residues of Veterinary Drugs in Foods (Codex) is a subsidiary body of the World Health Organization and the Food and Agriculture Organization. The purpose of Codex is to facilitate world trade in agricultural commodities through the establishment of internationally recognized standards, codes of practice, guidelines, and recommendations that are based on the consensus of expert scientific opinion. A primary function is the establishment of internationally recognized MRLs. Table 33.3 lists the proposed and adopted MRLs for antimicrobial drugs.

Epidemiologic Evidence of Adverse Reactions

Reports of acute adverse reactions in humans from ingestion of antimicrobial drug residues are rare. Of the few reports that document adverse reactions in people consuming residue-contaminated foods, the overwhelming majority are allergic reactions to penicillin. In reference to these allergic reactions, Burgat-Sacaze et al. (1986) stress the following:

1. Involvement of residues constitutes a very low number of cases (a small percentage) of food allergies. The major allergens involved are natural food constituents or human food additives.

TABLE 33.3. Maximum residue limits (MRLs) in mg/kg adopted or proposed for adoption by the Codex Alimentarius Commission

	Pen[a,b]	Ceff[c]	Tet[c]	Gent[c]	Neo[c]	Strep[c]	Spec[c]	SMZ[b]	Spir[b]	Til[c]	Thiam[c]	Carb[b]
Cattle												
Muscle	50	200	200	100	500	500	500		200	100	40	
Liver	50	2,000	600	2,000	500	500	2,000		600	1,000	40	
Kidney	50	4,000	1,200	5,000	10,000	1,000	5,000		300	300	40	
Fat		600		100	500	500	2,000		300	100	40	
Milk (μg/l)	4	100	100	200	500	200	200	25	200			
Pigs												
Muscle	50	200	200	100	500	500	500		200	100		5
Liver	50	2,000	600	2,000	500	500	2,000		600	1,500		30
Kidney	50	4,000	1,200	5,000	10,000	1,000	5,000		300	1,000		
Fat		600		100	500	500	2,000		300	100		
Sheep												
Muscle			200		500	500	500			100		
Liver			600		500	500	2,000			1,000		
Kidney			1,200		10,000	1,000	5,000			300		
Fat					500	500	2,000			100		
Milk (μg/l)			100							50		
Goats												
Muscle					500							
Liver					500							
Kidney					10,000							
Fat					500							
Poultry												
Muscle			200									
Liver			600									
Kidney			1,200									
Egg			400									
Chickens												
Muscle					500	500	500		200		40	
Liver					500	500	2,000		600		40	
Kidney					10,000	1,000	5,000		800		40	
Fat					500	500	2,000		300		40	
Eggs					500		2,000					

(continued)

TABLE 33.3. *Continued*

	Pen[a,b]	Ceft[c]	Tet[c]	Gent[c]	Neo[c]	Strep[c]	Spec[c]	SMZ[b]	Spir[b]	Til[c]	Thiam[c]	Carb[b]
Turkeys												
Muscle					500							
Liver					500							
Kidney					10,000							
Fat					500							
Ducks												
Muscle					500							
Liver					500							
Kidney					10,000							
Fat					500							
Fish												
Muscle			200									
Giant prawn												
Muscle			200									
Not specified												
Muscle								100				
Liver								100				
Kidney								100				
Fat								100				

Sources: 36th, 38th, 42nd, 43rd, 45th, 47th, 48th, and 50th Reports of the Joint FAO/WHO Expert Committee on Food Additives (1990–1998).

[a]Pen, benzylpenicillin; Ceft, ceftiofur; Tet, tetracycline/chlortetracycline/oxytetracycline; Gent, gentamicin; Neo, neomycin; Strep, streptomycin/dihydrostreptomycin; Spec, spectinomycin; SMZ, sulfadimidine; Spir, spiramycin; Til, tilmicosin; Thiam, thiamphenicol; Carb, carbadox.

[b]MRLs adopted by the Codex Alimentarius Commission.

[c]MRLs proposed for adoption at the 23rd Session of the Codex Alimentarius Commission, 1999.

2. The clinical observations report rashes the most frequently, but never, to our knowledge, has anaphylactic shock been noted.

3. In most cases, residues are implicated without sufficient diagnostic evidence. Most suspicions are established as follows: reaction of hypersensitivity observed following food intake, tests demonstrate that the individual is not allergic to the food eaten but is allergic to some drugs, and hence the possibility of the presence of residues of these drugs in the food, without checking the hypothesis. Thus "circumstantial evidence" is often the only criterion, and residues involvement is anecdotal in several reports.

BETA-LACTAM ANTIBIOTICS

Nearly all reports of acute adverse reactions from food-borne residues implicate penicillin as the offending agent, and the source of penicillin residues is most often milk or dairy products. These milk residues likely originated from intramammary infusion of penicillin used for the treatment of mastitis (Siegel, 1959). Although a substantial number of farm milk samples have been found to contain small amounts of penicillin, there have been relatively few published reports of adverse reactions from milk residues (Erskine, 1958; Vickers et al., 1958; Zimmerman, 1959; Borrie and Barrett, 1961; Wicher et al., 1969). In all instances, the victims reported a history of penicillin allergy or skin disease unrelated to penicillin allergy. Symptoms varied in intensity from mild skin rashes to exfoliative dermatitis. In an investigation of 252 patients with chronic recurrent urticaria, 70 (27.8%) were determined to be allergic to penicillin by dermal testing. When 52 of these penicillin-allergic patients were restricted to a diet containing no milk or dairy products, 30 experienced remission of symptoms, whereas only 2 out of a group of 40 patients with chronic urticaria and negative skin tests responded favorably to the milk-free diet (Boonk and Van Ketel, 1982). Many drugs other than penicillin—including other beta-lactams, streptomycin (and other aminoglycosides), sulfonamides, and to a lesser extent, novobiocin, and the tetracyclines—are known to cause allergic reactions in sensitive persons; however, with the exception of a single report of a reaction to meat suspected of containing streptomycin residues (Tinkleman and Bock, 1984), we are unaware of any reports of food-borne allergic reactions resulting from residues of any drug other than penicillin. Drug allergies are generally considered to be type 1 immune responses (Coombs and Gell, 1975). These reactions are mediated through IgE, and symptoms include anaphylaxis, urticaria, and angioedema.

CHLORAMPHENICOL

Chloramphenicol has never been approved in the United States for use in food-producing animals, and its use in food-producing animals is prohibited in most developed countries. Nevertheless, chloramphenicol gained wide popularity among food-animal veterinarians because of its effectiveness in treating bacterial infections. Despite its virtues as an antimicrobial agent (see Chapter 12), chloramphenicol has some inherent properties that render it a threat to human health. Most toxic effects attributed to chloramphenicol are dose dependent and would pose little public health risk from food-borne residues; however, one toxic effect, aplastic anemia in humans, may be dose independent and potentially could be induced by low concentrations of chloramphenicol in foods. Aplastic anemia in humans represents a true drug idiosyncrasy affecting 1 in 20,000 to 1 in 50,000 patients receiving a typical course of chloramphenicol therapy. The resulting disease is fatal in approximately 70% of the cases, and those who recover experience a high incidence of acute leukemia (Settapani, 1984). Evaluation of the safety of chloramphenicol by the FAO/WHO Joint Expert Committee on Food Additives led to the conclusion that no amount of chloramphenicol in human food could be considered to be without harmful effects (FAO/WHO, 1988).

Although there have been no reported cases of aplastic anemia that were attributable to consumption of chloramphenicol residues in food, the possibility of the occurrence of such an event may not be remote. Use of chloramphenicol in cattle is thought to be responsible for the death of a rancher in Kansas. The rancher was diagnosed as having aplastic anemia 4 months after he began treating his cattle with chloramphenicol (Settapani, 1984). In 1983, approximately 0.5% of all calves in the United States contained residues of chloramphenicol, but by 1984, the violation rate declined to 0.09%. Presently, the United States National Residue Program has suspended testing for chloramphenicol because no residues were detected for a period of several years. The food-animal producer in the United States must not use chloramphenicol for any purpose that would result in the presence of residues in food for consumption by humans. In the United States, use of chloramphenicol in food-producing animals is prohibited by law (21 CFR 530.41), and veterinarians have been sentenced to prison terms for its illegal use (Dols, 1986).

SULFAMETHAZINE

In the United States, efforts to control violative residues of sulfamethazine have been relatively successful, even though this drug still ranks among the top 10 drugs causing violative residues. During 1974 and 1975, approximately 10% of the swine slaughtered in the United States for food contained violative residues of sulfamethazine because of the routine use of sulfamethazine-medicated feeds. In 1976, the violation rate remained at 9.5% despite appeals to the swine industry, and by 1977, the violation rate rose to 13%. Because of the apparent inability of the swine industry to control sulfamethazine residues, the FDA seriously considered suspending the use of sulfonamides in swine feeds (Bevill, 1984). Instead, the FDA and USDA initiated an intensive educational and research program in 1978, which was designed to reduce the rate of violative sulfamethazine residues. In addition, the preslaughter withdrawal time was increased from 7 days to 15 days for all swine feeds containing sulfamethazine, and the drug manufacturing industry developed a granular form of sulfamethazine that left substantially less carryover in feed mixing equipment. The net result of these intensive efforts was a noticeable reduction in the rate of violative sulfamethazine residues, but in the early 1980s the residue violation rate began to increase once again, fluctuating between 3.7% and 6.7% between 1983 and 1986. Because a violation rate exceeding 1% is regarded as unacceptable by the FDA and FSIS, corrective measures were deemed necessary (Sulfamethazine, 1988).

In 1982, the FDA's National Center for Toxicological Research (NCTR) initiated a chronic toxicity and carcinogenesis study on sulfamethazine in both rats and mice. The results of those studies, released in early 1988, indicated that chronic dietary exposure to sulfamethazine produces a statistically significant increase in thyroid follicular cell adenomas in both rats and mice and a statistically significant increase in thyroid follicular cell adenocarcinomas in rats (Chronic Toxicity, 1988a,b). At approximately the same time that the NCTR results were announced, surveys of milk collected from various supermarkets in the northeastern United States revealed that sulfamethazine residues were present in approximately 40–70% of the samples (Paige and Kent, 1987; Collins-Thompson et al., 1988). Concerned by these findings, the FDA conducted a similar survey covering 10 major metropolitan cities throughout the United States. Their results showed that 73% of the supermarket milk samples contained sulfamethazine residues (Grassie, 1988). In response, a moratorium on sulfamethazine use in lactating cows was promoted by national organizations representing the dairy industry.

The effect of the moratorium on sulfamethazine in lactating dairy cattle led to a dramatic reduction in milk residues. The pork industry responded in a similar manner, resulting in a reduction in the rate of violative residues to less than 1% since 1990. An excellent review of the toxicology, residues, and metabolism of sulfonamides is by Rehm et al. (1986).

AMINOGLYCOSIDES

Although aminoglycosides produce nephrotoxic and ototoxic effects at high doses, the concentrations that occur as tissue residues would not be expected to cause adverse effects in humans. Allergic reactions following consumption of animal-derived foods containing aminoglycoside residues are limited to a single report in which a conclusive diagnosis was never established (Tinkleman and Bock, 1984). Nevertheless, the aminoglycosides rank among the top 10 drugs causing residue violations in the United States. The high incidence of residues results from the widespread use of these drugs and especially their extreme persistence in the kidneys of treated animals. Aminoglycosides are actively taken up by the renal proximal tubules through endocytosis and concentrated in lysosomes (Short et al., 1985). From the kidneys, aminoglycosides are excreted at a very slow rate, which may follow dose-dependent kinetics. The half-life of gentamicin in ovine kidneys is estimated to be 59 days, requiring a withholding time of 10 months or longer based on a MRL of 0.4 μg/g and a dose of 3 mg/kg given twice daily for 10 days (Brown and Baird, 1988). Residues of dihydrostreptomycin can be detected in the kidneys of cattle as long as 90 days after a single injection (Huber, 1988).

Although the bioavailability of aminoglycosides is limited when administered by routes other than injection, absorption following oral, intramammary, and intrauterine administration is often sufficient to cause violative tissue residues. Oral absorption may be substantial during the first 24 hours after birth because of the physiologic capacity of the small intestine to absorb macromolecules from colostrum. The common practice of incorporating neomycin into milk replacers probably accounts for a substantial percentage of residue violations in bob veal calves (Van Dresser and Wilcke, 1989; Wilson et al., 1991a,b). Following intramammary infusion, gentamicin can be detected in the blood of cattle, and residues persist in the kidneys for periods of 6 months or longer (RJ Erskine and R Wilson, pers. comm., 1991).

Information Sources for Controlling Residues

An information system is available that can assist veterinarians in estimating residue-depletion times for drugs or chemicals when the drugs are administered at dosages in excess of label recommendations, or when livestock are unintentionally exposed to environmentally persistent chemicals. The Food Animal Residue Avoidance Databank (FARAD) is a program designed to provide veterinarians with the most current information available on the disposition of drugs and other chemicals in livestock. The program is funded through the U.S. Department of Agriculture and was developed through the combined efforts of researchers at veterinary colleges in California, Florida, and North Carolina.

The FARAD system focuses on published pharmacokinetic information such as the biological half-lives, clearance rates, and volumes of distribution for those drugs, pesticides, and environmental contaminants that have the greatest potential for persisting in tissues of livestock at the time of slaughter. More than 15,000 records from 3,500 citations containing this type of information are presently available through FARAD, and the number of records increases daily. From these pharmacokinetic values, mathematical models are developed from which residue-depletion times can be estimated regardless of the drug dose.

Because the FARAD system uses data published in the scientific literature to estimate residue-depletion times for drugs used at extralabel doses, the FARAD estimates should be more accurate than those derived by the veterinary practitioner. Nevertheless, these estimates are not official withdrawal times, and whenever possible, the animal should be tested for residues prior to marketing.

In addition to pharmacokinetic data used to estimate residue-depletion times, the FARAD system also contains additional information:

1. FDA-approved drug trade name information for all drugs registered for food animals in the United States. This includes manufacturer, generic chemicals, species indications, disease indications, routes of administration, and official withdrawal times.
2. U.S. residue tolerances (MRLs) or action levels for more than 200 chemicals. Included are all established tissue, milk, and egg tolerances.
3. Residue screening tests available in the United States. Included are all drugs that are detected by the tests, the sensitivity of the assay, and the sample matrix.
4. Bibliographic references for all information contained in the FARAD system.

Veterinarians can learn more about FARAD and acquire direct access to information through the FARAD Web site < www.farad.org>.

Conclusions

Food safety is one of the most significant issues facing agriculture. Growing consumer health concerns about chemical residues continue to erode the demand for animal-derived foods. Globally, concerns over the safety of foods have resulted in disruption of international trade. Formal training in the area of residue prevention has been limited at a time when advances are rapidly reshaping the way that food safety programs operate. The development of rapid immunodiagnostic tests for drug residues has allowed the monitoring of much greater numbers of animal products prior to reaching the food supply. HACCP-like quality assurance programs are being developed that require the livestock producer and packer to verify that their animals and animal products are wholesome and free of drug residues. HACCP programs are being instituted at federally inspected abattoirs. Failure of the veterinary profession and the livestock industry to embrace and maintain currency in these emerging areas will ultimately undermine the public's confidence in the safety of the food supply. Clearly, at a time when consumer demand for a safe and wholesome food supply has never been greater, the need for national regulatory authorities, the veterinary profession, and the livestock industry to assert strong leadership in food safety has never been more critical.

Bibliography

Bevill RF. 1984. Factors influencing the occurrence of drug residues in animal tissues after the use of antimicrobial agents in animal feeds. J Am Vet Med Assoc 185:1124.

Boonk WJ, Van Ketel WG. 1982. The role of penicillin in the pathogenesis of chronic urticaria. Br J Dermatol 106:183.

Borrie P, Barrett J. 1961. Dermatitis caused by penicillin in bulked milk supplies. Br Med J 2:1267.

Brady MS, Katz SE. 1988. Antibiotic/antimicrobial residues in milk. J Food Prot 51:8.

Brown SA, Baird AN. 1988. Evaluation of renal gentamicin depletion kinetic properties in sheep, using serial percutaneous biopsies. Am J Vet Res 49:2056.

Burgat-Sacaze V, et al. 1986. Toxicological significance of bound residues. In: Rico A, ed. Drug Residues in Animals. Orlando, FL: Academic Press.

Chloramphenicol oral solution: opportunity for hearing. 1985. Fed Regist 50:27059.

Chronic Toxicity and Carcinogenicity Studies of Sulfamethazine in B6C3F$_1$ Mice. 1988a. NCTR Tech Rep Exp 418. Jefferson, AR: National Center for Toxicological Research.

Chronic Toxicity and Carcinogenesis Studies on Sulfamethazine in Fischer 433 Rats. 1988b. NCTR Tech Rep Exp 420. Jefferson, AR: National Center for Toxicological Research.

Collins-Thompson DL, et al. 1988. Detection of antibiotic residues in consumer milk supplies in North America using the Charm Test II procedure. J Food Prot 51:632.

Committee on Government Operations. 1985. 27th Report, Human Food Safety and the Regulation of Animal Drugs. 99th Congress, 1st Session, House Report 99—461:1.

Coombs RRA, Gell PGM. 1975. Classification of allergic reactions responsible for clinical hypersensitivity and disease. In: Gell PGM, ed. Clinical Aspects of Immunology. Oxford: Blackwell Scientific.

Dewdney JM, et al. 1991. Risk assessment of antibiotic residues of beta-lactams and macrolides in food products with regard to their immunoallergic potential. Food Chem Toxicol 29:477.

Dols P. 1986. Regulatory Highlights. FDA Vet 1:5.

Erskine D. 1958. Dermatitis caused by penicillin in milk. Lancet 1:431.

FAO/WHO. 1988. 32nd Report of the Joint FAO/WHO Expert Committee on Food Additives. Evaluation of Certain Veterinary Drug Residues in Food. WHO/FAO Tech Rep Ser 763:1.

FAO/WHO. 1989. 34th Report of the Joint FAO/WHO Expert Committee on Food Additives. Evaluation of Certain Veterinary Drug Residues in Food. WHO/FAO Tech Rep Ser 788:1.

FAO/WHO. 1990. 36th Report of the Joint FAO/WHO Expert Committee on Food Additives. Evaluation of Certain Veterinary Drug Residues in Food. WHO/ FAO Tech Rep Ser 799:1.

Grassie L. 1988. Eliminating sulfamethazine residues in milk. FDA Vet 3(4):1.

Huber WG. 1971. The impact of veterinary drugs and their residues. Adv Vet Sci Comp Med 15:101.

Huber WG. 1988. Aminoglycosides, macrolides, lincosamides, polymyxins, chloramphenicol, and other antibacterial drugs. In: Booth NH, McDonald LE, eds. Veterinary Pharmacology and Therapeutics, 6th ed. Ames: Iowa State Univ Press.

Paige JC, Kent R. 1987. Tissue residue briefs. FDA Vet 11:10.

Paige JC, et al. 1999. Federal surveillance of veterinary drugs and chemical residues (with recent data 1992–1996). Vet Clin North Am 15:45.

Patel BL, et al. 1997. USDA/FSIS Domestic Residue Data Book: National Residue Program 1995. Washington DC.

Rehm WF, et al. 1986. General aspects of metabolism, residues, and toxicology of sulfonamides and dihydrofolate reductase inhibitors. In : Rico A, ed. Drug Residues in Animals. Orlando, FL: Academic Press.

Schwartz HJ, Sher TH. 1984. Anaphylaxis to penicillin in a frozen dinner. Ann Allergy 52:342.

Settapani JA. 1984. The hazard of using chloramphenicol in food animals. J Am Vet Med Assoc 8:930.

Short CS, et al. 1985. The nephrotoxic potential of gentamicin in the cat: a pharmacokinetic and histopathologic investigation. J Vet Pharmacol Ther 9:325.

Siegel B. 1959. Hidden contacts with penicillin. Bull W H O 21:703.

Sponsored Compounds in Food-Producing Animals: Proposed Rule and Notice. 1985. Fed Regist 50:45530.

Sulfamethazine in Food-Producing Animals: Public Hearing before the Commissioner. 1988. Fed Regist 53:15886.

Tinkleman DG, Bock SA. 1984. Anaphylaxis presumed to be caused by beef containing streptomycin. Ann Allergy 53:243.

U.S. Food and Drug Administration. 1986. Extralabel Use of New Animal Drugs in Food-Producing Animals. Compliance Policy Guide 7126.06. Rockville, MD.

Van Dresser WR, Wilcke JR. 1989. Drug residues in food animals. J Am Vet Med Assoc 194:1700.

Vickers HR, et al. 1958. Dermatitis caused by penicillin in milk. Lancet 1:351.

Wicher K, et al. 1969. Allergic reaction to penicillin. J Am Med Assoc 208:143.

Wilson DJ, et al. 1991a. Antibiotic and sulfonamide agents in bob veal calf muscle, liver, and kidney. Am J Vet Res 52:1383.

Wilson DJ, et al. 1991b. Antibiotic and sulfonamide residues from Food Safety Inspection Service bob veal calf tissues by region, from October 1987 to September 1988. J Am Vet Med Assoc 199:341.

Zimmerman MC. 1959. Chronic penicillin urticaria from dairy products proved by penicillinase cures. Arch Dermatol 79:1.

34 Regulation of Antibiotic Use in Animals

M. A. MILLER and W. T. FLYNN

The use of antibiotics to treat disease in animals began in the 1940s. A few years later, producers began to use antibacterials to improve growth and feed efficiency. The introduction of commercially affordable antibiotics into feed for cattle, pigs, and chickens in the 1950s launched a new era in livestock management and meat production. Today antibacterial agents are used in animals to treat and prevent bacterial diseases as well as to improve growth and feed efficiency (National Research Council, 1998). Although a complete discussion of the laws that control antibacterial use by veterinarians and producers is beyond the scope of this chapter, this chapter highlights many of the regulatory changes that have an impact on veterinary use of antibacterials, with a focus on the United States.

International Standards

Most industrialized countries have laws, similar to those in the United States, governing the veterinary use of antibacterial products. Although drug approval requirements are similar, the differences add to the cost of drug development and thereby limit drug availability. Differences in the food safety assessments among countries also create trade barriers for edible products from treated animals. The preapproval requirements for veterinary medicinal products differ in the type and number of studies required, the study design, the study interpretation, and the risk management measures applied to ensure proper drug use. The United States, Japan, and the European Union are currently engaged in negotiations to standardize study requirements for veterinary medicinal products under the Veterinary International Cooperation on Harmonization (VICH). This effort is focusing on standardizing the study requirements for product approval, including the number and type of studies required for demonstrating efficacy and safety, and the design of these studies. Harmonizing the interpretation of the study and the risk management decisions associated with product approval is generally considered to be beyond the scope of this effort. It is believed that standardizing preapproval requirements will increase the number of approved products available to the veterinarian.

In 1962 the Codex Alimentarius Commission (Codex) was established as a subsidiary of the Food and Agricultural Organization (FAO) and the World Health Organization (WHO) of the United Nations. Codex was created to facilitate international trade by developing internationally accepted food standards. The Codex Commission on Residues of Veterinary Drugs in Foods provides expert advice on technical barriers to trade for veterinary products and is responsible for establishing maximum residue limits (MRLs) for veterinary drugs. Codex MRLs are not mandatory but are established as the standard for trade negotiations. In establishing the MRLs, the Codex Commission on Residues of Veterinary Drugs in Foods receives advice from the FAO/WHO Joint Expert Committee on Food Additives. This committee of international experts on toxicology, pharmacology, and metabolism reviews data similar to that reviewed by the FDA and establishes international acceptable daily intakes (ADIs) and MRLs for drug residues. Countries that do not have regulatory bodies overseeing animal drug use can adopt the Codex standard and be assured that their animal products are safe and permitted in international trade (Codex, 1995).

Animal Drug Approval Process in the United States

In the United States, antibacterial drugs used in animals for both therapeutic and growth promotion purposes are considered animal drugs. The federal Food, Drug, and Cosmetic Act (FD&C) defines animal drugs as articles intended for use in the diagnosis, cure, mitigation, treatment, or prevention of disease in animals and articles (other than food) intended to affect the structure or any function of the body of animals (FD&C 201(g)[1]). Before any animal drug can be legally marketed in the United States, the drug's sponsor must have a new animal drug application (NADA) approved by the Food and Drug Administration (FDA). To obtain a NADA approval, the drug sponsor must demonstrate to the FDA that the drug is effective and safe for the animal, is safe for the environment, and can be manufactured to uniform standards of purity, strength, and identity. If the animal drug is intended for use in food-producing animals, drug sponsors must also demonstrate that edible products produced from treated animals are safe for humans (FD&C 512).

To conduct investigational clinical studies with animal drugs before approval, the drug sponsor must request an investigational new animal drug (INAD) exemption from the FDA. Under the INAD exemption, the drug sponsor can conduct safety and efficacy studies required for approval of their product. Relatively early in the investigational process for a drug used in food animals, Center for Veterinary Medicine scientists review studies relating to human food safety and establish an appropriate period for drug withdrawal before slaughter to ensure that no unsafe residues are present in the food products. Once the human food safety is confirmed, the FDA may authorize the use in human food of products from animals treated in investigational studies (FD&C 512).

Animal Drug Availability Act

The Animal Drug Availability Act (ADAA) of 1996 changed the preapproval review process to facilitate the approval of animal drugs. The ADAA accomplished this by building flexibility into the animal drug review processes without decreasing FDA's authority to ensure that animal drug products are safe. FDA has implemented the spirit of the law, pending promulgation of implementing regulations. Thus, this discussion of the animal drug approval process reflects changes implemented since the enactment of ADAA (FD&C 512[d]). ADAA redefined *substantial evidence* as the term is used in the FD&C Act to describe the scientific evidence needed to establish that an animal drug is effective. The new definition provides FDA with flexibility in determining the type and amount of data needed to establish drug effectiveness. The ADAA also created a streamlined process for the approval of the combination use of animal drugs when each animal drug in the combination has been approved individually for the same use.

Marketing Status of Animal Drugs

During the evaluation of an animal drug application, FDA determines the marketing status (prescription, over-the-counter, or veterinary feed directive) of the animal drug product. This determination is based on whether or not it is possible to write directions adequate for a layperson to use the drugs safely and effectively. Products for which adequate directions for lay use can be written are labeled and marketed for over-the-counter use. If such directions cannot be written, the drug product is not considered safe for animal use except under the supervision of a licensed veterinarian. Such drugs are approved as prescription or veterinary feed directive products and can be dispensed only by or upon the lawful written order of a licensed veterinarian (FD&C 503–504).

Prior to ADAA, the use of animal drugs in animal feeds by veterinary prescription was considered impractical because many state pharmacy laws do not distinguish between human and veterinary products, and they require that prescription drugs be dispensed by licensed pharmacists. The ADAA created veterinary feed directives (VFDs), a new class of animal drugs for use in feed, similar to prescription animal drugs. VFD drugs are intended for use in or on animal feed under the professional supervision of a licensed veterinarian. VFD drugs and animal feeds containing them must be labeled with a cautionary statement. In addition, animal feed containing a VFD drug can be used only after a veterinary feed directive is issued by a licensed veterinarian in the course of the veterinarian's professional practice (FD&C 504[a]).

The VFD drug classification offers an alternative to prescription status, allowing FDA to approve drugs for use in feed that require supervision by a veterinarian while enabling the feed industry to maintain current feed distribution. A VFD drug can be fed to animals only in a manner consistent with the conditions of approval. Veterinarian participation in the decision to use one of these drugs satisfies FDA's concerns that the drug be used only in appropriate circumstances. In the future, all new antibacterial agents for therapeutic use in feed that require oversight by a veterinarian will be approved by FDA as VFD drugs.

Evaluation of Effectiveness

Prior to approval, a sponsor of an animal drug must provide substantial evidence that the drug is effective for the use indicated in proposed labeling. Traditionally, drug sponsors were required to establish a dose-response relationship by conducting dose titration studies. The lowest dose shown to produce the desired effect was typically selected for further testing in clinical trials. This effectiveness testing model resulted in product labels that included single fixed dosages and narrow indications. With the new flexibility provided with ADAA, FDA no longer requires dose titration studies for the approval of therapeutic antibacterial products. Although traditional dose titration studies are no longer required for therapeutic antibacterial products, drug sponsors are still required to provide a justification for the proposed dosage and to confirm effectiveness in clinical trials.

Professional Flexible Labeling

Veterinary prescription products labeled with single fixed dosages and indications directed against a narrow range of specific diseases and organisms often do not reflect current uses for therapeutic agents in veterinary medicine. Such restricted labeling limits the practical usefulness of veterinary prescription products. The passage of the ADAA provided for changes in the drug approval process that facilitate the approval of dose-ranged products, ie, professional flexible labeling (PFL). The basic concept of PFL is to provide prescription veterinary products that carry useful prescribing information for a range of clinical situations as part of their approved conditions of use. Implementation of PFL is based on the recognition that veterinarians can interpret diagnostic and prescribing medical information to develop appropriate therapeutic regimens. Thus, antibacterial product labels may now include more broadly written indications, expanded dosage ranges, more-detailed microbiological susceptibility information, pharmacokinetic and pharmacodynamic data, and the potential for dose-related withdrawal periods for dose-ranged products intended for food-producing animals (USFDA, 1998).

Evaluation of Animal Safety

Based on data collected in both effectiveness and animal safety studies, a range of drug concentrations is established at which the drug is both effective and nontoxic (ie, within the therapeutic window). To assess the safety limits of new products, drug tolerance testing is often conducted to characterize, under controlled conditions, the animal response to a potentially toxic dose or doses of a drug. Such testing is particularly important for systemically acting products that contain new chemical entities. However, conducting such provocative overdose studies may not be necessary if the new product contains approved chemical entities at concentrations for which the toxicity in the target animal is well established (USFDA, 1989).

Drug tolerance testing involves the administration of a range of doses of the test drug to a limited number of animals with the intent of inducing toxicity. Following drug administration, the test animals are closely monitored, and the clinical signs manifested by the animals are recorded. In addition, clinical pathologic and histologic data are collected. By characterizing the toxic effects associated with the drug, the results of the tolerance studies help focus the observations and endpoints in subsequent safety studies.

Additional animal safety studies are needed to establish the safety of the product when administered to the animal by the route and dosage defined in the proposed labeling. These studies are typically conducted using the class of animal that, based on the proposed labeling, will be the primary market for the product. For example, safety studies to support an antibacterial product for bovine respiratory disease would be conducted in cattle typical of U.S. feedlots. Animal safety studies are conducted using healthy animals; however, certain safety information is gleaned from clinical effectiveness trials in which diseased animals are administered the test drug. To evaluate the safety of new antibacterial products intended for use at a single point dose, safety studies are generally designed to include a number of test dose groups, including the label dose (X) and multiples of the label dose (eg, 3X, 5X). Overdose levels of drug are administered in these studies to assess the margin of safety relative to the indicated label dosage. Products that are labeled with a range of dosages are evaluated to assess safety of the highest dose in the range. With the advent of professional flexible labeling and the potential for broad dosage ranges, alternative approaches to establishing animal safety are being considered.

In addition to evaluating the systemic effects of antibacterial products, local effects of injectable dosage forms such as irritation, pain, and swelling at the injection site are investigated. For products intended for food-producing animals, this evaluation also includes assessment of injection sites and surrounding tissues for discoloration, drug residues, and other factors affecting carcass quality. The primary intent of obtaining such information is to inform the product's user of such effects through appropriate cautionary language on product labeling. Additional animal safety studies may be needed for products intended for use in pregnant animals or animals intended for breeding purposes. If reproductive safety is not determined, the product labeling must clearly identify that the safety of the product in breeding animals has not been established.

Finally, if the proposed antibacterial product belongs to a class of antibacterials that is known to cause adverse effects in certain breeds, classes, or age groups of the animal species, specific studies in these sensitive animals may be needed to assess the safety of the product. Based on the data provided on these suspected adverse effects, use of the product in the sensitive animals may be restricted or certain cautionary label language may be required.

Human Food Safety of Drug Residues

Whenever an animal is treated with an animal drug, some amount of the drug (residue) remains in edible tissue, at least for a certain time. *Drug residue* is defined as any compound present in edible tissue of the treated animals that results from the use of the drug, including the drug itself, its metabolites, and any substances formed in or on the food as a result of the use of the drug (21 CFR 500.82). *Substance* has been broadly defined to include everything from drug metabolites to endogenous compounds.

The hazard associated with an animal drug residue is assessed by having the drug's sponsor conduct a standard battery of toxicology tests. Each test is designed to determine a dose that causes an adverse effect and a dose that produces no observed effect for a specific toxicological endpoint. In determining the toxicological endpoints to be examined, the human food safety assessment generally focuses on the effect of chronic low-level exposure (USFDA, 1994).

The no observed effect level (NOEL) of the most sensitive effect from the most appropriate toxicology studies is divided by a safety factor to determine an acceptable daily intake (ADI). The ADI represents the total drug residues, of parent and all metabolites, that can be safely consumed daily throughout a person's lifetime. The amount of drug residue permitted in each of the edible tissues—ie, the safe concentration—depends upon the quantity of tissue that is consumed daily by the 90th-percentile consumer. Once the safe concentration is determined, the risk to consumers is minimized by controlling exposure. Generally, the tissue concentration of drug is highest immediately after treatment. Also, edible organ tissues—ie, liver and kidney—contain more drug residues than muscle. With time, the animal's normal metabolic and excretory processes remove the drug from the animal. The drug's sponsor conducts residue chemistry studies to determine when the level of drug in the animal reaches the calculated safe concentration for each of the different edible tissues.The first residue chemistry study conducted is the total residue and metabolism study. This study uses radiolabeled drug and is capable of monitoring all drug-derived residues resulting from the administration of the test compound. Metabolism of the drug is evaluated by extracting the radioactive material from the tissue, and chromatographic analysis follows. By analyzing the radiolabeled material isolated from the tissues collected at different times following treatment, it is possible to determine the drug residues that persist the longest and the edible tissue that eliminates the drug most slowly. The total drug residue consists of parent compound, free metabolites, and metabolites that are covalently bound to endogenous molecules, and it is very difficult to measure on a routine basis. Rather than measuring the total residues in all the edible tissues, FDA establishes one value, a tolerance, in one tissue, the target tissue, for monitoring drug residues. The tolerance is established so that when the measurable residue is below the tolerance in the target tissue, the whole carcass is safe. If an animal drug product requires time after the last treatment to allow the residues to deplete to the calculated safe concentration, the FDA establishes a withdrawal time for the product. Information about the withdrawal time is included on the drug label.

Residues of antibacterial animal drugs raise special human safety concerns with regard to allergenicity and effects on the human intestinal microflora (see Chapter 33). Allergic reactions are manifested in many ways, from life-threatening anaphylactic reactions to lesser reactions such as rashes. Animal drug residues do not cause primary sensitization of individuals, because exposures are too low and for short duration. Violative levels of animal drug residues in food—ie, levels that exceed an established tolerance—have caused allergic reactions in sensitive individuals. Violative levels of penicillin are the most frequently cited cause of allergic reactions in persons consuming drug residues. This is probably because a large number of individuals are allergic to penicillin, allergic reactions occur at low doses, and penicillin is extensively used in food-producing animals. Many other animal drugs, including tetracyclines, sulfonamides, and aminoglycosides, can cause allergic reactions in sensitive individuals. To date, there have been no documented cases of individuals having allergic reaction to these drugs following consumption of residues (Paige et al., 1997).

The indigenous bacteria that populate the gastrointestinal tract of humans provide protection against infections, metabolize toxins and carcinogens, produce vitamins, and aid in food digestion. Therapeutic levels of some antibiotics perturb the gut ecosystem, causing adverse health effects. There have been few studies to determine the lowest dose of antibiotic required to perturb the normal human flora. Although it is generally agreed that the very low tolerance levels of antibiotic residues in food are not sufficient to affect the flora, violative levels of antibiotics may perturb this ecosystem.

In the United States, the proper use of the animal drug product is ensured by providing appropriate use information on the label, educating animal producers and veterinarians about proper drug use, and monitoring the food supply for violative drug residues. The Food Safety Inspection Service of the U.S. Department of Agriculture oversees the residue monitoring program in the United States, and its monitoring data from random samples indicate that violative drug residues occur very infrequently, ie, in less than 1% of the nation's food supply. The FDA is responsible for taking regulatory action when a violative residue is identified. FDA prioritizes its regulatory action based on public health concerns. Whereas the health risk assessment for animal drug residues focuses on the chronic low-level exposure effects of drug residues, regulatory compliance actions on violative samples focus on the acute effects of drugs. FDA is particularly concerned about drug residues that elicit an "acute" toxic reaction at relatively low doses.

Microbial Human Health Safety Concerns

In recent years there has been increasing concern over the increase in food-borne disease resulting from the consumption of animal products contaminated with bacterial pathogens. Although the exact incidence of microbial food-borne disease in the U.S. human population is not known, a reasonable estimate is that there are 6.4 million to 33 million cases of human food-borne illness each year, with the number of deaths ranging as high as 9,000 per year (CAST, 1994). People are exposed to bacteria of animal origin via consumption of contaminated food, via direct contact, or through the environment. When animals are treated with antibacterial drugs, there may be an increase in the number of enteric bacteria that cause human disease (ie, pathogen load) or an increase in the quantity of resistant enteric bacteria in the animal's intestine (resistance). When these bacteria persist in the animal until slaughter, they can contaminant edible tissues. An estimated 1% of beef carcasses and 20% of the poultry carcasses are contaminated with *Salmonella* (USDA, 1996). If human illness is caused by pathogens resistant to antibiotics used for human therapy, medical treatment may be compromised.

Because of this safety concern, in the 1970s FDA began requiring specific microbiological studies as a condition of approval for antibacterial products used in feed. These studies were designed to examine the effect of an antibacterial drug product on pathogen load and on the level of drug-resistant bacteria in the animal. In 1996, FDA's Center for Veterinary Medicine, the Centers for Disease Control and Prevention, and the Department of Agriculture developed the National Antimicrobial Resistance Monitoring System (NARMS). The NARMS is a joint surveillance effort that prospectively monitors changes in antibacterial susceptibility patterns of some enteric pathogens from human and animal clinical specimens, from healthy farm animals, and from animal carcasses at slaughter. The goals of the NARMS are to facilitate the identification of resistant enteric pathogens (eg, *Salmonella, Campylobacter,* and *E. coli* 0157:H7) in humans and animals, to prolong the life span of drugs by promoting prudent drug use, and to identify areas for more-detailed investigations and research (Tollefson, 1996).

Animal Medicinal Drug Use Clarification Act

Prior to enactment of the Animal Medicinal Drug Use Clarification Act of 1994 (AMDUCA), all animal drug use was designated as unsafe unless approved by the FDA. In addition, an animal drug product could be used only in accordance with the approved labeling. Thus, extralabel use of drugs in animals was considered unsafe and a violation of the law (FD&C 512). To deal with extralabel drug use in animals, FDA outlined policies regarding the enforcement of such violations in two compliance policy guides (CPGs). These CPGs described circumstances under which FDA would likely take regulatory action against an extralabel use, and circumstances under which the agency would ordinarily exercise regulatory discretion. The passage of AMDUCA established provisions, similar to those in the CPGs, that allow veterinarians to prescribe extralabel uses of approved animal and human drugs for animals. The AMDUCA provisions were instituted when FDA promulgated the implementing regulations in December 1996 (21 CFR 530).

AMDUCA Regulatory Requirements

Extralabel use means the actual or intended use of a drug in a manner not in accordance with the approved labeling. This includes, but is not limited to, uses in species not listed in the labeling; use for indications (disease or other conditions) not listed in the labeling; use at dosage levels, frequencies, or routes of administration other than those stated in the labeling; and deviation from the labeled withdrawal time. The regulations implementing the extralabel use provisions of AMDUCA established certain conditions under which veterinarians are permitted to use approved animal or human drugs in an extralabel manner in animals. Understanding the AMDUCA regulations is important for veterinarians, to ensure appropriate extralabel use of drug products in animals.

An underlying premise for extralabel use is that such use must occur within the context of a valid veterinarian-client-patient relationship. Several conditions must be met to establish a valid veterinarian-client-patient relationship. First, the veterinarian must assume responsibility for making medical judgments regarding the health of the animal and the need for medical treatment, and the client (the owner or other caretaker of the animal) must agree to follow the instructions of the veterinarian. Next, there must be sufficient knowledge of the animal by the veterinarian to initiate at least a general or preliminary diagnosis of the medical condition of the animal. Finally, the veterinarian must be available for follow-up in case of adverse reactions or therapeutic failure. Thus, a veterinarian-client-patient relationship can exist only when the veterinarian has recently seen and is personally acquainted with the keeping and care of the animal by virtue of examination of the animal or by medically appropriate and timely visits to the premises where the animal is kept.

Veterinary Records and Labels

Under the AMDUCA regulations, FDA has access to a veterinarian's records. FDA requires specific information be recorded for every extralabel use, including the name of the drug, its active ingredient, the disease condition, the animal species, the dose administered, the duration of treatment, the number of animals treated, and the withdrawal or discard time. Veterinarians are required to maintain these records for 2 years or as required by state law, whichever is greater. In order to access a veterinarian's records, FDA must first determine that a particular extralabel use "may present a risk" to the public health. If FDA makes this determination, the finding is announced, and FDA surveys veterinary practices to gather information regarding such use. The regulations allow the practitioner to copy or reformulate records to provide FDA inspectors with only the information required by the regulations.

Any human or animal drug prescribed for extralabel use by a veterinarian or dispensed by a pharmacist on the order of a veterinarian must be accompanied by labeling information adequate to assure the safe and proper use of the product. This information includes the name and address of the veterinarian; the name of the drug; the directions for use, including animal or herd, flock, pen, lot, dosage, frequency, route of administration, and duration of therapy; cautionary statements; and the withdrawal or discard time.

Extralabel Use of Drugs in Food-producing Animals

Neither AMDUCA nor the implementing regulations lessen the responsibility of the drug's sponsor, the veterinarian, or the food producer with regard to causing violative drug residues or other adverse impacts on human health. For example, any amount of residue that "may present a risk to the public health" resulting from an extralabel use constitutes a violation of the FD&C Act and is subject to enforcement action.

Before using an animal or human drug in food-producing animals, the veterinarian must ensure that there is no approved animal drug containing the same active ingredient in the required dosage form and concentration. The veterinarian must also make a diagnosis, establish an adequate withdrawal period, and take measures to ensure that illegal drug residues do not occur. The extralabel use of an approved human drug in a food-producing animal is not permitted if an animal drug approved for use in food-producing animals can be used in an extralabel manner for the particular use.

Limitations on Extralabel Use of Antimicrobial Drugs

There are several situations in which the extralabel use of a drug in animals is not permitted. These include (1) extralabel use of an approved animal or human drug by a layperson; (2) extralabel use in animal feed of an approved animal or human drug; (3) extralabel use resulting in residues that "may present a risk" to the public health; and (4) extralabel use resulting in residues above the tolerance.

AMDUCA gives the FDA authority to prohibit specific extralabel uses in animals, provided the FDA finds that the extralabel use "presents a risk" to the public health. No specific extralabel uses have been prohibited in non-food-animal species at this time. In food-producing animals, the following antimicrobial drugs, families of drugs, and substances are currently prohibited for extralabel use: chloramphenicol; dimetridazole; ipronidazole; other nitroimidazoles; furazolidone, except for approved topical use; nitrofurazone, except for approved topical use; sulfonamide drugs in lactating dairy cattle, except for approved use of sulfadimethoxine, sulfabromomethazine, and sulfaethoxypyridazine; fluoroquinolones; and glycopeptides.

A new cautionary statement is added to the labeling of products that are approved for use in animals but prohibited from extralabel use in food-producing animals: "Federal law (USA) prohibits the extralabel use of this drug in food-producing animals."

Bibliography

Code of Federal Regulations. 1998. Title 21 (21 CFR) Food and Drugs, Parts 500 to 599. Washington, DC: Office of the Federal Register, National Archives and Records Administration.

Codex Alimentarius Commission. 1995. Implication of GATT and the World Trade Organization for the U.S. Washington, DC: Office of the U.S. Coordinator for Codex Alimentarius.

Council for Agricultural Science and Technology (CAST). 1994. Food-borne Pathogens Risks and Consequences. Ames, Iowa.

Food, Drug, and Cosmetic Act (FD&C). 1998. Washington, DC: U.S. Government Printing Office.

National Research Council. 1998. The Use of Drugs in Food Animals: Benefits and Risks. Washington, DC: National Academy Press.

Paige JC, et al. 1997. Public health impacts of drug residues in animal tissues. Vet Hum Toxicol 39:162.

Tollefson, L. 1996. FDA reveals plans for antimicrobial susceptibility monitoring. J Am Vet Med Assoc 208:459.

U.S. Department of Agriculture, Food Safety Inspection Service. 1996. Pathogen Reduction: Hazard Analysis and Critical Control Point (HACCP) Systems: Final Rule. Fed Regist 61:38806.

U.S. Food and Drug Administration. 1989. Target Animal Safety Guidelines for New Animal Drugs. Center for Veterinary Medicine, 7500 Standish Place, Rockville, MD.

U.S. Food and Drug Administration. 1994. General Principles for Evaluating the Safety of Compounds Used in Food-Producing Animals. Center for Veterinary Medicine, 7500 Standish Place, Rockville, MD.

U.S. Food and Drug Administration. 1998. Guidance for Industry: Professional Labelling of Antimicrobial Drugs. Center for Veterinary Medicine, 7500 Standish Place, Rockville, MD.

Index

For details of antimicrobial susceptibility of individual bacterial and fungal species, consult susceptibility
tables and antimicrobial activity sections for individual drugs.

Abamectin, 497
Abscesses, 97, 425, 657, 728
Acinetobacter, 153
Actinobacillus equuli, 310, 520, 521
Actinobacillus lignieresi, 204, 585
Actinobacillus pleuropneumoniae, 225, 226,
    260, 273, 285, 335, 606
Actinobacillus suis, 606, 613
Actinomyces, 306, 311, 362, 670
Actinomyces bovis, 587
*Actinomyces pyogenes. See Arcanobac-
    terium pyogenes*
Actinomyces viscosus, 311
Actinomycosis, 554, 587, 670
Acyclovir, 400–404, 412, 413, 635
Aditoprim, 300–304
Aditoprim-sulfonamides, 304–313. *See*
    Trimethoprim-sulfonamides
Adjunctive treatment, 97
Administration, drug, 50–60. *See also*
    Dosage
  intramammary, 592, 715
  intramuscular, 53–58, 541, 626, 681
  intraocular, 419
  intraosseous, 449, 627
  intratracheal, 627
  intravenous, 51–53, 541, 660
  local, 98–99, 627, 636

nebulization, 622, 630, 636
oral, 58–60, 542, 592, 603, 623–625,
    628–630, 639, 659–661, 681–683
routes, 50, 541, 603, 619, 639, 659
subcutaneous, 53–58, 541, 627, 660,
    681
topical, 630
water medication, principles, 646–647
Aeromonas hydrophila, 678, 687, 689, 705
Aeromonas salmonicida, 693, 705–706, 710
Aerosol therapy, 381
Age, and drug pharmacokinetics,
    437–448
Albendazole, 573
Alligator. *See* Crocodilians
Allometric scaling, 619, 658, 680,
    683–684
Allylamines, 375
Alternaria, 388
Amantadine, 399–400, 413
Amidopenicillins, 131
Amikacin, 211–214. *See also* Aminogly-
    cosides
  administration and dosage, 203, 535,
    568, 633, 664, 690
  antimicrobial activity, 211
  applications, clinical, 213, 517, 636,
    687–689
  toxicity and adverse effects, 197, 212
Aminocyclitols, 224–228
Aminoglycosides, 191–228. *See also* indi-
    vidual drugs
  administration and dosage, 198–199,
    203

773

Aminoglycosides (*continued*)
  antimicrobial activity, 198, 203
  chemistry, 192
  clinical usage, 199–200
  dosage considerations, 198–199
  drug interactions, 196
  mechanism of action, 192
  and meningitis, 425
  pharmacokinetic properties, 196
  renal failure, dosage, 456
  resistance, 195–196
  toxicity and adverse effects, 197–198,
    755–756
Aminobenzylpenicillins, 126–131
Amorolfine, 369
Amoxicillin. *See* Ampicillin; Clavulanic
    acid–amoxicillin
Amphotericin B, 376–382
  administration and dosage, 380–381,
    536, 568, 635, 663, 664
  antimicrobial activity, 376, 378
  applications, clinical, 381
  pharmacokinetic properties, 377
  toxicity and side effects, 379
Ampicillin, 126–131. *See also* Clavulanic
    acid–amoxicillin; Sulbactam-ampi-
    cillin
  administration and dosage, 129, 535,
    616, 632, 711
  antimicrobial activity, 126
  applications, clinical, 121, 129–130
    cattle, sheep, and goats, 129
    dogs and cats, 129
    fish, 711
    horses, 129
    poultry, 130
    reptiles, 687–689 (tables)
    rodents, rabbits and ferrets, 657,
      663, 665–677 (tables)
  pharmacokinetic properties, 56, 127
  sulbactam-ampicillin, 169–172
  toxicity and adverse effects,128, 657
Amprolium, 573, 649
Anaerobic infections, 132, 146, 148, 165,
    168, 171, 172, 233, 352, 458–461
  drugs, recommended, 460
Anaphylactic shock, 280

Anaplasma, 284, 589
Animal Drug Availability Act (United
    States), 763
Animal Medicinal Drug Use Clarifica-
    tion Act (AMDUCA), United
    States, 593, 768–771
Antagonism, 9–10
Anthelmintic chemotherapy, 490–508
  benzimidazoles, 500–502
  broad-spectrum anthelmintics,
    500–504
  cats, 496
  cattle, 491
  controlled drug delivery, 60, 497
  dogs, 495
  endectocides, 497–499
  horses, 494
  imidazothiazoles, 502–503
  narrow-spectrum anthelmintics,
    504–507
  organophosphates, 503–504
  pyridines, 502
  sheep and goats, 492
  swine, 493
  tetrahydropyrimidines, 502
Anthrax, 121
Antibacterial drugs. *See also* individual
    drugs
  classification, 4
  as growth promoters, 735–742
  history and development, 4, 5
  and human health, 39–46, 739–740,
    748–758, 765–767
  sites of action, 7
  spectrum of activity, 4,6
Antibiotic. *See also* Antibacterial drugs;
    individual antibiotics
  choice of, 88, 91–96
  definition of, 3
  as growth promoters, 735–742
  susceptibility, 12–26
Anticoccidials, 643–644, 649
Antifungal drugs, 8, 367–395, 575. *See
    also* individual drugs
  systemic, 373–395
  for topical application, 369–373, 375
Antimicrobial, 3. *See* Antibiotic; Antimi-

crobial treatment
Antimicrobial susceptibility. *See* Susceptibility
Antimicrobial treatment, 88–104
  adjunctive treatment, 97
  choice, 88, 91–96, 509–513, 540–541, 576–579, 603–605, 618–623, 638–642, 656–661, 679–681
  corticosteroid use, 98, 423
  cost effectiveness, 638
  dosage factors, 24, 79–80, 82, 93–96, 510–512, 543, 619–621, 658, 680–681, 697–699, 702
  drug combinations, 9, 99–100, 482–483
  drug formulations, 540–541
  drug incompatabilities, 90
  drug interactions, 9, 90, 640–641
  duration, 96–97, 434, 513, 543
  empirical use, 13, 91, 509, 543, 699
  failure, 23–25, 100, 434, 544
  immune system, 91
  neutropenia, 471–479
  principles of use, 93–103, 509–513, 540–544, 603–605
  prophylactic use, 101–103, 538–539
  rational use, 46
Antiprotozoals, 573
Antiviral drugs, 9, 396–415. *See also* individual drugs
  mechanisms of action, 396–397
Apramycin, 214–216
  administration and dosage, 203, 215, 616, 653
  antimicrobial activity, 211, 214
  applications, clinical, 215, 651
Aquaculture. *See* Fish
Arcanobacterium pyogenes, 121, 122, 141, 234, 242, 265, 293, 309, 583, 586, 614, 722
Area under the curve, AUC, 63, 68–71, 75, 328
Arsenicals, 360, 506, 616
Arthritis, septic, 222, 417–418, 513, 524, 554, 614
Ascaris suum, 493, 609
Aspergillosis, 371, 372, 381, 390, 393, 516, 548, 557, 627

Aspergillus, 371, 381, 385, 388, 394, 687, 688, 689
Avermectins, 497
Avoparcin, 43, 182, 186, 736, 737
Azalides, 238, 253. *See also* Azithromycin
Azidothymidine,
Azithromycin, 253–257
  antimicrobial activity, 253
  administration and dosage, 255, 571, 635
  applications, clinical, 256
  pharmacokinetic properties, 256
Azlocillin, 131
Azole antifungals, 371–372; *See also* individual drugs
Aztreonam, 175–176

Babesiosis, 284, 556, 564
Bacampicillin, 126
Bacillus anthracis, 121
Bacitracin, 187, 616, 653
  applications, 187
  and growth promotion, 187, 737
Bactericidal activity, 4, 81
Bacteriostatic activity, 4, 82
Bacteroides, 230. *See also* Anaerobic infections
Bacteroides asaccharolyticus. See Porphyromonas assacharolytica
Bacteroides fragilis, 132, 146, 149, 171, 172, 230, 352, 460
  and cephalosporins, 459
Baquiloprim, 300–304
Baquiloprim-sulfonamides, 304–313. *See* Trimethoprim-sulfonamides
Bartonella spp, 253, 287, 359
Benzenedisulfonamide, 505
Benzimidazoles, 500–502
Beta-lactam antibiotics, 105–177. *See also* individual drugs
  aminopenicillanic acid, 105
  betalactamase inhibitors, 160–172
  carbapenems, 172
  cephalosporins, 134–159
  cephamycins, 134–159
  chemistry, 107

Beta-lactam antibiotics (*continued*)
  introduction, 105
  mechanism of action, 107–110
  monobactams, 175
  penam penicillins, 111–133
  resistance, 110–111, 138
  structures, 106, 112
Beta-lactamases, 161–163
  cephalosporinases, 138
  classification, 161–163
  inhibitors, 160–172
  penicillinases, 110
Biapenem, 172–175
Bioavailability, 63–68
Bioequivalence, 65
Birds. *See* Pet birds
Blastomyces, 377, 392
Blastomycosis, 381, 386–387, 389–390,
  393, 557
Blood-brain barrier, 422, 442
Bones, infection, 416–417. *See also*
  Osteomyelitis
Bordetella bronchiseptica, 311, 336, 670,
  674
Borrelia burgdorferi, 121, 130, 286, 525
Brachyspira. *See Serpulina*
Brain abscesses, 425–426, 528
Breakpoints, 19
Brucella, 219, 253, 256, 308, 334, 358, 462,
  548, 615
Brucella abortus, 204, 284
Brucella canis, 286, 555
Brucella ovis, 204, 285, 597
Brucellosis, 462–463
Budgerigars. *See* Pet birds

Campylobacter fetus ssp. *fetus*, 596
Campylobacter fetus ssp. *venerealis*, 204,
  353
Campylobacter jejuni, 43, 242, 324, 550,
  562, 596
Candida, 370, 371, 377, 381, 382, 385, 387,
  388, 392–393, 652, 723
Carbadox, 360–361
Carbapenems, 172–175
Carbenicillin, 131–133
Carboxypenicillins, 131–133

Carfecillin, 131
Carindacillin, 131
Cats, 537–545, 559–565. *See also* individual drugs
  administration and dosage in (table),
    568–575
  amikacin, 213
  aminoglycosides, 205, 219, 222,
    227–228
  amoxicillin, 130
  amphotericin, 380–381
  ampicillin, 130
  anthelmintics, 496
  antimicrobial drug selection (Table),
    559–565
  azithromycin, 255–256
  Bartonella henselae, 256, 359, 563
  cephalosporins, 145, 154
  chlamydiosis, 256, 420, 560, 564
  chloramphenicol, 270
  clavulanic acid–amoxicillin, 168
  clindamycin, 235
  cryptococcosis, 383, 393, 559, 560
  dosage, usual drug, 568–575
  drug administration, routes of,
    541–542
  drugs, antifungal, 557–558
  ear infections, 560
  enrofloxacin, 336
  erythromycin, 243
  feline herpesvirus type 1, 402
  feline infectious anemia, 287, 564
  feline infectious peritonitis, 403, 408,
    411
  feline immunodeficiency virus, 404
  feline leukemia virus, 404
  fluconazole, 392–393
  flucytosine, 383
  fluoroquinolones, 336
  gastroenteritis, 562
  gentamicin, 222
  giardiasis, 353, 562
  griseofulvin, 374–375
  Haemobartonella felis, 287, 564
  Helicobacter gastritis, 130, 561
  herpesvirus keratoconjunctivitis, 402,
    560

infections, eye, 560
infections, respiratory, 560–561
infections, skin, 559–560
infections, urinary tract, 426–437, 563
itraconazole, 390
ketoconazole, 386–387
leprosy, 559
lincomycin, 235–236
marbofloxacin, 336
monensin, 341
Mycobacterium spp., 559
neomycin, 209
neutropenia, 471–489
nitrofurans, 347
nitroimidazoles, 353
oral infections, 561
orbifloxacin, 336
ormetoprim-sulfadimethoxine, 310
penicillin G, 123
polymyxins, 181
principles of antimicrobial therapy,
    537–545
pyothorax, 561
ribavirin, 403
rifampin, 359
ringworm, 375, 387
streptomycin, 202, 205
sulfonamides, 299
systemic mycoses, 557–558
tetracyclines, 286–287
therapeutic compliance, 543–544
tobramycin, 227
trimethoprim-sulfonamides, 310–311
tylosin, 246–247
urinary tract infections, 168, 426–437,
    552
zidovudine, 404
Cattle, 576–590. *See also* individual
    drugs
actinobacillosis (wooden tongue), 585
actinomycosis, 363, 587
aminoglycosides, 198
ampicillin, 129
anaplasmosis, 284, 589
anthelmintics, 491
apramycin, 215
baquiloprim-sulfadimidine, 309

blackleg, 587
bovine herpesvirus 1, 408, 410
brucellosis, 204, 284
campylobacteriosis, 353
cefoperazone, 157
ceftiofur, 153, 445, 578, 721
cefuroxime, 149
cephalosporins, 143, 149, 153, 157
chloramphenicol, 270
clavulanic acid–amoxicillin, 167
cowpox, 412
cystitis, 588
danofloxacin, 334–335
dermatophilosis, 586
digital dermatitis, 234, 284, 585
drug administration and dosage in
    (table), 590
drug selection (table), 583–589
endometritis, 586
enrofloxacin, 334–335, 582
erythromycin, 242
extralabel drug use, 580
florfenicol, 273, 578
fluoroquinolones, 331, 334–335
gentamicin, 221–22
griseofulvin, 375
infections, gastrointestinal, 583–584
infections, musculoskeletal, 586–587
infections, nervous system, 587–588
infections, reproductive tract, 586
infectious bovine keratoconjunctivitis,
    347, 421, 585. *See also Moraxella
    bovis*
injection site lesions, 581
interferon, use, 408
kanamycin, 198, 211
leptospirosis, 123, 471–472, 588
lincomycin, 234
listeriosis, 122, 587
mastitis, 712–734. *See also* Mastitis
metronidazole, 353
monensin, 340–342
neomycin, 208
nitrofurans, 347
nitroimidazoles, 352–353
novobiocin, 365
ormetoprim-sulfonamide, 309

Cattle (*continued*)
penicillin G, 121–122, 578
pharmacokinetic values, 73
pirlimycin, 237
pneumonia, 153, 576–579
polymyxins, 180
principles of antimicrobial use, 576–582
prophylactic antibiotics, 580
pseudocowpox, 412
residue avoidance, 580–581
respiratory disease, 309, 576–582, 583
rifampin, 358
ringworm, 370, 375, 395, 586
skin infections, 585
spectinomycin, 226
spiramycin, 248–249
streptomycin, 197, 204
sulbactam-ampicillin, 170
sulfonamides, 298
sulfonamides and trimethoprim, 309–310
tetracyclines, 283–285, 578
tiamulin, 259
tilmicosin, 251, 578
trimethoprim-sulfonamide, 309–310
tylosin, 245
undifferentiated bovine respiratory disease, 576–582
Cefachlor, 146–149
Cefadroxil, 143–146
Cefamandole, 146–149
Cefazolin, 140–143, 538
Cefepime, 158–159
Cefetamet, 155–156
Cefixime, 155–156
Cefmenoxime, 150–155
Cefmetazole, 146–149
Cefoperazone, 156–157, 690
Cefotaxime, 150–155, 632
Cefotetan, 146–149
Cefoxitin, 146–149, 460, 632
Cefpirome, 158–159
Cefquinome, 150–155
Cefsulodin, 156–157
Ceftazidime, 156–157, 687–690
Ceftiofur, 150–155, 444–445, 590, 616, 632, 653
Ceftizoxime, 150–155, 460
Ceftriaxone, 150–155, 632
Cefuroxime, 146–149
Center for Veterinary Medicine (US FDA), 45
"framework document", 45
Cephacetrile, 140–143
Cephalexin, 143–146
Cephaloglycin, 143–146
Cephaloridine, 140–143
Cephalosporins, Group 1, first-generation, 140–143
administration and dosage, 142, 535, 569
applications, clinical, 139, 142–143
pharmacokinetic properties, 142
Cephalosporins, Group 2, oral first-generation, 143–146
administration and dosage, 145, 159
antimicrobial activity, 144
applications, clinical, 145
pharmacokinetic properties, 144
Cephalosporins, Group 3, second-generation, 146–149, 535, 569
administration and dosage, 148
antimicrobial activity, 146
applications, clinical, 148–149
pharmacokinetic properties, 148
resistance, 148
Cephalosporins, Group 4, third-generation, 150–155, 535, 569
administration and dosage, 152
antimicrobial activity, 150
application, clinical, 152–153
pharmacokinetic properties, 151
Cephalosporins, Group 5, third-generation oral, 155–156
Cephalosporins, Group 6, antipseudomonal, 156–157, 687–689, 690
Cephalosporins, Group 7, fourth-generation, 158–159
clinical applications, 159
pharmacokinetic properties, 158
Cephalosporins and cephamycins, 134–159. *See also* Cephalosporins,

groups
antimicrobial activity, 137–138, 141
classification, 134–137
clinical usage, 139–140
generations, 135, 137
groups, 135
oral, 143, 155
pharmacokinetic properties, 138–139
resistance, 138
susceptibility testing, 137
toxicity and adverse effects, 139
Cephalothin, 140–143
Cephamycins, 134–159
Cephapirin, 140–143, 590
Cephradine, 143–146, 632
Chelonians. *See also* Reptiles
drug dosage, recommended (table),
690–691
drugs of choice (table), 687
Chickens. *See* Poultry
Chinchillas, 656–661
drug dosage, recommended (tables),
663, 664
drugs of choice (table), 673
Chlamydia, 246, 253, 256, 286, 298, 305,
308, 334, 359, 419, 557, 564, 596, 618
Chlamydia psittaci, 285, 564, 630, 636
Chlamydiosis, 286, 287, 309, 334, 630,
636
Chloramphenicol, 263–271
administration and dosage, 268–269,
535, 634, 663, 664, 690
antimicrobial activity, 264
applications, clinical, 269–270
dogs and cats, 270
horses, 270, 536
reptiles, 687–689 (tables)
rodents, rabbits and ferrets, 665–677
(tables)
chemistry, 263
drug interactions, 266–267
mechanism of action, 263
pharmacokinetic properties, 266,
619–620
toxicity and adverse effects, 267–268,
754
Chlortetracycline. *See* Tetracycline

and growth promotion,
Chronic respiratory disease (CRD),
poultry, 651. *See also Mycoplasma
gallisepticum*
Cilastatin, 173
Cilia-associated respiratory (CAR) bacil-
lus, 665, 667
Cilofungin, 394
Ciprofloxacin. *See* Fluoroquinolones
Citrobacter, 131, 156, 665, 687
Clarithromycin, 253–257. *See*
Azithromycin
Clavulanic acid–amoxicillin, 165–168
administration and dosage, 166, 568,
632
antimicrobial activity, 165, 460
applications, clinical, 167–168, 559
pharmacokinetic properties, 166
Clavulanic acid–ticarcillin, 168–169, 616
Clearance, ClB, 68–69
Clindamycin. *See* Lincomycin
Clioxanide, 504
Clofazimine, 635
Closantel, 504
Clostridial infections, 121, 122, 230, 284,
523, 587, 597
Clostridium colinum, 652
Clostridium difficile, 128, 152, 184, 232,
241, 281, 353, 459, 512
Clostridium perfringens, 123, 165, 187,
188, 343, 523, 597, 612, 652
Clostridium piliforme, 665, 667, 671, 674
Clostridium septicum, 587
Clostridium spiroforme, 128, 184, 187, 232,
657, 675
Clotrimazole, 371, 383
Cloxacillin, 124–125, 632
administration and dosage, 120
applications, 125
Coccidioides immitis, 381, 558
Coccidioidomycosis, 386–387, 390, 558
Coccidiosis, 300, 311, 313, 341–342, 598,
612, 643–644, 649–650
Codex Alimentarius Commission, 750,
761
Colibacillosis, 180, 208, 215, 584, 598,
607, 612

Colistin. *See* Polymyxins
Combinations, drug. *See* Antimicrobial
    treatment
Compliance, therapeutic, 543
Concentration-dependent killing effect,
    12, 81, 93
Conjunctivitis, 418–420
Corticosteroid use, 98, 425
Corynebacterium, 676
Corynebacterium kutcheri, 669
Corynebacterium pseudotuberculosis, 358,
    522, 599
Corynebacterium renale, 122, 588, 597
Cowdria ruminantium, 284
Coxiella burnetii, 242, 256, 283, 309, 334,
    359, 597, 672
Crocodilians. *See also* Reptiles
    dosage, recommended (table),
        690–691
    drugs of choice (table), 688
Cryptococcosis, 382, 386–387, 390,
    392–393, 558
Cryptococcus neoformans, 377, 380, 382,
    392, 558
Cryptosporidium, 556, 598, 671
Cytauxzoonosis, 564
Cytomegalovirus, 412, 413

Danofloxacin. *See* Fluoroquinolones
Dapsone, 299, 572
Deoxy-D-glucose, 409
Dermatophilus congolensis, 285, 525, 586,
    599
Diaminopyrimidines, antibacterial,
    300–304
Diaminopyrimidines, antiprotozoal,
    313–314
Diaminopyrimidines, antibacterial–sul-
    fonamide combinations, 304–313
Dichlorvos, 503, 704
Dicloxacillin. *See* Cloxacillin
Diethylcarbamazine, 505
Difloxacin. *See* Fluoroquinolones
Digital dermatitis, papillomatous, cattle,
    234, 284, 585
Dihydrostreptomycin. *See* Streptomycin
Dilution susceptibility testing, 18–19

Dimetridazole. *See* Nitroimidazoles
Dirofilaria immitis, 495, 498, 499
Disk diffusion testing, 16–17
Dogs, 537–558. *See also* individual drugs
    administration and dosage, in (table),
        568–575
    amikacin, 213
    aminoglycosides, 569–570
    amoxicillin, 130, 568
    amphotericin B, 380–381
    ampicillin, 130, 568
    anal sac infection, 547
    anthelmintics, 495
    antimicrobial therapy, principles of,
        537–545
    aspergillosis, 371, 372, 548, 557
    brucellosis, 205, 286, 552, 555
    canine herpesvirus (CHV), 403
    cephalosporins, 142–143, 145, 154, 569
    chloramphenicol, 270, 572
    clavulanic acid–amoxicillin, 168
    clindamycin, 235–236, 571
    clotrimazole, 371
    difloxacin, 336
    discospondylitis, 553
    dosage, usual drug, 568–575
    drug administration, routes of,
        541–542
    drug disposition kinetics in, 69
    drugs of choice (table), 546–558
    ehrlichiosis, 286, 557
    enilconazole, 371–372
    enrofloxacin, 336
    enteritis, 550–551
    erythromycin, 243
    fluoroquinolones, 336, 570
    gastroenteritis, 550–551
    gentamicin, 222
    giardiasis, 353, 550
    gingivitis, 549
    griseofulvin, 373–375
    infections, ear, 222, 546, 547
    infections, eye, 547–548
    infections, genital tract, 552–553
    infections, musculoskeletal, 553–554
    infections, oral, 549
    infections, respiratory, 548–549

infections, skin, 546
infections, urinary tract, 426–437, 552
itraconazole, 389
kanamycin, 210
kennel cough, 311, 336, 548
leptospirosis, 470, 555
lincomycin, 235–236, 571
marbofloxacin, 336
metronidazole, 352, 458–461, 546
    (tables), 574
neomycin, 209
neutropenia, 471–489
    infectious complications, 474–476
    prophylaxis, 476–479
    risk factors, 472–474
    treatment, 476–487
nitrofurans, 347
nitroimidazoles, 352
orbifloxacin, 336
ormetoprim-sulfadimethoxine, 310
penicillin G, 123, 568
penicillin V, 124, 568
polymyxins, 181
rickettsiosis, 286
ringworm, 375, 387, 546
spectinomycin, 226–227
streptomycin, 202, 205
sulfonamides, 299
systemic mycoses. *See* individual
    infections
tetracyclines, 286–287, 570–571
therapeutic compliance, 543
tinidazole, 353, 572
trimethoprim-sulfonamides, 310, 571
tylosin, 246–247
urinary tract infection. *See* Urinary
    tract infection
Dosage. *See also* Administration, drug
    allometric scaling, 619, 658, 680,
        683–684
    design, 79–80
    factors affecting, 79–82, 198–199
    interval, 80
    modification, 437–458
Doxycycline, 225, 289, 634, 690. *See also*
    Tetracyclines
Drug approval, United States, 748–750,

760–771. *See also* Regulation, veteri-
    nary drugs
Drug bioavailability, 50–87
Drug disposition, 50–62. *See also* Phar-
    macokinetics, applied clinical
Drugs, growth-promoting, 642, 735–742
    drugs used (tables), 737
    mechanisms of action, 737–739
    manufacturing issues, 740
    public health and environmental con-
        cerns, 39–45, 324–326, 740–742
    regulatory review criteria, 736
    usage practices and benefits, 739–740
Drug withdrawal, 103, 641–642
Dry-cow treatment, 729–731
Dysentery. *See* Swine; *Serpulina hyo-*
    dysenteriae

**For details of antimicrobial suscepti-
bility of individual bacterial and fungal species, consult susceptibility
tables and antimicrobial activity sections for individual drugs.**

E test, 17
Echinocandins, 394
Edwardsiella tarda, 705, 710
Ehrlichia, 283, 334, 557
Ehrlichia canis, 286, 557
Ehrlichia equi, 286, 534
Ehrlichia phagocytophilia, 598
Ehrlichia risticii, 243, 286, 359
Eimeria, 671. *See* Coccidiosis
Encephalitis, 422. *See also* Meningitis
Endophthalmitis, 421
Endotoxin, 180–181, 597, 718–719
Enilconazole, 371–372,516, 549, 635. *See*
    Azole antifungals; Antifungal
    drugs, for topical application
Enrofloxacin. *See* Fluoroquinolones
Enterobacter, 131, 147, 153, 155, 156, 168,
    171
Enterobacteriaceae, 133, 149, 152, 155, 156,
    172, 175, 199, 213
Enterococcus faecalis, 184, 189
Eperythrozoon, 286, 615

Equine protozoal encephalomyelitis, 310, 313, 529

Erysipelothrix rhusiopathiae, 121, 122, 285, 598, 613

Erythromycin, 238–244
  administration and dosage, 233, 535, 601, 633, 711
  antimicrobial activity, 239, 240
  applications, clinical, 242–243
    cattle, sheep, and goats, 242
    dogs and cats, 243
    fish, 704, 711
    horses, 242
    poultry, 243
    swine, 242
  pharmacokinetic properties, 239–240
  toxicity and adverse effects, 241

Escherichia coli, 35–36, 147, 152, 167, 170, 215, 220, 309, 334, 336, 584, 598, 651, 668, 674, 687, 720

Ethambutol, 465

Eubacterium suis, 615

Extralabel drug use, 97–98, 580, 593, 769–771

Eye, infections, 418–422
  drug dosages (table), 421

Famciclovir, 402

FARAD, 756–757

Feed additives. *See* Drugs, growth-promoting

Feedlot pneumonia, 576–579

Ferrets, 656–661
  antimicrobial drug toxicity, 657–658
  drug administration, routes of, 659–667
  drug dosage, recommended (tables), 663
  drugs of choice (table), 676–677

Fish, aquaculture, drug use, 692–711
  antimicrobial resistance, 705–707
  disease agents, 694–695
  drug classes, 703–705, 711 (table)
  drug selection, principles of, 698–699
  environmental constraints, 705–707
  florfenicol, 273, 705
  half-lives, antimicrobials, 72–73

pharmacokinectic considerations, 697–698
  principal bacterial pathogens, 710
  regulatory constraints, 695–697
  routes of application, 699–703
  sea lice treatment, 704
  tissue antimicrobial drug residues, 707
  topical disinfectants, 703

Flavobacterium psychrophilum, 693, 704

Fleroxacin. *See* Fluoroquinolones

Florfenicol, 272–274, 590, 705, 711

Fluconazole, 391–394, 519, 635

Flucytosine, 382–383

Flumequine, 704, 711

Fluoroquinolones, 315–338
  administration and dosage, 330–333, 535, 570, 590, 616, 634, 663, 664, 690, 711
  antimicrobial activity, 318–322
  applications, clinical, 333–337
    cattle, sheep, and goats, 334–335
    dogs and cats, 336
    fish, 704
    horses, 335–336,
    poultry, 336–337
    reptiles, 687–689 (tables)
    rodents, rabbits and ferrets, 665–677 (tables)
    swine, 335
  chemistry, 316–317
  drug interactions, 329
  mechanism of action, 317–318
  pharmacodynamic properties, 328–329
  pharmacokinetic properties, 326–327
  resistance, 15, 322–326
  toxicity and adverse effects, 330

Fomivirsen, 406, 412

Food
  Animal Residue Avoidance Databank, FARAD, 756–757
  antimicrobial drug residues, 744–771
  oral drug availability, effects on, 542–543, 567

Foscarnet, 404, 412, 413

Fosfomycin, 190

Framework document (United States, Food and Drug Administration, Center for Veterinary Medicine), 45
Francisella tularensis, 203, 672
Furazolidone, 653. *See* Nitrofurans
Furunculosis, 273, 525
Fusidic acid, 361–362
Fusobacterium necrophorum, 121, 585, 599, 614, 674

Gammaglobulin, 398
Ganciclovir, 413
Gentamicin, 216–224. *See also* Aminoglycosides
   administration and dosage, 218, 535, 569, 590, 616, 633, 653, 663, 664, 691
   antimicrobial activity, 216
   applications, clinical, 219–224
      cattle, sheep, and goats, 220–221
      dogs and cats, 222
      horses, 221–222
      poultry, 222
      reptiles, 687–689 (tables)
      rodents, rabbits and ferrets, 665–677 (tables)
      swine, 221, 607
   chemistry, 192
   drug interactions, 217
   mechanism of action, 192
   pharmacokinetic properties, 196, 217, 447–448
   resistance, 195,
   toxicity and adverse effects, 197, 217–218
Gerbils, 656–661
   antimicrobial drug toxicity, 657–658
   drug administration, routes of, 659–661
   drug dosage, recommended (tables), 662, 664
   drugs of choice (table), 668
Giardia lamblia, 344, 349, 352,
Giardia muris, 667
Glycopeptides, 182–187
Goats, 591–601. *See also* individual drugs

abortion, 596
ampicillin, 129, 601
anthelmintics, 492
antimicrobial drug selection (table), 596–600
Campylobacter abortion, 596
ceftiofur, 153
chlamydiosis, 596
clavulanic acid–amoxicillin, 167, 601
coccidiosis, 598
drug administration, routes of, 591–592
drug dosage (table), 601
drug use, extralabel, 593
drug use, in feed and water, 592
erythromycin, 242, 601
fluoroquinolones, 334
gastroenteritis, 597, 598
general considerations, 591–594
gentamicin, 220
infections, foot, 599
infections, skin, 599
infectious abortion, 596–597
mastitis, 600
monensin, 342, 592
pasteurellosis, 598
penicillin G, 121, 601
respiratory disease, 598–599
rifampin, 358
sulbactam-ampicillin, 170, 601
sulfonamides, 298, 601
tetracyclines, 283–285
tilmicosin toxicity, 251, 252, 601
trimethoprim-sulfonamides, 309, 601
tylosin, 245–246, 601
Griseofulvin, 373–375
Growth promotion, *See* Drugs, growth-promoting
Guinea pigs, 656–661
   ampicillin toxicity, 128, 657
   antimicrobial drug toxicity, 657–668
   drug administration, routes of, 659–661
   drug dosage, recommended (tables), 662, 664
   drugs of choice (table), 670–671
   penicillin toxicity, 658

Haemobartonella, 287,557, 564
Haemonchus, 499
Haemophilus paragallinarum, 336, 651
Haemophilus parasuis, 424, 613
Haemophilus pleuropneumoniae. See *Actinobacillus pleuropneumoniae*
Haemophilus somnus, 122, 170, 273, 309, 425, 588
Half-life, $t_{1/2}$, 72–75
Haloprogin, 369
Hamsters, 656–661
    antimicrobial drug toxicity, 657–658
    drug administration, routes of, 659–661
    drug dosage, recommended (tables), 662, 664
    drugs of choice (table), 667
Hedgehogs, 656–661
    drug administration, routes of, 659–661
    drug dosage, recommended (tables), 663
    drugs of choice (table), 672
Helicobacter hepaticus, 665
Helicobacter mustelae, 677
Helicobacter spp., 130, 253, 349, 550
Hepatozoonosis, 556
Herpesvirus, 412, 413
Hetacillin, 126. *See also* Aminobenzylpenicillins
Hexachlorphene, 369
Hexadepsipeptides, cyclic, 188
Hexamita meleagridis, 652
Histomonas meleagridis, 349, 652
Histoplasma capsulatum, 381, 386–387, 390, 558
Horses, 509–536. *See also* individual drugs
    acyclovir, 403
    amikacin, 213
    ampicillin, 129–130
    anthelmintics, 494
    bacterial pathogens, susceptibility, 511
    cefotaxime, 535
    ceftiofur, 153–154
    cephalosporins, 143, 153, 535

chloramphenicol, 270, 536
clavulanic acid–amoxicillin, 167
colitis, antibiotic-induced, 128, 512
colitis, treatment, 353, 519
contagious equine metritis, 532
cystitis, 527
drug administration, routes of, 512
drug dosage (table), 535–536
drug selection, 509–512
drugs of choice (table), 515–534
endocarditis, 527
enterocolitis, 519
equine herpesvirus 2, 402, 403
erythromycin, 242–243, 535
fluoroquinolones, 335, 535
gentamicin, 221, 535
guttural pouch mycosis, 391, 515
infections, eye, 529
infections, reproductive tract, 530–533, 536
infections, skin, 525
infections, upper respiratory tract, 515–516
itraconazole, 390
keratitis, 370, 371, 381, 390, 529
leptospirosis, 470–471, 534
lincomycin toxicity, 235, 512
mastitis, 532
meningitis, 310, 528
metritis, 530, 536
metronidazole, 353
monensin toxicity, 340
neomycin, 208
nitrofurans, 347
osteomyelitis, 524
penicillin G, 123, 535
peritonitis, 520
phycomycosis, 381, 526
pleuropneumonia, 353, 518
pneumonia, 517
polymyxins, 181
Potomac horse fever, 243, 519
protozoal encephalomyelitis, 310, 313, 529
pyrimethamine, 313
rhinitis, mycotic, 390, 516

rifampin, 358
ringworm, 375, 526
salmonellosis, 519. *See also* Salmonellosis
Sarcocystis neurona, 310, 313, 529
septicemia, 521
strangles, 310, 515
streptomycin, 10
sulfonamides, 299
tetracyclines, 286, 513
ticarcillin, 132
trimethoprim-sulfonamides, 310, 536
tylosin, 246

Idoxuridine, 400–404, 412
Imidazole antifungals, 383–388. *See* Itraconazole; Ketoconazole
Imidocarb, 473
Imipenem, 172–175
  antimicrobial activity, 172
  applications, clinical, 174
  drug interactions, 173
  pharmacokinetic properties, 173
Immunodeficiency. *See* Neutropenia, dogs and cats
Immunoglobulin, antiviral, 398
Influenza, 413
Injection, tissue damage, 581, 591, 603
Integrons, 33–34
Interactions, antibacterial drug. *See* Drug interaction
Interferons, 406–409
Intra-abdominal sepsis, 171. *See also* Peritonitis
Iodides, 394–395
Ionophores, 339–343. *See also* individual drugs
Ipronidazole. *See* Nitroimidazoles
Isoniazid, 362–363, 635
Isoquinolines, 507
Isospora, 550, 562
Itraconazole, 388–391
  administration and dosage, 389–390, 536, 575, 635, 691
  antimicrobial activity, 388–389

applications, clinical, 390–391, 689
  toxicity and adverse effects, 389
Ivermectin, 497, 704

Josamycin, 253
Johne's disease. *See Mycobacterium paratuberculosis*

Kanamycin, 209–211. *See also* Aminoglycosides
  administration and dosage, 203, 210, 711
  antimicrobial activity, 193, 209
  applications, clinical, 210
Kennel cough, 336
Keratitis
  fungal, 370, 390, 421
  herpetic, 412, 421
  ulcerative, 221, 370, 420
Keratoconjunctivitis sicca, 296,
Ketolides, 257
Ketoconazole, 371, 384–388
  administration and dosage, 386–387, 536, 575, 635, 691
  antimicrobial activity, 384–385
  applications, clinical, 387, 690
  pharmacokinetic properties, 385
  toxicity and side effects, 386
Kirby Bauer method (disk diffusion), 16
Kitasamycin, 253
Klebsiella pneumoniae, 131, 145, 147, 152, 181, 213, 221
Kudoa, 695

Lasalocid, 343, 649
Latamoxef (moxalactam), 150–155
Lawsonia intracellularis, 187, 226, 242, 260, 285, 519, 667
Legionella, 253
Leishmania, 556
Leptospira, 123, 188, 470
Leptospirosis, 123, 129, 202, 204, 205, 242, 285, 286, 470–471, 534, 596
Levamisole, 502
Lice, 615

Lincomycin (clindamycin), 229–237
administration and dosage, 233, 571, 616, 633, 653
antimicrobial activity, 230
applications, clinical, 233–236
cattle, sheep, and goats, 234
dogs and cats, 235–236
horses, 235
poultry, 236
swine, 234
chemistry, 229
drug interactions, 231–232
mechanism of action, 230
pharmacokinetic properties, 231
resistance, 231
toxicity and adverse effects, 232
Lincosamides, 229–237
Liposomes, 103, 196, 220
Listeriosis, 122, 129, 284, 303, 309, 425, 670
Liver failure, drug usage in, 566
Lizards. *See also* Reptiles
dosage, recommended (table), 690–691
drugs of choice (table), 689
Loading dose, 98
Lyme disease, 286, 555. *See also Borrelia burgdorferi*

For details of antimicrobial susceptibility of individual bacterial and fungal species, consult susceptibility Tables and Antimicrobial Activity sections for individual drugs.

Macrolactones, 188
Macrolides, 237–262. *See also* individual drugs
advanced generation, 253–257
Maduromicin, 343, 649
Malachite green, 687, 703–704
Malassezia pachydermatis, 370, 371, 372, 375, 546
Mange, 615
Mannheimia haemolytica. See Pasteurella haemolytica

Marbofloxacin. *See* Fluoroquinolones
Mastitis, 712–734. *See also* individual animal species; Milk
Arcanobacterium pyogenes, 722
assessing efficacy, 713–715
Candida, 370, 723
cefoperazone, 157
cefuroxime, 149
coliforms, 717–721
considerations before treatment, 713–717
dry cow therapy, 729–731
heifers, 731–733
lactating cow, antimicrobial therapy, 125, 153, 717–729
mild clinical mastitis, 724–725
Mycoplasma, 723
noncoliform acute mastitis, 721–725
pharmacokinetic considerations, 82–85, 715–717
Prototheca zopfii, 723
Pseudomonas spp., 721
Serratia spp., 722
Staphylococcus aureus, 725–729, 730
streptococcal, 724–728
subclinical mastitis, 725–729
therapeutic protocols, 734
Maximum residue limit, 699, 749–752, 761
MBC. *See* Minimum bactericidal concentration
Mean residence time, 75–76
Mecillinam, 131
Meglumine antimonate,
Meningitis, 422–425
drugs of choice, 151, 152, 170, 424, 587
treatment, 423
Meropenem, 172–175
Metabolic scaling. *See* Allometric scaling
Methenamine, 364
Methicillin, 124–126
Methisazone, 412
Metronidazole. *See* Nitroimidazoles
Mezlocillin, 132
MIC. *See* Minimum inhibitory concentration
Mice, 656–661

drug administration, routes of, 659–661
drug dosage, recommended (tables), 662, 664
drugs of choice (table), 665–666
Miconazole, 371
Microsporida, 695
Microsporum. See Ringworm
Milbemycins, 497
Milk. *See also* Mastitis
    passage into, 82–85
Minimum bactericidal concentration (MBC), 12, 423
Minimum inhibitory concentration (MIC), 12, 18, 28, 30
Minocycline, 275–289
MLS cross-resistance, 231
Monensin, 339–343
    applications, clinical, 341, 596, 649
    growth promotion, 737
    toxicity and adverse effects, 340–341, 592
Monobactams, 175–176. *See also* Betalactam antibiotics
Moraxella bovis, 122, 210, 284, 347
Morganella morganii, 687, 689
Moxalactam. *See* Latamoxef
Moxidectin, 497
Mucor, 378, 381, 687
Mupirocin, 363–364
Mycobacterial infections, atypical, 256, 358, 362, 463–466, 559
Mycobacterium, 253, 358, 559, 617
Mycobacterium avium, 172, 196, 253,465, 635
Mycobacterium bovis, 362–363, 564
Mycobacterium chelonae, 465, 687
Mycobacterium fortuitum, 465
Mycobacterium kansasii, 309, 362
Mycobacterium marinum, 309, 694
Mycobacterium paratuberculosis, 358, 363
Mycoplasma bovis, 226, 245, 259, 283, 347, 467, 587
Mycoplasma californicum, 245, 285
Mycoplasma conjunctivae, 285
Mycoplasma felis, 286, 518, 565
Mycoplasma gallisepticum, 236, 243, 247, 251, 287, 337, 645, 651
Mycoplasma hyopneumoniae, 246, 260, 285, 335, 467, 606
Mycoplasma hyorhinis, 235, 606, 612
Mycoplasma hyosynoviae, 235, 614
Mycoplasma infections, 234, 253, 256, 334, 420, 466–468, 678
    cattle, sheep, and goats, 599, 600, 723
    swine, 605–607
    tetracycline use, 467
Mycoplasma meleagridis, 651
Mycoplasma mycoides, 245–246, 248, 599, 600
Mycoplasma ovipneumoniae, 599
Mycoplasma pulmonis, 665, 669
Mycoplasma synoviae, 227, 287, 651, 652
Mycoses. *See* Antifungal drugs
Myxosporida, 695

Nafcillin, 124–126
Naftifine, 375
Nalidixic acid,
Narasin, 343, 649
Natamycin, 369–370
National Antimicrobial Resistance Monitoring System (NARMS), 43, 768
Nebulization, 622, 630, 636
Necrotic enteritis, poultry, 123, 652
Nematodirus, 499
Neomycin, 206–209. *See also* Aminoglycosides
    administration and dosage, 207, 616, 633, 662, 663, 711
    antimicrobial activity, 193
    applications, clinical, 207–209
    toxicity and adverse effects, 197, 207
Neonates, 437–452, 566. *See also* individual drugs
    drug disposition, 437–448
    drug selection and dosage, 448–450, 566
Neospora caninum, 236, 313, 556
Neosporosis, 313
Netilmicin, 228
Netobimin, 501
Neutropenia, dogs and cats, 471–489
    infections, complications, 472

Neutropenia, dogs and cats (*continued*)
  infections, documented, 487
  therapy, for febrile illness, 479–487
  therapy, prophylactic, 476–478
  treatment, empirical, 479–487
New antibacterial drugs, 8
Nicarbazin, 649
Niclosamide, 504
Nifuratel. *See Nitrofurans*
Nitrofurans, 343–348
  administration and dosage, 347, 634
  antimicrobial activity, 344–345
  applications, clinical, 347
  chemistry, 343
  pharmacokinetic properties, 346
  resistance, 345–346
  toxicity and adverse effects, 346–347
Nitrofurantoin. *See Nitrofurans*
Nitrofurazone. *See Nitrofurans*
Nitroimidazoles, 348–354
  administration and dosage, 351–352,
    536, 574, 616, 653, 662, 663, 691
  antimicrobial activity, 349, 460
  applications, clinical, 352–353
    cattle, sheep, and goats, 352–353
    dogs and cats, 353
    horses, 353
    poultry, 353
    reptiles, 687–689 (tables)
    rodents, rabbits and ferrets, 665–677
      (tables)
    swine, 353, 608
  mechanism of action, 349
  pharmacokinetic properties, 350
  resistance, 349
  toxicity and adverse effects, 350–351
Nocardia asteroides, 298, 299, 305, 308,
    468, 723
Nocardial infections, 468–470
Norfloxacin, *See* Fluoroquinolones
Novobiocin, 364–366, 653
Nystatin, 370–371, 635, 653, 690

Ofloxacin. *See* Fluoroquinolones
Olaquindox, 361
Oleandomycin, 253, 633
Orbifloxacin. *See* Fluoroquinolones

Organophosphates, 503–504
Ornithobacterium rhinotracheale, 651
Ormetoprim, 300–304
Ormetoprim-sulfonamide combinations.
  See Trimethoprim-sulfonamides
Osteomyelitis, 416–417, 524
Ostertagia, 499
Otitis externa, 222, 547
Oxacillin, 124–126
Oxolinic acid, 704, 711
Oxytetracycline. *See* Tetracycline

Paromomycin, 208
Parrot. *See* Pet birds
Passerines. *See* Pet birds
Pasteurella haemolytica, 122, 170, 226, 242,
    251, 273, 283, 298, 309, 334, 577, 598
Pasteurella multocida, 123, 170, 242, 251,
    273, 285, 309, 334, 577, 606, 651, 674
Pasteurella piscicida, 705, 710
Pasteurella pneumotropica, 665, 667, 669
Pasteurella testudinis, 687
Pefloxacin. *See* Fluoroquinolones
Penciclovir, 402
Penicillin G, 117–124
  administration and dosage, 119, 120,
    121, 535, 568, 590, 616, 654
  antimicrobial activity, 118
  applications, clinical, 121–123
    cattle, sheep, and goats, 121
    dogs and cats, 123
    horses, 123
    poultry, 123
    swine, 122
  chemistry, 107
  drug interactions, 116, 119
  mechanism of action, 107
  pharmacokinetic properties, 116
  resistance, 118
  toxicity and adverse effects, 117, 119
Penicillins, anti-staphylococcal, 124–125
Penicillins, penam, 111–133
  amidopenicillins, 131
  aminobenzylpenicillins, 126–131
  antimicrobial activity, 114
  antipseudomonal, 131–133
  anti-staphylococcal, 124–126

benzyl penicillin, 117–124
beta-lactamase resistant, 124–126
broad-spectrum, 126, 131
carboxypenicillins, 131–133
classification, 113
clinical usage, 117
dosage (table), 120
dosage considerations, 117
drug interactions, 116
extended spectrum, 126–131
isoxazolyl penicillins, 124–126
mechanism of action, 113–114
narrow-spectrum, 117
orally absorbed, 124
penicillinase-resistant, 124
pharmacokinectic properties, 116
resistance, 114–116
toxicity and adverse effects, 117
ureidopenicillins, 131–133
Penicillin-streptomycin, combination,
122, 203
Penicillin V, 124
Pentamidine, 556, 574
Peptide antibiotics, 177–190
Periodontal disease, 235, 286, 353, 549,
561, 672
Peritonitis, intestinal spillage, 171, 336,
352, 520, 551
Pet birds, 617–636
comparative digestive anatomy, 621
drug administration, methods of,
623–630
drug administration, routes of (table),
622–630
drug dosage, usual (table), 632–635
drug extrapolation, 619–621
general comments, 617
oral dosage forms, 623–625
parenteral dosage forms, 625
respiratory system, anatomy, 622
Pharmacokinetics, applied clinical,
60–85
bioavailability, 63–68
bioequivalence, 65
changes in drug disposition, 76–79
clearance, Cl_B, 68–69
development of antimicrobial prepa-

rations, 80–82, 93
distribution, volume of, 69–72
distribution and elimination, 61–62
dosage regimen, 79–80, 318–319
dosing rate, 79–80
half-life, 72–75
mastitis, 715–717
mean residence time, 75
neonatal animals, 437–452
parameters, 63–80
species differences, 619–620, 658, 680,
698
Pharmacodynamic parameters, 13,
93–96
Pharmacokinetic properties, 12, 13,
60–85, 93–96
Phenothiazine, 506
Pigeons, 619, 624, 626, 629, 632–635. *See
also* Pet birds
Pigs. *See* Swine
Piperacillin, 131–133, 535, 691
Piperacillin-tazobactam, 171
Piperazine, 505
Pirlimycin, 237
Piscirickettsia salmonis, 693, 710
*Pityrosporum. See Malassezia pachyderma-
tis*
Pivampicillin, 126
Plague, 203, 563
Plasmids, resistance, 31–33
Pleuromutilins, 257–262
Pneumocandins, 394
Pneumocystis carinii, 234, 298, 303, 305,
308, 676
Polymethyl methacrylate, PMMA
antibiotic beads, 220
Polymyxins, 177–181
administration and dosage, 180
antimicrobial activity, 178
applications, clinical, 180, 607
pharmacokinetic properties, 178–179
toxicity and adverse effects, 179
Porphyromonas asaccharolytica, 122, 165
Porphyromonas, 146
Post-antibiotic effect, PAE, 12, 13, 95
Post-antibiotic leucocyte enhancement,
PALE, 12, 95

Potomac horse fever, 286
Poultry, 637–655. *See also* individual
    drugs
  ampicillin, 130
  apramycin, 215, 655
  aspergillosis, 372
  bacitracin, 187
  ceftiofur, 154
  coccidiosis, control of, 643–644;
    (table), 649–650
  chronic respiratory disease, 227, 236,
    251, 651
  danofloxacin, 655
  drug administration, routes of,
    639–640
  drug dosage, usual (tables), 653–654
  drug interactions, 640–641
  drugs, nutritional (table), 642
  drugs of choice (table), 650–651
  drug use, for newly hatched chicks,
    645
  E. coli septicemia, 311, 336, 645
  egg treatments, 645
  enrofloxacin, 336, 653
  erythromycin, 243
  fluoroquinolones, 336
  general considerations, 638–642
  gentamicin, 222, 653
  growth promoters (table), 642
  infections, intestinal, 652
  infections, soft tissue, 651
  infections, upper respiratory, 651
  lincomycin, 236, 653
  monensin, 341, 649
  necrotic enteritis, 123, 187, 652
  neomycin, 209, 653
  nitrofurans, 347, 653
  novobiocin, 366, 653
  ormetoprim-sulfamethoxazole, 311,
    653
  penicillin, 654
  penicillin G, 123, 653
  probiotics, 641
  salmonellosis, 652
  sarafloxacin, 336, 654
  septicemias, 651
  spectinomycin, 227, 654
  spiramycin, 249, 654
  sulfonamides, 300, 654
  tetracyclines, 287
  trimethoprim-sulfonamides, 311, 654
  tylosin, 247, 654
  water medication, principles, 646–647
  withdrawal time, 641–642
Pregnancy, 386, 452–453, 566
Prevotella, 146
Pristinamycin, 188, 189
Probiotics, 641
Prophylaxis, antibiotic, 101–103, 125,
    143, 538–539, 580
Prostatic infections, 231, 303, 311, 336,
    435–436, 552
Protease inhibitors, antiviral, 409, 412
Proteus mirabilis, 130, 131, 689
Prototheca, 370, 381, 385, 393, 723
Pseudomonas aeruginosa, 131, 132, 153,
    156, 180, 199, 213, 219, 221, 222,
    227, 286, 299, 318, 420, 433, 687,
    714, 721–722
  drugs of choice, for bovine mastitis
    (table), 721–722
  infections, in bones and joints, 221
  infections, urinary tract, 286
Pseudomonas fluorescens, 705
Psittacines. *See also* Pet birds
  drug dosage, usual (table), 632–636
Psittacosis, suggested drugs in birds,
    636. *See also Chlamydia psittaci*
Pulpy kidney infection, 597
Pyrimethamine, 313
Pyoderma, staphylococcal, 235, 287
Pythiosis, 526

Q fever. *See Coxiella burnetii*
Quinipristin-dalfopristin, 44, 189
Quinolones. *See* Fluoroquinolones

**For details of antimicrobial suscepti-
bility of individual bacterial and fungal species, consult susceptibility
tables and antimicrobial activity sections for individual drugs.**

Rabbits, 656–661, 664, 674–675
  ampicillin toxicity, 128, 657
  antimicrobial drug toxicity, 657
  drug administration, routes of,
    659–661
  drug dosage, recommended (tables),
    663–664
  drugs of choice (table), 674–675
  penicillin toxicity, 658
  tilmicosin, 250
Rafoxanide, 504
Rats, 656–661
  drug administration, routes of,
    659–661
  drug dosage, recommended (tables),
    662, 664
  drugs of choice (table), 669
Reimerella anatipestifer, 651
Regulation, veterinary drugs
  animal drug approval process, United
    States, 761–768
  Animal Drug Availability Act, 762
  Animal Medicinal Drug Use Clarifica-
    tion Act, AMDUCA, 768–771
  evaluation of animal safety, 764–765
  human food safety, drug residues,
    765–767
  international standards, 760–761
  professional flexible labelling,
    763–764
  United States, 748–750, 760–771
Renal disease, dosage and, 453–458, 566
Renibacterium salmoninarum, 693, 704, 710
Reptiles, 678–691
  allometric scaling, 680, 683–684
  drug administration, principles of,
    681–683
  drug dosage, suggested (table),
    690–691
  drug selection, principles of, 679–681
  drugs of choice, for chelonians (tor-
    toises) (table), 687
  drugs of choice, crocodilians (table),
    688
  drugs of choice, for lizards and
    snakes (table), 689
Residues, drug, in food animals, 605,

    740, 744–759
  Food Animal Residue Avoidance
    Databank (FARAD), 756–757
  human health, effects on, 750–756,
    765–768
    aminoglycosides, 755–756
    beta-lactams, 753
    chloramphenicol, 754
    sulfamethazine, 754–755
  maximum residue limit, 749–752
  rapid screening, 745–746
  residue limits, maximum, 696, 707
  residue, violations, in U.S.A., 744–748
  tolerance values, 749–750
  withholding times (tables), 698
Resistance, antibacterial drug, 27–49,
    324–326
  acquired, 29
  agricultural use of antimicrobials,
    44–45, 706
  Campylobacter jejuni, 43
  chromosomal mutation, 29–30
  conjugation, 31–33
  constitutive, 28
  control of, 45–47
  cross-chromosomal, 35
  determination of, 16–19
  extent of, 35–39
  human health, 39–45, 324–326,
    740–742
  integrons, 33–34
  intinsic, 28
  mechanisms, 35
  multi-antibiotic resistance (MAR), 35
  National Antimicrobial Resistance
    Monitoring System (NARMS), 43,
    768
  plasmids, 31–33
  Salmonella typhimurium DT104, 37–38
  surveillance, 43, 47, 742
  Swann Report, 40–41
  transduction, 31
  transfer of, 30–35
  transformation, 31
  transposons, 33–34
  vancomycin-resistant enterococci, 43,
    742

Resistance, antifungal, 368
R factors. *See* Resistance, plasmids
Rhinitis, atrophic, 606
Rhinitis, mycotic, 371, 390, 516, 549, 635
Rhinovirus, 398, 408
Rhizopus, 378, 381
Rhodococcus equi, 130, 184, 242, 256, 358, 517
Ribavarin, 412, 413
Rickettsia, 256, 259, 334, 573, 599
Rickettsia rickettsii, 286, 292, 557
Rifampin, 354–360
    administration and dosage, 358, 536, 572, 635
    antimicrobial activity, 355–356
    applications, clinical, 358–359
        cattle, sheep, and goats, 359
        dogs and cats, 359
        horses, 358–359
    drug interactions, 357–358
    mechanism of action, 355
    pharmacokinetic properties, 356–357
    toxicity and adverse effects, 358
Rifamycins. *See* Rifampin
Rimantidine, 399–400
Ringworm, 369, 374–375, 386–387, 390
Risks, in antimicrobial therapy, 88–90
Ritonavir, 409, 413
Robenidine, 650
Rodents, 656–677. *See also* individual species
    ampicillin toxicity, 128
    drug dosage, recommended (tables), 662–664
    drug toxicity, in, 657–658
Ronidazole. *See* Nitroimidazoles
Rosaramicin, 253
Roundworms,
Roxithromycin, 253–257. *See* Azithromycin
Ruminal development, 439, 592

Salicylanilides, 504
Salinomycin, 343, 650
Salmonella arizona, 652, 678, 688, 689
Salmonella dublin, 344
Salmonella gallinarum, 651

Salmonella pullorum, 652
Salmonella typhimurium, 37–38, 215, 326. *See also* Salmonellosis
Salmonellosis, 215, 235, 310, 334, 519, 550, 562, 584, 596, 598, 609, 612, 668, 671, 672, 677, 687, 688, 689
Sanfetrinem cilexetil, 176
Saquinovir, 409, 413
Sarafloxacin. *See* Fluoroquinolones
Sarcocystis neurona, 310, 313, 529
Septicemia, 200, 513
Serpulina hyodysenteriae, 234, 349, 607
Serpulina pilosicoli, 607, 612
Serratia, 147, 156, 687, 688, 689, 722
Sheep, 591–601. *See also* individual drugs
    ampicillin, 129, 601
    anthelmintics, 492
    brucellosis, 597
    ceftiofur, 153, 601
    clavulanic acid–amoxicillin, 167, 601
    coccidiosis, 598
    drug administration, routes of, 591–592
    drug dosage (table), 601
    drug selection (table), 596–600
    drug use, extralabel, 593
    drug use, in feed and water, 592
    drug withdrawal periods, 593
    enzootic abortion, 596
    erythromycin, 242, 601
    fluoroquinolones, 335
    gastroenteritis, 597, 598
    general considerations, 591–594
    infections, foot, 599
    infectious abortion, 596–597
    infectious keratoconjunctivitis, 249, 259, 421, 599
    lincomycin, 234, 601
    mastitis, 600
    monensin, 342, 592
    pasteurellosis, 598
    penicillin G, 121, 601
    respiratory disease, 598–599
    spiramycin, 248–249
    sulbactam-ampicillin, 170, 601
    sulfonamides, 298, 601

tetracyclines, 283–285
tiamulin, 259
tilmicosin, 251, 601
toxoplasmosis, 249, 309, 596
trimethoprim-sulfonamides, 309, 601
tylosin, 245–246, 601
Sisomicin, 228
Snakes. *See also* Reptiles
  drug dosage, recommended (table),
    689–690
  drugs of choice (table), 689
Spectinomycin, 224–227
  administration and dosage, 203, 226,
    590, 633, 654
  antimicrobial activity, 224
  applications, clinical, 226
  toxicity and adverse effects, 225
Spectrum, antibacterial, 4, 6
Spiramycin, 248–249, 633, 654
Sporothrix schenckii, 388, 390, 394
Spotted fever, Rocky Mountain. *See*
  Rickettsia rickettsii
Staphylococcus aureus, 122, 124–125, 140,
    143, 145, 165, 182, 187, 189, 233,
    287, 320, 358, 362, 363, 365, 652,
    665, 667, 673, 712, 714, 725–729, 730
Staphylococcus hyicus, 615
Staphylococcus intermedius, 140, 247, 676.
  See also S. aureus
Streptobacillus moniliformis, 666
Streptococcus agalactiae, 713, 714, 726
Streptococcus canis, 330
Streptococcus dysgalactiae, 724, 726
Streptococcus equi, 515
Streptococcus pneumoniae, 667, 669
Streptococcus suis, 122, 261, 310, 614
Streptococcus uberis, 724, 726
Streptococcus zooepidemicus, 123, 515, 517,
    670, 676
Streptogramins, 44, 188–190
Streptomycin, 201–205. *See also* Amino-
  glycosides
  administration and dosage, 203, 535,
    569, 616, 633
  antimicrobial activity, 201
  applications, clinical, 202–206
    cattle, sheep, and goats, 204

dogs and cats, 205
horses, 205
poultry, 205
swine, 204
  pharmacokinetic properties, 196
  resistance, 201
  toxicity and adverse effects, 197, 202,
    657
Sub-MIC effect, 12, 13
Subtherapeutic, 735
Sulbactam, 169
Sulbactam-ampicillin, 169–171, 590. *See
  also* Clavulanic acid–amoxicillin
  applications, clinical, 170
Sulbactam-cefoperazone,
Sulfadiazine, 295
Sulfamethazine, 296–297
Sulfaquinoxaline, 654
Sulfasalazine, 296, 299
Sulfisoxazole, 297–298
Sulfonamides, 290–314
  administration and dosage, 296–298,
    571, 616, 711
  antimicrobial activity, 292–293
  applications, clinical, 298–300
    cattle, sheep, and goats, 298
    dogs and cats, 299
    fish, 711
    horses, 299
    poultry, 299, 650
    swine, 299, 754–755
  chemistry, 290
  drug interactions, 295
  mechanisms of action, 291
  pharmacokinetic properties, 294–295
  resistance, 293
  toxicity and adverse effects, 295,
    754–755
Surveillance, resistance, 47
Susceptibility, 12–26
  antifungal, 367
  antimicrobial, 12
  bacterial, 13–16
  break-points, 19
  defined, 18
  failure of testing, 16, 23–25
  guidelines, 19–23

Susceptibility (*continued*)
  indications, 13–16, 510
  interpretation of data, 19–24, 618
  NCCLS (National Committee for
    Clinical Laboratory Standards),
    19, 21–23
  testing, 16–19, 367–368, 618–619
  and urinary tract, 432–433
Swann Report, 40–41
Swine, 602–616. *See also* individual
    drugs
  anthelmintics, 493, 609–610
  apramycin, 215, 616
  arsenicals, 360
  arthritis, 614
  atrophic rhinitis, 606, 612
  bacitracin, 187, 616
  carbadox, 360–361, 616
  ceftiofur, 154, 616
  clavulanic acid–amoxicillin, 167, 616
  coccidiosis, 612
  colibacillosis, 612
  dimetridazole, 352
  drug administration, routes of, 603
  drug dosages (table), 616
  drug residues, 604–605, 745, 754–755
  drug selection (table), 612–615
  drug use, extralabel, 605
  drug withdrawal periods, 605
  dysentery, 234–235, 260, 342, 361,
    607–608, 612
  edema disease, 614
  enzootic pneumonia, 260, 605–607,
    612
  erythromycin, 242, 616
  fluoroquinolones, 331, 335
  gentamicin, 221, 616
  general considerations, 602–611
  infections, gastrointestinal, 607–609,
    612
  infections, skin, 615
  infections, urogenital tract, 615
  infectious arthritis, 614
  leptospirosis, 204, 242, 262, 471–472,
    615
  lincomycin, 234–235
  meningitis, 310, 614

  monensin, 342
  neomycin, 208, 614
  nervous diseases, 614
  nitrofurans, 347
  nitroimidazoles, 353, 616
  penicillin G, 122–123, 616
  penicillin V, 124
  pleuropneumonia, 260, 613
  polymyxins, 181, 607
  proliferative intestinal adenomatosis,
    187, 188, 226, 242, 251, 261, 285,
    342, 361, 608, 612
  respiratory diseases, 605–607, 612
  safety and efficacy, 604–605
  spectinomycin, 226
  spiramycin, 249
  streptomycin, 204
  sulfonamides, 299, 616
  tetracyclines, 285–286, 616
  tiamulin, 260–261, 616
  tilmicosin, 251, 252, 616
  trimethoprim-sulfonamides, 310, 616
  tylosin, 246, 616
Synergism, antibacterial drug, 9–10

Targeted drug delivery, 103
Tazobactam, 171–172
Teicoplanin, 184–186
Temocillin, 133
Terbinafine, 375
Tetanus, 528, 554, 614
Tetracycline, 275–289
  administration and dosage, 281–282,
    535, 570, 590, 616, 634, 653, 662,
    663
  antimicrobial activity, 276–278
  applications, clinical, 283–287
    cattle, sheep, and goats, 283–285
    dogs and cats, 286–287, 433
    fish, 711
    horses, 286, 513
    poultry, 287
    rabbits, 658
    rodents, rabbits and ferrets, 665–677
      (tables)
    swine, 285–286
  chemistry, 275

drug interactions, 280
mechanism of action, 276
pharmacokinetic properties, 278–279,
448
resistance, 278
toxicity and adverse effects, 280–281,
657, 660
Theileria, 284
Thiabendazole, 500
Thiamphenicol, 271–272, 711
Thienamycin. *See* Beta-lactam antibiotics
Thymol, 369
Tiamulin, 257–262
administration and dosage, 233, 616,
633
antimicrobial activity, 257
applications, clinical, 259–262
cattle, sheep, and goats, 259
poultry, 259
swine, 608
drug interactions, 258
toxicity and adverse effects, 259
Ticarcillin, 131–133
Tick-borne fever, 284, 598
Tigemonam, 175
Tilmicosin, 249–252
administration and dosage, 233,
250
antimicrobial activity, 240, 249
applications, clinical, 251–252
toxicity and adverse effects, 250–251
Time-dependent killing effect, 81, 93
Tinidazole. *See* Nitroimidazoles
Tobramycin, 227
Tolnaftate, 369
Tortoises. *See* Chelonians; Reptiles
Toxoplasma, 235, 249, 298, 313, 342, 408,
556, 564, 596
Transposons, 33
Treponema cuniculi, 658, 675
Treponema hyodysenteriae. See *Serpulina
hyodysenteriae*
Triazole antifungals, 388–394. *See* Flu-
conazole; Itraconazole
Tribactams, 176
Tritrichomonas foetus, 344, 349, 351, 352
Trichophyton. *See* Ringworm

Trichostrongylus, 491
Trichuris, 497
Trifluridine, 400–404, 412
Trimethoprim, 300–304
Trimethoprim-sulfonamides, 304–314
administration and dosage, 308, 535,
571, 616, 633, 653, 662, 663, 691,
711
antimicrobial activity, 305–306
applications, clinical, 308–313
cattle, sheep, and goats, 309–310
dogs and cats, 310–311
fish, 711
horses, 310
poultry, 311
reptiles, 687–689 (tables)
rodents, rabbits and ferrets, 665–677
(tables)
swine, 310
drug interactions, 307
pharmacokinetic properties, 307
toxicity and adverse effects, 307–308
Trovafloxacin. *See* Fluoroquinolones
Trypanosomiasis, 557
Tularemia, 203, 672
Turkeys. *See* Poultry
Tylosin, 244–248
administration and dosage, 233, 245,
571, 616, 654, 691
antimicrobial activity, 244
applications, clinical, 245
cattle, sheep, and goats, 245–246
dogs and cats, 246
horses, 246
poultry, 247
reptiles, 687–689 (tables)
rodents, rabbits and ferrets, 665–677
(tables)
swine, 246
pharmacokinetic properties, 244
toxicity and adverse effects, 244, 660
Tyzzer's disease, 520, 665

U.S. Food and Drug Administration,
regulations, 760–771
Ureaplasma, 226, 254, 318, 586
Ureidopenicillins, 131–133

Urinary tract infections, dogs and cats, 168, 426–437, 552
  bacteriuria, 426
  clinical manifestations, 429
  diagnosis, 430
  drug, selection, 433
  multiple episodes, 434
  pathogenesis, 427
  therapeutic failure, 435
  treatment, 432–435
  urine culture and susceptibility testing, 432–433
  urine sediment examination, 430
Urinary tract infections, other species, 527, 552, 563, 588, 615

Valaciclovir, 402
Valnemulin, 257, 608
Vancomycin, 182–184
  administration and dosage, 183
  antimicrobial activity, 182
  applications, clinical, 184
  resistance, 182–183
  toxicity and adverse effects, 183
Vancomycin-resistant enterococci (VRE), 43, 186
"Veterinary cascade" system, 696
Vibrio anguillarum, 693, 705
Vidarabine, 400–404, 412, 413
Virginiamycin, 44, 188–189, 441, 616, 654
Viruses. *See* Antiviral drugs
Volume of distribution, (Vd), 69–72
Voriconazole, 394

Water medication, principles of, 646–647
Withdrawal, drug. *See* Drug withdrawal
World Health Organization, agricultural antimicrobial recommendations, 44

Yeasts. *See* Antifungal drugs; individual yeast species
Yersinia enterocolitica, 308, 673
Yersinia pestis, 203
Yersinia pseudotuberculosis, 672
Yersinia ruckeri, 693, 710

Zidovudine (AZT), 404–405, 413
Zoalene, 650
Zoonotic pathogens, 37–45